Clinical Pain Management

Cancer Pain

Series editors

Andrew S C Rice MB BS MD FRCA
Senior Lecturer in Pain Research, Department of Anaesthetics, Faculty of Medicine, Imperial College, Chelsea & Westminster Hospital Campus, London, UK

Carol A Warfield MD
Edward Lowenstein Professor of Anesthesia, Harvard Medical School; Chairman, Department of Anesthesia and Critical Care, Beth Israel Deaconess Medical Center, Boston, Massachusetts, USA

Douglas Justins MB BS FRCA
Pain Management Centre, St Thomas' Hospital, London, UK

Christopher Eccleston PhD
Director, Pain Management Unit, University of Bath & The Royal National Hospital for Rheumatic Diseases, Bath, UK

Acute Pain
Edited by David J Rowbotham and Pamela E Macintyre

Chronic Pain
Edited by Troels S Jensen, Peter R Wilson, and Andrew S C Rice

Cancer Pain
Edited by Nigel Sykes, Marie T Fallon, and Richard B Patt

Practical Applications and Procedures
Edited by Harald Breivik, William Campbell, and Christopher Eccleston

Clinical Pain Management
Cancer Pain

Edited by

Nigel Sykes MA BM BCh FRCGP FRSA
Head of Medicine, Consultant in Palliative Medicine, St Christopher's Hospice, and Honorary Senior Lecturer in Palliative Medicine, King's College, University of London, London, UK

Marie T Fallon MBChB MD FRCP MBCGP DCH DRCOG
Senior Lecturer in Palliative Medicine, University of Edinburgh, Edinburgh, UK

and

Richard B Patt MD
President and Chief Medical Officer, The Patt Center for Cancer Pain and Wellness, and Medical Director, Inpatient Services, Hospice and the Texas Medical Center Houston, USA

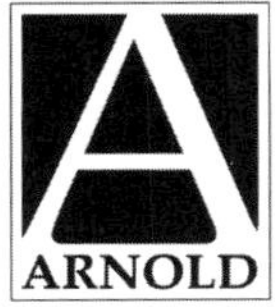

A member of the Hodder Headline Group
LONDON

First published in Great Britain in 2003 by
Arnold, a member of the Hodder Headline Group,
338 Euston Road, London NW1 3BH

http://www.arnoldpublishers.com

Distributed in the United States of America by
Oxford University Press Inc.,
198 Madison Avenue, New York, NY10016
Oxford is a registered trademark of Oxford University Press

British Library Cataloguing in Publication Data
A catalogue record for this book is available from the British Library

Library of Congress Cataloging-in-Publication Data
A catalog record for this book is available from the Library of Congress

ISBN 0 340 80994 9 (Cancer Pain)

ISBN 0 340 73152 4 (2-vol set: Cancer Pain/Practical Applications and Procedures)

ISBN 0 340 70635 X (4-vol set: Acute Pain/Chronic Pain/Cancer Pain/Practical Applications and Procedures)

1 2 3 4 5 6 7 8 9 10

Commissioning Editor: Joanna Koster
Development Editor: Sarah Burrows
Production Editor: James Rabson
Production Controller: Martin Kerans
Project Manager: Helen MacDonald
Cover Designer: Terry Griffiths

Typeset in 10 on 12 pt Minion by Prepress Projects Ltd, Perth

Printed and bound in Italy by Giunti Industrie Grafiche

Contents

Contributors

Julia Addington-Hall PhD HonMFPHM
Professor of Palliative Care Research and Policy and Head of Department, Department of Palliative Care and Policy, Kings College, London, UK

Ehud Arbit MD FACS
Professor of Surgery, Cornell University Medical College, New York, and Director of Neurosurgical Oncology, Staten Island University Hospital, Staten Island, NY, USA

Michael Ashby MD (Adel) MRCP (UK) FRCR FRACP FAChPM MRACMA
Professor and Head of Palliative Care Unit, Medicine Program, Southern Health and Southern Clinical School, Faculty of Medicine, Nursing and Health Sciences, Monash University, Clayton, Victoria, Australia

Charles Berde MD PhD
Professor of Anaesthesia and Pediatrics, Harvard Medical School, and Director, Pain Treatment Service, Children's Hospital, Boston, MA, USA

Eduardo Bruera MD
Chair, Department of Palliative Care and Rehabilitation, M.D. Anderson Cancer Center, University of Texas, Houston, TX, USA

Richard Burstal FANZCA FFPMANZCA
Staff Specialist, Department of Anaesthesia, Intensive Care and Pain Management, John Hunter Hospital, Newcastle, New South Wales, Australia

Colin Campbell MBChB DRCOG MRCGP
Consultant in Palliative Medicine, St Catherine's Hospice, Scarborough, UK

Hester M D Cardwell BHB MBChB
Research Fellow, Discipline of Anaesthesiology, Faculty of Medical and Health Sciences, University of Auckland, Auckland, New Zealand

John Cavenagh MB BS(Qld) DA FRCA FAChPM MMedSci(Epidemiology)
Staff Specialist in Palliative Care, Department of Palliative Care, Newcastle Mater Misericordiae Hospital, Warabrook, Australia

John J Collins, MB BS PhD FRACP
Head, Pain and Palliative Care Service, The Children's Hospital at Westmead, Westmead, New South Wales, Australia

Polly Edmonds MBBS FRCP
Consultant/Honorary Senior Lecturer, King's College Hospital NHS Trust, Denmark Hill, London, UK

Marie T Fallon MBChB MD FRCP MRCGP
Senior Lecturer in Palliative Medicine, University of Edinburgh, Western General Hospital, Edinburgh, UK

Betty Ferrell PhD FAAN
Research Scientist, Department of Nursing Research and Education, City of Hope National Medical Center, Duarte, CA, USA

Jacqueline Filshie MBBS FRCA
Consultant in Anaesthesia and Pain Management, Royal Marsden Hospital, Sutton, UK

Robert George MA MD FRCP
Director, Palliative Care Centre, Middlesex Hospital, London, UK

Margot Gosney MD FRCP
Senior Lecturer in Geriatric Medicine, Department of Geriatric Medicine, University Clinical Departments, Liverpool, UK

Julie Hearn BSc MSc
Senior Executive, National Cancer Research Institute, Clinical Studies Groups, London, UK

Irene Higginson BMedSci BMBS FFPHM PhD
Head, Department of Palliative Care and Policy, Guy's, King's and St Thomas' School of Medicine, King's College, London, UK

Peter J Hoskin MD FRCP FRCR
Reader in Oncology, Royal Free and University College London Medical Schools, London, and Consultant Clinical Oncologist, Centre for Cancer Treatment, Mount Vernon Hospital, Northwood, UK

Kate Jackson MB BS (Melb) DTM&H FRCA FAChPM
Senior Specialist and Senior Lecturer in Palliative Medicine, Consultant Anaesthetist, Palliative Care Unit, Medicine Program, Southern Health and Southern Clinical School, Faculty of Medicine, Nursing and Health Sciences, Monash University, Clayton, Victoria, Australia

Malgorzata Krajnik
Department of Palliative Care, The Ludwik Rydgier Medical University, Bydgoszcz, Poland

Maeve McKeogh MB MRCP
Consultant in Palliative Medicine, Sue Ryder Care Centre – Nettlebed, Henley-on-Thames, UK

Barbara Monroe BA BPhil CQSW
Chief Executive, St Christopher's Hospice, London, UK

Catherine Neumann MSc
Palliative Care Program, Grey Nuns Community Hospital and Health Care Centre, Edmonton, Alberta, Canada

Juan M Núñez Olarte
Research and Academic Co-ordinator, Palliative Care Unit, Hospital General Universitario Gregorio Maranon, Madrid, Spain

Victor Pace
Consultant in Palliative Medicine, St Christopher's Hospice, London, UK

Susan C Pannullo MD
Assistant Professor of Neurosurgery, Columbia University, New York, USA, and Director of Neuro-oncology, Staten Island University Hospital, Staten Island, NY, USA

Fiona Randall FRCP PhD
Consultant in Palliative Medicine, Christchurch Hospital, Macmillan Unit, Christchurch, UK

Peter J Ravenscroft MB BS MD FRACP FFPMANZCA FAChPM
University of Newcastle, Area Director of Palliative Care, Hunter Area Health Service, and Director of Division of Palliative Care, Newcastle Mater Misericordiae Hospital, Newcastle, New South Wales, Australia

Joanne E Ritchie MB ChB
Fellow, Department of Intensive Care Medicine, Middlemore Hospital, Otahuhu, Auckland, New Zealand

Vicky Robinson
Clinical Service Manager, Camden and Islington Palliative Care Centre, Middlesex Hospital, London, UK

Stephan A Schug MD FANZCA FFPMANZCA
Professor of Anaesthesia, Department of Pharmacology, and Director of Pain Medicine, Royal Perth Hospital, University of Western Australia, Perth, Western Australia, Australia

Catherine Stannard MB ChB FRCA
Consultant in Pain Medicine, Pain Clinic, Macmillan Centre, Frenchay Hospital, Bristol, UK

Michael Stevens MB BS FRACP
Head, Oncology Unit, The Children's Hospital at Westmead, Westmead, New South Wales, Australia

Nigel Sykes MA BM BCh FRCGP
Honorary Senior Lecturer in Palliative Medicine, King's College, University of London, and Head of Medicine and Consultant in Palliative Medicine, St Christopher's Hospice, London, UK

Robert Twycross DM FRCP FRCR
Emeritus Clinical Reader, Oxford University, and Sir Michael Sobell House, Churchill Hospital, Oxford, UK

Sharon Weinstein
Director, Pain Medicine and Palliative Care, Huntsman Cancer Institute, University of Utah, Salt Lake City, UT, USA

John Welsh BSc MbChB FRCP Ed FRCPS Glas
Professor, Glasgow University Division of Palliative Medicine, Beatson Oncology Centre, Western Infirmary, Glasgow, UK

Adrian R White MA BM BCh
Senior Lecturer, Department of Complementary Medicine, School of Postgraduate Medicine and Health Sciences, University of Exeter, Exeter, UK

John Williams MB BS FRCA
Pain Management Team, Royal Marsden NHS Trust, London, UK

Zbigniew Zylicz
Chair of Palliative Care, Ludwik Rydygier University of Medical Sciences, Bydgoszcz, Poland, and Medical Director, Hospice Rozenheuvel, Rozendaal, The Netherlands

Series preface

Clinical Pain Management is a brand new reference text, providing comprehensive coverage of this broad discipline for those training and practicing in pain management and related specialties. The work comprises four volumes, three covering the three major clinical disciplines of pain relief (acute, chronic, and cancer pain) accompanied by a fourth complementary volume discussing practical aspects of clinical management and clinical research that share a greater or lesser degree of communality with all three disciplines.

We believe that practice should be firmly based on the best available evidence. However, as things currently stand, a truly evidence-based textbook of pain management would be a relatively scant affair. We were anxious not to exclude discussion of clinical management strategies that are thought to represent reasonable practice by an appreciable body of clinicians, but for which there is currently a lack of evidence to either support or refute such a practice. Nevertheless, we were also concerned that the reader should be instantly aware of the quality of evidence that supports any recommendation for a clinical intervention. Therefore, we have encouraged authors to use a universal system for scoring quality of evidence. If no score is included in the text then the implication is that the supporting evidence is of very low quality.

As befits the multidisciplinary nature of modern pain management, both the authorship and editorship of *Clinical Pain Management* is drawn from a wide range of medical and paramedical clinical specialties. The team of contributors is truly international in nature, with a total of over 200 authors and editors practicing in 16 different countries. While we have attempted to ensure that each author has contributed a balanced discussion that crosses national boundaries, inevitably in a few chapters the authors' views will predominantly reflect the viewpoint as seen from a particular country or system of health care delivery.

Although the textbook of *Clinical Pain Management* is extensively referenced, we are also keen that the reader can easily identify key references. Accordingly, in the reference list at the end of each chapter important and seminal papers and key reviews are highlighted with special symbols.

Clinical Pain Management is not intended to replace the most prestigious and well-known textbook edited by Ronald Melzack and the late Patrick Wall. Instead it represents a complementary work, addressing the practical clinical aspects immediately relevant to those working on the 'factory floor' of clinical pain management rather than the equally important cutting edge of laboratory research into pain. We believe that there is a proper place for both titles on the bookshelves of pain management clinicians.

Finally, we are greatly indebted to the volume editors and chapter authors, without the considerable efforts of whom publication would not have been possible. We are also most grateful to the publishing team at Arnold, particularly the publisher, Joanna Koster, without whose Herculean efforts in holding together a team of editors and authors spanning the globe none of this would have seen the light of day. Thanks are also due to her predecessor, Annalisa Page, who was instrumental in conceiving and administering the early stages of the project, and to the production and project management teams.

Andrew S C Rice
Carol Warfield
Douglas Justins
Christopher Eccleston
London, Boston, and Bath
August 2002

Introduction to Clinical Pain Management: Cancer Pain

In the public mind, and often the professional mind too, cancer is perceived to be an especially painful disease. World wide, cancer is becoming more common as Western populations age and those of developing countries live long enough to enter the peak years of cancer risk. For these reasons it was decided to devote a volume of this textbook of pain to the management of cancer-related pain.

At the heart of cancer pain relief is the analgesic ladder of the World Health Organization. Naturally, the opioids and other analgesic modalities that are involved in the ladder are considered, as is the question of what is to be done when the ladder fails to produce the results hoped for. However, this volume takes a broad sweep of the issues that arise in the management of malignancy-related pain, from ethics to the use of complementary therapies.

Groups of cancer patients with special needs, such as children and the elderly, receive attention in this book. We also acknowledge that cancer raises strong emotions, and hence, unless the psychological needs of both patients and those close to them are understood, the quality of pain control will suffer. Yet it must be remembered that pain is only one of many symptoms that can arise from cancer, and most people who contract the disease will die of it. Accordingly, this volume includes coverage of palliative care in its own right, and briefly describes the management of symptoms other than pain.

The last 40 years have seen major strides in the control of cancer pain, but less clearly recognized even now is the pain that often arises from progressive nonmalignant conditions. This volume has attempted to include some of the better recognized pain problems arising in life-threatening diseases other than cancer, but there is much more still to be learnt. The editors hope that this book may not only be a help to clinicians in relieving their cancer patients' pain but that it may also inspire them to look afresh at the pain of those with advanced neurologic, cardiac, pulmonary, and other conditions. By the time of the second edition we expect to see much more evidence of how to ease the lives of these groups whose pain needs currently remain inadequately appreciated.

Nigel Sykes
Marie T Fallon
Richard B Patt
London, Edinburgh, and Houston

Cross-references, evidence scoring, and reference annotation

The four volumes of *Clinical Pain Management* incorporate the following special features to aid the readers' understanding and navigation of the text.

Cross-references

Cross-references to other chapters within *Clinical Pain Management* are prefixed by a code indicating the volume in which the chapter referred to is to be found. The codes are as follows:

A Acute Pain
Ch Chronic Pain
Ca Cancer Pain
P Practical Applications and Procedures

Evidence scoring

In chapters in which recommendations for surgical, medical, psychological and complementary treatment, and diagnostic tests are presented, the quality of evidence supporting authors' statements relating to clinical interventions is graded by insertion of the following symbols into the text:

*** systematic review or meta-analysis
** one or more well designed randomized controlled trials
* nonrandomized controlled trials, cohort study etc.

Where no * is inserted, the quality of supporting evidence, if any exists, is of low grade only (e.g. case reports, clinical experience).

Other textbooks devoted to the subject of pain include a tremendous amount of anecdotal and personal recommendations, and it is often difficult to distinguish these from those with an established evidence base. This text is thus unique in allowing the reader the opportunity to do this with confidence.

Reference annotation

The reference lists are annotated, where appropriate, to guide readers to key primary papers and major review articles as follows:

Key primary papers are indicated by a ◆
Major review articles are indicated by a ●

We hope that this feature will render extensive lists of references more useful to the reader and will help to encourage self-directed learning among both trainees and practicing physicians.

PART I

Basic considerations in cancer pain management

1

Cancer pain syndromes

ROBERT TWYCROSS

Pain is experienced by 20–50% of cancer patients at diagnosis (depending on the primary site) and by up to 75% of patients with advanced cancer.[1,2] Data for the common primary sites or conditions are listed in Table 1.1 Pain is:

- moderate or severe in 40–50% of patients;
- very severe or excruciating in 25–30% of patients.[2]

In a series of over 2,000 patients with advanced cancer and pain, it was observed that about:

- one-third had one site of pain;
- one-third had two sites of pain;
- one-third had three or more sites of pain.[3]

Further, not all pain was due to the cancer itself:

- 85% of pain was directly attributable to the cancer itself;
- 17% of pain was caused by treatment:
- 9% of pain was related to the cancer and/or debility;
- 9% was caused by a concurrent disorder.[3]

In 15% of the patients, none of the pain was caused directly by the cancer itself. Common individual causes are shown in Table 1.2.

Careful evaluation is necessary to prevent inappropriate treatment. For example, abdominal pain caused by constipation may be relieved by morphine but morphine is clearly inappropriate, as is the use of morphine for the treatment of cramp and myofascial pain.

Evaluation of pain in advanced cancer is based primarily on probability and pattern recognition. Awareness of common pain syndromes associated with advanced cancer is therefore important. It generally allows clinical diagnosis to be made much more rapidly and appropriate treatment started weeks, occasionally months, sooner than might otherwise have been the case – to the patient's obvious advantage.

Table 1.1 *Prevalence of pain in advanced or terminal cancer*[2]

	Patients with pain	
Primary site of cancer	**Mean**[a]	**Range**
Esophagus	87	80–93
Sarcoma	85	75–89
Bone (metastasis)	83	55–96
Pancreas	81	72–100
Bone (primary)	80	70–85
Liver/biliary	79	65–100
Stomach	78	67–93
Cervix uteri	75	40–100
Breast	74	56–100
Bronchus	73	57–88
Ovary	72	49–100
Prostate	72	55–100
CNS	70	55–83
Colon–rectum	70	47–95
Urinary organs	69	62–100
Oral–pharynx	66	54–80
Soft tissue	60	50–82
Lymphomas	58	20–69
Leukemia	54	5–76

a. Derived from 3–6 reports.

Table 1.2 *Top ten pains among 211 patients with advanced cancer (Sobell House, Oxford, UK)*

1	Bone	Caused by cancer itself
2	Visceral	
3	Neuropathic	
4	Soft tissue	
5	Immobility	Related to cancer and/or debility
6	Constipation	
7	Myofascial	
8	Cramp	
9	Esophagitis	
10	Degeneration of the spine	Concurrent disorder

VERTEBRAL METASTASES

Metastases to vertebral bodies often cause midline pain (Table 1.3).[2,4,5] Pain from a vertebral pedicle (a common site of metastasis) may be associated with unilateral nerve root pain. Epidural extension of a paravertebral tumor can also cause unilateral root pain. Disease progression may lead to vertebral body collapse, unilateral or bilateral root pain, and paraplegia or tetraplegia. Common differential diagnoses to consider in cancer patients complaining of neck or back pain are:

- degenerative disk disease;
- osteoporosis.

Degenerative disk disease is rare at C7, T1, or L1. Radiographic differentiation of osteoporosis from bone metastases may be difficult, particularly in the presence of vertebral body collapse. Ordinary and computed tomography (CT) usually allow a distinction to be made. In osteoporotic vertebral body collapse, tomography usually shows intact vertebral end plates and symmetrical collapse. In metastatic disease, there is:

- erosion of the vertebral end plates;
- destruction of one or more pedicles;
- asymmetrical collapse of the vertebral body.

Because the image is based on a signal that reflects tissue chemistry, magnetic resonance imaging (MRI) is the radiological investigation of choice to detect a metastasis that is not causing structural deformity (Fig. 1.1).

With C7–T1 metastases, an associated Horner's syndrome suggests paravertebral disease with involvement

Table 1.3 *Pain syndromes caused by vertebral metastases, spinal cord compression, and meningeal involvement*[2,4,5]

Syndrome	Pathophysiology	Characteristics of pain	Concomitants
Vertebrae			
Fracture of odontoid process of C1	Metastasis of odontoid process of C1 → pathological fracture and subluxation → compression of spinal cord	Severe neck pain radiating to occiput and vertex of skull, exacerbated by movements of neck, particularly flexion	Progressive sensory, motor, and autonomic dysfunction beginning in upper limb
C7–T1 metastasis	Hematogenous spread of cancer of breast and bronchus; or tumor in paravertebral space → spread to adjacent vertebra and epidural space	Constant aching pain in paraspinal area radiating to both shoulders; unilateral radicular pain (C7–T1) radiating to shoulder and medial aspect of arm	Often tenderness on percussion of spinous process; paresthesia and numbness in fingers 4 and 5; progressive weakness of triceps and hand
Lumbar metastasis	Common site of metastasis from breast, prostate, and other tumors	Aching pain in midback with reference to one or both sacroiliac joints; radicular pain in groins/thighs	Pain may be exacerbated by sitting or lying down and relieved by standing or vice versa
Sacral metastasis	Common site of metastasis from breast, prostate, and other tumors	Aching pain in the sacral and/or coccygeal region exacerbated by sitting and relieved by walking	Perianal sensory loss; bowel and bladder dysfunction; impotence; may be exacerbated by sitting or lying down and relieved by walking
Epidural spinal cord compression and meninges			
Epidural spinal cord compression	Tumor compression of spinal cord; generally related to vertebral metastasis and collapse	Aching pain and tenderness in the region of involved vertebrae, radicular pain, and garter or cuff distribution of pain in legs	Motor weakness progressing to paraplegia; sensory loss; loss of bowel and bladder function
Meningeal carcinomatosis	Tumor infiltration of the cerebrospinal meninges	Headache, with or without neck stiffness; and pain in the low back and buttocks	Malignant cells in cerebrospinal fluid

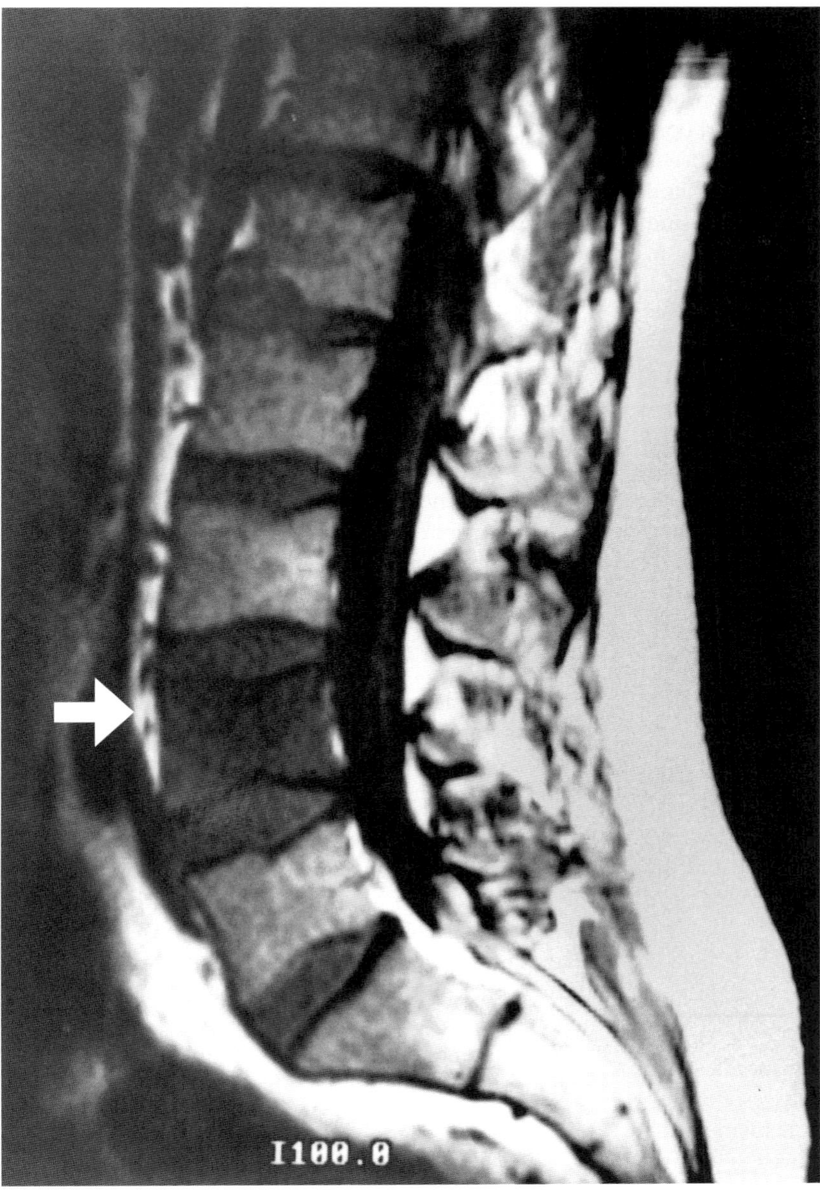

Figure 1.1 *An example of the ability of MRI to detect metastatic disease in bone marrow. This 28-year-old man presented with unremitting low back pain. Clinical examination and conventional radiographs were normal, as was CT. MRI shows an abnormal signal throughout the L4 vertebral body (arrow). Biopsy showed non-Hodgkin's lymphoma.*

of the sympathetic chain. With lumbar metastases, there is occasionally little local pain. Instead, pain is referred to the sacroiliac joint and/or superior posterior iliac crest. Thus, when investigating sacroiliac pain, it is important to take radiographs of the whole of the lumbar spine.

RIB METASTASES

Pathological fractures of the ribs are relatively common in cancers of the breast and prostate, and in multiple myeloma. A rib fracture may well be painless at rest, particularly if a patient is already taking analgesics. The rectus abdominis muscles, however, are attached to the inner aspect of the lower ribs. Thus, when the body is moved from a sitting to a lying position, or vice versa, these muscles tug on a fractured bone and cause transient severe pain. Deep breaths, coughing, laughing, and twisting the trunk also cause severe pain. However, the diagnosis may not be made because the patient simply complains of new severe chest pain. A doctor who is alert to the possibility of rib metastases will ask the appropriate questions and elicit the classical features of the syndrome.

BASE OF SKULL METASTASES

The base of the skull is roughly the area behind the nose and above the pharynx. There are several syndromes associated with metastases to this area. They share certain features:

- paresthesia, dysesthesia, or pain;

- dysfunction of one or more cranial nerves;
- limited diagnostic help from plain radiographs.

The cranial nerves are affected as they pass through or emerge from various foramina in the middle and posterior cranial fossae (Table 1.4). The commonest cause is a cancer spreading directly from the nasopharynx and metastases from cancers of the breast, bronchus, and prostate. Although headache features prominently in the classical descriptions of these syndromes (Table 1.5), some patients complain only of paresthesia or dysesthesia and numbness in the distribution of one or more cranial nerves. When pain is present, this may precede any other symptoms and signs by weeks or months. Sometimes the syndromes occur bilaterally.

Involvement of the hypoglossal nerve (XII) indicates involvement of the neighboring hypoglossal canal. An associated Horner's syndrome indicates extracranial involvement of the sympathetic nerves in proximity to the jugular foramen:

- ipsilateral ptosis;
- constricted pupil;
- exophthalmos;
- reduced facial sweating.

Radiographic investigation is often unrewarding. A plain radiograph is normally no help, but an isotope bone scan or CT may identify the skull metastases (Fig. 1.2). In about 25% of cases, neither of these is of use and the diagnosis has to be made on clinical evidence only.[6]

SPINAL CORD COMPRESSION

Spinal cord or cauda equina compression manifests in about 3% of all cancer patients.[7] It generally results from the distortion of a vertebral body or pedicle by metastasis. Collapse of the vertebral body is not always a feature. In some cases, the compression is caused by nonvertebral epidural metastasis. In about 70% of cases, compression occurs in the thoracic region, in 20% of cases in the lumbar spine, and in 10% of cases in the cervical spine.[7] Multiple sites of compression occur in about 20% of patients. Cancers of the breast, bronchus, and prostate account for over 60% of cases. Most others are associated with:

Table 1.4 *Foramina in base of skull through which cranial nerves pass*

Foramen	Cranial nerve
Middle fossa	
Rotundum	V^2
Ovale	V^3
Posterior fossa	
Jugular	IX, X, XI
Anterior condylar (hypoglossal) canal	XII

- lymphoma;
- melanoma;
- renal cell cancer;
- myeloma;
- sarcoma;
- head and neck and thyroid cancers.

Pain is the first symptom in >90% of cases and may be present for as little as 1 day to as long as 2 years. The nature of the pain varies according to the site of compression. Local pain is not always present and may be masked by previously prescribed analgesics. Local tenderness is common. Root pain is often unilateral in cervical or lumbar compression but is generally bilateral in patients with a thoracic lesion, particularly if associated with epidural spread.

Some patients experience more pain when lying flat (which is therefore worse at night), whereas in patients with peripheral nerve compression rest usually reduces pain intensity (nights not disturbed by pain). Almost all patients with thoracic cord compression have an upgoing plantar response. Pain may be caused by:[8]

- vertebral metastasis;
- root compression (radicular pain);
- compression of the long tracts of the spinal cord (funicular pain).

Radicular and funicular pains are often exacerbated by neck flexion or straight-leg raising, and by coughing, sneezing, or straining. Funicular pain is generally less sharp than radicular pain, has a more diffuse distribution (like a cuff or garter around the thighs, knees, or calves), and is sometimes described as a cold, unpleasant sensation.

More than one-quarter of all paraplegics complain of burning, tingling pain (dysesthesia) in areas of the body below the level of the lesion. These pains are sometimes replaced by:

> Severe crushing pressure. By vice-like pinching sensations, by streams of fire running down the leg to the feet and out of the toes, or by a pain produced by the pressure of a knife being buried in the tissue, twisted around rapidly, and finally withdrawn all at the same time.[9]

These pains may occur after total or partial spinal cord lesions at any level, and possibly more so after lesions of the cauda equina.[8] The onset of such pains may be immediate, but most occur only after months or years. Because of the long latent period, few patients with malignant paraplegia experience them.

A plain radiograph of the whole spine is essential. In 80% of cases it will reveal bone destruction at one or more levels, e.g. loss of a pedicle or vertebral body collapse (usually sparing the intervertebral disk). It may also reveal a soft-tissue mass adjacent to the vertebrae. However, an obvious collapsed vertebra may not be the site of

Table 1.5 *Pain syndromes caused by vertebral metastases, spinal cord compression, and meningeal involvement*[2,4,5]

Syndrome	Pathophysiology	Characteristics of pain	Concomitants
Cavernous sinus	Metastasis to cavernous sinus	Frontal headache	Dysfunction of cranial nerves III–VI (diplopia, ophthalmoplegia, papilledema)
Sphenoid sinus	Metastasis to sphenoid sinus	Frontal headache radiating to temple with intermittent retro-orbital pain	Dysfunction of cranial nerve VI (diplopia) and nasal stuffiness
Clivus syndrome	Metastasis to clivus of sphenoid bone and basilar part of occipital bone	Vertex headache exacerbated by neck flexion	Dysfunction of cranial nerves VII and IX–XII (facial weakness, hoarseness, dysarthria, dysphagia, trapezius muscle weakness). Begins unilaterally but extends bilaterally
Jugular foramen	Metastasis to jugular foramen	Occipital pain exacerbated by head movement, radiating to the vertex and to shoulder and arm	Dysfunction of cranial nerves IX–XII (hoarseness, dysarthria, dysphagia, trapezius muscle weakness)
Occipital condyle	Metastasis to occipital condyle	Localized occipital pain exacerbated by neck flexion	Dysfunction of cranial nerve XII (paralysis of tongue → dysarthria and buccal dysphagia), weakness of sternomastoid muscle, stiff neck

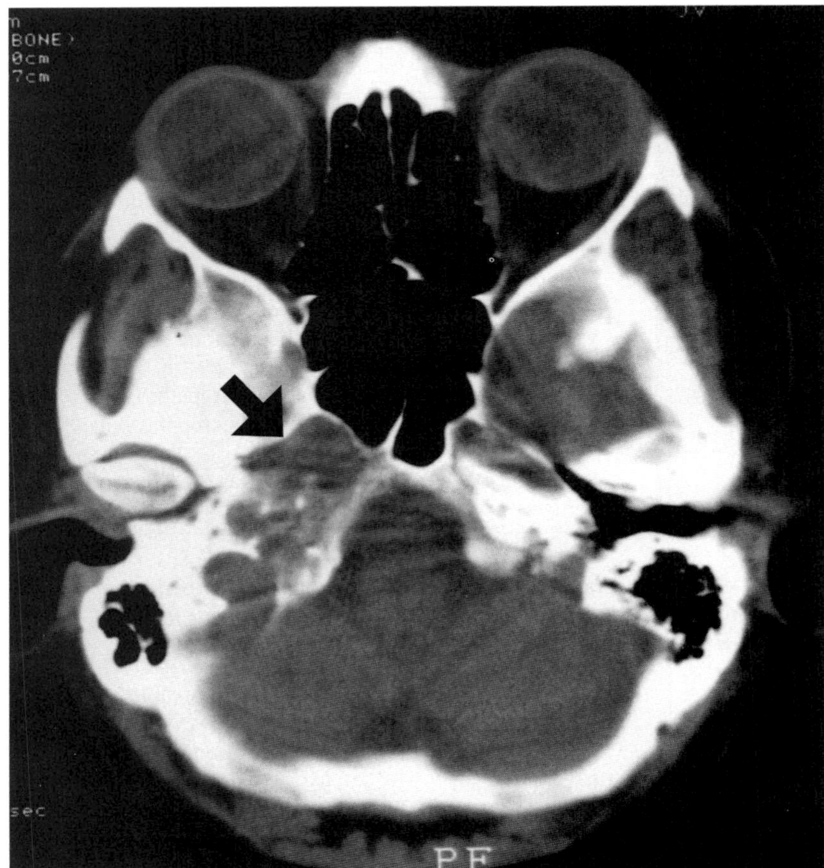

Figure 1.2 *This middle-aged woman who had had breast cancer 4 years earlier presented with paralysis of the right VI and XII nerves. CT shows metastatic erosion of the apex of the right petrous bone (arrow).*

the cord compression. A bone scan does not usually yield additional information. MRI is the investigation of choice (Fig. 1.3). This must not delay treatment, and to be helpful it needs to be readily available. CT with myelography may be helpful if MRI is not available.

MENINGEAL CARCINOMATOSIS

Meningeal carcinomatosis occurs as a result of metastatic spread into the cerebrospinal fluid. Numerous metastatic seedlings develop on the meninges of both the brain and the spinal cord. There may also be concomitant invasion of the central nervous system (CNS). In one survey, meningeal infiltration by cancer occurred in about 10% of patients with disseminated cancer.[10] In another survey, 90% of cases related to: [11]

- breast cancer (>50%);
- lung cancer (>25%)
- melanoma (12%).

Lymphoma is another relatively common cause.

Symptoms and signs can be grouped into those involving:

- brain (Table 1.6);
- cranial nerves (Table 1.7);
- spinal nerves (Table 1.8).

Most patients have symptoms and signs in more than one area at the time of diagnosis. Initial cytological examination of the cerebrospinal fluid was diagnostic in just

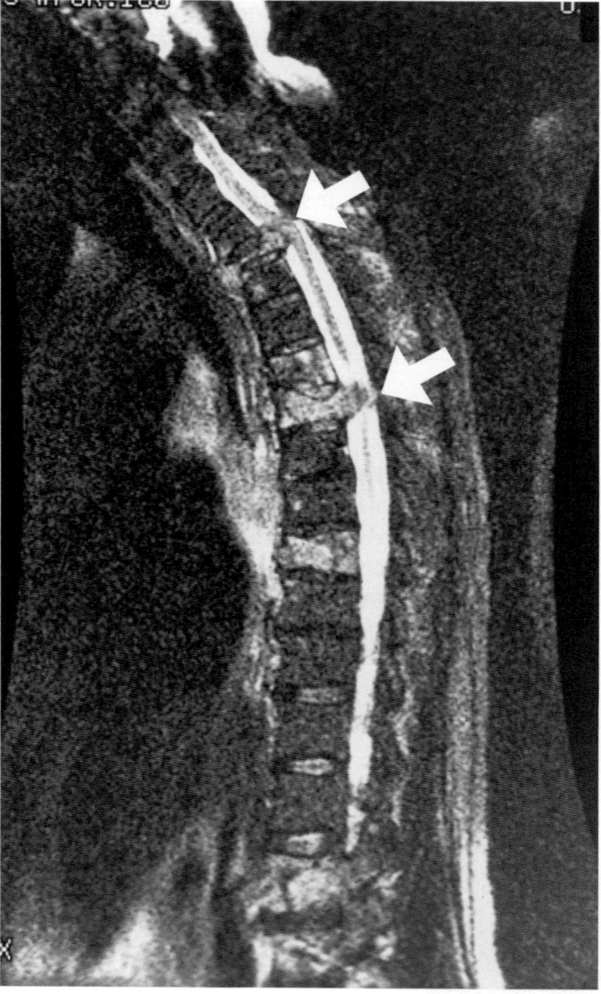

Figure 1.3 *An example of the value of MRI as a noninvasive alternative to myelography in patients with suspected spinal cord compression. This patient with cancer of the prostate had symptoms which appeared clinically to refer to the lower thoracic region. Sagittal MRI shows altered signal intensity in the bodies of T4, 7, 8, and 11. These indicate active metastases. At two levels (T4 and T8) there has been partial vertebral collapse and tumor extension into the canal, producing significant cord compression (arrows). The patient therefore required radiotherapy covering both levels.*

Table 1.6 *Cerebral symptoms and signs caused by meningeal metastases from solid tumors (45/90 patients)*

Symptoms		Signs	
Headache	30	Mental change	28
Mental change	15	Seizures	5
Difficulty walking	12	Generalized	3
Nausea/vomiting	10	Focal	2
Unconsciousness	2	Papilledema	5
Dysphasia	2	Diabetes insipidus	2
Dizziness	2	Hemiparesis	1

Table 1.7 *Cranial nerve symptoms and signs caused by meningeal metastases from solid tumors (50/90 patients)[11]*

Symptoms		Signs	
Diplopia	18	Ocular muscle paresis (III, IV, VI)	18
Hearing loss	7	Facial weakness (VII)	15
Visual loss	5	Diminished hearing (VIII)	9
Facial numbness	5	Optic neuropathy (II)	5
Decreased taste	3	Trigeminal neuropathy (V)	5
Tinnitus	2	Hypoglossal neuropathy (XII)	5
Hoarseness	2	Blindness	3
Dysphagia	1	Diminished gag (IX, X)	3
Vertigo	1		

Table 1.8 *Spinal symptoms and signs caused by meningeal metastases from solid tumors (74/90 patients)[11]*

Symptoms		Signs	
Lower motor neuron weakness	34	Reflex asymmetry	64
		Weakness	54
Paresthesia	31	Sensory loss	24
Back/neck pain	23	Straight-leg raising	11
Radicular pain	19	Decreased rectal tone	10
Bowel/bladder dysfunction	12	Neck rigidity	7

over half the cases, and eventually became positive in over 90%.[11]

Headache and back pain are the most common initial features. The headache is often severe and may well be associated with symptoms and signs of meningeal irritation, i.e. nausea, vomiting, photophobia, and neck rigidity. In one series, radicular pain in the buttocks and legs occurred in one-third of cases.[12] Helpful radiological investigations are:

- myelography;
- CT myelography;
- MRI with gadolinium enhancement (Fig. 1.4).

UNILATERAL FACIAL PAIN IN CANCER OF THE BRONCHUS

Unilateral ear and facial pain associated with cancer of the bronchus has been reported.[13] The characteristic features are:

- Pain is unilateral.
- It is initially localized in or around the ear.
- Later it becomes more diffuse.
- There is usually no detectable local cause.

The pain is a form of referred pain, relating to a sensory branch of the vagus (nerve of Arnold), which conveys impulses from part of the external auditory canal and a small area of skin behind the ear. In patients not previously known to have lung cancer, finger clubbing sometimes provides a clue to diagnosis.[14]

BRACHIAL PLEXOPATHY

Painful brachial plexopathy in cancer patients may be caused by:[15]

- stretch injury during surgery;
- transient inflammatory plexopathy (idiopathic or radiation induced);
- metastasis;
- progressive radiation fibrosis.

Brachial plexopathy is a common complication of Pancoast's tumor (superior pulmonary sulcus syn-

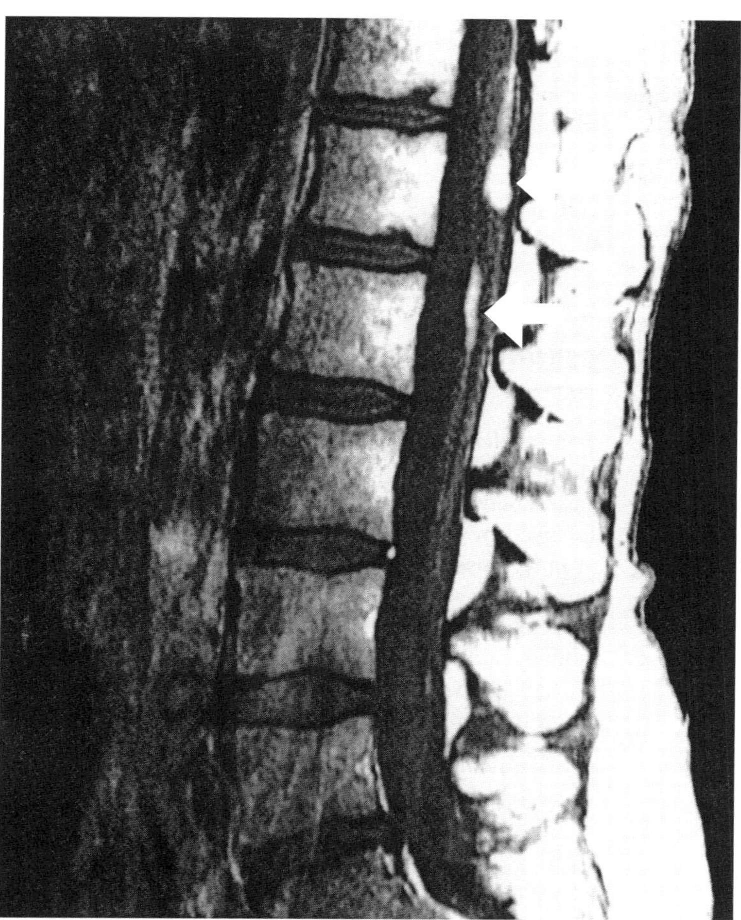

Figure 1.4 *MRI used to detect cauda equina infiltration. This patient with a previous history of carcinoma of the breast presented with severe sciatica. MRI was the investigation of choice, because of its ability to distinguish between degenerative disk disease and root compression by vertebral metastases. If neither possibility is demonstrated, gadolinium-enhanced MRI is required in case the symptoms are caused by metastases in the spinal canal. In this patient enhanced images showed two plaques of tumor (arrows) infiltrating the roots of the cauda equina.*

drome), breast cancer, and lymphoma. Compared with radiation plexopathy, recurrent tumor is more often associated with:

- earlier onset;
- severe pain
- Horner's syndrome.

The differential diagnosis is discussed further on p.16.

LUMBOSACRAL PLEXOPATHY

Lumbosacral plexopathy presents with sacral and leg pain and associated weakness. Additional inconstant features include:[16]

- leg edema;
- a mass palpable on rectal examination;
- hydronephrosis.

Three syndromes have been described:[16]

- upper (L1–L4) 31%
- lower (L4–S3) 51%
- upper and lower (L1–S3) 18%

Most patients report an insidious development of pelvic pain and nerve pain radiating into the leg, followed weeks or months later by sensory symptoms and weakness. Bladder dysfunction and impotence are uncommon.

Lumbar plexopathy ("upper lumbosacral plexopathy") may be caused by a tumor at one of several sites:

- intrathecal (meningeal carcinomatosis);
- epidural (epidural extension of paravertebral tumor, e.g. lymphoma, or associated with spinal cord compression);
- nerve root compression (vertebral collapse);
- paravertebral, i.e. at exit foramina from spinal canal (paravertebral tumor, e.g. lymphoma);
- psoas muscle (malignant psoas syndrome, e.g. melanoma, gynecological cancers, psoas muscle sarcoma);
- renal bed (recurrence of renal cancer);
- retroperitoneum (lymphadenopathy overlying psoas muscle associated with spread of cancer of colon, stomach, adrenal gland, and pancreas);
- retroperitoneum (sarcoma).

A similar range of possibilities exists for sacral plexopathy. CT is generally helpful. However, the density of muscle and of tumor is similar, and the diagnosis may be made on the basis of an enlarged "muscle" mass. MRI will clarify if the diagnosis is in doubt.

Renal bed recurrence

Local recurrence of renal cancer after nephrectomy may cause ipsilateral lumbar back pain and L1 and/or L2 nerve compression pain in the ipsilateral groin and/or upper thigh. There is often associated numbness and weakness of iliopsoas muscle manifesting as impaired flexion of the thigh. Activity typically exacerbates the pain. Radiographic investigation may be difficult. Bowel prolapses into the renal bed after nephrectomy and interferes with ultrasound. CT is the best imaging technique in this situation.

Malignant psoas syndrome

The features of this syndrome are:[17]

- clinical evidence of lumbar plexopathy;
- painful fixed flexion of the ipsilateral thigh with exacerbation of pain when extension of the hip is attempted (= a positive psoas test);
- CT evidence if ipsilateral psoas major muscle enlargement (Fig. 1.5).

Ultrasound is better than CT because muscle and cancer have different echogenicity. MRI will also distinguish. A painful fixed flexion deformity is also seen with more distal muscle infiltration, i.e. of the iliacus within the pelvis.

Proximally, the psoas major muscle is attached to vertebrae T12–L5. The ventral rami of nerves L1–3 and most of nerve L4 transverse the paravertebral belly of the psoas muscle. Branches give rise to iliohypogastric (L1), ilioinguinal (L1), and genitofemoral (L1–2) nerves, which descend superficially on the surface of the muscle posterior to the iliac fascia and the para-aortic and iliac lymph nodes.

PERIPHERAL NEUROPATHY

The incidence of peripheral neuropathy as a nonmetastatic (paraneoplastic) manifestation of malignant disease is between 1% and 5%.[15] It is highest in lung cancer, followed by cancer of the stomach, colon, and breast.[18] A pure sensory neuropathy may be caused by an autoimmune dorsal root ganglionitis. This is most commonly associated with small-cell lung cancer but is seen occasionally with cancer of the breasts, ovary, and colon.[15]

Cancer may also directly invade a peripheral nerve, for example:

- Chest wall or rib lesions may infiltrate intercostal nerves.
- Paraspinal masses may entrap one or more nerves as they emerge from intervertebral foramina. CT or MRI usually identifies the tumor. As already noted, paraspinal tumors may extend into the epidural space and lead also to progressive spinal cord compression.

A

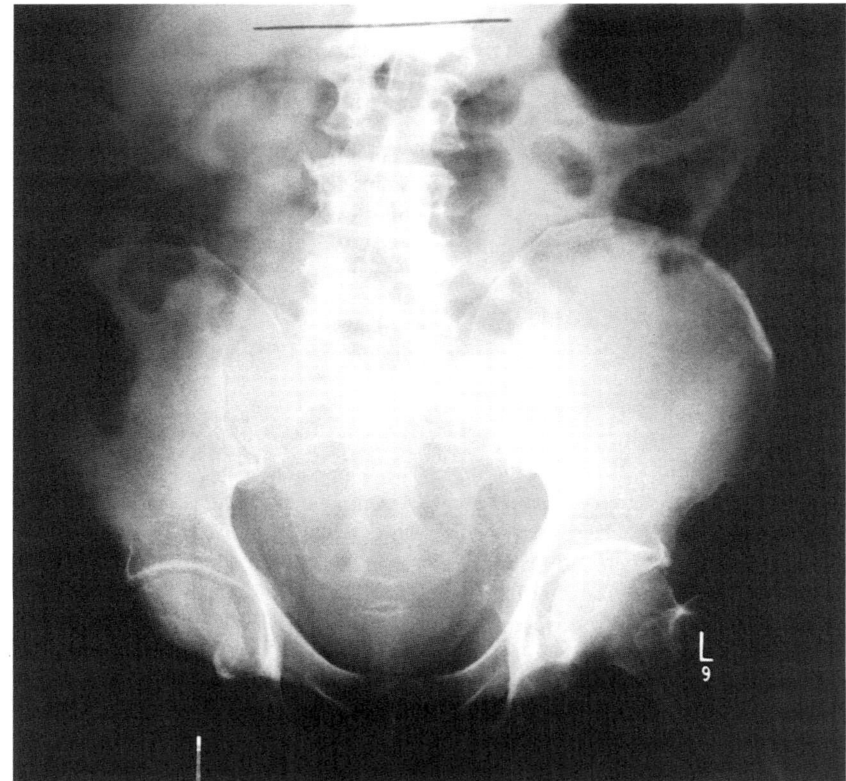

B

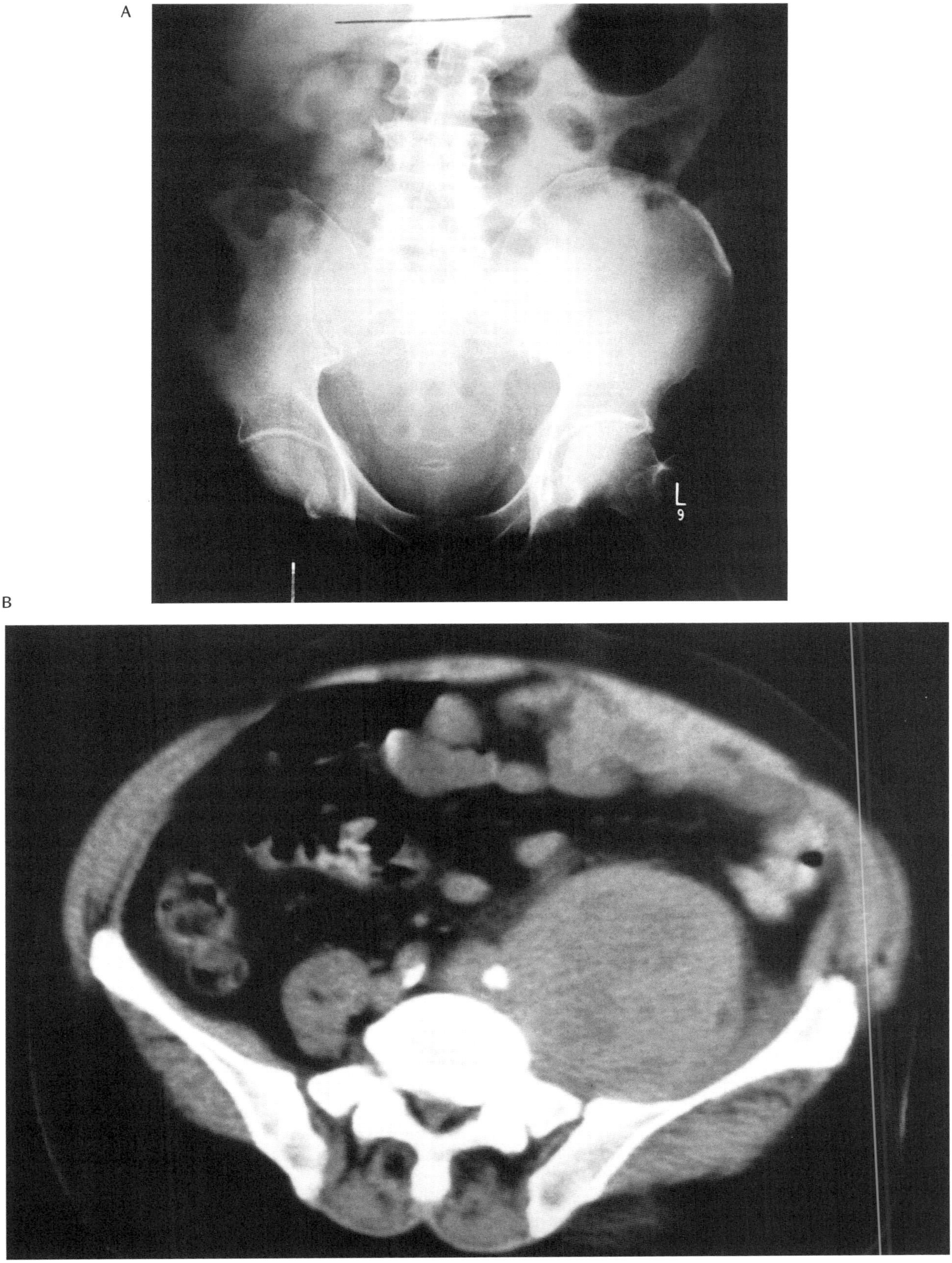

Figure 1.5 *Plain radiograph (A) and CT scan (B) in a patient with severe pain in the anterior left thigh and associated fixed thigh flexion. CT shows massive expansion of the left psoas muscle in the left iliac fossa caused by infiltration by tumor. No abnormality was detectable on the plain radiograph.*

HEPATIC PAIN

Pain is not a constant feature of hepatomegaly. Among 90 patients with advanced cancer and hepatomegaly, less than 40% had right hypochondrial pain (Table 1.9).[19] When pancreatic cancer patients are excluded (in whom the pain could be pancreatic rather than hepatic), the figure falls to about one-third. The most common pain associated with hepatomegaly is an aching pain in the right hypochondrium (Table 1.10). In some patients this is exacerbated by standing or prolonged walking. This is probably caused by traction on the hepatic ligaments.

Patients occasionally develop rapidly increasing right upper quadrant pain, and present with an "acute abdomen." In patients with advanced cancer, the most likely cause of such pain is hemorrhage into a hepatic secondary with acute distension of the pain-sensitive liver capsule. The pain will diminish as the hematoma resolves and/or the capsule adapts, and analgesic requirements generally return to prehemorrhage levels within a week.

Patients with gross hepatomegaly sometimes complain of discomfort in the lower rib cage, often bilaterally. This may relate to outward pressure on the rib cage. A non-opioid, e.g. acetaminophen (paracetamol), often provides significant relief. A few patients complain of intermittent sharp pains in the right hypochondrium. These are probably caused by the enlarged liver pinching the parietal peritoneum against the lower border of the rib cage. Explanation, a change of position, and local massage usually provide relief. Some patients with hepatomegaly also complain of backache. This is caused by postural factors and is similar to backache in pregnancy.

Table 1.9 *Right hypochondrial pain in 90 patients with hepatomegaly*[19]

Primary site	Number of patients	Percent with pain
Bronchus	19	26
Colon	14	36
Stomach	12	42
Breast	11	27
Rectum	8	25
Pancreas	5	100
Others	12	17
Unknown	9	89
Total	90	39

Table 1.10 *Origins of pains associated with hepatomegaly*

Stretching of hepatic capsule
Traction on hepatic ligaments (when standing or walking)
Intrahepatic hemorrhage
Outward pressure on rib cage
Pinching of abdominal wall
Lumbar spinal strain (as in pregnancy)

Table 1.11 *Site of pain in 32 patients with cancer of the pancreas*[21]

Site	Percentage[a]
Right upper quadrant	38
Left upper quadrant	28
Circumferential (at level of pancreas)	25
Epigastrium	19
Left lower quadrant	19
Right lower quadrant	13
Back only	6

a. Forty-one percent of patients had multiple sites of pain.

PANCREATIC PAIN

As with other primary sites, pain is not a constant feature in pancreatic cancer. Pain relates to obstruction of the pancreatic ducts and to infiltration of pancreatic connective tissue, capillaries, and/or afferent nerves. It occurs in about 90% of patients with cancer of the head of the pancreas, particularly if the growth is near the ampulla of Vater.[20] Jaundice is a common accompanying feature. On the other hand, pain occurs in only 10% of patients with cancer of the pancreatic body and tail and is generally a late feature.

Pancreatic pain usually occurs in the upper abdomen. It is often said that the pain will be on the right side with cancer of the head of the pancreas and on the left with cancer of the tail. This is not always the case (Table 1.11).[21] The patient usually experiences constant pain, which becomes increasingly severe over a period of time. As with other causes of epigastric pain, in some patients the pain is eased by bending forward and exacerbated by lying supine.

Pain may also be experienced in the back. It is typically midline in the upper lumbar and lower thoracic region. It may spread laterally to right and left, particularly if severe. Unless there is coexistent degenerative spinal disease, there is no bone tenderness or restriction of spinal movement. The presence of back pain may indicate:

- spread into the retroperitoneum and para-aortic nodes;
- penetration into paravertebral muscles;
- referred pain from the pancreas itself.

INTRAPELVIC PAIN

Intrapelvic pain was present in 11% of a series of 350 patients with advanced cancer.[19] In over half, the pain was associated with recurrent cancer of the colon or rectum. A quarter had malignancies of the female reproductive tract, and 1% had extra-abdominal primaries.

The pattern of pain associated with intrapelvic malignant disease varies (Table 1.12). Central hypogastric pain

Table 1.12 *Sites of pain associated with intrapelvic cancer*

Site	
Hypogastric/suprapubic	
Iliac fossae	
Upper thighs	
Rectal	
Unpleasant sensation of full rectum	
Pressure when sitting	
Dragging when standing	
Stabbing	
Back	
Lumbar spine	
Sacrum	
Perineum	Lumbosacral plexopathy
External genitalia	Lumbosacral plexopathy
Legs	Lumbosacral plexopathy

is relatively common in patients with cancers of the bladder and uterus. It is also seen in patients with colorectal cancer, particularly if adherent to or invading the bladder or uterus. More common is pain in the iliac fossae. This is typically unilateral and associated with local recurrence adherent to the lateral pelvic wall. Sometimes the patient becomes bedbound because walking exacerbates the pain. This suggests attachment to, or infiltration of, the ipsilateral iliopsoas muscle by the cancer.

Presacral recurrence often leads to lumbosacral plexopathy. Pain may be felt in the perineum or external genitalia rather than the legs. Severe intrapelvic pain often radiates to the upper thighs in a diffuse manner. Pain may also be referred to the lumbar region, as in some nonmalignant gynecologic disorders

Rectal pain is another type of intrapelvic malignant pain. It may be experienced even if the rectum has been excised surgically. If a local recurrence is present the patient may complain of discomfort on sitting. This may be mild and described as a feeling of "pressure," or it may be severe enough to prevent the patient from sitting down. The reverse is also seen: no pain when sitting but an increasingly severe dragging pain when standing for more than a few minutes or after walking some 50–100 m. This type of pain may relate to a deeper recurrence with adherence to myofascial structures.

A painful sensation of rectal fullness is occasionally a problem. It is similar to the discomfort felt by normal subjects when experiencing an intense urgent desire to defecate. Such pain is generally related to a local tumor in the unresected rectum or to involvement of the presacral plexus by recurrent tumor. Rarely, it is a phantom phenomenon after rectal excision. Severe stabbing pains ("like a red-hot poker") are occasionally reported. These may relate to spasm of the rectum or the pelvic floor. This type of pain can make the patient distraught.

After perineal resection for rectal cancer, most early-onset pains (within a few weeks of surgery) are postoperative neuropathic pains, and late-onset pain (after more than 3 months) almost invariably indicates recurrence.[22] In many patients, the pain may develop months before the recurrence becomes apparent (median 6 months).[23]

In one study, nearly two-thirds of patients described early-onset pain as shooting, bursting, or a tight ache. In most the pain was mild to moderate, intermittent, and spontaneous.[22] Less than 5% obtained good relief from nonopioids and opioids. The late-onset pain was mainly sharp, aching, and often severe and continuous, located deeper within the pelvis and was typically exacerbated by pressure and sitting.[22] In contrast to the early-onset group, over half of the patients responded well to nonopioids and opioids.

Phantom bladder pain is rare. It probably occurs only after cystectomy when the patient has had considerable preoperative bladder pain either from the tumor itself or from intractable cystitis. Phantom bladder symptoms (bladder distension and a desire to void) are described more frequently. They occur after cystectomy and cord transection and in patients on hemodialysis.[24]

Bladder spasm

Spasm of the detrusor muscle manifests as a deep painful sensation lasting several minutes or up to half an hour in the suprapubic region and/or referred to the tip of the penis. Frequency depends on the cause (Table 1.13). Irritation of the trigone by infection or cancer may act as a trigger. Investigation may include:

- bacterial cultures (to identify infection);
- cystoscopy (to detect intravesical cancer);
- MRI to detect intramural and extravesical cancer).

INFECTION

Infection was the cause of pain in 4% of nearly 300 patients referred to a pain relief service in a cancer hospital.[25] Infection in or around a tumor can lead to a rapid

Table 1.13 *Causes of bladder spasms in cancer*

Cause	
Cancer	
Intravesical	Of bladder or prostate or other intrapelvic tumors
Intramural	Of bladder or prostate or other intrapelvic tumors
Extravesical	Of bladder or prostate or other intrapelvic tumors
Cancer treatment	
Radiation fibrosis	
Indwelling catheter	
Without retention (mechanical irritation)	
With partial retention (catheter sludging)	
Secondary to infection	
Concurrent	
Infection (cystitis)	
Anxiety	

increase in pain but is not always thought of as a possible cause. However, one report describes seven patients with head and neck cancer in whom infection was responsible for some or all of their pain.[26] All the patients had large tumor masses with ulceration and necrosis, together with swelling, induration, and erythema of the surrounding tissue. In each case, pain had previously been well controlled with an oral opioid, and then increased considerably over a few days. In three of the patients there was a change in the appearance of the tumor, two had a leukocytosis and one was febrile. Empirical treatment with antibiotics resulted in pain relief within 3 days in all seven patients.[26]

TREATMENT-RELATED PAIN

Pains related to anticancer treatment are summarized in Table 1.14.

Chronic postoperative neuropathic pain

Chronic neuropathic pain is a rare complication of surgical treatment.[27] In most patients, nerve section causes only anesthesia. In a small portion, it may also result in pain (Table 1.14). This occurs mostly after:

- thoracotomy;
- mastectomy;
- radical neck dissection;
- amputation.

Post-thoracotomy pain

Pain develops 1 or 2 months after thoracotomy. Although neuropathic, it is commonly aching in character. The pain occurs in an area of sensory loss and the patient may complain of intermittent stabbing pains. Allodynia is usually present but may not be prominent.

Table 1.14 *Treatment-related cancer pain syndromes*[2,4,5]

Syndrome	Pathophysiology	Characteristics of pain	Concomitants
Postoperative			
Post-thoracotomy Postmastectomy Postradical neck resection	Severance of nerves during operation → neuropathic response	Continuous burning or aching pain ± spontaneous bouts of stabbing pain in the areas supplied by affected nerves, exacerbated by touch and movement	Allodynia in the scar; hyperesthesia in the adjacent area; neuroma uncommon
Postamputation pain	As above	Constant aching or burning pain in stump and/or in phantom limb	Palpation of trigger points in stump precipitates or exacerbates pain
Postchemotherapy			
Mucositis	Ulceration of buccal and pharyngeal mucosa	Severe pain exacerbated by talking, drinking, and eating	
Peripheral neuropathy	Caused by vinca alkaloids	Constant symmetrical burning pain in the hands and/or feet	Allodynia
Steroid pseudorheumatism	Caused by rapid withdrawal of corticosteroids	Diffuse myalgia and arthralgia	Fatigue and general malaise
Aseptic necrosis of humoral/femoral head	Complication of chronic corticosteroid therapy	Aching pain in shoulder or knee	Limitation of joint movement
Postradiation therapy			
Radiation fibrosis of brachial or lumbosacral plexus	Fibrosis of connective tissue surrounding nerves with consequent neural injury	Increasingly severe burning pain in the arm or leg	Allodynia; numbness, motor weakness (generally C5–6 distribution in the arm)
Radiation myelopathy	Damage to spinal cord; pain in less than 20%	Pattern similar to spinal cord compression; local back pain, radicular pain and/or neuropathic pain referred distally	Other sensory and motor symptoms and signs

Postmastectomy pain

Among a convenience sample of 95 women who had had breast cancer surgery, 20% had postmastectomy pain.[28] Although a temporal classification has been suggested (acute, subacute, and late[29]), it is more helpful to classify the pain according to cause:[30]

- postaxillary dissection pain;
- postmastectomy scar pain;
- phantom breast pain.

If recurrence is suspected, however, it is important to investigate with CT or MRI.

Postaxillary dissection pain usually develops less than 6 months after mastectomy and relates to the section of the intercostobrachial nerve (T1–2) close to the lateral chest wall during axillary lymph node dissection.[30,31] The pain is typically superficial and burning in character, and there is associated numbness (Fig. 1.6). The area affected is the inner aspect of the upper arm and a band around the ipsilateral chest wall at the level of the axilla. There may be intermittent stabbing pains, which occasionally are the dominant feature.

Some patients with postaxillary dissection pain have associated paresthesiae in the hand. These may be caused by an otherwise subclinical lesion to the brachial plexus. Postaxillary dissection pain accounts, however, for less than a quarter of cases of ipsilateral arm pain in breast cancer.

Postmastectomy pain that does not affect the axilla may be either a postoperative scar pain or a phantom breast sensation.[32] These affect the chest wall in the area of the amputated breast. With neuropathic postoperative scar pain, a woman may be unable to wear a breast prosthesis because of associated allodynia. Clothing often has to be loose for the same reason.

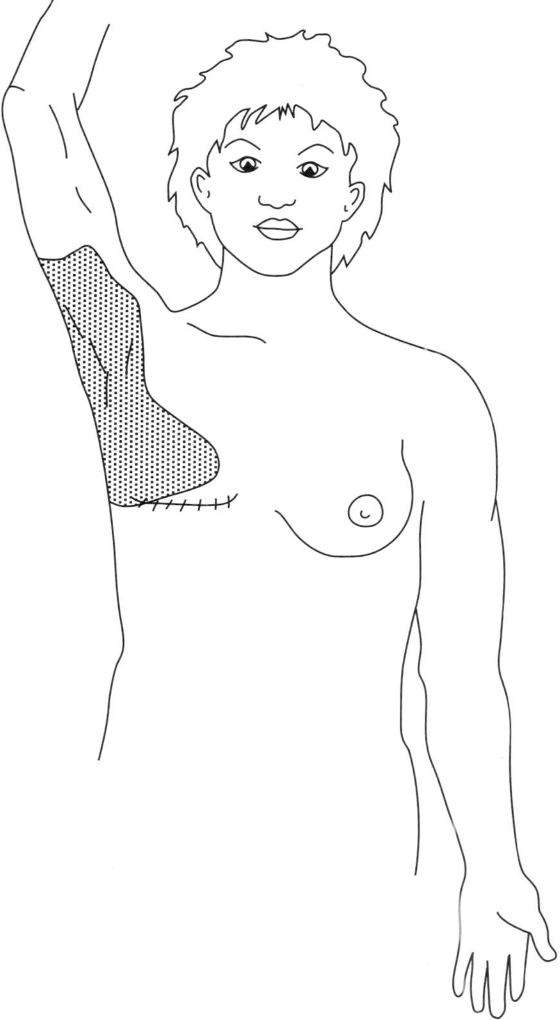

Figure 1.6 *The intercostobrachial nerve can be injured during breast surgery. The nerve has a variable distribution to the skin of the axilla and anterolateral chest wall.*

Postradical neck dissection pain

This is characterized by ipsilateral neck pain (C3 distribution) that is usually superficial and burning (in association with allodynia and with or without stabbing pains). Sometimes it is predominantly aching in character.

Postamputation pain

After amputation of a limb, the patient may complain of either stump pain or phantom limb pain. These are distinct from phantom limb sensation, which is experienced by all amputees.

Mucositis

Mucositis is a painful condition secondary to local radiotherapy or to some forms of chemotherapy caused by mucosal injury and inflammation of the mouth, pharynx, and sometimes the esophagus, with or without secondary infection. Occasionally the pain is so severe that ingestion of food and fluids is impossible. In one series of patients who had undergone bone marrow transplantation for aplastic anemia and leukemia, 62% had moderate to severe pain for 2–4 weeks and 22% had mild discomfort.[33] The pain develops 2–3 days after marrow transplantation. Local radiation can also cause colorectal mucositis (colitis, proctitis).

Steroid pseudorheumatism

Patients receiving corticosteroids for rheumatoid arthritis occasionally develop a syndrome comprising diffuse pains in muscles, tendons, joints, and bones, associated with malaise, asthenia, pyrexia, and, sometimes, neuropsychologic disturbances. Patients may experience cramps, and the muscular pain may have a burning quality about it, particularly in the intercostals. This syndrome, called steroid pseudorheumatism, is sometimes seen in cancer patients:

- who are receiving 100 mg of prednisolone daily (equivalent to about 14 mg of dexamethasone) for several days in association with chemotherapy;
- with spinal cord compression given dexamethasone 100 mg daily for several days;[34]
- on relatively high doses of dexamethasone to reduce intracranial pressure caused by brain metastases;
- undergoing reduction from high-dose to low-dose steroids;
- undergoing reduction of an average maintenance dose after prolonged course.

Avascular bone necrosis

Aseptic necrosis of the head of the humerus or femur may develop in patients receiving a corticosteroid. Pain in the shoulder or hip and leg is the most common presentation. There is progressive limitation of joint movements. Radiographic changes may not be apparent for weeks or months. MRI is the investigation of choice in the early stage (Fig. 1.7). Aseptic necrosis is more common in patients with lymphoma.

Radiation plexopathy

From time to time a patient presents with pain in the arm associated with other symptoms and signs that suggest compression of, or damage to, the brachial plexus. In the majority there is clear evidence of metastatic disease from a cancer of the head and neck, breast, or bronchus. Sometimes there is no such evidence and, in a patient who has had previous radiotherapy to this area, the question arises as to whether the plexopathy could be caused by postradiation fibrosis.[35]

The distinction is very important because, if metastatic, hormonal treatment or chemotherapy may be beneficial. Difficulty arises when evidence of postradiation tissue damage is present but recurrence is also possible. Only surgical exploration and/or the passage of time will confirm the cause. After 5 years of progressive plexopathy without evidence of metastasis, the likelihood of recurrence becomes progressively less and the value of the time factor as a criterion of radiation plexopathy becomes cor-

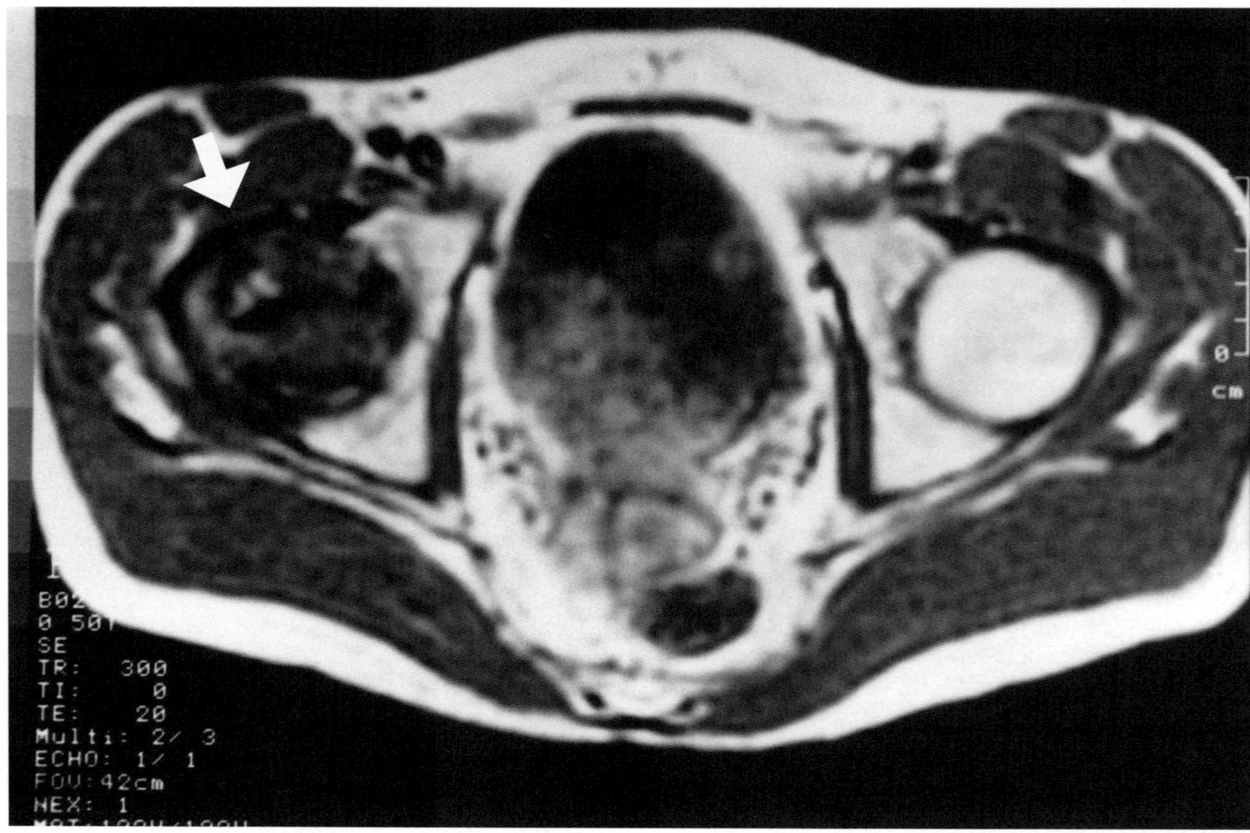

Figure 1.7 *This 32-year-old man developed pain in the right hip some months after chemotherapy for teratoma of the testicles. An axial MRI section of the pelvis shows normal medullary bone in the head of the left femur but a dramatically altered signal intensity in the right femoral head (arrow) because of replacement of normal fatty marrow by necrotic bone. MRI generally gives obvious and unequivocal findings in osteonecrosis, making it the technique of choice.*

Table 1.15 *Characteristics of pain in 100 patients with brachial plexopathy*[36]

	Tumor group (*n* = 78)	Radiation group (*n* = 22)
Presenting symptom	82%	18%
Location	Shoulder, upper elbow; radiates to fingers 4 and 5	Shoulder, wrist, hand
Nature	Aching pain in shoulder; lancinating pain in elbow and ulnar aspect of hand; occasional dysesthesia, burning, freezing sensations	Aching pain in shoulder; tightness and heaviness in arm and hand; paresthesiae in C5, 6 distribution
Severity	98% severe	35% severe
Course	Progressive neurological dysfunction, atrophy, and weakness C7–T1 distribution; pain persistent	Progressive weakness in C5, 6 distribution; pain stabilizes or improves with appearance of weakness

respondingly greater. However, the two conditions can differ in a number of respects (Table 1.15), including the presence or absence of pain.[36]

Radiation myelopathy

Pain is an early symptom in 15% of patients with radiation myelopathy (postradiation spinal cord ischemia).[37] The pain may be localized to the area of the spinal cord injury and may be referred pain, with dysesthesiae below the level of injury. Clinically, the neurological symptoms and signs usually begin with a Brown–Sequard syndrome (ipsilateral motor paresis with contralateral sensory loss at a cervical or thoracic level) and progress to a complete transverse myelopathy. Diagnosis is by exclusion. The differential diagnosis includes:

- intramedullary tumor;
- epidural spinal cord compression;
- arteriovenous malformation;
- transverse myelitis.

Investigation begins with plain radiographs of the spine; these are usually normal. Myelography is usually also normal. MRI will either be normal or show atrophic changes.

Radiation-induced peripheral nerve tumors

A painful enlarging mass in an area that has been irradiated some years before is likely to be a late local recurrence. Rarely it turns out to be a radiation-induced tumor of the nerve sheath (Schwannoma). Such tumors have been reported 4–20 years after radiation therapy.[38] They cause pain and progressive neurological deficit in the distribution of the involved nerve (usually the brachial or lumbar plexus). The diagnosis is established by biopsy. The most important differential diagnoses are:

- radiation fibrosis;
- recurrent tumor.

Ultrasound can often distinguish between a scar (contracted) and a tumor (expanded). If doubt persists, MRI should be performed.

FUNCTIONAL INTESTINAL PAINS

Constipation

Although severe constipation is often painless, in some patients it causes pain. Constipation can cause intestinal (abdominal) colic and, if there is fecal impaction, rectal (deep perineal) colic. Constipation can also cause pain in the right iliac fossa. In this situation, hard retained feces are usually palpable in the descending colon. Sometimes the transverse colon is palpable too. The cecum is distended and tender on palpation. The pain is caused by gaseous cecal distension secondary to constipation. Identical cecal symptoms and signs are also seen in obstruction of the colon. Careful history-taking and clinical evaluation usually enable the two conditions to be differentiated.

Irritable bowel syndrome

Irritable bowel syndrome (IBS) is the term used to describe several functional motility disorders of the gastrointestinal tract.[39,40] About 10% of the population are affected. This means that IBS will be seen in cancer patients from time to time. Common features are abdominal pain and a variable pattern of defecation:

- alternation between frequent passage of loose feces and constipation with small pellets or "ribbon" stools;
- more frequent and looser feces at the onset of bouts of pain;
- passage of mucus with feces.

There is often a feeling of incomplete rectal evacuation.

Upper gastrointestinal symptoms such as postprandial fullness and heartburn are also common, and stress the diffuse nature of the functional disturbance. Symptoms may be intermittent or continuous. Descriptions of the pain include colic, cramping, stabbing, aching, burning, and "like a blockage." Some patients complain of a continuous dull ache with intermittent attacks of colic. Defecation and the passage of flatus often ease the pain. Many patients have symptom-free periods.

Balloon distension of the pelvic colon produces pain more consistently in patients with IBS than in healthy control subjects.[41] IBS can be thought of as an oversensitive gastrointestinal tract in which normal alimentary sensations are perceived as pain. Most cancer patients with IBS will have had the condition diagnosed many years before and will probably not confuse the pain of IBS with cancer pain.

REFERENCES

1. Kane RL, Wales J, Bernstein L, *et al.* A randomised controlled trial of hospice care. *Lancet* 1984; **1:** 890–4.
● 2. Bonica JJ. Cancer pain: current status and future needs. In: Bonica JJ ed. *The Management of Pain*, 2nd edn. Philadelphia, PA: Lea & Febiger, 1990: 400–55.
◆ 3. Grond S, Zech D, Diefenbach C, *et al.* Assessment of cancer pain: a prospective evaluation in 2266 cancer patients referred to a pain service. *Pain* 1966; **64:** 107–14.
● 4. Foley KM. Pain syndromes in patients with cancer. In: Bonica JJ, Ventafridda VV eds. *Advances in Pain Research and Therapy*, vol. 2. New York, NY: Raven Press, 1979: 59–75.
● 5. Portenoy RK. Cancer pain: epidemiology and syndromes. *Cancer* 1989; **63:** 2298–307.
6. Greenberg HS, Deck MDF, Vikram B, *et al.* Metastasis to the base of the skull: clinical findings in 43 patients. *Neurology* 1981; **31:** 530–7.
● 7. Kramer JA. Spinal cord compression in malignancy. *Palliative Med* 1992; **6:** 202–11.
8. Guttman L. *Spinal Injuries: Comprehensive Management and Research*. Oxford: Blackwell Scientific Publications, 1973.
9. Davis L. Martin J. Studies upon spinal cord injuries. II. The nature and treatment of pain. *J Neurosurg* 1947; **4:** 483–91.
10. Posner JB, Chernik NL. Intracranial metastases from systemic cancer. *Advanc Neurol* 1978; **19:** 579–92.
◆ 11. Wasserstrom WR, Glass JP, Posner JB. Diagnosis and treatment of leptomeningeal metastases from solid tumours: experience with 90 patients. *Cancer* 1982; **49:** 759–72.
12. Olson ME, Chernik NL, Posner JB. Infiltration of the leptomeninges by systemic cancer: a clinical and pathologic study. *Archiv Neurol* 1974; **30:** 122–37.
13. Bindoff L, Heseltine D. Unilateral facial pain in patients with lung cancer: a referred pain via the vagus. *Lancet* 1988; **1:** 812–15.
14. Schoenen J, Broux R, Moonen G. Unilateral facial pain as the first symptom of lung cancer: are there diagnostic clues? *Cephalagia* 1992; **12:** 178–9.
15. Kelly JB, Payne R. Pain syndromes in the cancer patient. *Neurol Complic Systemic Cancer* 1991; **9:** 937–53.
16. Jaeckle KA, Young DF, Foley KM. The natural history of lumbosacral plexopathy in cancer. *Neurology* 1985; **35:** 8–15.
17. Stevens J, Gonet YM. Malignant psoas syndrome: recognition of an oncologic entity. *Australas Radiol* 1990; **34:** 150–4.
● 18. McLeod JG. Carcinomatous neuropathy. In: Dyck PJ, Thomas PK, Lambert EH, Bunge R eds. *Peripheral Neuropathy.* Philadelphia, PA: WB Saunders, 1984: 2180.
19. Bains M, Kirkham SR. Carcinoma involving bone and soft tissue. In: Wall PD, Melzack R eds. *Textbook of Pain*. Edinburgh: Churchill Livingstone, 1989: 590–7.
20. MacFarlane DA, Thomas LP. *Textbook of Surgery*. Edinburgh: Churchill Livingstone,1964.
21. Krech RL, Walsh D. Symptoms of pancreatic cancer. *J Pain Symptom Manage* 1991; **6:** 360–7.
22. Boas RA, Schug SA, Acland RH. Perineal pain after rectal amputation: a 5 year follow up. *Pain* 1993; **52:** 67–70.
23. Radbruch L, Zech D Grond S, *et al.* Perineal pain and rectal carcinoma – prevalence in local tumour recurrence. *Medizinische Klinik* 1991; **86:** 180–5.
24. Dorpat TL. Phantom sensations of internal organs. *Comprehen Psychiatry* 1971; **12:** 27–35.
25. Gonzalez GR, Foley KM, Portenoy RK. Evaluative skills necessary for a cancer pain consultant. American Pain Society Meeting, Phoenix, Arizona, 1989.
26. Bruera E, MacDonald RN. Intractable pain in patients with advanced head and neck tumours: a possible role of local infection. *Cancer Treat Rep* 1986; **70:** 691–2.
27. Perry H, Nash TP. Scar neuromata. *Pain Clin* 1992; **5:** 3–7.
28. Stevens PE, Dibble SL, Miaskowski C. Prevalence, characteristics, and impact of postmastectomy pain syndrome: an investigation of women's experiences. *Pain* 1995; **61:** 61–8.
29. IASP. Subcommittee on Taxonomy. Classification of chronic pain. *Pain* 1986 Suppl. 3: 1–225.
30. Vecht CJ. Arm pain in the patient with breast cancer. *J Pain Symptom Manage* 1990; **5:** 109–17.
31. Granek I, Ashikari R, Foley KM. Postmastectomy pain syndrome: clinical and anatomical correlates. *Proc Am Soc Clin Oncol* 1982; **1:** 152.
32. Jamison K, Wellish DK, Katz RL, O'Pasnau RO. Phantom breast syndrome. *Archiv Surg*1979; **114:** 93–5.
33. Sullivan KM, Syrjala K, Flournoy N, *et al.* Pain following intensive chemoradiotherapy and bone marrow transplantation. *Pain* 1984 (Suppl. 2): 215.
34. Greenberg HS, Kim J-H, Posner JB. Epidural spinal cord compression from metastatic tumour: results with a new treatment protocol. *Ann Neurol* 1979; **8:** 361–6.
◆ 35. Bates T, Evans RGB. *Brachial Plexus Neuropathy Following Radiotherapy for Breast Carcinoma* London: Royal College of Radiologists, 1995.
36. Kori SH, Foley KM, Posner JB. Brachial plexus lesions in

patients with cancer: 100 cases. *Neurology (NY)* 1981; **31:** 45–50.
37. Jellinger KM Sturm KW. Delayed radiation myelopathy in man. *J Neurol Sci* 1971; **14:** 389–408.
38. Foley KM, Woodruff JM, Ellis F, Posner JB. Radiation-induced malignant and atypical schwannomas. *Neurology* 1975; **25:** 354.
39. Read NW, *Irritable Bowel Syndrome*. London: Grune & Stratton, 1985.
40. Thompson WG. Irritable bowel syndrome: pathogenesis and management. *Lancet* 1993; **341:** 1569–72.
41. Ritchie J. Pain from distension of the pelvic colon by inflating a balloon in the irritable colon syndrome. *Gut* 1973; **14:** 125–32.

2

Epidemiology of cancer pain

IRENE J HIGGINSON, JULIE HEARN, AND JULIA ADDINGTON-HALL

Pain is defined as "an unpleasant sensory and emotional experience associated with actual or potential tissue damage, or described in terms of such damage."[1] Not only is pain a sensation in a part or parts of the body, but it is also "always unpleasant and therefore an emotional experience."[1] The perception of pain is subjective and is modulated by the patient's mood, the patient's morale, and the meaning of pain for the patient.[2] Moreover, pain is influenced by culture and ethnicity.[3]

Because of the multidimensional nature of pain, it is often useful to think in terms of "total pain," encompassing the physical, psychological, social, and spiritual aspects that influence a person's perception of pain.[4] The concept of "total pain" is pertinent to the understanding of cancer pain in epidemiology as well as in individual patients.

ASSESSING THE PREVALENCE OF PAIN

An estimated 6.6 million people worldwide die from cancer each year.[5,6] Despite major improvements in pain control over the last 15 years, cancer-related pain continues to be a significant global public health concern. Exactly how many patients experience pain is difficult to ascertain. Studies to date show a wide variation in the reported prevalence (e.g. Foley,[7] Bonica,[8] Portenoy[9]). This is because prevalence studies are reported in varied settings and patient groups.[10,11] Usually, prevalence estimates relate to a group of patients referred to a specific service, e.g. a pain clinic. This may mean that many studies concentrate on groups of patients with the most complex problems. Some studies include only those patients who have pain.

In addition, pain is assessed and defined in different ways, and the type of pain is often not well identified. There are no established easily recognized signs of pain, and much reliance is placed on effective communication with the person experiencing pain. In addition, in some instances the prevalence of pain is determined from records of analgesic use. These estimates are likely to be lower than would have been obtained if pain had been systematically assessed. Pain associated with cancer has features of both chronic and acute pain, and can be either the direct or indirect result of the cancer.[12,13] A patient may have several pains, which can have different causes. Although the site of the tumor influences the characteristics of the pain and the type of intervention,[14] the situation is complicated because the definition of cancer pain also incorporates the pathology of pain (i.e. nociceptive or neuropathic[12]), pain related to the cancer, pain related to the cancer treatment, or pain caused by a concurrent disorder.[15]

MEASUREMENT OF PAIN IN EPIDEMIOLOGY

Any measure of pain must be sufficiently graded to identify changes, clear to both subjects and investigators, easy to score, and have been demonstrated as valid and reliable. Visual analog scales, verbal descriptor scales, and numeric rating scales have been used in a clinical setting to assess pain severity and appear to be broadly equivalent.[16] Numerical rating scales have been endorsed for use in cancer clinical trial instruments because they are easier to understand and easier to score[17] than visual analog scales.

Some general assessment tools include pain alongside other symptoms and problems and thus can be valuable in monitoring pain. As more and more standardized assessment tools become available,[18] comparisons between settings may become feasible. Such measures include the Edmonton Symptom Assessment System (ESAS),[19] the Palliative Care Outcome Scale,[20] and the Support Team Assessment Schedule (STAS).[21]

Whether an assessment is carried out by the patient, the physician, the nurse, or the family will obviously affect the data collected. In a study validating an outcome measure for use in palliative care, staff were found to underrate the level of pain and family or carers over-rated the level of pain compared with the patient's self-report of pain.[21] However, feedback of patients' assessments may improve professional assessments and thereby improve treatment.

THE PREVALENCE OF CANCER PAIN

The prevalences reported here are based on a systematic literature review of prevalence reported elsewhere.[22] Although pain is common in all stages of cancer, it is most common in later rather than early disease, so early and advanced illness are considered separately.

The prevalence of pain in early disease

Table 2.1 shows studies that reported pain in the general adult population. It includes three low estimates which determined prevalence from analgesic use (Foley: 29% and 38%; Hiraga *et al.*: 33%). In addition, Elliott *et al.*[28] reported a prevalence of 18% among pediatric patients with current or past malignancy. As a result of the variation in methods of measuring and reporting the data, the values were simply combined to provide a crude overall mean prevalence based on the number of patients in each study and the number reported to be experiencing pain, i.e. a weighted estimate. Excluding these four studies with low estimates would provide a weighted (by sample size) mean prevalence of pain of 48% (range 38–100%).

There is little evidence on the prevalence of pain at or around the time of diagnosis. Vuorinen[30] reported that 35% of newly diagnosed patients had experienced pain in the past 2 weeks; Daut and Cleeland[24] reported 18–49% of patients had had pain as an early symptom of the disease. Ger *et al.*[41] found that 38% of newly diagnosed cancer patients had pain.

Prevalence of pain in advanced cancer

Table 2.2 shows studies that reported pain prevalence among patients with advanced or terminal cancer. In the majority of cases the data are point prevalence estimates, obtained at referral to a particular service. Period prevalence estimates mainly related to pain over the past week, and occasionally the past 2 weeks or 1 month. The combined weighted mean prevalence of pain was 74% (range 53–100%). There was no relationship between prevalence and study sample size. The various stages of disease considered and the methods of measurement make it difficult to summarize the data in the tables to provide valid estimates of the prevalence of severe pain, or the proportion of pain affecting or dominating the daily life of patients.

Five studies had used retrospective data collected from bereaved carers of patients with cancer, or from other informants who could provide information on particular patients.[47,64,69,74,78] Obviously there are limitations to these data in that the interviews with the bereaved carers or informants took place at least 6 months after the death of the patient. The data are therefore subject to some recall bias as well as being subjective assessments. Overall, the estimates were slightly higher than for patient reports (see Table 2.2).

The prevalence of pain by primary tumor site and the effect of metastatic disease

Table 2.3 combines some studies that provided prevalence data on pain in more than one cancer type in the general adult cancer population. These show a wide range in reported prevalence by tumor site. However, pain appears to be most consistently prevalent among patients with head and neck cancers, genitourinary cancers, cancer of the esophagus, and prostate cancer. In contrast Foley[7] reported that only 5% of patients with leukemia experienced pain. In some instances the estimates were very varied, e.g. the pain prevalence values for lymphoma ranged from 20% to 87%.

Daut and Cleeland[24] found that more pain is usually associated with metastatic than nonmetastatic disease. For example, 64% of patients with metastatic breast cancer had pain compared with 40% of patients with nonmetastatic disease, a pattern that is consistent throughout cancer types.

RELATIONSHIPS BETWEEN PAIN AND OTHER FACTORS

For many patients pain is the most feared consequence of cancer.[10,75,76] Unrelieved pain causes unnecessary suffering and can be psychologically devastating for the cancer patient.[75] Physical and mental exhaustion may result, along with the loss of hope and undermining of the value of life.[77,78]

In reviewing the effects of cancer pain on the patient, Bonica[79] summarizes thus "the physiologic, psychologic, emotional, and sociologic impacts of cancer pain on the patient and family are greater than that of nonmalignant chronic pain." Bonica goes on to state that, if acute pain

Table 2.1 *The prevalence of cancer pain in general cancer populations (studies are listed in date order of publication)*

Study type	Disease definition and tumor type	Sample size	Prevalence[a]	Reference
Prospective survey	General cancer population	1. 540	29% (specified by site)	Foley (1979)[7]
		2. 397	38% (60% of the terminal patients)	
Prospective survey	General cancer population	237	72%	Trotter *et al.* (1981)[23]
Prospective survey	Breast, prostate, colon, or rectum and three gynecological tumors	667	18–49% had had pain as an early symptom (specified by site); 48% had had pain in the past month Pain was due to the cancer in 56% and 17% of patients with metastatic and nonmetastatic disease respectively Mean scores for worst pain: 4.0 (SD 3.6) to 6.7 (SD 7.1)[b] Mean scores for average pain: 2.5 (SD 3.5) to 5.7 (SD 2.1)[b]	Daut and Cleeland (1982)[24]
Prospective survey	Lung, pancreas, prostate, and uterine cervix	536	64% with typical pain (specified by site) 30% slight pain, 30% moderate pain, 4% very bad pain 19% had worst pain possible	Greenwald *et al.* (1987)[25]
Prospective survey	General cancer population	240	45% Mean score for present intensity: 2.9 (SD 2.5)[b] Mean score for most severe pain in past week: 7.2 (SD 2.4) 28% maximal interference, 55% extensive interference	Dorrepaal *et al.* (1988)[26]
Quasi-meta-analysis	General cancer population	14,417	51% patients at all stages 74% patients with advanced/terminal disease	Bonica (1990)[27]
Prospective study	Pediatric cancer patients with current or past malignancy	160	18%, of which 21% cancer-related, 58% treatment-related, 21% unrelated 39% of those with pain were inpatients, 13% outpatients 7% severe (staff reported)	Elliott *et al.* (1991)[28]
Retrospective patient record survey	General cancer population	35,683	32.6% overall In 11.4% before treatment, 24.9% in curative stage, 48.7% in conservative stage, 71.3% in terminal stage	Hiraga *et al.* (1991)[29]
Prospective survey	Newly diagnosed general cancer population	240	35%; a total of 28% still had pain 46% pain related to the cancer, 67% had pain secondary to cancer or its treatment, 18% had unrelated pain	Vuorinen (1993)[30]
Prospective survey	General cancer population with intractable pain	1,635	99% with continuous pain, 1% with incident or breakthrough pain 3% mild, 11% moderate, 33% severe, 49% very severe/maximal	Grond *et al.* (1994)[10]
Prospective study	Prostate, colon, breast, or ovarian cancer patients	243	64% (specified by site)	Portenoy *et al.* (1994)[31]

Table 2.1 *Continued*

Study type	Disease definition and tumor type	Sample size	Prevalence[a]	Reference
Prospective survey	Ovarian cancer patients	151	42% 62% had had pain preceding diagnosis or recurrence Mean severity of pain in general was moderate; mean severity for worst pain was severe 40% experienced any pain almost constantly, 21% experienced worst pain almost constantly Median duration of worst or only pain 2 weeks (range <1–756)	Portenoy *et al.* (1994)[32]
Prospective survey	Advanced general cancer population	369	54% with cancer-related pain Mean score for average daily pain: 3.6 (SD 2.2) (between mild and moderate) Mean number of hours per day in pain: 9.2 (SD 9.1) Mean number of days per week in pain: 4.2 (SD 2.8)	Glover *et al.* (1995)[33]
Prospective cross-sectional multicenter survey	General cancer population	605	57% (specified by site), 65% of whom had metastatic disease 69% rated pain as significant (score of 5 or more)[b] 54% rated average pain significant	Larue *et al.* (1995)[34]
Descriptive survey (unclear if it was cross-sectional or prospective)	Ambulatory patients with breast cancer	97	64%, of which 7 3% was cancer-related Mean score for average daily pain: 3.4 (SD 2.3) (mild to moderate) Mean number of hours per day in pain: 8.9 (SD 10.1) Mean number of days per week in significant pain: 3.8 (SD 3.0)	Miaskowski and Dibble (1995)[35]
Prospective survey	Pain clinic cancer population	2,266	85% caused by cancer, 17% treatment-related, 9% associated with cancer disease, 9% unrelated 77% had an average pain intensity of severe or worse on previous day 30% had one pain, 39% had two pains, 31% had three or more	Grond *et al.* (1996)[36]
Prospective study	General cancer population all with pain	383	Patients had a mean of 1.8 pain locations and a mean pain duration of 14.2 months (SD 33.4) Mean present pain intensity on a numeric rating scale (maximum score 10) was 3.3 (SD 2.3); mean average pain intensity over previous week was 4.9 (SD 2.1)	De Wit *et al.* (1997)[37]
Randomized controlled trial	General cancer population	438	Pain score – mean 9.9 in treatment group and 11.1 in control group (range 0–40) Prevalence – 42% in treatment group and 36% in control group at pretest and 39% in both groups at post test.	Elliott *et al.* (1997)[38]
Retrospective cross-sectional study	General cancer population	13,625	29% reported daily pain	Bernabei *et al.*(1998)[39]
Prospective survey	Patients with recurrent breast or gynecologic cancers	114	70% of patients with breast cancer and 63% of patients with gynecologic cancer had had at least a little pain over the past 4 weeks 51% had mild to moderate pain 62% stated that their pain interfered with their ability to function	Rummans *et al.* (1998)[40]

Prospective study	Newly diagnosed general cancer population	296	38% had cancer-related pain; of these, 65% had significant worst pain (i.e. worst pain level scores ≥ 5 on a 10-point scale) and 31% had significant average pain (i.e. average pain level scores ≥ 5 on a 10-point scale)	Ger *et al.* (1998)[41]
Cross-sectional study	General cancer population	217	64% had pain at some time in the previous 2 weeks	Wells *et al.* (1998)[42]
Prospective cross-sectional international survey	General cancer population all with pain requiring opioid medication	1,095	Mean duration of pain: 5.9 months (SD 105)	Caraceni and Portenoy (1999)[43]
			67% reported worst pain intensity over past day was ≥ 7 on a 10-point numeric scale 25% experienced two or more pains 80% had pain due to the cancer, 18% had treatment-related pain	
Prospective longitudinal study	Patients with cancers of the head and neck	93	48% had pain at admission, 8% severe, 14% in the shoulder 25% had pain at 12 months, 3% severe, 37% in the shoulder 26% had pain at 24 months, 3% severe, 26% in the shoulder	Chaplin and Morton (1999)[44]
Prospective study	General cancer population all with pain	593	64% had nociceptive pain, 5% neuropathic pain, 31% mixed Mean intensity on a numeric rating scale (maximum score 100) at admission was 66 (nociceptive), 70 (neuropathic), and 65 (mixed), reducing to 26, 28, and 30 after 3 days, and 18, 21, and 17 at the end of the survey	Grond *et al.* (1999)[45]
Secondary analysis of prospective data from four studies including a clinical trial	Patients with primary lung cancer or cancer metastatic to bone	125	72% had pain McGill Pain Questionnaire total score – mean 19.7 (SD 12.5); range 0–53	Berry et al. (1999)[46]
Prospective study	Patients with pancreas cancer all with pain	50	The 36 patients in group 1 scored 5.4 (SD 0.54) on a pain visual analog scale (maximum score possible 10) The 14 patients in group 2 scored 7.6 (SD 0.88)	Rykowski and Hilger (2000)[47]

a. Percentages for severity breakdowns may not equal overall percentages quoted because of missing values.
b. 0 = no pain, 10 = worst pain as assessed by a pain rating scale.

Study types
Survey – the main purpose of the study was to survey pain or symptom prevalence.
Study – there may have been other reasons for the study, e.g. service evaluation or evaluation of management/control.

Table 2.2 *The prevalence of cancer pain in patients with advanced or terminal disease, or at the end of life (studies are listed in date order of publication)*

Study type	Disease definition and tumor type	Sample size	Prevalence[a]	Reference
Retrospective record review and interviews with general practitioners and carers	Patients who had died from cancer of the pharynx, breast, bronchus, stomach, colon, rectum	279	62%	Ward (1974)[48]
Retrospective interview study	Bereaved carers of advanced general cancer population	165	36% had none to mild pain, 31% moderate, 33% had severe to very severe pain	Parkes (1978)[49]
Prospective survey	Far-advanced general cancer population, all in pain	100	In only 41% was all pain caused directly by the cancer 90% had had pain for >4 weeks, 57% of these for >16 weeks Of those who had pain for >8 weeks, 77% severe to excruciating 80% had more than one pain, 34% of these had four or more	Twycross and Fairfield (1982)[50]
Prospective study	Terminal general cancer population or their primary care persons	1,754	69% 19% mild, 21% discomfort, 16% distressing, 7% horrible, 5% excruciating	Morris *et al.* (1986)[51]
Prospective evaluation study	Advanced general cancer population	256	53%	McIllmurray and Warren (1989)[52]
Prospective study	Terminal general cancer population	60	Mean scores 53.5 (SD 37.5) and 41.9 (SD 29.1) for home care and hospital care patients respectively[c]	Ventafridda *et al.* (1989)[53]
Retrospective record review but with prospective data collection	Advanced clinically challenging cancer patients	90	100%, of which 27% mild, 19% mild to moderate, 34% moderate, 20% moderate to severe Major limitation for 94% of those rating pain as moderate to severe	Coyle *et al.* (1990)[54]
Prospective study	Advanced general cancer population	65	68% pain rated as a problem	Higginson *et al.* (1990)[55]
Prospective study	Terminal general cancer population	120	100%	Ventafridda *et al.* (1990)[56]
Prospective survey	Advanced general cancer population	78	71% (specified by site) 24% mild, 40% moderate, 36% severe 60% had one main site of pain, 35% two, 5% three or more	Simpson (1991)[57]
Retrospective record review	Advanced cancer population	110	69% 34% related to the primary cancer, 43% related to metastatic disease	Chan and Woodruff (1991)[58]
Retrospective record review	Advanced general cancer population who died on the unit	100	99%	Fainsinger *et al.* (1991)[59]
Retrospective interview study	Bereaved carers or informants of people who had died from cancer	383	87% in 1969 84% in 1987	Cartwright (1991)[60]
Retrospective record review	Advanced general cancer population over 65 year of age	239	58% with discomfort/pain 12% mild, 18% discomfort, 17% distress, 7% horrible, 6% excruciating	Stein and Miech (1993)[61]
Prospective study	Lung cancer patients	52	88%	Mercadante *et al.* (1994)[62]
Prospective study	General advanced cancer population	1,000	83% with pain Ranked as most severe symptom out of 30 common symptoms	Donnelly *et al.* (1995)[63]

Prospective survey	Advanced general cancer population	125	74% over 25%	Ellershaw (1995)[64]
Retrospective interview study	Bereaved carers of general cancer population	2,018	88%	Addington-Hall and McCarthy (1995)[65]
Prospective study	Far-advanced general cancer population	98	64%	Shannon *et al.* (1995)[66]
Prospective survey	Advanced general cancer population, all in pain	111	46% had all pain caused by the cancer, 29% had associated pains, 5% had pain related to the treatment	Twycross *et al.* (1996)[67]
			Median score 4 for average pain, median score 6 for worst pain[b] 85% had >1 pain, >40% of these had four or more	
Prospective study	Advanced cancer population	1,640	72% (specified by site)	Vainio *et al.* (1996)[68]
			24% mild, 30% moderate, 21% severe	
Prospective study	Advanced general cancer population	695	70% (specified by site) 54% mild or moderate, 16% severe or overwhelming	Higginson and Hearn (1997)[69]
Retrospective study	Caregivers of general cancer population	170	86% stated pain was a problem; 61% reported a great deal or quite a bit of pain; 25% some or a little	Bucher *et al.* (1999)[70]
			82% reported data on pain relief intervention, 46% of which made pain stop/get better and 56% of which made pain a little better or had no effect or made it worse	
Retrospective cross-sectional survey	Advanced general cancer population	100	77% had current pain	Chung *et al.* (1999)[71]
			Majority had mild pain	
			76% had regular analgesics for their pain	
Prospective study	Advanced general cancer population	3,577	70.3% had pain at referral Mean intensity on a visual analog scale (maximum score 10) was 4.4 at referral, 2.5 at 1 week, 2.3 in the last week of life	Mercadente (1999)[72]
Retrospective cohort study	Advanced cancer patients who subsequently died	223	Pain reported in 66% of all abstracted patient visits 13.2% of patients never had a documented pain complaint 19% had pain complaints documented at each visit Presence of metastases not significantly associated with presence of pain Hospice programs differed in the proportion of visits for which pain was reported (75%, 64%, and 48%)	Nowels and Lee (1999)[73]

a. Percentages for severity breakdowns may not equal overall percentages quoted because of missing values.
b. 0 = no pain, 10 = worst pain as assessed by a pain rating scale.
c. Scores relate to hours of pain multiplied by a severity coefficient; values can range from 0 to 240.

Study types
Survey – the main purpose of the study was to survey pain or symptom prevalence.
Study – there may have been other reasons for the study, e.g. service evaluation or evaluation of management/control.

Table 2.3 *Prevalence of pain by primary tumor site*[a]

Tumor site	Foley (1979)[7]	Daut and Cleeland (1982)[24b]	Greenwald *et al.* (1987)[25]	Simpson (1991)[57]	Portenoy *et al.* (1994)[31]	Donnelly *et al.* (1995)[63]	Larue *et al.* (1995)[34]	Vainio and Auvinen *et al.* (1996)[68]	Higginson and Hearn (1997)[69c]	Number of studies	Range of %
Breast	52%	64%; 40%		50%	60%	89%	56%	78%	76%	8	40–89
Lung	45%		71%	17%			58%	74%	71%	6	17–74
Prostate		75%; 30%	56%		68%	94%		83%		5	56–94
Genitourinary	70–75%			88%			58%	90%	74%	5	58–90
Lymphoma	20%			50%			35%	87%	74%	5	20–87
Colo-(rectal)		47%; 40%			62%	79%		79%		4	40–79
Gastrointestinal	40%			50–71%			56%		68%	4	40–68
Cervix[d]		0%; 35%	56%			87%				3	33–87
Head and neck						91%	67%	83%		3	67–91
Ovary		59%; 39%			67%	71%				3	46–71
Esophagus						77%		71%		2	71–77
Pancreas			72%			85%				2	72–85
Uterine corpus		40%; 14%				90%				2	30–90
Bladder						85%				1	–
Bone	85%									1	–
Carcinomatosis				83%						1	–
CNS				50%						1	–
Kidney						83%				1	–
Leukemia	5%									1	–
Melanoma				20%						1	–
Multiple myeloma						100%				1	–
Oral cavity	80%									1	–
Sarcoma				100%						1	–
Stomach								74%		1	–

a. See Tables 2.1 and 2.2 for further details on each study (Donnelly *et al.*,[67] Simpson,[61] Vainio and Auvinen,[72] and Higginson and Hearn[69] report on advanced cancer populations).
b. Metastatic disease; nonmetastatic disease. NB An overall percentage was determined for each cancer type from the original article, not given here.
c. A special further analysis of the data was undertaken from this study for this chapter.
d. Cervix/cervix–vagina/uterine cervix.

is the initial symptom of cancer, it is considered the harbinger of a serious illness, and is consequently associated with severe anxiety. However, if the pain is the result of antineoplastic therapy, the physical and emotional reactions are significantly less because of the promise of a successful outcome.

The relation between pain and psychological well-being is complex. Mood disturbance and beliefs about the meaning of pain in relation to illness can exacerbate perceived pain intensity,[80,81] and the presence of pain is a major determinant of function and mood.[24] The relation between pain and psychological distress among patients with cancer has been demonstrated in a range of tumor types.[82–85] Cancer patients have been reported to develop greater emotional reactions to pain – anxiety, depression, hypochondriasis, somatic focusing, and neuroticism – than patients with nonmalignant chronic pain, presumably because the effects of chronic pain are superimposed on the effects of the cancer itself.[27]

There is evidence that the cancer patient with pain has significantly increased levels of depression, anxiety, hostility, and somatization than the cancer patient without pain.[86] Evidence from an early study showed that patients with pain were significantly more emotionally disturbed than those without pain, and that they responded less well to the treatment and died sooner.[87] Personality factors may be distorted by cancer pain.[80,88]

Evidence that pain may cause psychological distress rather than the reverse comes from a study by Spiegel *et al.*,[89] who examined both current and lifetime psychiatric disturbances among 96 patients with cancer from two studies who had high and low pain symptoms. The results suggested that pain in patients with cancer causes substantial depression and anxiety, thereby reducing the patient's capacity to cope with pain and other aspects of the illness. This is unrelated to prior depression.

One of the most extreme consequences of unrelieved pain in cancer is that uncontrolled pain is a major risk factor in cancer-related suicide.[90–93] Every attempt should also be made to diagnose and treat depression if it exists.[89] Psychiatric symptoms in patients with cancer frequently disappear with adequate pain relief.[94]

FUTURE CHALLENGES

The need to improve cancer pain control, coupled with the increasing number of people living to older ages and living longer with cancer, makes reducing the prevalence of pain at any stage of the disease process of paramount importance. Much more work is needed to study the epidemiology and natural history of pain in general and community populations, rather than in specialist centers. Standardized assessment tools should be used. Work is also needed to better understand and treat pain in different cultural populations and among older people. As cancer treatments change, so the nature and prevalence of pain in cancer may change, and this will require careful assessment.

Clinicians often do not recognize how frequently pain remains untreated or inadequately managed.[8] It should not be assumed, just because a person has been receiving cancer care or treatment in a health care setting, that their pain is being adequately controlled.[69] Continual assessment of the response of the patient's pain complaint is essential to ensure continual pain control and to prevent breakthrough pain. There is also a need for training and education for doctors and nurses at all stages of their careers. The monitoring of pain and knowledge of how to treat cancer pain effectively needs to be extended to all health care settings.

REFERENCES

1. International Association for the Study of Pain. Subcommittee on taxonomy of pain terms: a list with definitions and notes on usage. *Pain* 1979; **6:** 249–52.
2. Twycross R. Cancer pain classification. *Acta Anaesthesiol Scand* 1997; **41:** 141–5.
3. Cleeland CS, Nakamura Y, Mendoza TR, *et al.* Dimensions of the impact of cancer pain in a four country sample: new information from multidimensional scaling. *Pain* 1996; **67:** 267–73.
4. Saunders CM. *The Management of Terminal Illness.* London: Arnold, 1985.
5. World Health Organization. *The World Health Report 1996.* Fighting disease, fostering development, executive summary. Geneva: The World Health Organization, 1996.
6. World Health Organization. *Cancer Pain Relief and Palliative Care*, 2nd edn. Geneva: World Health Organization, 1996.
7. Foley KM. Pain syndromes in patients with cancer In: Bonica JJ, Ventafridda V eds. *Advances in Pain Research and Therapy.* New York, NY: Raven Press, 1979: 59–75.
8. Bonica JJ. Treatment of cancer pain: current status and future needs In: Fields HL ed. *Advances in Pain Research and Therapy.* New York, NY: Raven Press, 1985: 589–616.
9. Portenoy R. Epidemiology syndromes and cancer pain. *Cancer* 1989; **63:** 2298–307.
10. Grond S, Zech D, Diefenbach C, Bischoff A. Prevalence and pattern of symptoms in patients with cancer pain: a prospective evaluation of 1635 cancer patients referred to a pain clinic. *J Pain Symptom Manage* 1994; **9:** 372–82.
11. Field GB, Chamberlain C, Urch C, *et al.* Evaluation of the support team assessment schedule for the in-patient setting – and its further development. In: de Conno F ed. *Proceedings of the IV Congress of the Euro-*

pean Association for Palliative Care. Milan: European Association of Palliative Care, 1997: 99–108.

12. Portenoy R. Cancer pain: pathophysiology and syndromes. *Lancet* 1992; **39:** 1026–31.
13. Welsh Office NHS Directorate. *Pain, Discomfort and Palliative Care.* Cardiff: Welsh Health Planning Forum, Welsh Office, 1992.
14. Spross JA, McGuire DB, Schmitt RM. Oncology nursing forum position paper on cancer pain: Part 1. *Oncol Nurs Forum* 1991; **17:** 595–614.
15. World Health Organization. *Cancer Pain Relief and Palliative Care.* Geneva: World Health Organization, 1990.
16. Jensen MP, Karoly P, Braver S. The measurement of clinical pain intensity: a comparison of six methods. *Pain* 1986; **27:** 117–27.
17. Moinpour CM, Feigl P, Metch B, *et al.* Quality of life end points in cancer clinical trials: review and recommendations. *J Natl Cancer Inst* 1989; **81:** 485–95.
18. Hearn J, Higginson IJ. Outcome measures in palliative care for advanced cancer patients: a review. *J Publ Hlth Med* 1997; **19:** 193–9.
19. Bruera E, Kuehn N, Miller MJ, *et al.* The Edmonton Symptom Assessment System (ESAS): a simple method for the assessment of palliative care patients. *J Palliative Care* 1991; **7:** 6–9.
20. Hearn J, Higginson IJ, on behalf of the Palliative Care Audit Project Advisory Group. Development and validation of a core outcome measure for palliative care – The Palliative Care Outcome Scale. *Quality in Healthcare* 1999; **8:** 219–27.
21. Higginson IJ, McCarthy M. Validity of the Support Team Assessment Schedule: do staffs' ratings reflect those made by patients or their families. *Palliative Med* 1993; **7:** 219–28.
22. Hearn J, Higginson IJ. Cancer pain epidemiology: a systematic literature review. In: Portenoy RK, Bruera E eds. *Cancer Pain.* New York, NY: Cambridge University Press, 2003: in press.
23. Trotter JM, Scott R, Macbeth FR, *et al.* Problems of oncology outpatients: role of the liaison health visitor. *Br Med J Clin Res Ed* 1981; **282:** 122–4.
24. Daut RL, Cleeland CS. The prevalence and severity of pain in cancer. *Cancer* 1982; **50:** 1913–18.
25. Greenwald HP, Bonica JJ, Bergner M. The prevalence of pain in four cancers. *Cancer* 1987; **60:** 2563–9.
26. Dorrepaal KL, Aaronson NK, van Dam FS. Pain experience and pain management among hospitalised cancer patients. *Cancer* 1989; **63:** 593–8.
27. Bonica JJ. Cancer pain In: Bonica JJ ed. *The Management of Cancer Pain.* Philadelphia, PA: Lea & Febiger, 1990: 400–60.
28. Elliott SC, Miser AW, Dose AM, *et al.* Epidemiologic features of pain in pediatric cancer patients: a co-operative community based study. North Central Cancer Treatment Group and Mayo Clinic. *Clin J Pain* 1991; **7:** 263–8.
29. Hiraga K, Mizuguchi T, Takeda F. The incidence of cancer pain and improvement of pain management in Japan. *Postgrad Med J* 1991; **67:** S14–S25.
30. Vuorinen E. Pain as an early symptom in cancer. *Clin J Pain* 1993; **9:** 272–8.
31. Portenoy R, Thaler HT, Kornblith AB, *et al.* Symptom prevalence, characteristics and distress in a cancer population. *Quality Life Res* 1994; **3:** 183–9.
32. Portenoy RK, Kornblith AB, Wong G, *et al.* Pain in ovarian cancer patients – prevalence, characteristics and associated symptoms. *Cancer* 1994; **74:** 907–15.
33. Glover J, Dibble SL, Dodd MJ, Miaskowski C. Mood states of oncology outpatients: does pain make a difference? *J Pain Symptom Manage* 1995; **10:** 120–8.
34. Larue F, Colleau SM, Brasseur L, Cleeland CS. Multicentre study of cancer pain and its treatment in France. *Br Med J* 1995; **310:** 1034–7.
35. Miaskowski C, Dibble SL. The problem of pain in outpatients with breast cancer. *Oncol Nursing Forum* 1995; **22:** 791–7.
36. Grond S, Zech D, Diefenbach C, *et al.* Assessment of cancer pain: a prospective evaluation in 2266 cancer patients referred to a pain service. *Pain* 1996; **64:** 107–14.
37. de Wit R, van Dam F, Zandbelt L, *et al.* A Pain Education Program for chronic cancer pain patients: follow-up results from a randomized controlled trial. *Pain* 1997; **73:** 55–69.
38. Elliott TE, Murray DM, Oken MM, *et al.* Improving cancer pain management in communities: main results from a randomized controlled trial. *J Pain Symptom Manage* 1997; **13:** 191–203.
39. Bernabei R, Gambassi G, Lapane K, *et al.* for the SAGE study group. Management of pain in elderly patients with cancer. *JAMA* 1998; **279:** 1877–82.
40. Rummans TA, Frost M, Suman VJ, *et al.* Quality of life and pain in patients with recurrent breast and gynecologic cancer. *Psychosomatics* 1998; **39:** 437–45.
41. Ger LP, Ho ST, Wang JJ, Cherng CH. The prevalence and severity of cancer pain: a study of newly-diagnosed cancer patients in Taiwan. *J Pain Symptom Manage* 1998; **15:** 285–93.
42. Wells N, Johnson RL, Wujick D. Development of a short version of the Barriers Questionnaire. *J Pain Symptom Manage* 1998; **15:** 285–93.
43. Caraceni A, Portenoy RK, a working group of the IASP Task Force on Cancer Pain. An international survey of cancer pain characteristics and syndromes. *Pain* 1999; **82:** 263–74.
44. Chaplin JM, Morton RP. A prospective, longitudinal study of pain in head and neck cancer patients. *Head & Neck* 1999; **21:** 531–7.
45. Grond S, Radbruch L, Meuser T, *et al.* Assessment and treatment of neuropathic cancer pain following WHO guidelines. *Pain* 1999; **79:**15–20.
46. Berry DL, Wilkie DJ, Huang HY, Blumenstein BA. Cancer pain and common pain: a comparison of patient-

reported intensities. *Oncol Nursing Forum* 1999; **26:** 721–6.

47. Rykowski JJ, Hilger M. Efficacy of neurolytic celiac plexus block in varying locations of pancreatic cancer. *Anesthesiology* 2000; **92:** 347–54.
48. Ward AWM. Terminal care in malignant disease. *Soc Sci Med* 1974; **8:** 413–29.
49. Parkes CM. Home or hospital? Terminal care as seen by surviving spouses. *J Roy Coll Gen Pract* 1978; **28:** 19–30.
50. Twycross R. Pain in far-advanced cancer. *Pain* 1982; **14:** 303–10.
51. Morris JN, Mor V, Goldberg RJ, *et al.* The effect of treatment setting and patient characteristics on pain in terminal cancer patients: A report from the National Hospice Study. *J Chron Dis* 1986; **39:** 27–35.
52. McIllmurray MB, Warren MR. Evaluation of a new hospice: the relief of symptoms in cancer patients in the first year. *Palliative Med* 1989; **3:** 135–40.
53. Ventafridda V, De Conno F, Vigano A, *et al.* Comparison of home and hospital care of advanced cancer patients. *Tumori* 1989; **75:** 619–25.
54. Coyle N. The last four weeks of life. *Am J Nursing* 1990; **90:** 75–8.
55. Higginson I, Wade A, McCarthy M. Palliative care: views of patients and their families. *Br Med J* 1990; **301:** 277–81.
56. Ventafridda V, Ripamonti C, De Conno F, *et al.* Symptom prevalence and control during cancer patients' last days of life. *J Palliative Care* 1990; **6:** 7–11.
57. Simpson M. The use of research to facilitate the creation of a hospital palliative care team. *Palliative Med* 1991; **5:** 122–9.
58. Chan A, Woodruff RK. Palliative care in a general teaching hospital. 1. Assessment of needs. *Med J Aust* 1991; **155:** 597–9.
59. Fainsinger RL, Miller MJ, Bruera E, *et al.* Symptom Control during the last week of life on a palliative care unit. *J Palliative Care* 1991; **7:** 5–11.
60. Cartwright A. Changes in life and care in the year before death 1969–1987. *J Publ Hlth Med* 1991; **13:** 81–7.
61. Stein WM, Miech RP. Cancer pain in the elderly hospice patient. *J Pain Symptom Manage* 1993; **8:** 474–82.
62. Mercadante S, Armata M, Salvaggio L. Pain characteristics of advanced lung cancer patients referred to a palliative care service. *Pain* 1994; **59:** 141–5.
63. Donnelly S, Walsh D, Rybicki L. The symptoms of advanced cancer: identification of clinical and research priorities by assessment of prevalence and severity. *J Palliative Care* 1995; **11:** 27–32.
64. Ellershaw JE, Peat SJ, Boys LC. Assessing the effectiveness of a hospital palliative care team. *Palliative Med* 1995; **9:** 145–52.
65. Addington-Hall JM, McCarthy M. Dying from cancer: results of a national population-based investigation. *Palliative Med* 1995; **9:** 295–305.
66. Shannon MM, Ryan MA, D'Agostino N, Brescia FJ. Assessment of pain in advanced cancer patients. *J Pain Symptom Manage* 1995; **10:** 274–8.
67. Twycross R, Harcourt J, Bergl S. A survey of pain in patients with advanced cancer. *J Pain Symptom Manage* 1996; **12:** 273–82.
68. Vainio A, Auvinen A. Prevalence of symptoms among patients with advanced cancer: an international collaborative study. Symptom Prevalence Group. *J Pain Symptom Manage* 1996; **12:** 3–10.
69. Higginson IJ, Hearn J. A multi-centre evaluation of cancer pain control by palliative care teams. *J Pain Symptom Manage* 1997; **14:** 29–35.
70. Bucher JA, Trostle GB, Moore M. Family reports of cancer pain, pain relief, and prescription access. *Cancer Pract* 1999; **7:** 71–7.
71. Chung JW, Yang JC, Wong TK. The significance of pain among Chinese patients with cancer in Hong Kong. *Acta Anaesthesiol Sin* 1999; **37:** 9–14.
72. Mercadante S. Pain treatment and outcomes for patients with advanced cancer who receive follow-up care at home. *Cancer* 1999; **85:** 1849–58.
73. Nowels D, Lee JT. Cancer pain management in home hospice settings: a comparison of primary care and oncologic physicians. *J Palliative Care* 1999; **15:** 5–9.
74. Parkes CM. Terminal care as seen by surviving spouses. *J Roy Coll Gen Pract* 1978; **28:** 19–30.
75. Breitbart W. Cancer pain management guidelines: implications for psycho-oncology. *Psycho-oncology* 1994; **3:** 103–8.
76. Foley KM. The treatment of cancer pain. *N Engl J Med* 1985; **313:** 84–95.
77. Twycross RG; Lack SA. *Symptom Control in Far Advanced Cancer.* London: Pitman, 1983.
78. Cherny NI, Coyle N, Foley KM. The treatment of suffering when patients request elective death. *J Palliative Care* 1994; **10:** 71–9.
79. Bonica JJ. Evolution and current status of pain programs. *J Pain Symptom Manage* 1990; **5:** 368–74.
80. Bond MR, Pearson IB. Psychosocial aspects of pain in women with advanced cancer of the cervix. *J Psychosomat Res* 1969; **13:** 13–21.
81. Barkwell DP. Ascribed meaning: a critical factor in coping and pain attenuation in patients with cancer-related pain. *J Palliative Care* 1991; **7:** 5–14.
82. Heim HM, Oei TP. Comparison of prostate cancer patients with and without pain. *Pain* 1993; **53:** 159–62.
83. Kaasa S, Malt U, Hagen S, *et al.* Psychological distress in cancer patients with advanced cancer. *Radiother Oncol* 1993; **27:** 93–197.
84. Lancee WJ, Vachon ML, Ghadirian P, *et al.* The impact of pain and impaired role performance on distress in persons with cancer. *Can J Psychiatry* 1994; **39:** 617–22.
85. Kelsen DP, Portenoy RK, Thaler HT, *et al.* Pain and depression in patients with newly diagnosed pancreas cancer. *J Clin Oncol* 1995; **13:** 748–55.
86. Ahles TA, Blanchard EB, Ruckdeschel JC. The multidi-

mensional nature of cancer-related pain. *Pain* 1983; **17:** 277–88.
87. Woodforde JM, Fielding JR. Pain and cancer In: Weisenberg M ed. *Pain, Clinical and Experimental Perspectives*. St Louis, MO: Mosby, 1975: 326–35.
88. Bond MR. Psychologic and emotional aspects of cancer pain In: Bonica JJ, Ventafridda V eds. *Advances in Pain Research and Therapy*. New York, NY: Raven Press, 1979: 81–8.
89. Spiegel D, Sands S, Koopman C. Pain and depression in patients with cancer. *Cancer* 1994; **74:** 2570–8.
90. Bolund C. Medical and care factors in suicides by cancer patients in Sweden. *J Psychosomat Oncol* 1985; **3:** 31–52.
91. Breitbart W. Suicide in the cancer patient. *Oncology* 1987; **1:** 49–54.
92. Cleeland CS. The impact of pain on the patient with cancer. *Cancer* 1984; **54:** 2635–41.
93. Baile WF, Di Maggio JR, Schapira DV, Janofsky JS. The requests for assistance in dying: the need for psychiatric consultation. *Cancer* 1993; **72:** 2786–91.
94. Breitbart W. Cancer pain and suicide In: Foley KM, Bonica JJ, Ventafridda V eds. *Second International Congress on Cancer Pain: Advances in Pain Research and Therapy*. New York, NY: Raven Press, 1990: 399–412.

3

Clinical pharmacology – including tolerance

STEPHAN A SCHUG AND HESTER M D CARDWELL

Therapy of cancer pain usually involves quite sophisticated pharmacotherapy with combinations of potent drugs. Such use of medication requires a profound knowledge of pharmacologic principles and detailed familiarity with the clinical pharmacologic properties of the medications used. The purpose of this chapter is to summarize pharmacologic knowledge relevant to the management of cancer pain.

For this purpose, we divided analgesics into three groups, based on the analgesic ladder promoted by the World Health Organization (WHO):[1]

1 Nonopioids – analgesic drugs whose effect is not mediated via opioid receptors:
   a acetaminophen (paracetamol);
   b nefopam (international availability is limited, e.g. it is not available in the USA);
   c nonsteroidal anti-inflammatory drugs (NSAIDs).
2 Opioids – analgesic drugs whose effect is mediated via opioid receptors.
3 Adjuvant analgesics – any drug that has a primary indication other than pain but is analgesic in some painful conditions. (Details of these drugs will be discussed elsewhere in this book.)

NONOPIOID ANALGESICS

Acetaminophen (paracetamol)

Acetaminophen is a para-aminophenol derivative. As such, it is the active metabolite of acetanilide and phenacetin. It has virtually replaced these two because of its relative lack of toxicity. It is used primarily as an analgesic and antipyretic and should be the nonopioid of choice for mild to moderate pain, unless contraindicated. Used properly, it is a very effective analgesic and widely underestimated.

Mechanism of action

Acetaminophen has dose-dependent analgesic and antipyretic activity but is almost devoid of anti-inflammatory effect.

Acetaminophen easily crosses the blood–brain barrier. One mechanism of action is in the central nervous system (CNS), where it inhibits cyclo-oxygenase, and therefore the production of prostaglandins.[2] Here it has a particular effect on the E series of prostaglandins, which elevate the set point for body temperature (it acts on both COX-1 and COX-2, but only in an environment low in peroxides).[3] Prostaglandins are generated in the hypothalamus after stimulation by interleukin 1 (IL-1), which is released from macrophages in response to bacterial endotoxins. This mechanism most likely accounts for the antipyretic effect of acetaminophen.

The analgesic effect is not clearly understood but may also be due to central inhibition of cyclo-oxygenase and modulation of CNS pain pathways. It has also been postulated, mainly from animal studies, that the analgesic effect of acetaminophen involves spinal cord receptors for *N*-methyl-D-aspartate (NMDA) or substance P and the inhibition of nitric oxide synthesis.[4,5] Other animal studies have shown the central serotonergic system to be indirectly involved in the antinociceptive effect of acetaminophen.[6–8]

Acetaminophen is generally thought to exhibit little peripheral activity, which would explain its lack of anti-inflammatory effect.

Pharmacokinetics

Acetaminophen is well absorbed orally with a bioavailability of 70–90% as a result of limited first-pass metabolism. Rectal bioavailability is variable and 54–88% of oral bioavailability.[9]

Acetaminophen is quickly absorbed from the upper gastrointestinal tract and achieves it peak plasma concentration in 30–60 min and its peak concentration in cerebrospinal fluid (CSF) 1–2 h later.[10] The rate of absorption varies with gastric emptying and can be prolonged if gastric emptying is delayed. Acetaminophen is very lipid soluble, crosses the blood–brain barrier easily, and is rapidly distributed throughout total body water. Its volume of distribution is 1 l/kg. Protein binding is less than 10%.[11,12]

CSF kinetics reflect effect compartment kinetics more closely than do plasma kinetics, but there is still a lag time from peak CSF concentration to effect, possibly reflecting the time required for acetaminophen to act on spinal cord receptors and the hypothalamus.[12] Maximum analgesic and antipyretic effect occur 1–2 h after peak plasma concentration.

Acetaminophen is chiefly metabolized in the liver, with less than 5% excreted unchanged in the urine. At therapeutic doses, glucuronide and sulfate conjugate approximately 80%, and the resulting inactive metabolites are renally excreted. Children have less capacity for glucuronidaton than adults.[12] Ten percent is metabolized by the cytochrome P450 enzyme system to the toxic metabolite *N*-acetyl-*p*-benzoquinone imine (NAPQI), which is in turn inactivated by conjugation with glutathione to form mercapturic acid and cysteine conjugates.[11]

Clearance shows a large amount of interindividual variability but is lower in children than in adults. The elimination half-life is 2–4 h; this can increase with toxic doses.

Acetaminophen is excreted in breast milk in small amounts but there are no documented problems with its use in lactating humans.[11]

Adverse effects

Hepatotoxicity

Acetaminophen is a dose-related hepatotoxin. Fulminant hepatic necrosis occurs when the formation of the active metabolite NAPQI exceeds the binding capacity of glutathione, i.e. when excess NAPQI is formed or when glutathione is depleted. NAPQI binds covalently to nucleophilic proteins in the liver cell, causing cell death. Excess NAPQI can occur through overdose or by cytochrome P450 enzyme induction caused by chronic alcohol use or coadministration of isoniazid, omeprazole, carbamazepine, or phenobarbital.[13] In addition, chronic alcohol use and fasting can lead to reduced glutathione stores.[14]

Doses of acetaminophen over 10 g in adults can cause hepatic injury, and 15–20 g can be fatal.[10] There is a risk of inadvertent overdose if acetaminophen-containing combinations are used with acetaminophen.[15]

Treatment should be instituted early and constitutes methionine to increase conjugation reactions and *N*-acetylcysteine to replenish glutathione.[10,13]

There is no evidence that pre-existing chronic liver disease increases the risk of acetaminophen-induced hepatotoxicity at therapeutic doses, despite prolongation of the elimination half-life. Exceptions include alcoholic liver disease and methotrexate toxicity.[14,16]

Nephrotoxicity

There is no convincing evidence that analgesic nephropathy occurs with chronic therapeutic doses of acetaminophen alone. Therefore, in a 1996 position paper, the National Kidney Foundation recommended acetaminophen as the nonopioid of choice "for episodic use in patients with underlying renal disease."[17] Evidence is conflicting as to whether acetaminophen combination preparations cause analgesic nephropathy.[18]

In about 2% of cases of massive acetaminophen overdose, acute tubular necrosis occurs, probably as a result of the same mechanisms that lead to hepatic cell death.[19]

Phenacetin, the prodrug of acetaminophen can, however, cause renal papillary necrosis if used chronically. All phenacetin-containing analgesics are associated with analgesic nephropathy. It is also associated with cardiovascular toxicity, cancer, and methemoglobinemia.[18]

Other adverse effects

Acetaminophen is well tolerated with few adverse effects at therapeutic doses. Hypersensitivity reactions are rare, with little cross-sensitivity with NSAIDs. Acetaminophen does not cause gastric irritation, does not precipitate bronchospasm, and does not inhibit platelet aggregation. It causes neither CNS depression nor tolerance and dependence. There is no association with Reye's syndrome.

Gastrointestinal upset and skin disorders occur occasionally. Idiosyncratic hematopoietic disturbances such as thrombocytopenia, neutropenia, and pancytopenia have been reported in a few isolated cases at therapeutic doses.

A minor phenacetin metabolite can cause methemoglobinaemia and hemolytic anemia in patients with genetic glucose 6-phosphate deficiency.[11]

Drug interactions[20]

The following drug interactions may occur:

- Barbiturates: chronic use leads to enzyme induction and increased production of the toxic metabolite NAPQI.
- Zidovudine is inactivated by glucuronidation. Acetaminophen can interfere with this mechanism and inhibit elimination of zidovudine.
- Warfarin may be potentiated by prolonged high doses of acetaminophen.
- Metoclopramide affects gastric emptying and may thereby affect acetaminophen absorption.
- Cholestyramine reduces acetaminophen absorption.

Presentations

Acetaminophen is available in several formulations, as follows:

- tablets and suppositories of various strengths;
- syrup or sugar-free solutions, particularly for children;
- as part of many combination preparations (with weak opioids, antiemetics, antihistamines, caffeine, etc.);
- in some countries, as a water-soluble prodrug, propacetamol, as an intravenous preparation.

Recommended doses

Recommended doses in children and adults are as follows:

- adults: 1 g 4-hourly (up to a maximum of 6 g in 24 h);
- children: 15–20 mg/kg 4-hourly.

Acetaminophen achieves antipyresis in children with lower steady-state plasma concentrations than are needed for analgesia.[21,22] However, a few recent studies have shown that conventional dosing regimens of 15 mg/kg 4-hourly do not always achieve the necessary steady-state plasma concentrations. These studies in children suggest loading doses of 50 mg/kg with 6-hourly maintenance doses of 30 mg/kg for antipyresis and loading doses of 70 mg/kg with maintenance of 50 mg/kg 8-hourly for analgesia.[22]

The proper use of acetaminophen is crucial to optimizing its effectiveness.** Doses should be regular in order to maintain steady-state plasma concentrations. This provides analgesia that is far more effective for chronic pain than p.r.n. dosing.[9,16] If used acutely, acetaminophen should be given 1–2 h before anticipated pain or fever.[12]

Conclusions

At therapeutic doses acetaminophen has very few adverse effects compared with NSAIDs and is equally efficacious for relief of mild to moderate pain that has a minimal inflammatory component.[23,24]

It has a very high therapeutic ratio in children, in whom it should be used in preference to nonsteroidal anti-inflammatory drugs (NSAIDs). Infants and newborns also tolerate acetaminophen without problems.[25]**

Nefopam

Nefopam is a centrally acting analgesic used for the treatment of mild to moderate pain.

Mechanism of action

Its mode of action is unclear, but it is possible that serotonergic mechanisms are involved.[26]

Pharmacokinetics

Nefopam hydrochloride is rapidly absorbed and hepatically metabolized by oxidation and glucuronidation. Oral bioavailability is around 60%. The half-life is about 4 h.[27]

Adverse effects

Nefopam has significant anticholinergic activity, which is largely responsible for its unpleasant side-effect profile, particularly in the elderly. Side-effects include dry mouth, blurred vision, tachycardia, headache, nausea, urinary retention, hallucinations, drowsiness, and confusion.

Presentations

It is available in oral and intramuscular forms. The medication is not recommended for use in children.

Dose recommendations[20]

Recommended doses in adults are as follows:

- Adults: 30–90 mg p.o. three times daily or 20 mg i.m. 6-hourly.
- Elderly: 30 mg p.o. three times daily.

Conclusions

There is little to recommend this drug, particularly as randomized controlled trials have shown other nonopioids to be equianalgesic to nefopam for mild to moderate pain while causing fewer side-effects.[28]**

Nonsteroidal anti-inflammatory drugs (NSAIDs)

Mechanism of action

Nonsteroidal anti-inflammatory drugs have analgesic, antipyretic, and anti-inflammatory activity. Most of their actions can be explained by their interference in arachidonic acid metabolism by inhibition of cyclo-oxygenase and subsequent formation of the unstable prostaglandin endoperoxides, PGG_2 and PGH_2[29] (Fig. 3.1).

The end products of arachidonic acid metabolism can be different depending on the individual tissue. The lung and spleen synthesize a wide range of prostaglandins, whereas in vascular endothelium prostacyclin is the main product and in platelets thromboxane A_2 is the main result.[30]

There are two isoforms of cyclo-oxygenase, COX-1 and COX-2. COX-1 is a constitutive enzyme with clear physiological functions. Its activation leads to the production of many substances, such as prostacyclin, which is a vasodilator and has antithrombogenic activity. It is also cytoprotective when released by the gastric mucosa.[29,31]

Inflammatory stimuli and cytokines in migratory and other cells induce COX-2.[32] Both forms of cyclo-

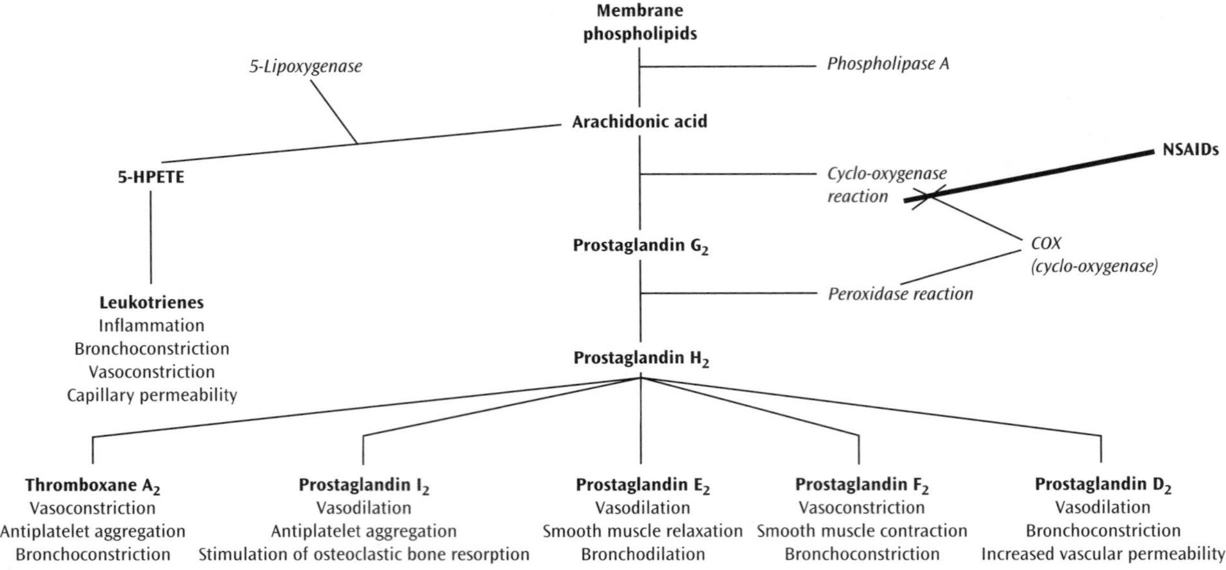

Figure 3.1 *Arachidonic acid metabolism.*

oxygenase are inhibited by NSAIDs, which compete in a dose-dependent manner with arachidonate to modulate cyclo-oxygenase activity. Some drugs inhibit one form more than the other. The adverse effects of NSAIDs are thought to be due to the inhibition of COX-1, and the anti-inflammatory actions to COX-2 inhibition. It is hoped that the recent identification of selective COX-2 inhibitors will lead to therapeutic benefits and safer NSAIDs.[29,33]

NSAIDs are believed to act mainly in the periphery, although there is evidence that spinal NSAIDs can act centrally, providing analgesia at very low doses.[34,35] Their antipyretic activity is due to inhibition of prostaglandins in the hypothalamus. NSAIDs can also exhibit nonprostaglandin effects such as free radical scavenging, inhibition of lipo-oxygenase, and hydrogen peroxide. Other effects have been demonstrated, such as inhibition of chemotaxis, downregulation of IL-1, and interference with calcium-mediated intracellular events.[10,30,35]

Aspirin and its main metabolite, salicylate, act as oxygen radical scavengers and irreversibly inhibit cyclo-oxygenase by acetylating its serine residue.[36] This irreversible inhibition accounts for its effect on platelets, which cannot synthesize new proteins. The duration of this effect is therefore dependent on new platelet formation, which can take over 1 week.

Aspirin and other NSAIDs also inhibit some of the chemical mediators of the kallikrein system and therefore granulocyte adherence to damaged blood vessels, stabilize lysosomes, and inhibit phagocyte migration to sites of inflammation.[10]

Pharmacokinetics

Most NSAIDs are weak organic acids. They are divided into different chemical classes with differing pharmacokinetic parameters (Table 3.1).

Oral NSAIDs are well and rapidly absorbed. Time to peak plasma concentration varies from 0.5 h for ketorolac to 3 h for piroxicam and 4 h for mefenamic acid. However, the majority reach peak plasma concentration in 1–2 h. There is a high degree of protein binding and small volume of distribution. They have variable lipid solubility dependent on their pH. The more lipid-soluble drugs will have greater CNS effects.[37] NSAIDs diffuse slowly into synovial fluid and their effect persists long after synovial drug concentration has become undetectable.[33] Most NSAIDs are extensively metabolized in the liver and their water-soluble metabolites excreted in the urine.

It would probably require significant hepatic impairment to affect the pharmacokinetics of the many NSAIDs metabolized in the liver, but caution should be exercised in those patients known to have hepatic dysfunction.[30]

NSAIDs differ in their renal elimination, but their clearance is reduced in the elderly and those with impaired renal function. NSAIDs are not absolutely contraindicated in impaired renal function but they should be used with caution and at appropriate doses with regular monitoring for adverse effects. Renal excretion is particularly important for indomethacin and ketorolac.[38]

Pregnancy and lactation

Most NSAIDs cross the placenta and are excreted in milk.[39] They are not generally recommended in pregnant or nursing mothers. Consequences to newborns of mothers treated with NSAIDs in pregnancy can include renal failure, fetal hemorrhages, and cardiac abnormalities. However, NSAIDs have been used in lactating women with no documented ill-effects.

Adverse effects

Gastrointestinal toxicity

Gastrointestinal toxicity accounts for most morbidity and mortality due to NSAIDs, particularly with chronic use and in the elderly and debilitated.[40,41] Symptoms can be overt or silent. They range from nausea and vomiting to occult bleeding, gastric perforation, and catastrophic hemorrhage.

Prostaglandins in the gut are important in the repair of gastric epithelium, reducing acid secretion, and, overall, exert a cytoprotective effect. They also increase bicarbonate secretion, mucus synthesis, mucosal thickness, and mucosal blood flow.[30] NSAIDs cause gastrointestinal toxicity by inhibition of prostaglandin synthesis and by direct acid action on the mucosa (e.g. in the case of acetylic salicylic acid).

Prophylactic therapy is possible with prostaglandin analogs such as misoprostol, which offers significant protection against gastric ulceration.[42]** However, this approach is expensive, with unpleasant side-effects such as diarrhea, abdominal pain, and stimulation of uterine contractions. Alternatively, proton pump inhibitors such as omeprazole are proving to be efficacious for decreasing the incidence of NSAID-induced gastroduodenal ulceration and alleviating dyspeptic symptoms.[43]** H_2-receptor antagonists are effective in reducing symptoms due to mucosal injury, but only high-dose famotidine has so far been shown to reduce the incidence of gastric ulcers.[43]

Nephrotoxicity

Prostaglandins have a major protective role in the kidney. They act as vasodilators to improve renal perfusion in patients with reduced renal plasma flow. Thromboxane A_2 (TxA_2) acts as a cortical vasoconstrictor. At the glomeruli, prostaglandins and TxA_2 modulate the filtration rate and regulate renal vascular resistance and renin secretion. In the tubules, prostaglandins influence sodium excretion and antidiuretic hormone activity.[30]

Those at risk of increased nephrotoxicity with NSAIDs are patients with an acute renal insult, pre-existing renal disease, gout, diabetes, arteriopathy, or hypertension, as well as the elderly and patients taking other potentially nephrotoxic medications such as diuretics. NSAIDs are implicated in papillary necrosis, acute and chronic interstitial nephritis, and generalized vasculitis associated with glomerulonephritis.[30,38] The risks of analgesic nephropathy increase with chronic dosing.

However, acute renal failure can occur within hours of a single dose and is then due to interference in the prostaglandin-mediated autoregulation of renal blood flow.[38] This renal ischemia is usually reversible after withdrawing the NSAID but draws attention to acute risk factors such as hypotension and hypovolemia.

NSAIDs can also cause peripheral edema and worsen congestive cardiac failure, hypertension, and hyperkalemia.[30,32]

Asthma

Aspirin and most NSAIDs can precipitate acute and sometimes fatal bronchospasm in asthmatic patients. This syndrome can occur in 8–20% of adult asthmatics. There is cross-sensitivity for bronchospasm between NSAIDs, but not with acetaminophen. Asthma should be regarded as a relative contraindication for NSAIDs. The mechanism may involve the shunting of arachidonate metabolism away from bronchodilator prostaglandins to the synthesis of bronchoconstrictor leukotrienes.[30]

Hematostasis and hematopoiesis

All NSAIDs inhibit platelet aggregation. This is significant in patients with genetic clotting disorders, concurrent anticoagulant use, or history of peptic ulcer disease.[44]

Rarely, severe blood dyscrasias can develop. These have been reported particularly with the pyrazolones.[10]

Immune system

Most NSAIDs can cause anaphylaxis. They impair leukocyte functions *in vitro* and have been associated with necrotizing fasciitis.[30]

Hepatic dysfunction

NSAIDs can cause a variety of liver problems, including asymptomatic raised liver enzymes, mild hepatitis, or, rarely, fatal acute fulminant hepatitis.[45]

Other

Neurological and psychiatric reactions ranging from dizziness to delirium have been reported. Aspirin has a controversial role in the etiology of Reye's syndrome, an acute microvascular encephalopathy associated with a recent viral illness.[46] Its use is not recommended in children who have had a viral illness, but there are no data to show that other NSAIDs should be avoided.

Ibuprofen has been implicated, rarely, in angioedema, thrombocytopenia,[47] and aseptic meningitis.[48] Diclofenac has been associated with thrombocytopenia,[49] hemolytic anemia, and hepatitis.[50] Intramuscular diclofenac can cause local tissue damage and abscess formation.[51]

Drug interactions

NSAIDs show many drug interactions which are relevant for their use and their rate and severity of adverse effects (Table 3.2).

Choice of NSAID

There are many different NSAIDs, from many different chemical classes. However, the same broad principles apply to their pharmacodynamics, and they differ mainly in their pharmacokinetic parameters.[52] Flexible dosing is easier to achieve with those drugs that have short half-lives as maintenance therapy is facilitated. NSAIDs exhibit a ceiling effect, but maximum recommended doses are reported to be more effective than lower ones, although predictably with a significant increase in side-effects. Treatment should start at the lowest recommended dose to minimize toxicity. Patients vary in their

Table 3.1 *Nonsteroidal anti-inflammatory drugs: chemical classes and pharmacokinetic properties (modified from Rang HP, Dale MM.* Pharmacology, *2nd edn. Edinburgh: Churchill Livingstone, 1991: 281–306)*

Chemical class and drug	Plasma half-life (h)	Protein binding (%)	Metabolism	Urinary excretion (% unchanged)	Comments
Salicylic acid derivatives					
Aspirin[a,b]	0.25 (varies with dose)	80–90 (increases with dose)	Hydrolysis by plasma and tissue esterases to salicylic acid and acetic acid. Metabolites are conjugated in the liver. Metabolic pathways are saturable	<5	Irreversible inhibition of cyclo-oxygenase by acetylation. Inhibits osteolytic activity of some malignant cell lines. Dose-dependent hepatotoxicity[14]
Diflunisal	5–20 (dose dependent)	>99	Hepatic glucuronidation	3–9	
Choline magnesium trisalicylate	9–17			2–30 (increases with urinary pH)	
Acetic acids					
Ketorolac[b]	5	>99	Significant renal clearance of unchanged drug	60	Used primarily as a postoperative analgesic
Diclofenac[b]	1.5	>99	Hepatic oxidation then renal excretion. Idiosyncratic hepatotoxin[14]	<5	Also inhibits lipo-oxygenase pathway and therefore leukotriene production. Topical formulation available
Indomethacin[b]	5	>90	Hepatic oxidation and glucuronidation. Enterohepatic recycling. Some renal clearance	15	Very potent but higher incidence of adverse effects
Sulindac[a]	7 (active metabolite 18)	>95	A pro-drug metabolized in liver. Idiosyncratic hepatotoxin[14]	<5	Can cause severe skin disorders and blood dyscrasias
Propionic acids			*Glucuronide conjugates accumulate in renal insufficiency and are cleaved back to the parent drug*		*Racemic mixtures. S-isomer is the active form. Variable interisomeric conversion in humans*
Ibuprofen	2–2.5	>99	Hepatic oxidation and glucuronidation	<5	Lowest incidence of adverse effects, particularly in gastrointestinal tract, but also lower efficacy. Topical formulation available
Naproxen	14	>99	Hepatic glucuronidation	5–10	The only NSAID sold as the *S*-isomer. All others are racemic mixtures
Fenbufen[a]	10 (metabolites)	>99	Prodrug activated in the liver	<5	Skin rashes occur, mild to severe, e.g. Stevens–Johnson syndrome
Ketoprofen[b]	2	>99	Hepatic glucuronidation and some renal clearance	25	Some ability to inhibit lipo-oxygenase

Fenamic acids					*Gastrointestinal tract upsets, particularly diarrhea, common*
Mefenamic acid	4	>99		10	
Oxicams					*Time taken to reach steady state too long to allow for flexible dosage adjustments*
Tenoxicam[b]	60–75	>98		<5	
Piroxicam	45–50	>99	Hepatic oxidation	10	Inhibits the production of hydrogen peroxide by activated neutrophils
Pyrazalones					*Blood dyscrasias a concern*
Phenylbutazone[a]	50–95	>99		<5	
Dipyrone[b]	7	Low	Hydrolyzed to active metabolites		Agranulocytosis a risk. Silent fatal toxic effects and no analgesic efficacy over other NSAIDs, therefore not recommended for use
Nonacidic					
Nabumetone[a]	20–30 ($t_{1/2}$ of active metabolite)	99	A prodrug activated in the liver.	<5	Active metabolite has high selectivity for COX-2. Low incidence of side-effects

a. Active metabolites.
b. Available for parenteral use.

tolerance to different NSAIDs and they will have different concurrent organ dysfunction and pre-existing medical problems, which may influence the choice of medication. It is important to reassess patients regularly, and to anticipate and treat any side-effects.[53,54]

Conclusions

Like acetaminophen, NSAIDs can be used for management of cancer pain and breakthrough pain. NSAIDs are particularly useful analgesics for pain with an inflammatory component and pain due to bony metastases. There is often a high local concentration of prostaglandins in the affected bone, produced by tumor cells, and these are felt to be at least partially responsible for the spread and pain of metastatic bone disease.[55***,56***] However, incidence of adverse effects and the side-effect profile with use of NSAIDs require caution in their use, in particular in at-risk patients and the elderly.

OPIOIDS

Terminology

Opioid is a broad term that applies to any substance which produces its effects by binding to opioid receptors and which is stereospecifically antagonized by naloxone. It includes naturally occurring, semisynthetic, and synthetic opioids.

The term *endogenous opioids* refer to the families of opioid peptides: *enkephalins, endorphins, endomorphins,* and *dynorphins.*

Opiates are drugs derived from opium. They include naturally occurring drugs such as morphine, codeine, and thebaine, as well as their semisynthetic derivatives. *Opium* is an extract of poppy juice, *Papaver somniferum.* It is a mixture of more than 20 different alkaloids including morphine (9–20%), codeine (up to 4%), thebaine, and papaverine.

Narcotics is a loose term derived from the Greek word *narke*, meaning numbness or stupor. The word has unfortunate connotations in that it is used worldwide to describe drugs of abuse. Regrettably, it is still used in textbooks and by health workers to describe morphine-like drugs. This does not help the persistent opiophobia that hampers the therapeutic use of opioids for managing pain. The term should be avoided in medical literature.

Mechanism of action

Opioid receptors

There are three principal types of opioid receptor, OP3 (μ), OP1 (δ), and OP2 (κ). They are coupled to G-proteins and exert both inhibitory and stimulatory effects by acting on adenyl cyclase synthesis, ion channels, and intracellular calcium stores.[57–59] Opioid receptors are found both pre- and postsynaptically; about 75% are thought to be presynaptic.[60] There is still no firm evidence as to the existence of the opioid receptor subtypes for μ, κ, and δ.[61] A fourth receptor, ORL-1, has recently been discovered; its role as an opioid receptor and in pain pathways looks exciting, but is as yet unclear.[59,60,62]

Opioid receptors and endogenous opioid peptides are widely distributed throughout the CNS[63] and gastrointestinal tract[64] and at peripheral sites in inflammatory states.[65–67] Supraspinal receptors are most densely populated in the periaqueductal gray matter of the midbrain, the locus ceruleus, and the nucleus raphe magnus in the rostral ventromedial medulla.[63,68] Spinal opioid receptors are predominantly μ (65%) and δ (20%) and are found in the substantia gelatinosa of the superficial dorsal horn.[60,63]

Opioids affect many different systems throughout the body, influencing neurotransmitter and peptide release and the immune system. In the CNS, the systems primarily affected are:

1. Ascending and descending pain pathways. In the ascending pathway μ-, δ-, and κ-receptors modulate sensory transmission. All three receptor types are located in the spinal cord, but μ and κ are more prominent in the thalamus. In the descending pathways, mainly μ and κ are involved at higher levels in the periaqueductal gray and nucleus raphe magnus, and all three receptors types are expressed in the gigantocellular reticular nuclei.[63]
2. Nigrostriatal and mesolimbic dopamine systems.
3. Hypothalamic and pituitary axes.

Opioid receptors are also widely distributed in the gastrointestinal tract. Mu- and κ-receptors have been identified in animal studies on nerve fibers and neurons in the myenteric and submucosal plexus, and on interstitial cells.[64]

Endogenous opioids

The opioid peptides derive from three common precursors molecules, proenkephalin, prodynorphin, and pro-opiomelanocortin. Particular endogenous opioids display a binding preference for certain opioid receptors but are not completely selective for each receptor type. However, two opioid peptides, endomorphin 1 and endomorphin 2, recently identified in the human brain,[69] show high affinity and selectivity for μ-receptors.[70]

The endogenous opioids, their preferred receptor, and actions mediated by agonist activity at that receptor are depicted in Table 3.3.

Classification of opioids

Opioids can be classified according to their source or, more usefully, their activity at opioid receptors (Table 3.4).

Table 3.2 *Pharmacological interactions of nonsteroidal anti-inflammatory drugs (modified from Bowdle TA ed.,* The Pharmacologic Basis of Anaesthesiology: Basic Science and Practical Applications. *Edinburgh: Churchill Livingstone, 1994)*

NSAID	Drug affected	Effect	Management
Pharmacokinetic			
Aspirin (high dose)	Warfarin	Potentiation of anticoagulant effects	Monitor carefully.
	Sodium valproate	Inhibition of valproate metabolism	Avoid aspirin. If another NSAID used, monitor plasma valproate concentrations carefully
Salicylate	Phenytoin Sodium valproate	Competition for plasma protein binding sites	Monitor phenytoin levels carefully
Pyrazolones	Oral anticoagulants	Inhibition of metabolism of *S*-warfarin, increasing anticoagulant effect	Avoid these NSAIDs if possible or monitor carefully
	Sulfonylureas	Inhibition of metabolism, prolonging half-life and risk of hypoglycemia	Avoid these NSAIDs or monitor blood glucose closely
	Phenytoin	Inhibition of metabolism. Increased plasma levels and risk of toxicity	Avoid these NSAIDs or monitor phenytoin levels very closely
	Sodium valproate	Inhibition of valproate metabolism. Increased plasma levels	Avoid these NSAIDs or monitor closely
All	Digoxin	No interaction if renal function normal. Potential reduction in kidney function thereby reducing renal clearance and increasing plasma digoxin levels	Avoid NSAIDs if possible or monitor plasma digoxin levels and creatinine frequently
Except possibly sulindac and aspirin	Lithium	As above. Can increase plasma lithium concentrations	Monitor lithium levels carefully and adjust dose accordingly
	Aminoglycosides	Reduction in renal function in susceptible people. Decrease clearance and increase plasma aminoglycoside concentrations	Monitor levels and adjust dose accordingly
	Methotrexate (high doses)	Reduced clearance, increasing risk of toxicity	NSAIDs contraindicated. May be safe between cycles of chemotherapy
Pharmacodynamic			
Salicylates	Sulfonylureas	Potentiates hypoglycemic effects	Avoid these NSAIDs if possible or monitor blood glucose levels carefully
All	Antihypertensive drugs β-Blockers Diuretics Angiotensin-converting enzyme inhibitors	Reduced antihypertensive effect due to salt and water retention and vasoconstriction	Avoid all NSAIDs if possible
	Anticoagulants	Mucosal damage to gastrointestinal tract and platelet inhibition increase risk of gastrointestinal bleeding	Avoid all NSAIDs if possible
All (but particularly indomethacin)	Diuretics	Reduced natriuresis and diuresis, may exacerbate congestive heart failure, and potentiate nephrotoxicity. Increased risk of renal failure and hyperkalemia	Avoid combination. Check plasma potassium
All	Cyclosporine	Increased risk of nephrotoxicity	Monitor renal function

NB: Other drugs can affect NSAIDs, mainly by pharmacokinetic interactions. Barbiturates increase NSAID metabolism and metoclopramide, cholestyramine, and caffeine can affect the rate of absorption of NSAIDs. These interactions are seldom of any clinical importance.

Opioid activity at receptors is based on the theory that receptors are specific membrane-bound proteins that interact selectively with extracellular substances to initiate biochemical events within the cell. These substances may be endogenous or exogenous, such as opioid drugs. They can exhibit pure agonist activity, antagonist activity or act as partial agonists or agonist–antagonists.

An *agonist* acts at a receptor to initiate changes in cell function. Traditionally, an agonist produces the normal biological response of the cell.

A *partial agonist* binds to the receptor but causes less response than a full agonist, i.e. it has a lower efficacy. It may, however, have a higher affinity for the receptor and act as a competitive antagonist in the presence of a full agonist. A typical example would be the partial agonist buprenorphine, which has a greater affinity for opioid receptors than morphine.

An *agonist–antagonist* acts as an antagonist at some receptors and an agonist or partial agonist at others. Pentazocine is a μ-receptor antagonist but exerts its opioid effect by agonist activity at the κ-receptor.

Antagonists occupy the receptor but have no biological activity. A competitive antagonist such as naloxone binds reversibly to the receptor and can displace and is displaced by the agonist. A noncompetitive antagonist binds irreversibly to the receptor.

Drugs have two separate attributes at receptor sites, affinity and efficacy. *Affinity* is the tendency or ability to bind to a receptor to produce a stable complex. A drug with high affinity binds to a receptor more strongly than does one with lower affinity. Buprenorphine, for example, has a higher affinity for opioid receptors than morphine (although it is not as efficacious).

Efficacy, or intrinsic activity, is the ability of the drug, once bound, to produce a certain effect. Efficacy can range from zero, for an antagonist, to a potential maximum effect for that particular receptor. A partial agonist may be more potent than a full agonist at the lower end of the effect range; however, even at maximal doses, a partial agonist cannot achieve the full effect of an agonist. Partial agonists exhibit a ceiling effect that does not occur with a full agonist, the maximum dose of which is limited not by lack of analgesic effect, but by adverse effects.

The *potency* of a drug is its ability to produce a certain effect, in other words the relative dose required to achieve an effect. The drug's absorption, distribution, metabolism, excretion, and affinity for its receptor influence potency.

Dose–response curves describe the relationships between the dose of a drug and the subsequent response (Fig. 3.2). Curves are characterized by their position on the *x*-axis (potency), maximal height (efficacy), and slope (number of receptors that must be bound to produce a response).

Partial agonists or agonist–antagonists have only limited usefulness as analgesics in cancer pain;[71] if they are regarded as useful, then they should be used before a pure agonist such as morphine. Animal studies suggest that, if given to a patient who has received morphine analgesia for even a short period, withdrawal symptoms can be precipitated, possibly accompanied by a decline in analgesic effect.[72]

Pharmacokinetics

Knowledge of the disposition of opioids in the body is vital in prescribing correct doses and achieving the desired therapeutic effect, analgesia.

Terminology

Most of the following definitions are applicable to oral analgesia, the most common form of drug administration for patients with cancer pain.

Absorption is the extent to which the intact drug is absorbed from the gut lumen into the portal circulation. It is expressed as a fraction of the dose that is absorbed from the gut. Factors affecting absorption are dissolution of the drug, gastric emptying rate, intestinal motility, drug interactions in the lumen, and passage through the gut wall.

Table 3.3 *Receptors, response on activation, and their preferred opioid peptides*

Receptor	Response on activation	Endogenous opioid
OP3 (μ)	Analgesia, respiratory depression, euphoria, sedation, miosis, reduced gastrointestinal motility, nausea, vomiting, pruritus, skeletal muscle rigidity, biliary spasm, urinary retention, most cardiovascular effects, changes in neurotransmitter turnover, and endocrine effects	Endomorphin 1 and 2 β-Endorphin Met-enkephalin
OP1[a] (δ)	Analgesia, nausea, vomiting, dopamine turnover	Enkephalins
OP2 (κ)	Analgesia, dysphoria, psychotomimetic effects, miosis,[b] respiratory depression,[b] sedation,[b] neurotransmitter turnover, endocrine effects, urinary retention	Dynorphins
ORL-1[a] (orphan)	Supraspinal hyperalgesia, spinal analgesia, affects acoustic information processing, lacks motivation and reward properties	Nociceptin (orphanin FQ)

a. Less intense than with OP3 activation.
b. Animal studies only.

Table 3.4 *Classification of opioids by their action at receptors (modified from Rang HP, Dale MM.* Pharmacology, *2nd edn. Edinburgh: Churchill Livingstone, 1991: 714–36)*

Class	Drug	Action at opioid receptor		
		OP3 (μ)	**OP1** (δ)	**OP2** (κ)
Agonists				
Morphine and its congeners (epoxymorphinans)	Morphine (naturally occurring)	+++	++	++
(Phenanthrene derivatives)	Diamorphine (semisynthetic)	Prodrug		
	Papaveretum (mixture of naturally occurring opioids)	++	++	++
	Codeine (naturally occurring)	+	+	+
	Dihydrocodeine (semisynthetic)	+	+	+
	Hydromorphone	+++	++	++
	Oxycodone	+++	++	++
	Oxymorphone	+++	++	++
Morphinan derivative	Levorphanol	+++	+++	+++
Methadone and its congeners	Methadone (synthetic)	+++	++	++
	Dextropropoxyphene	+	+	+
Phenylpiperidines (all synthetic)	Meperidine (pethidine)	++	+	+
	Fentanyl	++++	+	
Other	Tramadol (synthetic)	++		
Agonist–antagonists				
Benzmorphan derivatives	Pentazocine	•	+	+++
Morphinan derivative	Butorphanol	•		++
Epoxymorphinan	Nalbuphine	•	+	++
Partial agonists				
Thebaine derivative	Buprenorphine	(+++)		
Antagonists				
Epoxymorphinans	Naloxone	•••	••	••
	Naltrexone	•••	••	••

+, Agonist; •, antagonist; ( ), partial agonist.

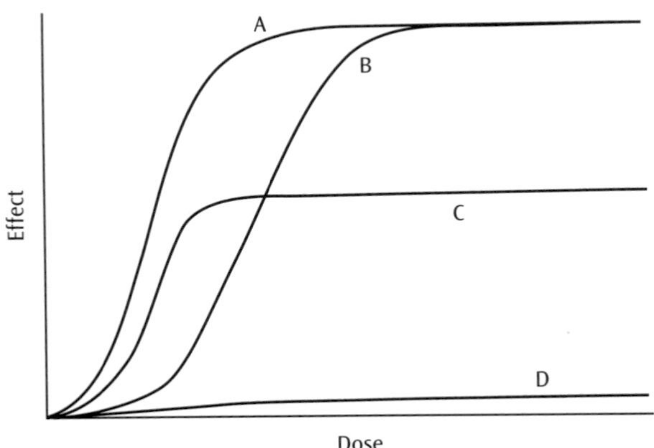

Figure 3.2 *Dose–response curves for hypothetical opioids (A and B are full agonists and A is more potent than B, C is a partial agonist and D an antagonist).*

First-pass clearance is the extent to which the drug is removed by the liver in its first pass in the portal blood through the liver to the systemic circulation. Changes in hepatic extraction are due to changes in microsomal enzyme activity and liver blood flow.

Bioavailability (*F*) is the fraction of the dose that reaches the systemic circulation intact and is available at the effect site. Bioavailability depends on the fraction of drug absorbed and how much escapes first-pass metabolism in the liver. The route of administration obviously has a significant effect on bioavailability. The i.v. route has a bioavailability of 100%. Most opioids are well absorbed from the gut but undergo substantial first-pass metabolism. The bioavailability of oral morphine varies from 15% to 35%, and that of meperidine and codeine is about 50%.

Bioavailability = absorption × fraction escaping first-pass metabolism

Volume of distribution (V_d) is the pharmacokinetic parameter used to determine the loading dose of a drug. It is an imaginary volume, relating the total amount of drug in the body, to the plasma concentration of the drug.

V_d = total amount of drug in the body/plasma concentration of drug

Opioids have an initial V_d of 20–50 l, but after some time the drugs will distribute from more vascularized regions to fat tissues, thereby increasing the initial V_d to a steady-state V_d of 150–250 l.

Clearance (Cl) describes the efficiency of irreversible elimination of a drug from the body, by excretion or metabolism. It is defined as the volume of blood cleared of the drug in time. Total body clearance is the sum of the clearances of all the organs, e.g. liver, kidney, lung. Almost all opioids are extensively metabolized in the liver, and clearance is approximately equal to hepatic blood flow. In the case of systemic, chronically administered opioids that have reached steady state, changes in hepatic blood flow can have major effects on the steady-state concentrations of these highly extracted drugs. The situation is a little different for chronic oral dosing of opioids. Changes in hepatic blood flow make little difference, but alterations in hepatic enzyme activity can alter bioavailability. For example, assuming 100% absorption, inducing hepatic enzymes will have a small effect on the amount extracted by the liver, as this is already large, e.g. increase from 90% to 95% extraction. However, the small amount escaping extraction can decrease by a relatively large amount, e.g. from 10% to 5%. Alternatively, if drugs or seriously impaired liver function inhibits hepatic enzymes, bioavailability can be increased by a comparatively large amount.

Elimination half-life ($t_{1/2\beta}$) is the time taken for the amount of drug in the body to fall by half; for most opioids it is in the range of several hours. Clearance and volume of distribution determine half-life.

$$t_{1/2\beta} = \frac{V_d \times \ln 2}{Cl}$$

Half-life is important in determining the duration of action after a single dose, the time required to reach steady state, and the dosing interval with chronic dosing: It takes five half-lives to reach steady state, and the dosing interval required to avoid excessive fluctuations in plasma concentration is in the range of one half-life. It also takes about five half-lives to completely remove a drug from the body.

Calculating a dosing regimen of a drug

When designing a dosing regimen it is important to remember the loading dose. Without one, it could take five half-lives to achieve an adequate therapeutic effect. Morphine has a $t_{1/2\beta}$ of 1–4 h, so that a poor dosing regimen could result in a 5- to 20-h wait for adequate pain relief.

The values used here are approximate only, and vary considerably between patients.

For an intravenous infusion and intermittent bolus dosing the formula is:

Loading dose = effective plasma concentration × V_d

As mentioned above, the initial V_d is not the same as the steady-state V_d, and this must be taken into account. For example, the initial V_d of morphine is 25 l. If the required plasma concentration is 0.05 mg/l, then the initial bolus is 25 × 0.05 = 1.25 mg. If the V_d at steady state reaches 250 l, then the above initial loading dose needs to be followed by a loading infusion over 1 h of (250–25) × 0.05 = 11.25 mg.

Following this loading dose, the dose needed to maintain the target concentration over time should be calculated as follows:

Maintenance dose = target plasma concentration × Cl

Returning to the above example, the clearance of morphine is about 1 l/min, so the hourly maintenance dose is 0.05 × 60 = 3 mg.

For oral administration, the same principles apply, with two differences. The slower absorption of an oral dose means that plasma concentration fluctuates less between doses. Sustained-release formulations show an even better concentration–time profile, approaching that of a continuous infusion. Further on, the dose reaching the effect compartment is affected by the bioavailability, so that at steady state the calculation is:

Oral maintenance dose rate = target plasma concentration × Cl/*F*

Factors influencing pharmacokinetics

Renal and hepatic disease can alter the pharmacokinetic parameters of opioids, with clinical consequences.

Hepatic disease

The liver is the main site of opioid metabolism, and alterations in hepatic function may be expected to have an effect on drug clearance.[73] Liver blood flow, enzyme activity, and protein binding all influence opioid clearance. Severe hepatic cirrhosis can cause alterations in blood flow due to intra- and extrahepatic shunting. Alcoholic cirrhosis and acute hepatitis, which affect the pericentral regions, impair oxidative metabolism. Diseases affecting the periportal regions have little effect on drug metabolism. The conjugating enzymes are only affected in end-stage liver disease. Low albumin levels due to malnutrition or renal, or hepatic disease can lead to decreased protein binding and hence increase the response to opioids. The metabolism of i.v. opioids is flow limited, and a decrease in liver blood flow can decrease the clearance and prolong the half-life of opioids.

Morphine clearance is reduced, and terminal half-life prolonged, in severe hepatic dysfunction.[74] Significant extrahepatic conjugation of morphine makes the effect of hepatic cirrhosis less important in the metabolism of this drug than is the case for highly extracted drugs, such as meperidine, that are cleared by oxidation.[75–77]

Chronic liver disease can also cause a large increase in the bioavailability of oral opioids, and caution must be used with dosing regimens.[78] The rate of clearance is decreased, and in conjunction with the rise in bioavailability can lead to increased intensity and duration of action of opioids at relatively low doses.

Meperidine (pethidine) and pentazocine have been studied in patients with cirrhotic liver disease. Both show large increases in bioavailability as a result of decreased enzyme activity and portosystemic shunting, over 30% for meperidine and greater than 200% for pentazocine.[79,80]

Renal impairment

Although the kidneys play a minor role in the elimination of most opioids, renal disease can lead to build-up of active or toxic metabolites, which are normally excreted in the urine. The active metabolite of morphine, morphine 6-glucuronide (M6G), is excreted by the kidneys and can accumulate in severe renal impairment as its excretion is directly related to creatinine clearance. It has a high affinity for opioid receptors, its half-life varies between 2.5 and 7.5 h, and it is responsible for the prolonged analgesia and sedation seen in patients with renal failure. Morphine 3-glucuronide (M3G) also accumulates and is possibly proalgesic by antagonizing the effects of morphine and M6G.[81,82] M3G may also cause hyperalgesia by nonopioid mechanisms at spinal cord level. Increased amounts of the toxic metabolite normorphine may be responsible for myoclonic activity.[83] Morphine can still be used in patients with renal failure, but caution should be exercised as prolonged sedation can occur.

Fentanyl metabolites may accumulate in patients with renal failure, but this is unlikely to have clinical consequences, as such metabolites are pharmacologically inactive. Prolonged sedation may occur with i.v. infusions in renal failure.[84]

The terminal half-life of meperidine is unaffected in renal failure, as meperidine undergoes extensive hepatic metabolism. The potentially toxic metabolite of meperidine, normeperidine (norpethidine), is excreted in the urine, and its half-life can increase from 20 to 40 h in patients with renal failure. Normeperidine is a proconvulsant and causes significant adverse neurological effects, including tremors, myoclonus, and generalized seizures. Although the administration of a single dose appears to carry little risk for patients with renal impairment, the regular use of meperidine should be avoided.[82] This property makes meperidine even more unsuitable for cancer patients with renal failure who need long-term opioids.

Methadone is mainly metabolized in the liver, and the metabolite excreted in the feces, but 20% is excreted unchanged in the urine. There are few studies regarding methadone in renal failure, but also no reports of specific problems. In one report of three patients with chronic renal disease receiving chronic methadone treatment, there was no evidence for the accumulation of methadone or its metabolites.[85] It is speculated that in renal failure more methadone is metabolized in the liver and excreted as its primary metabolite in the feces. Methadone can probably be safely used in renal failure, but there are few conclusive data one way or the other.

There are no specific changes in the pharmacokinetic parameters of buprenorphine in patients with renal insufficiency and normal doses can be used.[82]

Codeine can cause CNS and respiratory depression and hypotension at normal doses. Its half-life can increase from to 4 to 18 h in renal failure and it can produce excessive sedation.[86] It is recommended that doses are reduced or an alternative opioid used in patients with renal impairment. Dihydrocodeine has also caused prolonged narcosis in some patients with renal failure, and a reduction in dose may be advisable.

Dextropropoxyphene and its main metabolite, norpropoxyphene accumulate in renal failure, causing CNS and respiratory depression and cardiotoxicity in animals. It is probably better to avoid this drug in patients with renal impairment. There have been several reports in the literature associating dextropropoxyphene with hypoglycemia in patients with renal failure.[87]

Neither hepatic nor renal impairment is a contraindication to the use of opioids for cancer pain. Monitoring is needed, as is awareness of the potential need to reduce doses, increase dosing intervals, or switch to alternative opioids or routes of administration.

Adverse effects

There are many adverse effects associated with opioids, the most common being nausea, vomiting, constipation, and sedation. Side-effects tend to be dose related, and show a large amount of variability between different opioids and different patients, depending on many pharmacokinetic and pharmacodynamic factors. Tolerance can occur to many of these side-effects, particularly in patients with chronic pain and cancer, who can be on opioids for long periods. If side-effects become unbearable and intractable with a particular opioid, at doses required for analgesia, it is often useful to rotate to another opioid. This is discussed in Chapter Ca12.

Central nervous system effects

Sedation is common on initiation of therapy but gradually resolves within a week as tolerance develops.[81] Interaction with other CNS depressants, such as alcohol and benzodiazepines, is additive. If sedation persists, or is severe, the opioid dose could be decreased and the frequency of intake increased, to decrease peak plasma levels while maintaining therapeutic plasma concentrations. Patients could also be switched to another opioid. The use of CNS stimulants, such as caffeine, dextroamphetamine, and methylphenidate, has been advocated for morphine-induced sedation,[88,89] although such substances are felt to have a minor role in reducing daytime sedation and improving sleep.[90]

Cognitive impairment is also common, at least initially. Patients may experience significant cognitive impairment after starting opioids, or after a recent dose increase, but tolerance can develop rapidly. However, patients are not always aware of any decline in function.[91] Consideration must be given to these factors when advising patients on driving, work, and decision-making while taking opioids. Some data support the view that patients on stable doses of morphine do not show significantly impaired cognitive and psychomotor function and may restart activities, such as driving, when opioid doses have stabilized.[92] Persistent confusion due solely to opioids is rare, and other causes, such as drug interactions or disease processes, should be actively sought.

Other central effects associated with chronic morphine use include miosis, sleep disturbances, hallucinations, nightmares, dizziness, euphoria, dysphoria, hyperalgesia, and allodynia. Myoclonus also occurs with chronic high-dose opioid use.[93] This is a sign of toxicity and the need to reduce peak plasma opioid levels, or an indication for opioid rotation. If severe, myoclonus can be managed with clonazepam, dantrolene, barbiturates, or sodium valproate. It is mainly a problem with repeated large doses of parenteral meperidine, due to the accumulation of its toxic metabolite, normeperidine.[94] Normeperidine accumulates even more in renal impairment. Myoclonus can proceed to generalized seizures, which can be fatal.[95]

Pruritus is a common opioid side-effect and can be very unpleasant for the patient and intractable to therapy. It is more common with parenteral opioid administration, even more so with neuraxial opioids. It is thought to be a μ-receptor effect at the level of the medullary dorsal horn and is not associated with histamine release or allergy.[96,97] However, because many different pharmacologic therapies are helpful to a greater or lesser degree the mechanisms of opioid-induced pruritus are still unclear. Antihistamines, opioid antagonists, ondansetron, and propofol can be used successfully, but none are universally effective. Two small case reports have described the effect of opioid rotation on pruritus. In one report, morphine-induced pruritus responded to a change to hydromorphone.[98] In the other, six patients with opioid-induced pruritus that was unresponsive to antihistamines gained significant relief within 60 min from intranasal butorphanol.[99]

Respiratory depression is potentially the most serious adverse central effect of all strong opioids.[100] Opioids act directly on the medullary respiratory center to produce dose-related depression of all phases of respiratory activity. Apnea is the commonest cause of death from opioids. Opioid-naive patients in particular, and those with preexisting respiratory disease, are more at risk of significant respiratory depression.

Where the opioid dose has been titrated against pain in the cancer patient, tolerance is rapid and respiratory depression is rare. Care must be taken, however, if the opioid dose is suddenly increased by a large amount, the route of administration is changed, or the patient is switched to a different opioid that is more potent or longer acting. Also, if pain is suddenly and completely relieved, respiratory arrest is a potential problem if patients are continued on the same dose of opioid.[100] If pain that has formerly been controlled by opioids is suddenly and completely relieved by nerve block or cordotomy, there is the danger of severe respiratory depression at opioid doses that had previously caused no adverse effects; pain acts as a physiological antagonist to the central depressant effects of opioids.[101] It has been postulated that the medullary respiratory center receives nociceptive input.[102]

Sedation, mental clouding, and a slowed respiratory rate always accompany clinically significant respiratory depression.[100] Naloxone is the standard treatment for opioid-induced respiratory depression, but should be used with caution as it can precipitate sudden, severe withdrawal symptoms and a recurrence of pain. Suppression of the cough reflex is a potentially useful side-effect, unless it decreases the ability to clear secretions. Non cardiogenic pulmonary edema is also associated with opioid use, including opioid antagonists.[100]

Nausea and vomiting are debilitating and very distressing common effects of all opioids. They can occur in up to two-thirds of patients taking oral morphine but vary in intensity between patients. Like most opioid effects, nausea and vomiting are centrally mediated by effects on receptors in the chemoreceptor trigger zone in the area postrema. Increased vestibular sensitivity and delayed gastric emptying are also important factors in the development of opioid-induced emesis. It is worse in ambulating patients, and with parenteral administration. This is a side-effect that should be anticipated and, if it occurs, antiemetics should be readily available and used regularly until tolerance to this opioid effect develops, usually within a week. Persistent nausea despite treatment warrants a change in dose, opioid, or route of administration.

Gastrointestinal effects

These are due mainly to binding to peripheral opioid receptors in the gut, leading to delayed gastric emptying, reduced gastric secretions, decreased gastrointestinal motility, and increased sphincter tone. The result is *constipation*, which can range in severity from mildly troublesome to bowel obstruction. Tolerance to these effects does not occur, therefore constipation should be treated prophylactically in patients on long-term opioids, with peristaltic agents and stool softeners.[81]

Others

Urinary retention can be a problem, particularly in the elderly, due to opioid-induced increased smooth muscle tone.[100]

Postural hypotension is centrally mediated, and due to the action of opioids on the vasomotor center and a fall in sensitivity of baroreceptor reflexes. Bradycardia is due to a central vagotonic action. Meperidine produces tachycardia due to an atropine-like effect. Opioids can also cause histamine release, which in turn leads to localized urticaria and peripheral vasodilation. Sweating and dry mouth are also observed with opioid use.[100]

Adverse effects with long-term use

Tolerance, physical dependence, and addiction

Pain is the most common symptom in over 70% of patients with advanced cancer,[103,104] and opioids are the mainstay of pain management.[1,105] Some patients with cancer would rather die than experience unrelieved, escalating, severe pain.[106] However, many cancer patients with pain are consistently undertreated, enduring an unnecessary, living hell of uncontrolled pain.[107–110]

The reasons for this are multiple, including absence of national policies on cancer pain relief and palliative care, lack of financial resources and health care delivery systems, and legal restrictions on the use and availability of opioids due to the misconception that increased medical use will increase illicit drug traffic. There is a lack of awareness on the part of health workers that cancer pain can, and should, be relieved, and concern that medical use of opioids will produce dependence and drug abuse.

Many physicians and nursing staff underprescribe and underadminister opioid analgesia for moderate to severe pain through fear and ignorance: fear of tolerance and addiction,[107,110] and of escalating dose requirements and adverse effects, and ignorance of the pharmacokinetics and pharmacodynamics of opioids and the meaning and mechanisms of tolerance, physical dependence, and substance abuse.[111,112]

Patients also fear opioids, the stigma attached to their use, loss of control over their disease, and the potential for addiction. Patients and their families also fear that opioids are being used as a kind of surreptitious euthanasia.[113,114]

Particularly at risk from physician opiophobia and poor pain control are patients in perceived “minority” groups[115] and those whose first language is not that of their health workers or of the pain assessment tools available, such as the BPI (Brief Pain Inventory).[116,117] The Single Convention on Narcotic Drugs stated in 1961 that “the medical use of narcotic drugs continues to be indispensable for the relief of pain” and “addiction to narcotic drugs constitutes a serious evil.”[1] Unfortunately, while paying lip service to the first statement, health workers and legislative authorities still seem to have an irrational attachment to the idea that the use of opioids causes addiction. This opiophobia is widespread and persistent, possibly as common today as when it was discussed over 20 years ago.[107,108]

A good understanding of the terms surrounding addiction, dependence, and tolerance is necessary to avoid suboptimal management of cancer patients with pain.

Tolerance

When tolerance occurs, higher doses of a drug are required to produce the same effect or the same dose has decreasing efficacy.[118] Tolerance is a biological effect due to prior exposure to a drug, and this exposure drives the diminution in effect. Tolerance has been reliably shown to occur in both human and animal models both *in vivo* and *in vitro*.[119]

Acquired tolerance can be acute or chronic. *Acute* tolerance (tachyphylaxis) is a phenomenon that typically occurs within minutes.

Pharmacokinetic tolerance refers to changes in distribution or metabolism of a drug such that concentrations of the drug are reduced in the plasma and at the effect site. A common cause would be an increase in the rate of metabolism of a drug, as a result of hepatic enzyme induction, and therefore lessening of effect by more rapid removal of the drug from the circulation.

Pharmacodynamic tolerance occurs at a receptor level in the system acted on by the drug.

Learned tolerance is a reduction in the effects of a drug due to learned compensatory mechanisms. For example, behavioral tolerance is involved in learning how to function in a mild state of intoxication or conditioned tolerance when environmental cues are constantly paired with drug administration.

Cross-tolerance occurs when repeated doses of a drug in a given category confer tolerance to that drug and to other drugs in similar structural and mechanistic categories.[118]

Tolerance to opioids is predominantly pharmacodynamic, receptor selective, and reversible.[119,120] It has also been shown to be dose dependent. The major factor in tolerance development is thought to be the uncoupling of opioid receptors from second-messenger systems, possibly by the decoupling of the receptors from G-proteins.[121,122] Opioid tolerance is characterized by a shortened duration and decreased intensity of analgesia, euphoria, and central nervous system depressant effects and a significant elevation in the potentially lethal dose.[118]

Most studies on tolerance have been conducted in animals. Other systems have been shown to be involved in the development of tolerance. NMDA antagonists and nitric oxide synthase inhibitors can prevent morphine tolerance in rodents.[123] Rats in chronic pain self-administered a stable dose of morphine and reduced their intake when a nonsteroidal anti-inflammatory drug was added. When the pain was removed the rats rapidly increased their opioid intake in a similar manner to pain-free rats, theoretically for the positive reinforcing properties of euphoria or withdrawal prevention.[124] Dopamine has long been thought to be involved in the reward mechanisms of opioid dependence. Recent studies on rats in chronic pain have found decreased levels of dopamine in the brain, and administration of morphine raised the dopamine levels toward normal. If morphine was given to pain-free rats, dopamine levels increased above normal.[125,126]

Human studies and observations on opioid dependence and tolerance have mainly been carried out in recreational addicts and volunteers. Studies on patients with chronic pain are rare. There is conflicting evidence as to the existence of acute tolerance.[127,128]

Differing opioid effects manifest tolerance at different rates.[118,123] Tolerance to respiratory depression develops rapidly and is rapidly reversible. Respiratory depression in patients in pain who are not opioid naive is infrequent. Tolerance to the sedative and cognitive effects of opioids also develops rapidly, although it has been suggested that some patients are less aware of cognitive impairment.[91] Nausea and vomiting occur in a significant proportion of patients on opioids, but tolerance usually develops within a week. Until then, they should take regular antiemetics.

Unfortunately, tolerance to constipation develops rarely, if at all. It must therefore be anticipated and treated prophylactically.

Fear of tolerance to analgesic effects and escalating dose requirements frequently limit the prescribing of opioids for cancer pain. Some physicians feel that increasing the dose too soon will result in severe side-effects and leave no analgesic options for when the pain gets "really bad!"** However, despite all the publicity and animal studies, clinical evidence has shown that true analgesic tolerance to opioids in patients with pain is extremely rare. Patients with cancer can be maintained on a steady level of opioids for prolonged periods.[129–131] It is useful to remember that a decline in analgesic effect has a differential diagnosis, with true tolerance only one of the possible diagnoses.[119]

The main reason for a reduced analgesic effect in such patients, however, is increased nociceptive input.[129,132,133] If dose requirements increase and pain is no longer controlled, the patient should be carefully evaluated for disease progression. Other causes of decreasing analgesic effect are more likely to be psychological, such as increasing anxiety, depression, change in cognitive state, or conditioned pain behavior.

In both animals and humans, *cross-tolerance* to opioids occurs and has been shown to be incomplete because of selective tolerance at different subpopulations of opioid receptors.[120] When initially managing severe pain, there is probably a clinical advantage in using a relatively selective μ-agonist first, such as morphine. Rats and mice that have been chronically treated with levorphanol (an agonist at μ-, κ-, and δ-receptors) and methadone show significant tolerance to morphine (which has mainly μ-agonist activity), but when treated with morphine alone they develop tolerance to morphine but minimal tolerance to methadone or levorphanol.[134,135]

Cross-tolerance has an important role in patients who have their pain controlled by opioid agonists, particularly when considering opioid rotation. Patients whose pain is poorly controlled with escalating doses of morphine and who are experiencing unbearable adverse effects can be rotated to an opioid that may provide a more tolerable balance between analgesia and side-effects.

Physical dependence

Physical dependence is a physiological state that develops as a result of the adaptation produced by a resetting of homeostatic mechanisms in response to repeated drug use.[118] It is a predictable effect that can be seen in both animals and humans and is characterized by the appearance of signs and symptoms of withdrawal syndrome after sudden dose reduction or discontinuation of a drug on which a patient is physically dependent. It can also be precipitated by administration of an antagonist.

Withdrawal symptoms are typical for a given category of drugs, and they tend to be the opposite of the original effects of the medication. The symptoms are due to removal of the drug of dependence; such effects can be observed with many drugs and are not limited to CNS effects. Examples are rebound tachycardia after β-blocker withdrawal and rebound hypertension after clonidine withdrawal. On a CNS level, hyperarousal of the central nervous system by readaptation to absence of the drug of dependence occurs.

The time to onset, duration, and severity of withdrawal symptoms after opioid use depends on the pharmacokinetics of the drug of dependence. Physical dependence probably starts after the first dose, and symptoms will become noticeable after 1–2 weeks of exposure.[100] The shorter the duration of administration of a drug and the smaller the dose, the less pronounced the withdrawal symptoms when it is stopped. A drug such as methadone, which is slowly eliminated, will produce less severe withdrawal symptoms, with a later onset of 36–48 h, than a drug with a shorter half-life such as morphine, with an onset 6–12 h after the last dose. If the dosing interval for short-acting opioids is too long, symptoms of withdrawal can be apparent between doses.

When reducing or discontinuing chronic opioid therapy a tapering schedule is recommended. Prevention of withdrawal symptoms can be managed by decreasing the dose by 25% each day.[136] This rule can be used to titrate down to a lower dose or to eventually discontinue a drug when pain relief has been achieved by other means, such as radiotherapy or surgery.

Chronic agonist use can also increase sensitivity to even weak antagonists such as agonist–antagonists.[137] Therefore, if these opioids are going to be used in patients with cancer, they should be initiated before regular use of an opioid agonist. Even more care is required when using a full antagonist in patients on opioids; it can precipitate withdrawal after only one or two doses of an agonist.

Addiction (psychological dependence/substance dependence)

Addiction, also called psychological dependence, is the most complex of these terms; it is distinct from physical dependence and tolerance.[138] It is used to describe a pattern of drug use characterized by a continued craving for the drug leading to an overwhelming involvement with the use and procurement of the drug. There is continued use of the substance despite knowledge and evidence that it causes physical and/or psychological harm.

Substance dependence is the alternative term used by the American Psychiatric Association (APA in DSM-IV, 1994).[138] According to the APA, substance dependence is defined as a maladaptive pattern of substance use, leading to clinically significant impairment or distress, as manifested by three or more symptoms of dependence occurring at any time in the same 12-month period. This diagnostic system further classifies substance dependence as dependence with physiological dependence (evidence of tolerance or withdrawal) or without physiological dependence (no evidence of tolerance or withdrawal).

Obviously, neither tolerance nor withdrawal is necessary or sufficient for a diagnosis of substance dependence. It is extremely important to realize that patients with cancer pain may develop tolerance to prescribed opioids and show signs of withdrawal without any evidence of compulsive use. These patients may well be physically and therapeutically dependent on opioids, but they are not addicted.

Therapeutic dependence is another important term here. When specific pharmacological therapy is needed to control or cure a disease process or a symptom of that disease, the patient is essentially dependent on it, e.g. antibiotics for sepsis, insulin for insulin-dependent diabetes, and opioids for pain.[136] Some patients with good pain control may seem to be too obsessed with ensuring an adequate and regular supply of medication. This is indicative not necessarily of addiction but of an understandable fear of running out of analgesic, of not having enough to deal with breakthrough pain, or of withdrawal symptoms. The term "pseudoaddiction," defined as an iatrogenic syndrome due to poorly managed and uncontrolled pain, has been used in such a situation.[139] It is characterized by behavioral changes very similar to those of drug addiction. The patient endures and complains of constant pain, which is, at best, only partially relieved. Drug-seeking behavior, such as obtaining medication from multiple sources, repeated episodes of prescription loss, and requests for early refills from health workers for larger or more frequent doses of opioids are often met with mistrust and, all too frequently, refusal. This can lead to a spiral of increasing demands and "clock watching," with anger and distrust on all sides.[123] It is vitally important that this disastrous failure of care is recognized and avoided. Failure to do so can lead to lengthy periods of unacceptable pain for a patient and years of resentment and stress for their families.

Management should start with acknowledgment that the pain is real, followed by appropriate analgesia, "by the clock," with rescue medication for breakthrough pain and frequent review.

Routes of administration

It is important to be familiar with the different routes of opioid administration. Although the oral route for analgesia in cancer pain is the most common, up to 70% of patients with cancer-related pain require an alternative route of opioid administration before death.[140,141] The reasons for change of route are usually to improve pain relief, reduce toxicity, or both, and to make life as tolerable as possible for the patient.[141] It is wise to remember that there is a difference in analgesic potency when the route of administration is changed, and dose adjustment is necessary to avoid under- or overdosing. However, the dose of any opioid is the same when given subcutaneously, intramuscularly, or intravenously. Oral to parenteral potency ratios for some opioids are in Table 3.5 – however inter- and intraindividual variability limits the usefulness of such tables. The ideal technique for switching opioids and routes of administration remains individual titration – the ratios documented here are only average approximations.

Oral

The oral route is the preferred route and is recommended as such by WHO.[1] It is well tolerated by most cultures, easy for anyone to administer, and comparatively cheap. A variety of opioid analgesics are available as oral formulations: immediate release, enteric coated, and sustained release. Sustained-release preparations are designed to produce slow uniform absorption for 8 h or more. These preparations allow a reduction in frequency of administration, therapeutic effect overnight, and a decrease in undesirable side-effects by elimination of peaks in plasma concentration.

Opioids undergo extensive hepatic metabolism and, when given orally, succumb to significant first-pass clearance. They therefore have a variable, relatively low, bioavailability. The oral route is unsuitable in patients with severe vomiting, dysphagia, bowel obstruction, or severe confusion, or when rapid dose escalation is necessary.

Nasogastric tube

If a patient is unable to ingest medication but has normal gastrointestinal function, the nasogastric tube is an alternative.[142] This is more invasive than oral medication and used only for those patients who are receiving enteral feeding. However, it is more suitable for administration of analgesics long term than the rectal route. Liquid preparations are preferred as they can be administered unaltered and do not clog the tube. Immediate-release tablets can be dissolved or crushed. This method is unsuitable for most sustained-release formulations, sublingual or buccal preparations, and enteric-coated tablets. Morphine sulfate elixir and immediate-release tablets are suitable to give by this route and are compatible with many different enteral formulas.[142]

Sublingual

The sublingual route avoids hepatic first-pass metabolism as the blood vessels in the area drain directly into the superior vena cava. Absorption is best for those drugs that are highly lipid soluble and potent and of which a high proportion is unionized in the alkaline medium of the mouth. The absorption of morphine by this route is 18%, compared with 51% for fentanyl, 34% for methadone, and 55% for buprenorphine.[143] Buprenorphine is the only opioid currently available via this route. Morphine's efficacy via this route is minimal.[144]

Transmucosal (buccal and intranasal)

Absorption by the transmucosal route is rapid and opti-

Table 3.5 *Approximate oral to parenteral potency ratios for some commonly used opioids (compiled from multiple sources)*

Agonist drug	Oral to parenteral ratio	*Oral* analgesic potency compared with *oral* morphine
Morphine	6 acute dosing; 3 chronic dosing	1
Codeine	1.5	<0.1
Hydromorphone	5	5
Oxycodone	≈2.5	1–2
Oxymorphone	No oral preparation available	10
Methadone	2	≈8–11
Levorphanol	2	5
Meperidine	4	0.1
Fentanyl	–	80–100
Buprenorphine	(sublingual to parenteral)	25–50
Pentazocine	3	0.16–0.3
Butorphanol	No oral preparation available	5
Nalbuphine	No oral preparation available	≈1
Tramadol	≈1	0.25

mum with low-molecular-weight, highly lipid-soluble, and potent drugs. The high first-pass effect of the oral route is avoided. Oral transmucosal fentanyl citrate (OTFC) is now available as a lozenge for the treatment of breakthrough pain.[145,146] Butorphanol is available as an intranasal spray. Fentanyl can also be given intranasally, although no commercial preparations are available.[147,148]

Transdermal

Transdermal delivery also avoids the problem of first-pass metabolism. Again, lipid-soluble, low-molecular-weight drugs are more appropriate for this route.[149] A patch containing a depot of the drug is usually applied to the torso. Patches do not stick well to hairy or sweaty skin. The rate-limiting step is dissolution from the patch, not absorption from the skin. The absorption rate will vary with the vehicle and local conditions.[150] Absorption is slow and, although therapeutic levels can be maintained for many days, this is an unsuitable route for rapid pain control or in opioid-naive patients. It is also unsuitable in the presence of generalized edema. The removal of the delivery system does not terminate the effect of the drug as a depot forms in subcutaneous tissue. Fentanyl is currently the only opioid available as a transdermal patch. Compliance is usually good, and this route offers the advantage of continuous administration of a potent opioid without the need for cannulae, infusion pumps, or skilled personnel, and is very useful in ambulatory patients.[151]

Iontophoresis

Iontophoresis, a new method of rapid transdermal delivery of drugs in an ionized state, by electric current, is still under investigation. Studies have been done on fentanyl and morphine, with promising results.[147]

Rectal

The rectal route is cheap and requires no specialized skills. It is useful in a vomiting or unconscious patient. Absorption is often irregular and incomplete and local irritation can occur. The rectal veins drain to both the hepatic portal vein and the inferior vena cava, thus some first-pass metabolism is avoided. However, the variability of drainage makes uptake unpredictable. It has been shown that analgesia is of more rapid onset and longer duration than that achieved via the oral route.[149] Many opioids can be administered by this route; most commonly given are morphine, hydromorphone, oxycodone, and oxymorphone. Even slow-release tablets can be given by this route. If suppositories are not available, morphine can be given as an enema. This route should not be used in patients with diarrhea or fecal incontinence. Immunosuppressed patients are at risk of localized infection. Administration of opioids via colostomy has been shown not to be useful, probably because of comparatively poor vascularity.

Subcutaneous

The subcutaneous route is only suitable for opioids that are soluble, nonirritating, and well absorbed. The rate of absorption via this route is usually sufficiently slow and constant to provide sustained effect. Battery operated syringe drivers can deliver continuous infusions and intermittent boluses. Infusion rates should not exceed 5ml/h, as higher volumes cause problems and discomfort at the site of injection. This method of opioid administration has been used successfully for many years for morphine, hydromorphone, and oxymorphone, in both the home and hospital setting. If a syringe driver is not available, a butterfly cannula can be left *in situ* and intermittent boluses given.

The subcutaneous route has proven to be both safe and efficacious, with a low incidence of acute side-effects, and it avoids repeated injections.[152] Bioavailability is often more than 90% but depends on the solubility of the drug, cardiovascular conditions, peripheral perfusion, the injection site, and physical exercise. Drugs with a short half-life reach steady state more quickly. Methadone causes inflammatory skin reactions at the site of administration and its administration by this route is not recommended.[153] Meperidine is also an irritant and should not be given subcutaneously.

Intravenous

The intravenous route allows 100% bioavailability and produces rapid-onset, short-lived analgesia. This route is difficult to maintain at home. However, it is very useful for swift control of severe pain in the hospital setting. Intermittent boluses, continuous infusions, and patient-controlled analgesia are the usual options.

Intramuscular

Intramuscular administration is painful and carries the risk of tissue damage and infection. Subsequent absorption depends on local blood flow and body habitus. Absorption is therefore unpredictable, and this route is not generally recommended unless nothing else is available.

Epidural and intrathecal

Epidural and intrathecal routes are used for the management of severe intractable pain and allow the use of small doses of opioid to produce profound analgesia. They are also useful routes of administration for those who experience intolerable side-effects at the doses required for oral analgesics. When changing from chronic oral opioids to the much lower doses required for the spinal route, withdrawal symptoms could be avoided by progressively reducing the oral dose.

Intraventricular opioids are rarely used, but can provide analgesia for patients who have a CSF reservoir *in situ*.

Individual opioids

Opioids for mild to moderate pain

These opioids are currently recommended by WHO as step 2 of the analgesic ladder.[1] They can be used alone or in conjunction with nonopioids. There is currently some debate as to their usefulness, except for tramadol.[154,155] The majority of patients with cancer will eventually progress to "strong" opioids for pain relief, so it might be advantageous just to use low doses of "strong" opioids in the first place.

Nonpharmacologic reasons for use of these drugs are a wide patient acceptance and better and easier availability than strong opioids.[154] No special permission or documentation is needed to write prescriptions. In some countries, strong opioids are virtually unobtainable by legal means, making the "weak" opioids both useful and essential.[1] Codeine is the representative on the model list of essential drugs.[156]

Codeine

Codeine is a naturally occurring alkaloid of opium. It has analgesic, antitussive, and constipating effects. The recommended dose is 30–60 mg 4-hourly. Its oral bioavailability is variable, and the duration of action of the oral dose is 4–6 h. The half-life in plasma is 2–4 h.

Codeine is metabolized in the liver; 6–15% is biotransformed to morphine, to which codeine owes most, if not all of its analgesic properties. Between 7% and 10% of Caucasians are poor metabolizers of codeine, rendering it a useless analgesic for such people.[157]

Codeine is often used in combination preparations with nonopioids at possibly ineffective small doses, such as 8 mg combined with 500 mg of acetaminophen. More useful combination preparations contain 30–60 mg per dose. In such combinations with ibuprofen or acetaminophen codeine produces valuable supplementary analgesia, even with single doses,[158***] but with an increase in side-effects.[154] Sustained-release codeine preparations are available in some countries.

Dihydrocodeine

Dihydrocodeine is a synthetic codeine derivative. It has similar effects and oral potency to codeine, greater parenteral potency, and a narrower therapeutic range.[159] It is metabolized in the liver and its clearance is decreased in renal failure. Its main advantage over codeine is its availability as a sustained-release preparation in many countries.[160]

Dextropropoxyphene

Dextropropoxyphene is a synthetic derivative of methadone. It has a μ-receptor affinity similar to that of codeine. It is well absorbed from the gastrointestinal tract and reaches peak plasma levels after 2 h. Dextropropoxyphene undergoes extensive, dose-dependent, first-pass metabolism to an active metabolite, norpropoxyphene, which is associated with CNS excitation. The elimination half-life is long (15 h), but it can increase up to 50 h, particularly in the elderly.[161]

Dextropropoxyphene is more effective when given regularly than as a single dose, probably because of its prolonged half-life and active metabolites.[155] Increased bioavailability and decreased clearance occur in patients with cirrhosis. The toxic metabolite, norpropoxyphene, has a half-life of 30 h and accumulates in patients with renal failure.[161]

Dextropropoxyphene can form part of many combination analgesics with acetaminophen 325 mg, aspirin 325 mg, and caffeine. There is little evidence to support the analgesic efficacy of these drug mixtures.[154] The amount of dextropropoxyphene in these preparations ranges from 32.5 to 100 mg. The dose of each component is often too small to be effective, and the pharmacokinetic differences are too great for safe regular use. The half-life of acetaminophen (2–4 h) is shorter than that of dextropropoxyphene, which consequently can accumulate, causing adverse effects such as confusion, and even respiratory depression. Parenteral administration is not recommended because of severe tissue irritation.[161]

Tramadol

Tramadol is a centrally acting analgesic with a moderate affinity for μ-receptors and a very weak affinity for δ- and κ-receptors. Tramadol also inhibits neuronal reuptake of norepinephrine (noradrenaline) and serotonin, which enhances the activity of the descending modulating pain pathways.[162]

Although better tolerated, tramadol is not always as efficacious as morphine for moderate to severe malignant pain. Thus, it has a greater role to play on step 2 of the analgesic ladder, in the treatment of mild to moderate pain. Its analgesic effect is only partially reversed by naloxone.[163]

Tramodol is available as capsules, soluble tablets, and suppositories of 50 mg and as a solution of 50 mg/ml for i.m. or i.v. injection. Sustained-release formulations are also available in some countries, and have been shown to be well tolerated and efficacious.[154] The usual oral dose is 50–100 mg, 4- to 6-hourly.

Oral bioavailability is 70% for a single dose and 90–100% after multiple doses. When given orally it is about one-quarter as potent as morphine, and parenterally it is about one-tenth as potent as morphine. Peak plasma concentrations are achieved in 2–4 h. Tramadol is metabolized in the liver, mainly to an active metabolite, *O*-desmethyltramadol, which has a greater affinity for opioid receptors than tramadol itself, and may well be mainly responsible for its opioid effects.[164] Ninety percent of the oral dose is excreted in the urine.

The elimination half-life of tramodol is 5 h and is doubled in hepatic cirrhosis, in which setting the maximum dose should be reduced. The dose should also be reduced in renal failure. Tramadol has minimal abuse potential and is therefore not registered as a controlled drug in most countries.[165]

Adverse effects include nausea, vomiting, constipation, sedation, dry mouth, and sweating, but these are less than with morphine, especially constipation.[166] Respiratory depression is also uncommon, but can occur, e.g. in a patient with impaired renal function.[167]

Opioids for moderate to severe pain

Full agonists

Morphine Morphine is the best-known and most commonly used opioid in the world and is included in the WHO essential drug list.[156] It is a naturally occurring alkaloid of opium, and was first isolated in the mid-1800s in Germany. It is still extracted from poppies, as the laboratory synthesis is difficult. Morphine is available for therapeutic use as the sulfate, tartrate, or hydrochloride.

Oral preparations include an elixir, immediate-release tablets, controlled-release tablets using different release mechanisms, and controlled-release suspensions.*** Despite the many different formulations available, an extensive review of 69 studies on the plasma concentrations of oral morphine found that, within formulations, there was little pharmacokinetic difference between brands or salts.[168] Immediate-release formulations had a mean time to maximum concentration (T_{max}) of 1.1 h. Controlled-release morphine 12-hourly had a mean T_{max} of 2.7 h. Controlled-release preparations registered for once-daily dosing showed a mean T_{max} of 8.5 h. The presence of food seemed to make a difference only with once-daily morphine, increasing T_{max} by 2 h. There was a large degree of variability between patients. However, although useful, these are only pharmacokinetic values and no information is given on efficacy and patient satisfaction.

Controlled-release preparations of morphine contain morphine sulfate either in a matrix, which slowly releases the drug after ingestion,[169] or in multiple polymer granules. Each granule is designed to release morphine at a different rate, providing very stable, precise, plasma concentrations with a 12-hourly dosing schedule.[170] The granules can be sprinkled onto food but should not be crushed, chewed, or broken. This preparation can also be used 24-hourly, showing a better pharmacokinetic profile than other controlled-release formulations, but no clinically significant difference in patient satisfaction.[171] However, a once-daily dose may well be more tolerable for patients.

Oral preparations of morphine can also be given rectally, but pharmacokinetic parameters show greater variability than with oral administration. Absorption is slower but greater. Specially formulated controlled-release suppositories have a rectal bioavailability of 42%.[170]

In common with other opioids, morphine absorption varies greatly between patients. Absorption of morphine through the small intestine is nearly 100%, but bioavailability varies from 15% to 35% owing to extensive first-pass metabolism.[172,173] Morphine equilibrates slowly between the plasma and CSF, and there is no interindividual correlation between the degree of analgesia and plasma concentration.[174] Morphine is metabolized in the liver to M6G, M3G, and normorphine. M6G is a more potent opioid than morphine and has significant analgesic effect at opioid receptors. M3G is the major metabolite and is thought to cause hyperalgesia and CNS excitability and antagonize morphine. The glucuronide conjugates are mainly excretion in the urine and accumulate in renal failure as previously discussed. Approximately 10% appears in the feces as conjugated morphine. The elimination half-life is 1.7–4.5 h in patients with normal renal function and the duration of analgesia 4–6 h.[173] These parameters are very similar for oral, s.c., and i.m. administration.[161]

Parenteral formulations are obviously available for s.c., i.m., i.v., epidural, and intrathecal use. Morphine is relatively hydrophilic, and this results in a prolonged half-life in cerebrospinal fluid when it is given via the epidural or intrathecal route.

Oxycodone Oxycodone is a potent thebaine derivative that is similar to morphine in its pharmacologic actions.[175] Oral bioavailability is 60–70%. It can be given orally, rectally, i.m., i.v., and s.c. but is not recommended for spinal use.[175,176] The half-life is 2–3 h and duration of effect 4–5 h. Oxycodone is demethylated in the liver to oxymorphone. Oral oxycodone is used in combinations with acetaminophen and aspirin. These can be useful for mild to moderate pain, but increasing doses for effect may lead to nonopioid toxicity. Oxycodone pectinate is the form for rectal administration and has a longer duration of action than the oral formulation.

Oxycodone is also available as a single-agent tablet or syrup as an immediate-release preparation.

An oral controlled-release formulation is also available designed for twice-daily dosing. This has a biphasic absorption pattern characterized by an initial rapid onset followed by a prolonged phase. Controlled-release oxycodone every 12 h is as effective as immediate-release oxycodone four times daily.[177,178]

Studies so far have shown oxycodone to provide a rational, effective alternative to morphine for the management of moderate to severe pain.[179]

Methadone Methadone is a potent synthetic opioid with μ-receptor agonist activity and limited NMDA antagonist activity.[180] It is lipophilic, can be given by the oral, rectal, and parenteral routes, and has a high oral bioavailability of 80–90%. The distribution half-life of 2–3 h and the long terminal half-life of 15–55 h make it essentially a sustained-release preparation.[181] Methadone is highly protein bound and can be displaced from α_1-acid glycoprotein by some drugs, but it is unlikely that this will cause any enhancement of methadone effect.[182] Methadone has low hepatic extraction. It undergoes oxidative metabolism and the inactive metabolites are excreted in the bile and urine. Approximately 20% is excreted unchanged in the urine and some is reabsorbed by the tubules, therefore changes in urinary pH can alter methadone excretion. The few studies to date on methadone in disease states show that methadone dosage need not be changed in patients with stable chronic liver disease or renal failure.[85,182] However, as the studies are very limited, it is probably wise to consider small dose decreases in patients with severe disease.

Methadone is cheap, has no active metabolites, and shows incomplete cross-tolerance with other μ-receptor agonists.

The main disadvantage of methadone is a large amount of interindividual variability in methadone kinetics, making it virtually impossible to predict accurate dosing regimens.[182] Overdose and toxicity are a very real risk. Dosing intervals are generally recommended as 8- to 12-hourly, but the half-life can be greater than 100 h. This makes careful, personalized dose titration for each patient starting methadone extremely important. It is safer, particularly when converting from a short half-life analgesic to a much longer one, to start at low doses and titrate to analgesic effect as needed.[180] Opioid rotation is discussed in Chapter Ca12, but it is worth pointing out that methadone is considerably more potent than shown by previously published equianalgesic tables. If some of the currently recommended ratios for conversion from other opioids are used, severe toxicity may occur.[181] Two recent studies have shown dose ratios to depend on individual patients and on the time course of previous opioid use. Median dose ratios for morphine to methadone vary from 7.75:1 to 11.36:1.[183,184]

Fentanyl Fentanyl is a potent μ-receptor agonist closely related to meperidine. Its primary use in the past has been as an anesthetic agent, but it has recently gained increasing use in the management of cancer pain.[185]

Fentanyl can be administered intravenously, particularly for brief, invasive procedures. The usual dose is 1–2 μg/kg 5 min before the procedure. Rapid administration of > 3 μg/kg may produce chest wall rigidity and severe respiratory embarrassment.

Time to onset of effect is 5 to 8 min, peak effect about 30 min, and duration of effect 1–2 h. The volume of distribution is 60–300 l, and the elimination half-life is 3–12 h when given intravenously. Fentanyl is metabolized in the liver to inactive metabolites including norfentanyl. Less than 6% is excreted unchanged in the urine. Fentanyl causes less pruritus than morphine, but does cause transient, irritating facial itching.[186]

Fentanyl is also available in a transdermal preparation that delivers 25, 50, 75, or 100 μg/h.[187] As a highly lipid-soluble, low-molecular-weight drug it is well suited to this formulation. The fentanyl patch is of no value in patients with acute pain or opioid-naive patients, or for the treatment of rapidly escalating pain. However, it is very useful for the management of chronic pain, particularly in those patients unable to tolerate oral medication. The patch is well tolerated and compliance is usually very good. It has proved both safe and efficacious, if expensive, in the management of malignant pain. Bioavailability is high as fentanyl is absorbed into the circulation. The time from application to peak plasma concentration is about 12–24 h and the terminal half-life is 17–21 h.[185] A depot remains in the skin for about 24 h after removal of the patch.[188,189] Rescue medication may be necessary during the first 24 h, until plasma levels have stabilized at a therapeutic concentration. Steady-state concentrations are proportional to dose. Each patch lasts for approximately 72 h but, as with all opioids, there is a large amount of interindividual pharmacokinetic variability, and some patients may need another patch after 48 h. Empirical observations suggest that a 100-μg fentanyl patch is roughly equal in analgesic effect to 2–4 mg/h intravenous morphine.[136] The patch does not work well on hairy or sweaty skin, or if there is local or generalized edema. Neither age nor location of the patch makes any difference to fentanyl absorption, but it would seem sensible to place the patch in an area with limited skin movement.

Fentanyl lends itself to transmucosal administration by virtue of its physical properties. It is highly lipid soluble and has a low molecular weight, and favors the alkaline medium of the mouth. Intranasal fentanyl has been suggested to be efficacious via this route but there are limited studies on its use.[147]

Oral transmucosal fentanyl citrate (OTFC) offers a unique way of treating breakthrough and incident pain. Most patients being treated for cancer pain experience episodic acute pain. Compared with sufferers, caregivers tend to perceive pain intensity, duration, and relief as much lower.[190] Commonly available oral analgesics are not particularly suitable for the rapid relief of breakthrough pain. Time to peak analgesia can be as long as 45–60 min, and duration of effect far in excess of that needed, leading to accentuation of adverse opioid effects. The transmucosal route is ideal for rapid pain relief and can be used for the control of incident and breakthrough pain.

OTFC has recently been approved by the Food and Drug Administration for the treatment of breakthrough cancer pain. It is available in 200-, 400-, 600-, 800-, 1,200-, and 1,600-μg dosage units as a flavored lozenge on a stick. All OTFC units are of equal size. When sucked, the lozenge matrix dissolves and 25% is absorbed through the buccal and sublingual mucosa, and some is swallowed. This delivery system avoids some first-pass metabolism, and the overall bioavailability is 50%. Because of its rapid absorption, analgesic effect is perceived 5–15 min after administration, with peak plasma concentrations at 22 min.[145,191,192] The V_d is about 280 l and the terminal half-life 460 ± 313 min. However, the duration of effect is short because of the drug's widespread distribution into tissues.[185] The best dose of OTFC is determined by titration and is not predicted by the previous daily opioid use.[146] It is probably advisable to start with a low initial dose until the patient has worked out an effective dose. Side-effects are those commonly associated with opioids, but OTFC appears to be well tolerated,[146] perhaps because it is not used in opioid-naive patients.

Oxymorphone Oxymorphone is the metabolite of oxycodone. It is widely available in the rectal form but not as an oral preparation. Its half-life is 1–2 h and the duration of action 3 to 5 h. It is less likely to cause histamine release than morphine.[189]

Hydromorphone Hydromorphone is a pure opioid agonist. It is very lipid soluble, with a short duration of action of 3–4 h and a half-life of 1.5 to 3 h.[136] It is more potent than morphine[193] and can be given orally, rectally, s.c., i.m., i.v., and spinally.

Diamorphine Diamorphine is a prodrug of morphine, being biotransformed to morphine and 6-acetylmorphine. It is twice as potent as morphine because of its high lipid solubility, but it has limited legal availability worldwide. It is of little value over morphine as it is equally efficacious to morphine[194] and exerts its analgesic effect only once it is converted to morphine.[195] Its only advantage is its high solubility, which makes it possible to give large doses in small volumes and offers potential advantages in neuraxial use.

Papaveretum Papaveretum is a standardized mixture of the anhydrous alkaloids of opium. One of the alkaloids, noscapine, is thought to be genotoxic, and some preparations are now made without noscapine. Papaveretum contains 50% morphine hydrochloride and is essentially weak morphine. It is available for parenteral use only, and therefore is rarely used in cancer patients. It is not recommended for spinal use owing to the presence of preservatives.

Levorphanol Levorphanol is a potent morphinan derivative. It is a strong agonist at μ-, κ-, and δ-receptors, which makes it potentially useful for opioid rotation when tolerance to morphine has developed. It has a long half-life of 12–16 h but a comparatively short duration of action of 4–6 h, therefore levorphanol has the potential to accumulate and cause sedation when repeated doses are given.[196]

Meperidine (pethidine) Meperidine is a synthetic opioid that is less potent than morphine. It has an elimination half-life of 2–4 h and duration of action of only 2 to 3 h. Accumulation of normeperidine can occur with impaired renal function and has been seen in patients with normal kidneys.[94] Normeperidine is neurotoxic and can lead to muscle fasciculations, involuntary movements, and, finally, tonic–clonic seizures; naloxone does not reverse meperidine-induced seizures. Severe drug interactions can occur with monoamine oxidase inhibitors, which can precipitate hypertensive crisis, and phenobarbital and chlorpromazine, which can increase meperidine toxicity. Its lack of potency, short duration of action, and adverse side-effect profile with repeated doses means that there is little to recommend this drug. It is not a useful analgesic and is contraindicated for the management of chronic cancer pain.

Partial agonists

Buprenorphine Buprenorphine is a partial agonist at μ-receptors. It is 25–50 times more potent than morphine.[161] Its principal advantage it is that it is available as sublingual preparations, which contain 0.2 mg or 0.4 mg. Doses between 0.4 mg and 0.8 mg provide analgesia for moderate pain.[197] Sublingual bioavailability is 55%, onset of action 30 min, and peak plasma concentration variable and slow, at about 3 h.[143,198] Duration of effect is 6–9 h owing to slow dissociation from opioid receptors. Thus, buprenorphine has a role in patients who cannot take oral medication, but progression to morphine is usually needed.

Buprenorphine can also be given i.v. and i.m., and 0.4 mg sublingually is equivalent to 0.3 mg parenterally. The terminal half-life is 3–5 h and the duration of action of the i.m. dose about 4–5 h. Ten milligrams of morphine is equivalent to 0.4 mg of i.m. buprenorphine.[197] There is no change in the pharmacokinetics of buprenorphine in renal failure.

Administration of buprenorphine to patients who are already taking high-dose opioid agonists may precipitate withdrawal. There is an increased risk of psychotomimetic side-effects, and respiratory depression is difficult to reverse with naloxone.[197]

Mixed agonist–antagonists

Mixed agonist–antagonists are not generally recommended for the control of moderate to severe cancer pain because of their low maximal efficacy and the potential to reverse analgesia, resulting in withdrawal.

Pentazocine Pentazocine is an agonist at κ-receptors and a weak competitive antagonist at μ-receptors. It is less potent than morphine and closer in analgesic efficacy to acetaminophen and aspirin than the weak opioids.[199,200] The adult oral dose is 50–100 mg 3- to 4-hourly; the parenteral dose is 30–60 mg 3- to 4-hourly. Onset of action of the i.v. dose is 2–3 min and of the i.m. dose 20 min. The drug is irritating when given subcutaneously or intramuscularly. The terminal half-life is 2–4 h. There is a ceiling effect for analgesia and respiratory depression at 30–60 mg.[189]

There is a high incidence of psychotomimetic effects with repeated high doses, which makes this drug unsuitable for long-term management of malignant pain. Patients who have received regular opioids may experience withdrawal when given pentazocine. High doses produce adverse cardiac effects.[161]

Nalbuphine Nalbuphine is an agonist at κ-receptors and a weak antagonist at μ-receptors. It is approximately as potent as morphine. It has poor oral bioavailability and is not available in the oral form. The adult dose is 10–20 mg i.v., i.m., or s.c. Onset of action is 2–3 min when given i.v. and 15 min when given i.m. The duration of action is 2–4 h and the terminal half-life is 3–5 h. Nalbuphine has a ceiling effect for respiratory depression and analgesia and it can precipitate withdrawal in patients who have developed physical dependence on a pure agonist.[161,189]

Butorphanol Butorphanol is a mixed agonist–antagonist and is usually only available for parenteral use. An intranasal form is also on the market. The terminal half-life is 2.5–3.5 h and the duration of action 3–4 h. Again, psychotomimetic effects are greater and there is a ceiling effect for analgesia and the risk of precipitating withdrawal in chronic opioid users.[199]

Antagonists

Naloxone Naloxone is a competitive opioid antagonist at μ-, κ-, and δ-receptors. It is the drug of choice for reversing the effects of opioids; its primary indication is reversing respiratory depression caused by opioids. Naloxone is ineffective orally as its bioavailability is only 2% owing to extensive first-pass metabolism. It can also be given subcutaneously and intramuscularly. The half-life of naloxone is about 1 h, much shorter than that of most opioids.[201] Onset of action is 1–2 min, and its duration of effect is dose dependent and ranges from 30 min to over 1 h.

Care must be employed when using naloxone in patients taking chronic opioids. Overzealous doses can precipitate severe withdrawal and a recurrence of pain, which may prove difficult to treat. For adults, 0.04–0.08 mg intravenously is a reasonable titration dose. Its duration of action is usually shorter than the effect of the offending opioid, and repeated boluses or an infusion may be necessary.

Recently, attention has been drawn to the use of naloxone to control other adverse effects of opioids. While not absorbed orally, an intestinal effect with reduction in opioid-induced constipation has been reported.[202] Even more challenging are findings that low-dose naloxone reduces not only opioid-induced nausea and vomiting but also opioid requirements.[203]

Naltrexone and nalmefene Naltrexone is a long-acting pure opioid antagonist at μ-, κ-, and δ-receptors. Its half-life ranges from 4 to 10 h. It is only available as an oral preparation and its primary use is in the treatment of opioid abuse.

Nalmefene is also a pure opioid antagonist. It is available as a parenteral formulation. Its half-life is 8–11 h, the onset of action of a 2-mg dose i.v. is 2 min, and its duration of action is up to 8 h.[201]

The long duration of action of naltrexone and nalmefene makes these drugs particularly unsuitable for patients who use opioids chronically, such as cancer patients.

REFERENCES

◆ 1. WHO. *Cancer Pain Relief: With a Guide to Opioid Availability*, 2nd edn. Geneva: World Health Organization, 1996.

2. Flower RJ, Vane JR. Inhibition of prostaglandin synthetase in brain explains the anti-pyretic activity of paracetamol (4-acetamidophenol). *Nature* 1972; **240:** 410–11.

3. Landolfi C, Soldo L, Polenzani L, *et al.* Inflammatory molecule release by B-amyloid-treated T98G astrocytoma cells: role of prostaglandins and modulation by paracetamol. *Eur J Pharmacol* 1998; **360:** 55–64.

4. Bjorkman R, Hallman KM, Hedner J, *et al.* Acetaminophen blocks spinal hyperalgesia induced by NMDA and substance P. *Pain* 1994; **57:** 259–64.

5. Gordh T, Karlsten R, Kristensen J. Intervention with spinal NMDA, adenosine, and NO systems for pain modulation. *Ann Med* 1995; **27:** 229–34.

6. Pelissier T, Alloui A, Caussade F, *et al.* Paracetamol exerts a spinal antinociceptive effect involving an indirect interaction with 5-hydroxytryptamine3 receptors: in vivo and in vitro evidence. *J Pharmacol Exp Ther* 1996; **278:** 8–14.

7. Pini LA, Sandrini M, Vitale G. The antinociceptive action of paracetamol is associated with changes in the serotonergic system in the rat brain. *Eur J Pharmacol* 1996; **308:** 31–40.

8. Raffa RB, Codd EE. Lack of binding of acetaminophen to 5-HT receptor or uptake sites (or eleven other binding/uptake assays). *Life Sci* 1996; **59(2):** L37–40.

9. Anderson B, Holford N, Woollard G, *et al.* Perioperative pharmacodynamics of acetaminophen analgesia in children. *Anesthesiology* 1999; **90:** 411–21.

10. Insel PA. Analgesic–antipyretic and antiinflammatory agents and drugs employed in the treatment of gout. In: Goodman JGG, Gilman A, Limbird LL eds. *Goodman and Gilman's the Pharmacological Basis of Therapeutics*, 9th edn. New York: McGraw-Hill, 1996: 617–58.

● 11. Clissold SP. Paracetamol and phenacetin. *Drugs* 1986; **32** (Suppl. 4): 46–59.

12. Anderson BJ, Holford NH, Woollard GA, Chan PL. Paracetamol plasma and cerebrospinal fluid pharmacokinetics in children. *Br J Clin Pharmacol* 1998; **46:** 237–43.

● 13. Fry SW, Seeff LB. Hepatotoxicity of analgesics and anti-inflammatory agents. *Gastroenterol Clin N Am* 1995; **24:** 875–905.

● 14. Tolman KG. Hepatotoxicity of non-narcotic analgesics. *Am J Med* 1998; **105(1B):** 13S–19S.

● 15. Strom BL. Adverse reactions to over-the-counter analgesics taken for therapeutic purposes. *JAMA* 1994; **272:** 1866–7.

● 16. Schnitzer TJ. Non-NSAID pharmacologic treatment options for the management of chronic pain. *Am J Med* 1998; **105:** 45S–52S.

● 17. Henrich WL, Agodoa LE, Barrett B, *et al.* Analgesics and the kidney: summary and recommendations to the Scientific Advisory Board of the National Kidney Foundation from an Ad Hoc Committee of the National Kidney Foundation. *Am J Kidney Dis* 1996; **27:** 162–5.

● 18. Gault MH, Barrett BJ. Analgesic nephropathy. *Am J Kidney Dis* 1998; **32:** 351–60.

● 19. Bowmer CJ, Yates MS. Pathophysiology and diseases of the renal system. In: Page C, Curtis M, Sutter M, *et al.* eds. *Integrated Pharmacology*. London: Mosby, 2002: 345–60.

20. Anonymous. *British National Formulary*, 32nd edn. London: British Medical Association and The Pharmaceutical Press, 1996.

21. Anderson BJ, Woolard GA, Holford NH. Pharmacokinetics of rectal paracetamol after major surgery in children. *Paediatr Anaesth* 1995; **5:** 237–42.

22. Anderson BJ, Holford NH. Rectal paracetamol dosing regimens: determination by computer simulation. *Paediatr Anaesth* 1997; **7:** 451–5.

23. Bradley JD, Brandt KD, Katz BP, *et al.* Comparison of an antiinflammatory dose of ibuprofen, an analgesic dose of ibuprofen, and acetaminophen in the treatment of patients with osteoarthritis of the knee. *N Engl J Med* 1991; **325:** 87–91.

24. Williams HJ, Ward JR, Egger MJ, *et al.* Comparison of naproxen and acetaminophen in a two-year study of treatment of osteoarthritis of the knee. *Arthr Rheum* 1993; **36:** 1196–206.

◆ 25. WHO. *Cancer Pain Relief and Palliative Care in Children*. Geneva: World Health Organization, 1998.

26. Hunskaar S, Fasmer OB, Broch OJ, Hole K. Involvement of central serotonergic pathways in nefopam-induced antinociception. *Eur J Pharmacol* 1987; **138:** 77–82.

● 27. Heel RC, Brogden RN, Pakes GE, *et al.* Nefopam: a review of its pharmacological properties and therapeutic efficacy. *Drugs* 1980; **19:** 249–67.

28. Minotti V, Patoia L, Roila F, *et al.* Double-blind evaluation of analgesic efficacy of orally administered diclofenac, nefopam, and acetylsalicylic acid (ASA) plus codeine in chronic cancer pain. *Pain* 1989; **36:** 177–83.

● 29. Vane JR, Botting RM. Mechanism of action of nonsteroidal anti-inflammatory drugs. *Am J Med* 1998; **104(3A):** 2S–8S; discussion 21S–22S.

● ◆ 30. Merry A, Power I. Perioperative NSAIDs: Towards greater safety. *Pain Rev* 1995; **2:** 268–91.

31. Bjorkman DJ. The effect of aspirin and nonsteroidal anti-inflammatory drugs on prostaglandins. *Am J Med* 1998; **105(1B):** 8S–12S.

32. Xie W, Robertson DL, Simmons DL. Mitogen-inducible prostaglandin G/H synthase: A new target for nonsteroidal antiinflammatory drugs. *Drug Dev Res* 1992; **25:** 249–65.

● 33. Brooks P. Use and benefits of nonsteroidal anti-inflammatory drugs. *Am J Med* 1998; **104(3A):** 9S–13S; discussion 21S–22S.

◆ 34. Malmberg AB, Yaksh TL. Antinociceptive actions of spinal nonsteroidal anti-inflammatory agents on the formalin test in the rat. *J Pharmacol Exp Ther* 1992; **263:** 136–46.

● 35. McCormack K. Non-steroidal anti-inflammatory drugs and spinal nociceptive processing. *Pain* 1994; **59:** 9–43.

● 36. Patrono C, Ciabattoni G, Patrignani P, *et al.* Clinical pharmacology of platelet cyclooxygenase inhibition. *Circulation* 1985; **72:** 1177–84.

● 37. Sunshine A, Olson N. Nonnarcotic analgesics. In: Wall PD, Melzack R eds. *Textbook of Pain*. London: Churchill Livingstone, 1994: 923–42.

● 38. Murray MD, Brater DC. Renal toxicity of the nonsteroidal anti-inflammatory drugs. *Annu Rev Pharmacol Toxicol* 1993; **33:** 435–65.

● 39. Schoenfeld A, Bar Y, Merlob P, Ovadia Y. NSAIDs: maternal and fetal considerations. *Am J Reprod Immunol* 1992; **28:** 141–7.

40. Fries JF, Williams CA, Bloch DA, Michel BA. Nonsteroidal anti-inflammatory drug-associated gastropathy: incidence and risk factor models. *Am J Med* 1991; **91:** 213–22.

41. Griffin MR. Epidemiology of nonsteroidal anti-inflammatory drug-associated gastrointestinal injury. *Am J Med* 1998; **104(3A):** 23S–29S; discussion 41S–42S.

42. Silverstein FE, Graham DY, Senior JR, *et al.* Misoprostol reduces serious gastrointestinal complications in patients with rheumatoid arthritis receiving nonsteroidal anti-inflammatory drugs. A randomized, double-blind, placebo-controlled trial. *Ann Intern Med* 1995; **123:** 241–9.

● 43. Scheiman J, Isenberg J. Agents used in the prevention and treatment of nonsteroidal anti-inflammatory drug-associated symptoms and ulcers. *Am J Med* 1998; **105(5A):** 32S–38S.

● 44. Schafer AI. Effects of nonsteroidal anti-inflammatory therapy on platelets. *Am J Med* 1999; **106(5B):** 25S–36S.

● 45. Bjorkman D. Nonsteroidal anti-inflammatory drug-associated toxicity of the liver, lower gastrointestinal tract, and esophagus. *Am J Med* 1998; **105(5A):** 17S–21S.

● 46. Hurwitz ES. Reye's syndrome. *Epidemiol Rev* 1989; **11:** 249–53.

47. Jain S. Ibuprofen-induced thrombocytopenia. *Br J Clin Pract* 1994; **48:** 51.

48. Horn AC, Jarrett SW. Ibuprofen-induced aseptic meningitis in rheumatoid arthritis. *Ann Pharmacother* 1997; **31:** 1009–11.

49. Kim HL, Kovacs MJ. Diclofenac-associated thrombocytopenia and neutropenia. *Ann Pharmacother* 1995; **29:** 713–15.

50. Bhogaraju A, Nazeer S, Al-Baghdadi Y, *et al.* Diclofenac-associated hepatitis. *South Med J* 1999; **92:** 711–13.

51. Rygnestad T, Kvam AM. Streptococcal myositis and tissue necrosis with intramuscular administration of

diclofenac (Voltaren). *Acta Anaesthesiol Scand* 1995; **39:** 1128–30.

● 52. Willkens RF. The selection of a nonsteroidal antiinflammatory drug. Is there a difference? *J Rheumatol* 1992; **19** (Suppl. 36): 9–12.

● 53. Sharma S, Prasad A, Anand KS. Nonsteroidal anti-inflammatory drugs in the management of pain and inflammation: a basis for drug selection. *Am J Ther* 1999; **6:** 3–11.

● 54. Kaplan B, Swain RA. NSAIDs. Are there any differences? *Arch Fam Med* 1993; **2:** 1167–74.

● 55. Bennett A, Charlier EM, McDonald AM, *et al.* Prostaglandins and breast cancer. *Lancet* 1977; **2**: 624–6.

● 56. Ventafridda V, Fochi C, De Conno D, Sganzerla E. Use of non-steroidal anti-inflammatory drugs in the treatment of pain in cancer. *Br J Clin Pharmacol* 1980; **10** (Suppl. 2): 343S–346S.

● 57. Jordan B, Devi LA. Molecular mechanisms of opioid receptor signal transduction. *Br J Anaesth* 1998; **81:** 12–19.

● 58. Harrison C, Smart D, Lambert DG. Stimulatory effects of opioids. *Br J Anaesth* 1998; **81:** 20–8.

59. Standifer KM, Pasternak GW. G proteins and opioid receptor-mediated signalling. *Cellular Signalling* 1997; **9:** 237–48.

60. Taylor F, Dickenson A. Nociceptin/orphanin FQ. A new opioid, a new analgesic? *Neuroreport* 1998; **9(12):** R65–70.

61. Lambert DG. Recent advances in opioid pharmacology. *Br J Anaesth* 1998; **81:** 1–2.

62. Darland T, Grandy DK. The orphanin FQ system: an emerging target for the management of pain? *Br J Anaesth* 1998; **81:** 29–37.

63. Mansour A, Fox CA, Akil H, Watson SJ. Opioid-receptor mRNA expression in the rat CNS: anatomical and functional implications. *Trends Neurosci* 1995; **18:** 22–9.

64. Bagnol D, Mansour A, Akil H, Watson SJ. Cellular localization and distribution of the cloned mu and kappa opioid receptors in rat gastrointestinal tract. *Neuroscience* 1997; **81:** 579–91.

65. Stein C, Yassouridis A. Peripheral morphine analgesia. *Pain* 1997; **71:** 119–21.

66. Likar R, Sittl R, Gragger K, *et al.* Peripheral morphine analgesia in dental surgery. *Pain* 1998; **76:** 145–50.

● 67. Dickenson AH. Mechanisms of the analgesic actions of opiates and opioids. *Br Med Bull* 1991; **47:** 690–702.

68. Gutstein HB, Mansour A, Watson SJ, *et al.* Mu and kappa opioid receptors in periaqueductal gray and rostral ventromedial medulla. *Neuroreport* 1998; **9:** 1777–81.

69. Hackler L, Zadina JE, Ge LJ, Kastin AJ. Isolation of relatively large amounts of endomorphin-1 and endomorphin-2 from human brain cortex. *Peptides* 1997; **18:** 1635–9.

70. Zadina JE, Hackler L, Ge LJ, Kastin AJ. A potent and selective endogenous agonist for the mu-opiate receptor. *Nature* 1997; **386:** 499–502.

● 71. Hanks GW. The clinical usefulness of agonist–antagonistic opioid analgesics in chronic pain. *Drug Alcohol Depend* 1987; **20:** 339–46.

72. Walker EA, Zernig G, Woods JH. Buprenorphine antagonism of mu opioids in the rhesus monkey tail-withdrawal procedure. *J Pharmacol Exp Ther* 1995; **273:** 1345–52.

● 73. Tegeder I, Lotsch J, Geisslinger G. Pharmacokinetics of opioids in liver disease. *Clin Pharmacokinet* 1999; **37:** 17–40.

74. Mazoit JX, Sandouk P, Zetlaoui P, Scherrmann JM. Pharmacokinetics of unchanged morphine in normal and cirrhotic subjects. *Anesth Analges* 1987; **66:** 293–8.

75. Mazoit JX, Sandouk P, Scherrmann JM, Roche A. Extrahepatic metabolism of morphine occurs in humans. *Clin Pharmacol Ther* 1990; **48:** 613–18.

76. Crotty B, Watson KJ, Desmond PV, *et al.* Hepatic extraction of morphine is impaired in cirrhosis. *Eur J Clin Pharmacol* 1989; **36:** 501–6.

77. Patwardhan RV, Johnson RF, Hoyumpa A, Jr, *et al.* Normal metabolism of morphine in cirrhosis. *Gastroenterology* 1981; **81:** 1006–11.

● ◆ 78. Sawe J. High-dose morphine and methadone in cancer patients. Clinical pharmacokinetic considerations of oral treatment. *Clin Pharmacokinetics* 1986; **11:** 87–106.

79. Neal EA, Meffin PJ, Gregory PB, Blaschke TF. Enhanced bioavailability and decreased clearance of analgesics in patients with cirrhosis. *Gastroenterology* 1979; **77:** 96–102.

80. Pond SM, Tong T, Benowitz NL, Jacob P. Enhanced bioavailability of pethidine and pentazocine in patients with cirrhosis of the liver. *Austral NZ J Med* 1980; **10:** 515–19.

● 81. Lawlor PG, Bruera E. Side-effects of opioids in chronic pain treatment. *Curr Opin Anaesthesiol* 1998; **11:** 539–45.

● ◆ 82. Davies G, Kingswood C, Street M. Pharmacokinetics of opioids in renal dysfunction. *Clin Pharmacokinet* 1996; **31:** 410–22.

● 83. Sear JW. Recent advances and developments in the clinical use of i.v. opioids during the peroperative period. *Br J Anaesth* 1998; **81:** 38–50.

84. Davies G, Kingswood C, Street M. Pharmacokinetics of opioids in renal dysfunction. *Clin Pharmacokinet* 1996; **31:** 410–22.

● 85. Kreek MJ, Schecter AJ, Gutjahr CL, Hecht M. Methadone use in patients with chronic renal disease. *Drug Alcohol Depend* 1980; **5:** 197–205.

86. Guay DR, Awni WM, Findlay JW, *et al.* Pharmacokinetics and pharmacodynamics of codeine in end-stage renal disease. *Clin Pharmacol Ther* 1988; **43:** 63–71.

87. Almirall J, Montoliu J, Torras A, Revert L. Propoxyphene-induced hypoglycemia in a patient with chronic renal failure. *Nephron* 1989; **53:** 273–5.

88. Bruera E, Chadwick S, Brenneis C, *et al.* Methylphenidate associated with narcotics for the treatment of cancer pain. *Cancer Treat Rep* 1987; **71:** 67–70.

89. Bruera E, Fainsinger R, MacEachern T, Hanson J. The use of methylphenidate in patients with incident cancer pain receiving regular opiates. A preliminary report. *Pain* 1992; **50:** 75–7.

90. Wilwerding MB, Loprinzi CL, Mailliard JA, *et al.* A randomized, crossover evaluation of methylphenidate in cancer patients receiving strong narcotics. *Support Care Cancer* 1995; **3:** 135–8.

● 91. Bruera E, Macmillan K, Hanson J, MacDonald RN. The cognitive effects of the administration of narcotic analgesics in patients with cancer pain. *Pain* 1989; **39:** 13–6.

◆ 92. Vainio A, Ollila J, Matikainen E, *et al.* Driving ability in cancer patients receiving long-term morphine analgesia. *Lancet* 1995; **346:** 667–70.

● 93. Mercadante S. Pathophysiology and treatment of opioid-related myoclonus in cancer patients. *Pain* 1998; **74:** 5–9.

94. Marinella MA. Meperidine-induced generalized seizures with normal renal function. *South Med J* 1997; **90:** 556–8.

95. Jiraki K. Lethal effects of normeperidine. *Am J Forensic Med Pathol* 1992; **13:** 42–3.

96. Thomas DA, Williams GM, Iwata K, *et al.* The medullary dorsal horn. A site of action of morphine in producing facial scratching in monkeys. *Anesthesiology* 1993; **79:** 548–54.

97. Thomas DA, Hammond DL. Microinjection of morphine into the rat medullary dorsal horn produces a dose-dependent increase in facial scratching. *Brain Res* 1995; **695:** 267–70.

98. Katcher J, Walsh D. Opioid-induced itching: morphine sulfate and hydromorphone hydrochloride. *J Pain Symptom Manage* 1999; **17:** 70–2.

99. Dunteman E, Karanikolas M, Filos KS. Transnasal butorphanol for the treatment of opioid-induced pruritus unresponsive to antihistamines. *J Pain Symptom Manage* 1996; **12:** 255–60.

●◆100. Schug S, Zech D, Grond S. Adverse effects of systemic opioid analgesics. *Drug Safety* 1992; **7:** 200–13.

101. Hanks GW, Twycross RG. Pain, the physiological antagonist of opioid analgesics [letter]. *Lancet* 1984; **1:** 1477–8.

●102. McQuay HJ. Opioids in chronic pain. *Br J Anaesth* 1989; **63:** 213–26.

●103. Cleeland CS, Gonin R, Hatfield AK, *et al.* Pain and its treatment in outpatients with metastatic cancer. *N Engl J Med* 1994; **330:** 592–6.

104. Bonica JJ. *The Management of Pain*, 2nd edn. Philadelphia, PA: Lea & Febiger, 1990.

◆105. WHO. *Cancer Pain Relief*. Geneva: World Health Organization, 1986.

106. Sullivan M, Rapp S, Fitzgibbon D, Chapman CR. Pain and the choice to hasten death in patients with painful metastatic cancer. *J Palliative Care* 1997; **13:** 18–28.

107. Marks RM, Sachar EJ. Undertreatment of medical inpatients with narcotic analgesics. *Ann Internal Med* 1973; **78:** 173–81.

◆108. Morgan JP. American opiophobia: customary underutilization of opioid analgesics. *Advanc Alcohol Substance Abuse* 1985; **5:** 163–73.

109. Janjan N, Payne R, Gillis T, *et al.* Presenting symptoms in patients referred to a multidisciplinary clinic for bone metastases. *J Pain Symptom Manage* 1998; **16:** 171–8.

●110. Lander J. Fallacies and phobias about addiction and pain. *Br J Addiction* 1990; **85:** 803–9.

111. Kaasalainen V, Vainio A, Ali-Melkkila T. Developments in the treatment of cancer pain in Finland: the third nation-wide survey. *Pain* 1997; **70:** 175–83.

112. Mercadante S, Salvaggio L. Cancer pain knowledge in Southern Italy: data from a postgraduate refresher course. *J Pain Symptom Manage* 1996; **11:** 108–15.

113. Gaylin W, Kass LR, Pellegrino ED, Siegler M. Doctors must not kill. *JAMA* 1988; **259:** 2139–40.

114. Wall PD. The generation of yet another myth on the use of narcotics. *Pain* 1997; **73:** 121–2.

115. Cleeland CS, Gonin R, Baez L, *et al.* Pain and treatment of pain in minority patients with cancer. The Eastern Cooperative Oncology Group Minority Outpatient Pain Study. *Ann Intern Med* 1997; **127:** 813–16.

116. Saxena A, Mendoza T, Cleeland CS. The assessment of cancer pain in North India: The validation of the hindi brief pain inventory – BPI-H. *J Pain Symptom Manage* 1999; **17:** 27–41.

117. Uki J, Mendoza T, Cleeland CS, *et al.* A brief cancer pain assessment tool in Japanese: the utility of the Japanese Brief Pain Inventory – BPI-J. *J Pain Symptom Manage* 1998; **16:** 364–73.

118. O'Brien CP. Drug addiction and drug abuse. In: Goodman JGG, Gilman A, Limbird LL eds. *Goodman and Gilman's the Pharmacological Basis of Therapeutics*, 9th edn. New York, NY: McGraw-Hill, 1996: 557–77.

119. Portenoy RK. Opioid tolerance and responsiveness: research findings and clinical observations. In: Gebhart GF, Hammond DL, Jensen TS eds. *Proceedings of the 7th World Congress on Pain, Progress in Pain Research and Management*. Seattle, WA: IASP Press,1994: 595–619.

120. Stevens CW, Yaksh TL. Studies of morphine and D-ala2-D-leu5-enkephalin (DADLE) cross-tolerance after continuous intrathecal infusion in the rat. *Anesthesiology* 1992; **76:** 596–603.

●121. Nestler EJ. Molecular mechanisms of opiate and cocaine addiction. *Curr Opin Neurobiol* 1997; **7:** 713–19.

122. Christie MJ, Williams JT, North RA. Cellular mechanisms of opioid tolerance: studies in single brain neurons. *Mol Pharmacol* 1987; **32:** 633–8.

●123. Collett BJ. Opioid tolerance: the clinical perspective. *Br J Anaesth* 1998; **81:** 58–68.

124. Lyness WH, Smith FL, Heavner JE, *et al.* Morphine self-administration in the rat during adjuvant-induced arthritis. *Life Sci* 1989; **45:** 2217–24.

●125. Balleine BW, Dickenson A. Goal-directed instrumental

action: contingency and incentive learning and their cortical substrates. *Neuropharmacology* 1998; **37:** 407–19.

●126. Kreek MJ. Opiates, opioids and addiction. *Mol Psychiatry* 1996; **1:** 232–54.

127. McQuay HJ, Bullingham RES, Moore RA. Acute opiate tolerance in man. *Life Sci* 1981; **28:** 2513–17.

128. Inturrisi CE, Portenoy RK, Max MB, *et al.* Pharmacokinetic–pharmacodynamic relationships of methadone infusions in patients with cancer pain. *Clin Pharmacol Ther* 1990; **47:** 565–77.

◆129. Schug S, Zech D, Grond S, *et al.* A long-term survey of morphine in cancer pain patients. *J Pain Symptom Manage* 1992; **7:** 259–66.

130. Brescia FJ, Portenoy RK, Ryan M, *et al.* Pain, opioid use, and survival in hospitalized patients with advanced cancer. *J Clin Oncol* 1992; **10:** 149–55.

131. Arner S, Rawal N, Gustafsson LL. Clinical experience of long-term treatment with epidural and intrathecal opioids – a nationwide survey. *Acta Anaesthesiol Scand* 1988; **32:** 253–9.

132. Kanner RM, Foley KM. Patterns of narcotic drug use in a cancer pain clinic. *Ann NY Acad Sci* 1981; **362:** 161–72.

133. Foley KM. Controversies in cancer pain. Medical perspectives. *Cancer* 1989; **63** (Suppl. 11): 2257–65.

134. Moulin DE, Ling GS, Pasternak GW. Unidirectional analgesic cross-tolerance between morphine and levorphanol in the rat. *Pain* 1988; **33:** 233–9.

135. Neil A. Morphine- and methadone-tolerant mice differ in cross-tolerance to other opiates. Heterogeneity in opioid mechanisms indicated. *Naunyn-Schmied Archiv Pharmacol* 1982; **320:** 50–3.

136. Hanks GWC, Cherny N. Opioid analgesic therapy. In: Doyle D ed. *Oxford Textbook of Palliative Medicine*, 2nd edn. Oxford: Oxford University Press, 1998: 331–54.

137. Kreek MJ, Koob GF. Drug dependence: stress and dysregulation of brain reward pathways. *Drug & Alcohol Dependence* 1998; **51:** 23–47.

138. Anonymous. Substance related disorders. In: *American Psychiatric Association Diagnostic and Statistical Manual of Mental Disorders DSM-IV*. Washington, DC: American Psychiatric Publishing, 1994.

139. Weissman DE, Haddox JD. Opioid pseudoaddiction – an iatrogenic syndrome. *Pain* 1989; **36:** 363–6.

140. Coyle N, Adelhardt J, Foley KM, Portenoy RK. Character of terminal illness in the advanced cancer patient: pain and other symptoms during the last four weeks of life. *J Pain Symptom Manage* 1990; **5:** 83–93.

141. Cherny NJ, Chang V, Frager G, *et al.* Opioid pharmacotherapy in the management of cancer pain: a survey of strategies used by pain physicians for the selection of analgesic drugs and routes of administration. *Cancer* 1995; **76:** 1283–93.

●142. Gilbar PJ. A guide to enteral drug administration in palliative care. *J Pain Symptom Manage* 1999; **17:** 197–207.

143. Weinberg DS, Inturrisi CE, Reidenberg B, *et al.* Sublingual absorption of selected opioid analgesics. *Clin Pharmacol Ther* 1988; **44:** 335–42.

●144. Coluzzi PH. Sublingual morphine: efficacy reviewed. *J Pain Symptom Manage* 1998; **16:** 184–92.

145. Fine PG, Marcus M, De Boer AJ, Van Der Oord B. An open label study of oral transmucosal fentanyl citrate (OTFC) for the treatment of breakthrough cancer pain. *Pain* 1991; **45:** 149–153.

146. Christie JM, Simmonds M, Patt R, *et al.* Dose-titration, multicenter study of oral transmucosal fentanyl citrate for the treatment of breakthrough pain in cancer patients using transdermal fentanyl for persistent pain. *J Clin Oncol* 1998; **16:** 3238–45.

●147. Alexander-Williams JM, Rowbotham DJ. Novel routes of opioid administration. *Br J Anaesth* 1998; **81:** 3–7.

148. Worsley MH, MacLeod AD, Brodie MJ, *et al.* Inhaled fentanyl as a method of analgesia. *Anaesthesia* 1990; **45:** 449–51.

●149. Ripamonti C, Zecca E, De Conno F. Pharmacological treatment of cancer pain: alternative routes of opioid administration. *Tumori* 1998; **84:** 289–300.

150. Gupta SK, Southam M, Gale R, Hwang SS. System functionality and physicochemical model of fentanyl transdermal system. *J Pain Symptom Manage* 1992; **7** (3 Suppl.): S17–26.

●◆151. Payne R. Transdermal fentanyl: suggested recommendations for clinical use. *J Pain Symptom Manage* 1992; **7** (Suppl. 3): S40–4.

●152. Bruera E, Brenneis C, Michaud M, *et al.* Use of the subcutaneous route for the administration of narcotics in patients with cancer pain. *Cancer* 1988; **62:** 407–11.

153. Bruera E, Fainsinger R, Moore M, *et al.* Local toxicity with subcutaneous methadone. Experience of two centers. *Pain* 1991; **45:** 141–3.

154. Grond S, Meuser T. Weak opioids – an educational substitute for morphine? *Curr Opin Anaesthesiol* 1998; **11:** 559–65.

155. Mercadante S, Salvaggio L, Dardanoni G, *et al.* Dextropropoxyphene versus morphine in opioid-naive cancer patients with pain. *J Pain Symptom Manage* 1998; **15:** 76–81.

156. WHO. *The use of Essential Drugs*. Eighth report of the WHO Expert Committee. Technical report series 882. Geneva: World Health Organization, 1998.

157. Eckhardt K, Li S, Ammon S, *et al.* Same incidence of adverse drug events after codeine administration irrespective of the genetically determined differences in morphine formation. *Pain* 1998; **76:** 27–33.

◆158. Moore A, Collins S, Carroll D, McQuay H. Paracetamol with and without codeine in acute pain: a quantitative systematic review. *Pain* 1997; **70:** 193–201.

159. Keats AS, Telford J, Kurosu Y. Studies of analgesic drugs: dihydrocodeine. *J Pharmacol Exp Ther* 1957; **120:** 354–60.

160. Wotherspoon HA, Kenny GN, McArdle CS. Analgesic efficacy of controlled-release dihydrocodeine. A com-

parison of 60, 90 and 120 mg tablets in cold-induced pain. *Anaesthesia* 1991; **46:** 915–17.

161. Reisine T, Pasternak G. Opioid analgesics and antagonists. In: Goodman JGG, Gilman A, Limbird LL eds. *Goodman and Gilman's the Pharmacological Basis of Therapeutics*, 9th edn. New York, NY: McGraw-Hill, 1996.

◆162. Raffa RB, Friderichs E, Reimann W, *et al.* Opioid and nonopioid components independently contribute to the mechanism of action of tramadol, an "atypical" opioid analgesic. *J Pharmacol Exp Ther* 1992; **260:** 275–85.

●163. Dayer P, Desmeules J, Collart L. The pharmacology of tramadol. *Drugs* 1997; **53** (Suppl. 2): 18–24.

●164. Duthie DJ. Remifentanil and tramadol. *Br J Anaesth* 1998; **81:** 51–7.

165. Preston KL, Jasinski DR, Testa M. Abuse potential and pharmacological comparison of tramadol and morphine. *Drug Alcohol Dependence* 1991; **27:** 7–17.

●166. Cossmann M, Kohnen C. General tolerability and adverse event profile of tramadol. *Revis Contemp Pharmacother* 1995; **6:** 513–31.

167. Barnung SK, Treschow M, Borgbjerg FM. Respiratory depression following oral tramadol in a patient with impaired renal function. *Pain* 1997; **71:** 111–12.

168. Collins SL, Faura CC, Moore RA, McQuay HJ. Peak plasma concentrations after oral morphine: a systematic review. *J Pain Symptom Manage* 1998; **16**: 388–402.

169. Savarese JJ, Goldheim PD, Thomas GB, Kaiko RF. Steady state pharmacokinetics of controlled release oral morphine sulphate in healthy subjects. *Clin Pharmacokinet* 1986; **11:** 505–10.

170. Gourlay GK. Sustained relief of chronic pain. Pharmacokinetics of sustained release morphine. *Clin Pharmacokinet* 1998; **35:** 173–90.

171. Gourlay GK, Cherry DA, Onley MM, *et al.* Pharmacokinetics and pharmacodynamics of twenty-four-hourly Kapanol compared to twelve-hourly MS Contin in the treatment of severe cancer pain. *Pain* 1997; **69:** 295–302.

172. Hoskin PJ, Hanks GW, Aherne GW, *et al.* The bioavailability and pharmacokinetics of morphine after intravenous, oral and buccal administration in healthy volunteers. *Br J Clin Pharmacol* 1989; **27:** 499–505.

◆173. Sawe J, Dahlstrom B, Paalzow L, Rane A. Morphine kinetics in cancer patients. *Clin Pharmacol Ther* 1981; **30:** 629–35.

174. Neumann PB, Henriksen H, Grosman N, Christensen CB. Plasma morphine concentrations during chronic oral administration in patients with cancer pain. *Pain* 1982; **13:** 247–52.

●175. Poyhia R, Vainio A, Kalso E. A review of oxycodone's clinical pharmacokinetics and pharmacodynamics. *J Pain Symptom Manage* 1993; **8:** 63–7.

176. Poyhia R, Seppala T, Olkkola KT, Kalso E. The pharmacokinetics and metabolism of oxycodone after intramuscular and oral administration to healthy subjects. *Br J Clin Pharmacol* 1992; **33:** 617–21.

177. Parris WC, Johnson BW, Jr, Croghan MK, *et al.* The use of controlled-release oxycodone for the treatment of chronic cancer pain: a randomized, double-blind study. *J Pain Symptom Manage* 1998; **16:** 205–11.

178. Kaplan R, Parris WC, Citron ML, *et al.* Comparison of controlled-release and immediate-release oxycodone tablets in patients with cancer pain. *J Clin Oncol* 1998; **16:** 3230–7.

179. Bruera E, Belzile M, Pituskin E, *et al.* Randomized, double-blind, cross-over trial comparing safety and efficacy of oral controlled-release oxycodone with controlled-release morphine in patients with cancer pain. *J Clin Oncol* 1998; **16:** 3222–9.

180. Foley KM, Houde RW. Methadone in cancer pain management: individualize dose and titrate to effect. *J Clin Oncol* 1998; **16:** 3213–15.

●◆181. Ripamonti C, Zecca E, Bruera E. An update on the clinical use of methadone for cancer pain. *Pain* 1997; **70:** 109–15.

●182. Fainsinger R, Schoeller T, Bruera E. Methadone in the management of cancer pain: a review. *Pain* 1993; **52:** 137–47.

183. Ripamonti C, Groff L, Brunelli C, *et al.* Switching from morphine to oral methadone in treating cancer pain: what is the equianalgesic dose ratio? *J Clin Oncol* 1998; **16:** 3216–21.

184. Lawlor PG, Turner KS, Hanson J, Bruera ED. Dose ratio between morphine and methadone in patients with cancer pain: a retrospective study. *Cancer* 1998; **82:** 1167–73.

●185. Fine PG. Fentanyl in the treatment of cancer pain. *Semin Oncol* 1997; **24** (Suppl. 5): 16–27.

186. Willens JS, Myslinski NR. Pharmacodynamics, pharmacokinetics, and clinical uses of fentanyl, sufentanil, and alfentanil. *Heart Lung* 1993; **22:** 239–51.

●187. Jeal W, Benfield P. Transdermal fentanyl. A review of its pharmacological properties and therapeutic efficacy in pain control. *Drugs* 1997; **53:** 109–38.

188. Lehmann KA, Zech D eds. *Transdermal Fentanyl. A New Approach to Prolonged Pain Control.* Berlin: Springer-Verlag, 1991.

●189. Cherny NI. Opioid analgesics: comparative features and prescribing guidelines. *Drugs* 1996; **51:** 713–37.

190. Fine PG, Busch MA. Characterization of breakthrough pain by hospice patients and their caregivers. *J Pain Symptom Manage* 1998; **16:** 179–83.

191. Cleary JF. Pharmacokinetic and pharmacodynamic issues in the treatment of breakthrough pain. *Semin Oncol* 1997; **24** (5 Suppl. 16): 9–13.

192. Ashburn MA, Fine PG, Stanley TH. Oral transmucosal fentanyl citrate for the treatment of breakthrough cancer pain: a case report. *Anesthesiology* 1989; **71:** 615–17.

193. Coda B, Tanaka A, Jacobson RC, *et al.* Hydromorphone

analgesia after intravenous bolus administration. *Pain* 1997; **71:** 41–8.

●194. Twycross RG. Opioid analgesics in cancer pain: current practice and controversies. *Cancer Surveys* 1988; **7:** 29–53.

195. Inturrisi CE, Max MB, Foley KM, *et al.* The pharmacokinetics of heroin in patients with chronic pain. *N Engl J Med* 1984; **310:** 1213–17.

196. Dixon R, Crews T, Inturrisi C, Foley K. Levorphanol: pharmacokinetics and steady-state plasma concentrations in patients with pain. *Res Commun Chem Pathol Pharmacol* 1983; **41:** 3–17.

●197. Heel RC, Brogden RN, Speight TM, Avery GS. Buprenorphine: a review of its pharmacological properties and therapeutic efficacy. *Drugs* 1979; **17:** 81–110.

198. Bullingham RES, McQuay HJ, Dwyer D, *et al.* Sublingual buprenorphine used postoperatively: clinical observations and preliminary pharmacokinetic analysis. *Br J Clin Pharmacol* 1981; **12:** 117–22.

●199. Hoskin PJ, Hanks GW. Opioid agonist-antagonist drugs in acute and chronic pain states. *Drugs* 1991; **41:** 326–44.

200. Daniel JR, Wilkins RD, Nicholson PA. Two comparisons of the analgesic activity of orally administered pentazocine, dihydrocodeine and placebo. *Br J Anaesth* 1971; **43:** 392–9.

201. Wang DS, Sternbach G, Varon J. Nalmefene: a long-acting opioid antagonist. Clinical applications in emergency medicine. *J Emergency Med* 1998; **16:** 471–5.

202. Jurna I, Baldauf J. Oral administration of slow-release naloxone for prevention of constipation but not analgesia following oral morphine. *Der Schmerz* 1993; **7:** 314–21.

203. Gan TJ, Ginsberg B, Glass PSA, *et al.* Opioid-sparing effects of a low-dose infusion of naloxone in patient-administered morphine sulfate. *Anesthesiology* 1997; **87:** 1075–81.

4

History and clinical examination of the cancer pain patient: assessment and measurement

EDUARDO BRUERA AND CATHERINE M NEUMANN

Pain occurs in 60–80% of patients with advanced cancer before death.[1,2] During the 1970s and early 1980s, a number of authors demonstrated that patients with cancer pain were inadequately managed.[3,4] As a result, organizations such as the International Association for the Study of Pain, the World Health Organization, and other intergovernmental and nongovernmental organizations launched major initiatives promoting the education of health care professionals and the lay public on cancer pain management.[4–6] Initial guidelines and scholarly reviews focused on dispelling existing myths and on proposing simple yet effective treatments. The assessment of pain was generally discussed in a very simple way, with emphasis on the need for an appropriate assessment of the "mechanics" of pain: location, radiation, character, intensity, syndromal presentation, and nerve pathways involved in the conduction of nociceptive stimuli.

During recent years, it has become more evident that the optimal evaluation of the patient with cancer pain requires a multidimensional assessment of the pain syndrome, the patient's clinical, psychological, and psychiatric characteristics, and a number of social and family variables. A number of prognostic factors have been identified that have a major impact on the nature of the pain complaint and on the response to treatment.

In the following, we will initially discuss the evaluation of patients with cancer pain along with the different aspects of the assessment of the pain syndrome and the need to integrate the pain with other common symptoms in patients with advanced cancer. Finally, areas for future research will be discussed.

EVALUATION OF PATIENTS WITH CANCER PAIN

History

Table 4.1 summarizes the main components of the medical history in patients with cancer pain. It is crucial to have a good understanding of the underlying cancer (primary site, histology, and anatomical extent) as well as the current disease status. In patients with advanced cancer the likelihood is higher that the pain is due to locally advanced or metastatic cancer. However, in up to one-fifth of these patients the pain is due to other causes, such as cancer treatments or unrelated, often premorbid, problems.[1] In addition, some specific primary sites and histologies are more likely to metastasize to specific areas of the body than others (e.g. prostate cancer to bones, small-cell lung cancer to the brain).

Previous cancer treatments should be reviewed in depth. Some antineoplastic treatments, such as aggressive surgery, chemotherapy, or radiation therapy, are capable of causing chronic pain syndromes. Alternatively, some patients may potentially benefit from specific antineoplastic interventions such as hormonal therapy or radiation therapy.

Most patients with cancer pain have advanced disease and a variety of other devastating physical symptoms and psychosocial sequelae,[7] some of which, such as anxiety or depression, may impact on the expression of pain intensity. Other symptoms, such as nausea and confusion, will

Table 4.1 *Medical history in patients with cancer pain*

Cancer stage
• Primary site
• Histology
• Anatomical extent
Previous cancer treatment
Cancer pain syndrome
Other physical symptoms
Previous pain syndromes and treatment
Psychosocial assessment
History of alcoholism/drug abuse
Assessment of cognitive function/delirium
Other medical conditions

influence the choice of therapeutic interventions for pain treatment. Therefore, it is of great importance to consider pain within the context of the other physical and psychosocial symptoms and to monitor the effects of pain and its treatment on these other symptoms.

The presence of other pain syndromes, due either to cancer or to chronic nonmalignant pain, may provide important information about patients' coping strategies and their prior responses to analgesic therapies.

A history of alcohol or drug abuse is an independent poor prognostic factor for pain control.[8] Patients should routinely undergo screening assessments for alcohol, such as the CAGE questionnaire,[9] and an assessment of a history of drug use.

One of the most important aspects of the psychosocial assessment is the presence or significant history of mood disorders.[10] Depression occurs in approximately 25% of patients with advanced cancer.[11] Mood disorders are likely to be intensified by cancer pain. On the other hand, the expression of pain and other somatic symptoms can be higher in patients with mood disorders.[8] A number of tools can be used for the assessment of the presence and intensity of depression.[12] Recent research suggests that simple assessments such as a visual analog scale (VAS) or the question "Are you depressed?" can be as reliable as more complex and time-consuming instruments in cancer patients.[13]

Cognitive failure is a frequent finding in patients with advanced cancer,[14] occurring in more than 80% of patients before death.[15,16] The presence of cognitive failure makes the assessment of intensity and other dimensions of pain very difficult. In addition, cognitive failure may be aggravated by pharmacological interventions for the management of pain, and, therefore, a regular screening of cognitive function and delirium should be performed.[16]

Three of the more commonly applied tools are the Folstein Mini-Mental State Exam (MMSE), the Memorial Delirium Assessment Scale (MDAS), and the Delirium Rating Scale (DRS). No single tool is relied on exclusively to establish a definitive diagnosis of delirium in all cases. An individual patient's score, whether normal or abnormal, must be correlated with the clinical situation.

The MMSE, devised by Folstein *et al.*,[17] comprises 11 questions that assess five general areas of cognition: orientation, registration, attention and calculation, recall, and language. A score of <24 out of 30 is generally indicative of cognitive dysfunction, although this score is generally corrected to reflect age and educational level.[18] The MMSE has several advantages in that it is among the most frequently used tests in the clinical evaluation of delirium and has been validated for use in patients with advanced cancer. It is familiar to many clinicians, and can be administered with very little training by most health care professionals. It is quick to complete, taking an average of 5–10 min, and its numerical score quantifies cognitive impairment, which can then be compared over time in a given patient, allowing evaluation of the efficacy of various management strategies. With routine use, it may increase clinician interest and competence in assessing and managing delirium, as was suggested in early studies.[17] The MMSE is limited by the fact that it is simply a screen for cognitive dysfunction and therefore cannot differentiate between delirium and other cognitive disorders such as dementia. It may also miss subtle degrees of cognitive impairment. Finally, as the MMSE does not characterize the presence of perceptual abnormalities or psychomotor agitation, two patients with equal scores may look quite different clinically, one being in severe distress with multiple hallucinations and severe agitation and the other being hypoactive in appearance.

The MDAS, developed by Breitbart *et al.*,[19] is a 10-item observer-rated scale that assesses disturbances in arousal, level of consciousness, psychomotor activity, and cognition. It is designed more specifically to address delirium than most other tools in that the assessed items reflect current *Diagnostic and Statistical Manual for Mental Disorders* vol. IV (DSM-IV) diagnostic criteria for delirium. Although reported to take approximately 10 min to administer, additional time is required for review and discussion with family members and nursing staff. Studies have shown that the MDAS is able to distinguish patients with delirium from those with other cognitive or noncognitive psychiatric disorders.[19] Although it has been suggested that the MDAS may be useful for diagnosis of delirium, currently it has only been validated as a measurement of delirium severity. As with the MMSE, the MDAS may miss mild cases of delirium and, although it is designed for repeated administration over time, it has not been tested in this manner. Its successful use requires the interviewer to apply clinical judgment and, therefore, it is not readily performed by all levels of health care professionals.

The DRS is a 10-item rating scale assessing a broad range of delirium symptomatology. It is suitably easy to administer and, although suggested as a suitable scale for the assessment of delirium severity, it has been validated more for use as a diagnostic tool. A limitation is its failure to assess some features considered essential to the diagnosis of delirium, including inattention, disorganized thinking, and clouding of consciousness.

An ideal clinical tool will be used regularly and repetitively on all patients. A "perfect tool," if used only rarely, is of no practical benefit. Regular assessment, even of patients who appear cognitively intact, is essential for timely identification and management, especially as mild delirium of recent onset has the greatest potential for reversibility.

Finally, a number of other medical conditions influence optimal pain management. The presence of renal failure may have implications for the accumulation of active opioid metabolites or the safe administration of nonsteroidal anti-inflammatory drugs. Patients with borderline cognitive function or dementia may have difficulties tolerating opioids or adjuvant drugs such as tricyclic antidepressants or anticonvulsants. Patients with acute or chronic infection or diabetes may be poor candidates for corticosteroids. In summary, clinicians need to have a complete understanding of the patient's medical and psychiatric condition in order to establish a safe and effective therapeutic plan.

Physical examination

Patients with cancer pain should undergo a complete physical examination, the results of which, when combined with those of a thorough history, are sufficient to reach an appropriate diagnosis of the cause of pain in the majority of patients.[20] In addition, the physical examination reveals important information about the anatomic extent of tumor spread and the overall physical condition of the patient. For example, patients who are confused, profoundly cachectic, and who are nonambulatory are unlikely to benefit from aggressive orthopedic reconstruction of the spine or long bones and are probably more appropriately treated with less aggressive, essentially pharmacologic, interventions.

Investigations

Even in seriously ill patients, ancillary laboratory and imaging investigations are sometimes extremely useful in clarifying the causes of pain and aiding the selection of analgesic interventions. Plain radiographs and bone scans contribute to decision-making regarding the appropriateness of radiation therapy and orthopedic procedures in patients with bone pain. Computed tomography and magnetic resonance imaging can help determine the cause of intrathoracic and intra-abdominal pain syndromes, and magnetic resonance imaging is essential to confirm the early diagnosis of epidural spinal cord compression.

CHARACTERIZATION OF THE CANCER PAIN SYNDROME

Table 4.2 summarizes the main factors that should be considered in characterizing the cancer pain syndrome. The location, radiation, descriptors, duration, and onset of the pain syndrome will provide important clues as to the pathophysiology and underlying cause of pain. Nociceptive pain is defined as pain that arises from activation of peripheral nociceptors. The nervous system is fundamentally intact, and complaints of pain usually correlate well with the extent of tissue damage (i.e. tumor invasion of bone or soft tissue[21]). Two subgroups of nociceptive pain are recognized:

1 Somatic: patients usually describe a discrete pain location and commonly use descriptors such as "aching," "sharp," "stabbing," or "throbbing." Typical examples of somatic nociceptive pains are those related to bone metastases or infiltration of the skin and soft tissues by cancer.
2 Visceral: because of the distribution and convergence of nociceptors, these pain syndromes are usually described more vaguely with regards to both location and quality. Patients usually use descriptors such as "tugging," "cramping," or "pressure." Pain is usually associated with tumor invasion of intra-abdominal or intrathoracic organs, distension, or compression, and pain signals are conducted by the afferent autonomic nervous system.

Neuropathic pain is defined as pain caused by aberrant somatosensory processing,[21] and in cancer patients this is most frequently due to tumor involvement of peripheral nerves, roots, or spinal cord. Patients most commonly describe this pain as "burning," "numb," shock-like," or "electrical." Pain is usually located in the trajectory of the involved nerves and is frequently accompanied by corresponding motor and/or sensory abnormalities. For example, a patient with lung cancer and burning pain in the right hemithorax radiating along the intercostal space arising after a thoracotomy is likely to be experiencing neuropathic pain due to a post-thoracotomy syndrome. Alternatively, continuous stabbing pain that is well localized and with no radiation which preceded the thoracotomy is more likely to reflect nociceptive pain due to involvement of the pleural space or bone by the primary tumor.

Table 4.2 *Cancer pain syndrome assessment*

Cause (tumor, treatment, unrelated)
Location(s) – radiation
Descriptors
Intensity – aggravating factors, relieving factors
Duration and onset
Previous analgesic treatments
Functional and psychological impairment

Careful assessment of previous therapies decreases the likelihood of using drugs or interventions that were previously found to be ineffective or poorly tolerated. Specifically, common opioid side-effects such as sedation, constipation, and nausea should be assessed.

In patients with multiple sites of pain, it is particularly important to assess each site separately and to record carefully the different characteristics. Often, the pathophysiology and cause of each pain is quite different, and this will require different approaches in a given patient.

Table 4.3 *Instruments for the measurement of pain intensity*

Edmonton Symptom Assessment System[25]
Brief Pain Inventory[26]
Memorial Pain Assessment Card[27]
McGill Pain Questionnaire[28]
Verbal descriptors
Numerical scales
Visual analog scales
Facial scales (pediatrics)[29]

PAIN EVALUATION

In recent years, it has become evident that the appropriate evaluation of pain requires the regular assessment of intensity, insight into its multidimensional features, an appreciation of the patient's clinical and psychosocial characteristics, and consideration of prognostic factors that may have a major impact on treatment outcome, thus helping to focus care. It has also become apparent that the features should be considered in the context of the other major symptom complexes that are also very common in patients with advanced cancer. Unfortunately, there is evidence that pain is usually poorly assessed by clinicians.[22–24] The following sections focus on the assessment of intensity and the multiple dimensions of pain.

Intensity

It is crucial to assess and monitor the intensity of pain. This can be accomplished using visual analog scales, verbal scales, and numerical scales or more complex pain questionnaires. Table 4.3 summarizes some of the most commonly used instruments for the measurement of pain intensity.[25–29] Most of these instruments and techniques are considered reliable for the assessment of the intensity of pain. The choice of instrument depends largely on the patient population and the setting in which care is delivered. In some regions of the world where the rate of illiteracy is high, facial scales, colored circles, or pictures of fruits of different size can be used to describe the intensity of pain at a given time.

The commonly used instruments described above measure the intensity of pain at a given time only. Of the more comprehensive instruments, we will describe the Brief Pain Inventory,[26] the McGill Pain Questionnaire,[27] and the Memorial Pain Assessment Card.[28]

The Brief Pain Inventory (BPI) can be administered by a health care professional or may be self-administered. The longer version takes approximately 15 min to complete while a shorter version requires just a few minutes. The BPI includes a graphic representation of the location of pain and a group of qualitative pain descriptors. The severity of pain is assessed using visual analog scales for pain at its best and worst, and on average. The perceived level of interference with normal activities (life enjoyment, work, mood, sleep, walking, relationships with others) is also reported. There is ample evidence that the BPI is cross-culturally valid.[26,30]

The McGill Pain Questionnaire (MPQ) is one of the oldest and best-established pain assessment instruments.[27] Patients are required to select terms used to describe pain from a list. The descriptors are then organized into sensory, affective, or evaluative dimensions. The MPQ also provides a graphic display of pain location. This instrument has been used in patients with cancer pain,[31] and in recent years a short form of the MPQ has been found to be a valuable tool in patients with chronic cancer pain.[32]

The Memorial Pain Assessment Card can be completed in less than 1 min and is easily understood by patients.[28] It consists of a small card that is folded so that four separate measures can be performed. It contains scales intended for the measurement of pain intensity, pain relief, and mood as well as a set of descriptors. It is valid and effective for clinical use and is recommended both for the clinical assessment of individual patients and as an outcome measure for clinical trials.[28]

The Edmonton Symptom Assessment System (ESAS) is a group of nine visual analog scales for nine different symptoms, including pain intensity. This tool allows for a very rapid (approximately 1 min) assessment of pain, mood, and other physical symptoms. The results are reported in a graph that is kept in the patient's chart. This tool has been found to be reliable for individual patient treatment,[25,33] as well as for clinical research and program evaluation.[34]

One major limitation of the more complex instruments is that, because of their length, they cannot easily be administered repeatedly. The appropriate frequency of measurement of pain has not been determined in prospective research. In acute care settings, assessment takes place usually once or twice a day. In chronic care settings, in which patients are assumed to be more stable, assessment is usually performed three times a week. Finally, in patients managed by home care or ambulatory care, assessment usually takes place at the time of the patient's clinic or hospital visit. Some simple instruments such as numerical scales can also be utilized reliably by telephone.

An important aspect of effective pain assessment and monitoring is a graphic display of pain intensity in the patient's chart.[25] In the past, it became apparent that a regular graphic display of the patient's vital signs greatly assisted in recognizing abnormalities that required correction. Regular reporting of laboratory results and radiographs in the medical records also make visible the number of factors not readily accessible to physical examination. An appropriate format for recording pain and other symptoms renders the patient's distress more visible and assists the team in the overall planning and monitoring of quality of care.[34,35]

Multidimensional pain assessment

At the present time, nociception occurring at the level of the primary or metastatic cancer site cannot be measured. Cortical perception of pain is also not measurable. Thus, all pain measurement is based on the patient's expression of pain intensity and distress. This expression is influenced by factors that modulate the level of nociception, perception, and expression. Therapeutic interventions can be conceived of as targeting pain production at each level of nociception perception and expression.

In the past, cancer pain and hospice groups used a more unidimensional methodology. This approach considered that "pain is what the patient calls pain and has the intensity the patient reports." This was frequently considered to mean that 100% of a given patient's expression of pain was due to nociception and, therefore, treatable with analgesic drugs. This rather simplistic approach could result in massive doses of opioids, opioid-related toxicity, and excessive reliance on pharmacological approaches compared with that which may result when nonpharmacological approaches to pain control are integrated.

Table 4.4 summarizes the components of pain expression in two different patients reporting bony metastatic pain with an intensity of 8/10. In the case of patient 1, in whom the overwhelming majority of the pain expression relates to nociception, opioid analgesics are likely to be highly effective. In the case of patient 2, a major part of the pain expression is due to somatization related to depression and to severe aggravation of pain with minimal movements. This second patient is much less likely to respond to simple increases in opioid doses. A combination of counseling, with or without antidepressant therapy, and the consideration of radiation therapy or orthopedic procedures to the painful bony area will likely be required in order to achieve a significant decrease in the expression of pain. These cases are examples of how multidimensional assessment can help in the recognition of the relative contribution of different dimensions to the patient's expression, thereby assisting in the planning of care.

A positive history of alcoholism or drug abuse indicates a higher risk for coping chemically. Alcoholism occurs in 5–15% of the general population and in approximately 20% of hospitalized patients.[36] Unfortunately, in more than two-thirds of patients the diagnosis is not made in a timely manner.[9,36] Four-item questionnaires such as the CAGE are extremely simple and result in an accurate diagnosis of alcoholism.[9,36] A history of alcoholism is a major prognostic factor for the development of rapid opioid dose escalation and the occurrence of opioid-related neurotoxicity.[8] However, when patients undergo regular screening for alcoholism and are offered multidimensional and multidisciplinary support, both pain intensity and overall opioid use are not significantly different among alcoholic patients compared with those with no history of alcoholism.[9]

Table 4.4 *Components of pain expression in two different patients*

	Patient 1 (intensity 8/10)	Patient 2 (intensity 8/10)
Nociception (%)	80	30
Somatization (%)	5	30
Chemical coping (%)	5	10
Incidental component (%)	10	30
	100	100

Somatization, either as a primary coping strategy or as a result of affective disorders such as anxiety or depression, is also an independent poor prognostic factor in patients with cancer pain.[8] The appropriate assessment and management of affective disorders with both pharmacological and nonpharmacological techniques, including appropriate counseling of patients with a history of somatization, can result in improved symptom control and satisfaction with care.

In noncommunicative patients with delirium or dementia, behavioral scales and third-party assessments have been proposed for the assessment of pain.[37] Unfortunately, validation of these tools following traditionally accepted criteria is elusive because of the characteristics of the patient population. Communicative patients with dementia are probably less able to recall, interpret, and articulate their experience and, consequently, are less likely to report pain[38] than patients without delirium. One of the main potential confounders for the measurement of pain in people with delirium and dementia is memory impairment, as pain experienced at one moment may soon be forgotten.[39,40] A comprehensive study in 51 control subjects and 44 patients with dementia concluded that dementia is capable of influencing not only the report but also the experience of pain.[40]

A number of authors have reported cases of communicative demented patients who appeared to have diminished or absent self-reporting of pain.[39] Behaviors displayed by the patients suggested that decreased pain perception rather than expression was the main reason for decreased self-reporting.[39,41]

Agitated behavior based on factors other than pain may be misinterpreted as pain and mistakenly treated with opioid analgesics, a phenomenon that has been observed in patients with agitated delirium related to cancer.[42] Decreased or absent self-reporting of pain may make the diagnosis of acute complications such as fractures, dental problems, urinary retention, or other acute intercurrent events difficult. Finally, the presence of cognitive failure significantly increases the likelihood of neurotoxicity from both opioids and most adjuvant analgesic drugs.

Neuropathic pain has been described as a syndrome in which there is commonly a reduced responsiveness to opioid analgesics.[8,43] The recognition of neuropathic pain should assist clinicians in deciding on the use of adjuvant analgesic drugs and early referral to specialized pain services.

Incident pain or "breakthrough" pain has been defined as a transitory increase in pain that occurs in one context of ongoing pain of moderate intensity or less. Opioid titration in patients with pain or breakthrough pain is typically difficult because of rapidly changing levels of pain and dose requirements.

Staging of pain (the development of a common language)

After the recognition of the poor quality of pain control in diverse populations,[3] intensive educational efforts have resulted in significant improvement in the management of cancer pain during recent years, although results reported by different groups remain variable. Some original papers describe extremely good results after the use of relatively low doses of opioids.[44–46] More recent studies have suggested that, even after using doses of opioids five or six times higher, 10–30% of patients are still unable to achieve adequate pain control.[47–50] One likely explanation for such varied results is the absence of a homogeneous method for the assessment of pain intensity and pain relief. Another explanation for some diverse findings is the differing characteristics of patients treated by different groups. The relative prevalence of patients with more severe or otherwise distinct pain syndromes in a given sample could have a major impact on treatment outcome.

The recognition of poor prognostic features has led to the development of staging systems for different primary tumors, which has been a major advance in cancer research and treatment.[51,52] These systems have required frequent changes as knowledge of the biology of cancer developed, but have allowed researchers to speak a common language and practitioners to apply the results of their research in a logical and predictable fashion.

The precise definition of patient characteristics in clinical research trials results in an accurate interpretation of data, successful application of therapies, and the subsequent formulation of more advanced clinical research studies. In the clinical field, the early recognition of patients with poor prognostic features results in better planning of care by ensuring faster referral to specialized services.

Unfortunately, such systems are not available for cancer pain. Most publications describe patients as having "pain due to cancer," although this statement is probably as simplistic and difficult to assess and interpret as "carcinoma of the breast." In patients with breast cancer, we know that estrogen and progesterone receptors, positive or negative axillary nodes, histological characteristics of the primary tumor, neoplastic status, and pattern of dissemination are all of prognostic importance. In pain, too, the factors described in Table 4.4 can influence prognosis and management. The presence or absence of these and perhaps other factors will have a major effect on the results of treatment.

The ESAS classifies patients as having a relatively good or poor prognosis for pain control with analgesics according to the presence of five known prognostic factors (Table 4.5). In a multicenter study in 271 consecutive evaluable patients with cancer pain, 85/91 patients with stage I disease achieved good pain control (93%) compared with 69/143 patients with stage II disease (48%, $P<0.0001$). A more specific assessment of each of the different prognostic factors would probably result in higher accuracy of staging systems. However, this would be significantly more time-consuming and might eventually discourage practitioners from the routine use of such a staging system. A more likely useful development would be the identification of new independent prognostic factors that might influence the response. These and other staging systems need independent validation. It is through development of staging systems that a common language and methodology for both clinical research and treatment planning can be established.

Table 4.5 *New Edmonton Staging System for cancer pain*[a]

Prognostic factor	Present
Neuropathic pain	No Yes
Incident pain	No Yes
Somatization	No Yes
Rapid opioid tolerance	No Yes
History of drug addiction or alcohol abuse	No Yes

a. "No" score in all categories = stage I (good prognosis); one or more "yes" scores = stage II (poor prognosis).

INTEGRATION OF PAIN AND OTHER SYMPTOMS

Pain is only one of many symptoms experienced by cancer patients.[7] It is important to assess pain within the context of other symptoms for a number of reasons. Pain may not necessarily be the symptom that is having the greatest impact on a patient's quality of life at a given point in time. Pain intensity may have an impact on other physical symptoms such as fatigue or mobility or on psychosocial symptoms such as depression or anxiety. Alternatively, psychosocial symptoms may have an impact on the patient's expression of pain.[8]

The treatment of pain may lead directly to a worsening of other symptoms such as nausea, constipation, and delirium. The ESAS,[25] STAS,[53] and a number of other tools allow for simultaneous assessment and monitoring of multiple symptoms. These tools involve the completion of a panel of visual analog scales or numerical scales at regular intervals by the patient or, if the patient is cognitively impaired, a nurse.

One of the pivotal clinical challenges in cancer pain management is to maximize the impact on the patient's pain expression while minimizing the worsening of coexisting symptoms and production of new symptoms.

SUMMARY AND CONCLUSIONS

In recent years, there has been increased emphasis on the importance of appropriate clinical assessment of patients with cancer pain. All patients complaining of cancer pain should undergo a complete medical history and physical examination. It is important to determine the cancer stage and previous treatments, to characterize each pain syndrome, and to assess contextual psychosocial issues and other medical conditions. Even in very ill patients, imaging studies may contribute important information for clinical decision-making. There are excellent and simple instruments for assessing and monitoring pain intensity. The most useful instruments for cancer patients are those that assess multiple symptoms and allow for a graphic display of data. The multiple dimensions that modulate the nociceptive production, cortical perception, and expression of pain should be considered in each patient. Clinicians should remember that the expression of pain intensity is a multidimensional construct that results from the relative contribution of many factors. Appropriate multimodal pain management will consider the relative contribution of these factors in a given patient at a given time. Finally, in cancer patients, pain occurs within the context of a number of devastating physical and psychosocial symptoms. Some of those symptoms are more common and may be more intense than pain itself. Because of the relative impact of pain and its treatment on other symptoms, they should be regularly measured.

Unfortunately, the available body of knowledge on the appropriate assessment of pain is not applied in the routine treatment of cancer patients. The main future challenge in this area is to ensure that patients have access to these evaluations on a regular basis.

REFERENCES

1. Levy MH. Pharmacologic treatment of cancer pain. *N Engl J Med* 1996; **335:** 1124–32.
2. Bruera E, Watanabe S. New developments in the assessment of pain in cancer patients. *Supportive Care Cancer* 1994; **2:** 312–18.
3. Marks RM, Sachar EJ. Undertreatment of medical inpatients with narcotic analgesics. *Ann Intern Med* 1973; **78:** 173–81.
4. ● World Health Organization Expert Committee Report 1990, *Cancer Pain Relief and Palliative Care*. Technical Series 804. Geneva: World Health Organization.
5. US Department of Health and Human Services. *Management of Cancer Pain. Clinical Practice Guidelines*. AHCPR Publications, No. 94-0592, March 1994.
6. World Health Organization. *Cancer Pain Relief*, 2nd edn. Geneva: World Health Organization, 1996: 43.
7. Bruera E, Neumann CM. Respective limits of palliative care and oncology in the supportive care of cancer patients. *Supportive Care Cancer* (in press).
8. ◆ Bruera E, Schoeller T, Wenk R, *et al.* A prospective multi-centre assessment of the Edmonton Staging System for cancer pain. *J Pain Symptom Manage* 1995; **10:** 348–55.
9. Bruera E, Moyano J, Seifert L, *et al.* The frequency of alcoholism among patients with pain due to terminal cancer. *J Pain Symptom Manage* 1995; **10:** 599–603.
10. ● Breitbart W, Bruera E, Chochinov H, Lynch M. Neuropsychiatric syndromes and psychological symptoms in patients with advanced cancer. *J Pain Symptom Manage* 1995; **10(2):** 131–41.
11. ● Breitbart W, Chochinov HM, Passik S. Psychiatric aspects of palliative care. In: Doyle D, Hanks GWC, MacDonald N eds. *Oxford Textbook of Palliative Medicine*, 2nd edn. Oxford: Oxford University Press, 1998: 933–54.
12. Lynch ME. The assessment and prevalence of affective disorders in advanced cancer. *J Palliative Care* 1995; **11(1):** 10–18.
13. ◆ Chochinov HM, Wilson KG, Enns M, Lander S. "Are you depressed?" Screening for depression in the terminally ill. *Am J Psychiatry* 1997; **154:** 674–6.
14. Pereira J, Hanson J, Bruera E. The frequency and clinical course of cognitive impairment in patients with terminal cancer. *Cancer* 1997; **79:** 835–42.
15. Massie MJ, Holland J, Glass E. Delirium in terminally ill cancer patients. *Am J Psychiatry* 1983; **140:** 1048–50.
16. Pereira J, Hanson J, Bruera E. The frequency and clini-

cal course of cognitive impairment in patients with terminal cancer. *Cancer* 1997; **79:** 835–42.

◆ 17. Folstein MF, Folstein S, McHugh PR. "Mini-mental state": a practical method for grading the cognitive state of patients for the clinician. *J Psych Res* 1975; **12:** 189–98.

18. Crum RM, Anthony JC, Bassett SS, Folstein MF. Population-based norms for the mini-mental state examination by age and educational level. *JAMA* 1993; **269:** 2386–91.

◆ 19. Breitbart W, Rosenfeld B, Roth A, *et al.* The Memorial Delirium Assessment scale. *J Pain Symptom Manage* 1997; **13(3):** 128–37.

● 20. Cherny N. Cancer pain: principles of assessment and syndromes. In: Berger A, Portenoy RK, Weissman DE eds. *Principles and Practice of Supportive Oncology.* Philadelphia, PA: Lippincott-Raven, 1998: 3–42.

21. Portenoy RK. The physical examination in cancer pain assessment. *Semin Oncol Nursing* 1997; **13(1):** 25–9.

22. Sloan PA, Donnelly MB, Schwartz RW. Cancer pain assessment and management by housestaff. *Pain* 1996; **67:** 475–81.

23. Grossman SA. Assessment of cancer pain: a continuous challenge. *Supportive Care Cancer* 1994; **2:** 105–10.

24. Grossman SA, Sheidler VR, Swedeen K, *et al.* Correlation of patient and caregiver ratings of cancer pain. *J Pain Symptom Manage* 1991; **6:** 53–7.

◆ 25. Bruera E, Kuehn N, Miller MJ, *et al.* The Edmonton symptom assessment system (ESAS): a simple method for the assessment of palliative care patients. *J Palliative Care* 1991; **7(2):** 6–9.

◆ 26. Cleeland CS, Ryan KM. Pain assessment: global use of the Brief Pain Inventory. *Ann Acad Med* 1994; **23(2):** 129–38.

◆ 27. Melzack R. The short-form McGill pain questionnaire. *Pain* 1987; **30:** 191–7.

28. Fishman B, Pasternak S, Wallenstein SL, *et al.* The memorial pain assessment card: a valid instrument for the evaluation of cancer pain. *Cancer* 1987; **60:** 11514–18.

●◆ 29. McGrath PA. Pain control. In: Doyle D, Hanks GWC, MacDonald N eds. *Oxford Textbook of Palliative Medicine,* 2nd edn. Oxford: Oxford University Press, 1998; 1013–31.

30. Caraceni A, Mendoza TR, Mencaglia E, *et al.* A validation study of an Italian version of the Brief Pain Inventory (Breve Questionario per al Valutazione del Dolore). *Pain* 1996; **65:** 87–92.

31. Graham C, Bond SS, Gerkovich MM, Cook MR. Use of the McGill Pain Questionnaire in the assessment of cancer pain: replicability and consistency. *Pain* 1980; **8:** 377–87.

32. Dudgeon D, Raubertas RF, Rosenthal SN. The short-form McGill Pain Questionnaire in chronic cancer pain. *J Pain Symptom Manage* 1993; **8:** 191–5.

33. Glare P, Virik K. Independent prospective validation of the PaP score in terminally patients referred to a hospital-based palliative medicine consultation service. *J Pain Symptom Manage* 2001; **22:** 891–8.

● 34. Bruera E, MacDonald S. Audi Methods: the Edmonton symptom assessment system. In: Higginson I ed. *Clin Audit in Palliative Care.* Oxford: Radcliffe Medical Press, 1993; 61–77.

● 35. Foley KM. Supportive care and quality of life. In: De Vita VT, Hellman S, Rosenberg SA eds. *Cancer Principles and Practice of Oncology,* 5th edn. Philadelphia, PA: Lippincott-Raven, 1997; 2807–41.

36. Moore RD Bone LR, Geller G, *et al.* Prevalence, detection, and treatment of alcoholism in hospitalized patients. *JAMA* 1989; **261:** 403–7.

37. Baker A, Bowring L, Brignell A, Kafford D. Chronic pain management in cognitively impaired patients: a preliminary research project. *Perspectives* 1996; **20(2):** 4–8.

38. Farrell MJ, Katz B, Helme RD. The impact of dementia on the pain experience. *Pain* 1996; **67:** 7–15.

◆ 39. Fisher-Morris M, Gelletly A. The experience and expression of pain in Alzheimer patients. *Age Aging* 1997; **26:** 497–500.

40. Porter FL, Malhotra KM, Wolf CM, *et al.* Dementia and response to pain in the elderly. *Pain* 1996; **68:** 413–21.

41. Robinson D, Bucci J, Fenn H. Pain assessment in the Alzheimer's patient. *J Am Gerontol Soc* 1995; **43:** 318–19.

42. Bruera E, Fainsinger R, Miller MJ, Kuehn N. The assessment of pain intensity in patients with cognitive failure: a preliminary report. *J Pain Symptom Manage* 1992; **7:** 267–70.

43. Portenoy RK, Foley KM, Inturrisi CE. The nature of opioid responsiveness and its implications for neuropathic pain: new hypothesis derived from studies of opioid infusion. *Pain* 1990; **43:** 273–86.

44. Lamerton R. *Care of the Dying.* New York, NY: Penguin, 1980.

45. Mount B. Medical applications of heroin. *CMAJ* 1979; **120:** 405–7.

46. Twycross R. Opioids. In: Wall P, Melzack R eds. *Textbook of Pain.* Edinburgh: Churchill Livingstone, 1984: 686–701.

47. Banning A, Stugren P, Henriksen H. Treatment outcome in a multidisciplinary cancer pain clinic. *Pain* 1991; **47:** 129–34.

48. Bruera E, Brenneis C, Michaud M, MacDonald RN. Influence of the pain and symptom control team (PSCT) on the patterns of treatment of pain and other symptoms in a cancer center. *J Pain Symptom Manage* 1989; **4:** 112–16.

◆ 49. Coyle N, Adelhart J, Foley KM, Portenoy RK. Character of terminal illness in the advanced cancer patient: pain and other symptoms during the last four weeks of life. *J Pain Symptom Manage* 1990; **5:** 83–93.

◆ 50. Grond S, Zech D, Schug SA, *et al.* Validation of World Health Organization guidelines for cancer pain relief during the last days and hours of life. *J Pain Symptom Manage* 1991; **6:** 411–22.

51. American Joint Committee for Cancer Staging and End Result Reporting. *Manual of Staging of Cancer.* Chicago, IL: American Joint Committee for Cancer Staging and End Result Reporting.

52. Paterson AHG. Clinical staging and its prognostic significance. In: Stall B ed. *Pointers to Cancer Prognosis.* Dordrecht: Nijhoff, 1988: 37–48.

● 53. Higginson I. Audit methods: validation and in-patient use. In: Higginson I ed. *Clinical Audit in Palliative Care.* Oxford: Radcliffe Medical Press, 1993: 48–54.

5

Psychological evaluation of patient and family

BARBARA MONROE

The individual's experience of pain is a multidimensional phenomenon with physiological, sensory, behavioral, cognitive, and affective components and therefore demands a multidimensional assessment. To acknowledge the role of psychological factors in pain in no way denies the physical component and the need to treat. It is, however, increasingly recognized that physical modalities alone may not be sufficient to help those who fear the meaning of pain and feel a sense of decreased control over their lives. Gamsa's[1] thorough review of the psychological factors in chronic pain concludes that: "systematic studies show that anxiety and depression contribute to pain, that certain personality disorders and cognitive styles are associated with chronic pain and that in some cases pain is maintained by psychological rewards." There is evidence that psychological approaches have added useful interventions to physical treatments in multidisciplinary pain clinics[2] and in oncology and palliative care settings.[3] Psychological distress is key in the patient's experience of cancer.[4–6] It interacts with physical distress and perhaps survival.[7,8] It is influenced by perceptions of family and social support, attributions of meaning and hope, and the perceived degree of personal control.

An acknowledgement of the links between psychological state and pain should not be used to manage the frustrations of health care providers at the failure of pharmacological efforts by shifting the "blame" to the patient with an alternative diagnosis that attributes pain to psychological causes. It is clear, however, that attention to the emotional and psychological distress that forms part of the cancer experience for patients and those close to them can diminish suffering, improve quality of life, and prevent problems in bereavement. It is also important that health care professionals can distinguish between normal reactions of adjustment to a life-threatening illness and symptoms of clinical psychiatric disorders that are amenable to treatment.

WHAT IS SPECIAL ABOUT CANCER PAIN?

Public attitudes to cancer pain are important.[9] There is a widespread understanding that cancer is potentially fatal and inevitably painful alongside an expectation that any pain may be untreatable. There is evidence that the belief that pain signifies disease progression is associated with elevated pain intensity.[10,11] The process by which pain is appraised and interpreted is likely to be a function of psychological as well as physical factors. Turk *et al.*[12] conclude that the variability in the occurrence of pain in patients with metastases as well as across cancer diagnoses seems to suggest that disease progression is only one of the factors accounting for the pain experienced by cancer patients. Beliefs, meaning, expectations, and mood will play an important role in modulating the pain experience of cancer patients. In Barkwell's[13] study, patients with cancer were divided into three groups according to the meaning they attributed to their disease: challenge, punishment, enemy. Those who saw their illness as a punishment experienced more pain and depression. Another study demonstrated a link between high levels of hope and high levels of coping.[14] Evidence suggests that patients who believe they can control their pain, avoid catastrophizing about their condition, and believe they are not severely disabled appear to function better than those who do not.[15]

In general, it is clear that social support is a key factor in maintaining coping and promoting adaptation in the cancer patient. Higher mortality rates have been recorded for cancer patients in the first year after the loss of a spouse, and it was noted that those who were married survived longer than single patients.[16,17] There is substantial evidence for links between patient and family functioning. Patients with high pain scores tend to express more anxiety about the future of their families,[18] and in turn there is concordance between levels of anxiety in family and patient.[19] There are also links between family depression and patient disability and symptoms.[20] A 2-year follow-up of over 600 newly diagnosed cancer patients found a strong relationship between the number and severity of unresolved concerns in the patients and the later development of anxiety disorder and depressive illness.[21] Another study found that the majority of cancer patients express most concern about their family's future and their own loss of independence, the number of concerns being clearly related to the degree of their psychological distress.[22] This is in contrast to an earlier study of hospice patients in which pain and symptom control were found to be the most important concern,[23] a difference that might be partly explained by deficits in communication skills. Evidence showed that hospice patients had a strong bias to selectively disclose physical symptoms and that nurses did not elicit or register patients' concerns accurately.[24] Unsatisfactory pain relief has also been correlated with relatives who had limited information about the death and found it hard to discuss the issues with clinical staff.[25] There are suggestions that longer illness duration is related to lessened mood disturbance and that a rapid course of terminal illness may lead to diminished well-being.[26] When pain in dying persons is lessened, their ability to adapt psychologically is increased. This cluster of results clearly highlights the necessity to assess patients' social and familial networks and any concerns they may have about them. It also emphasizes that, as the quality of life of patients and families is intertwined, it is evident that patient and family should be treated as the unit of care.

All of the studies confirm that pain is a complex phenomenon and that helping people with cancer pain needs much more than skilled drug prescribing.[27] Good pain control will take into account the society and culture of the patient, will seek to understand the psychological processes of the individual in coping with stress, and will provide excellent communication and support where appropriate to patient and family. It is important to remember that with appropriate pain and symptom interventions and good social support, some dying people score levels of self-esteem and well-being similar to those of healthy populations.[28]

COPING AND ADAPTATION

A diagnosis of cancer brings huge losses, both actual and potential, not only for the individual with cancer, but also for those close to him or her: loss of physical health, body image, independence, career and status, normal family life, predictability, self-esteem, motivation, meaning, and sometimes interpersonal relationships. Most profoundly, patients will experience a draining diminution in their self-confidence and their ability to control their own lives.[29] Saunders[30] created the concept of total pain (social, emotional, physical, spiritual) to describe the experience of suffering. It is usefully extended in the World Health Organization (WHO) components of pain diagram (Fig. 5.1).

The individual exists in a context in which body, mind, and spirit combine with family and broader relationship networks, community, and society. This framework is helpfully encapsulated in Fig. 5.2.

Lazarus and Folkman[33] defined coping as individuals' efforts to manage demands that are perceived as likely to exceed their resources. Behaviors are usually aimed at problem-solving by altering the relationship between the person and his or her environment, changing the perception of events, or changing the environment itself. Denial, anger, avoidance, regression, rationalization, intellectualization, and attachment are all common coping mechanisms. Whether a coping strategy is determined to be helpful or unhelpful is often a question of viewpoint.[34] No one way of coping is inherently more desirable; the important issue is whether it is effective for patients and not damaging to those close to them. Weisman[35] suggests that adaptive coping involves confronting problems, revising plans, keeping communication open, a willingness to use the assistance of others, and the ability to maintain an appropriate sense of optimism and hope. The ability to cope successfully with any crisis depends on having various kinds of resources, for example personal, social, medical, and financial. The extent and availability of such resources will influence adaptation. Variables such as social class, socioeconomic status, culture and ethnicity, age, gender, phase and nature of illness, and the behavior of health care providers will also influence the availability and choice of coping mechanisms and styles.[36]

ASSESSMENT

The National Council for Hospice and Specialist Palliative Care Services[37] provides a helpful definition of psychosocial care, stating that it is "concerned with the psychological and emotional wellbeing of the patient and their family/carers, including issues of self esteem, insight into, and adaptation to the illness and its consequences, communication, social functioning and relationships." The objective of the psychological assessment is to maximize

Cancer
Noncancer pathology
Side-effects of therapy
Symptoms of debility
Chronic fatigue
Physical source
Loss of social position
Loss of job, income
Role in family
Helplessness
Disfigurement/body image
Insomnia
Depression
Total pain
Anger
Bureaucratic bungles
Friends – let down
Delays in diagnosis
Unavailable doctors
Therapeutic failure
Anxiety
Fear of pain
Fear of hospital
Loss of dignity
Loss of control
Loss of bodily function
Uncertainty – future
Worry about family
Guilt and sadness
Spiritual unrest
Fear of death

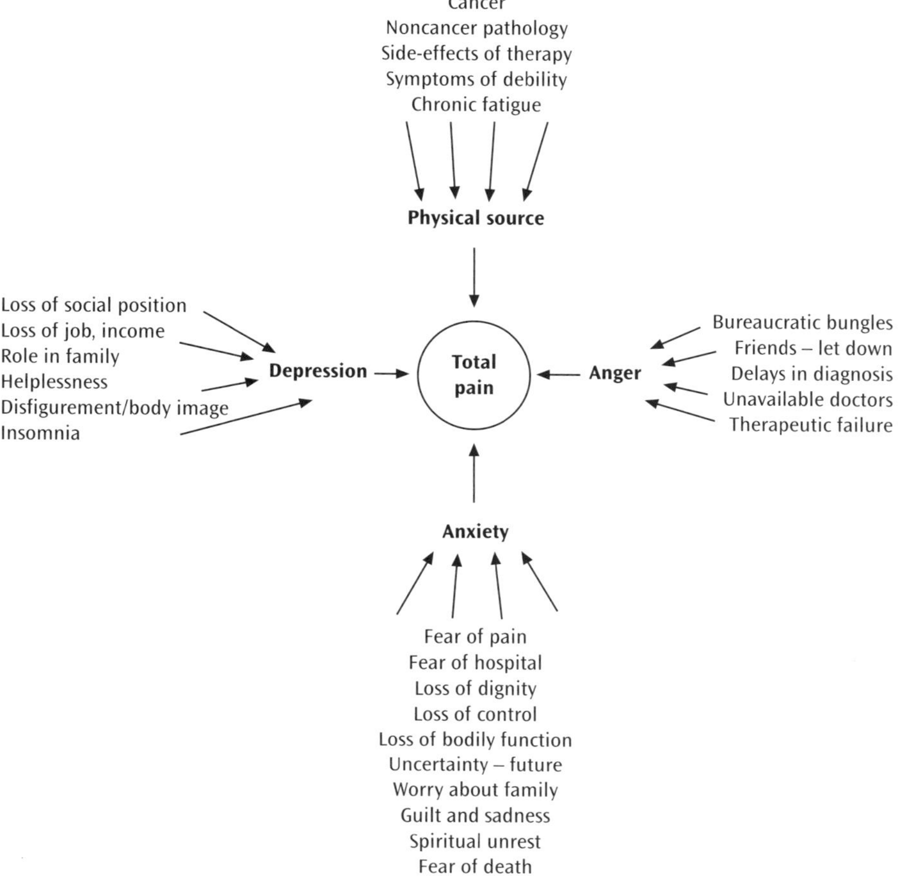

Figure 5.1 *Components of pain (after WHO[31]).*

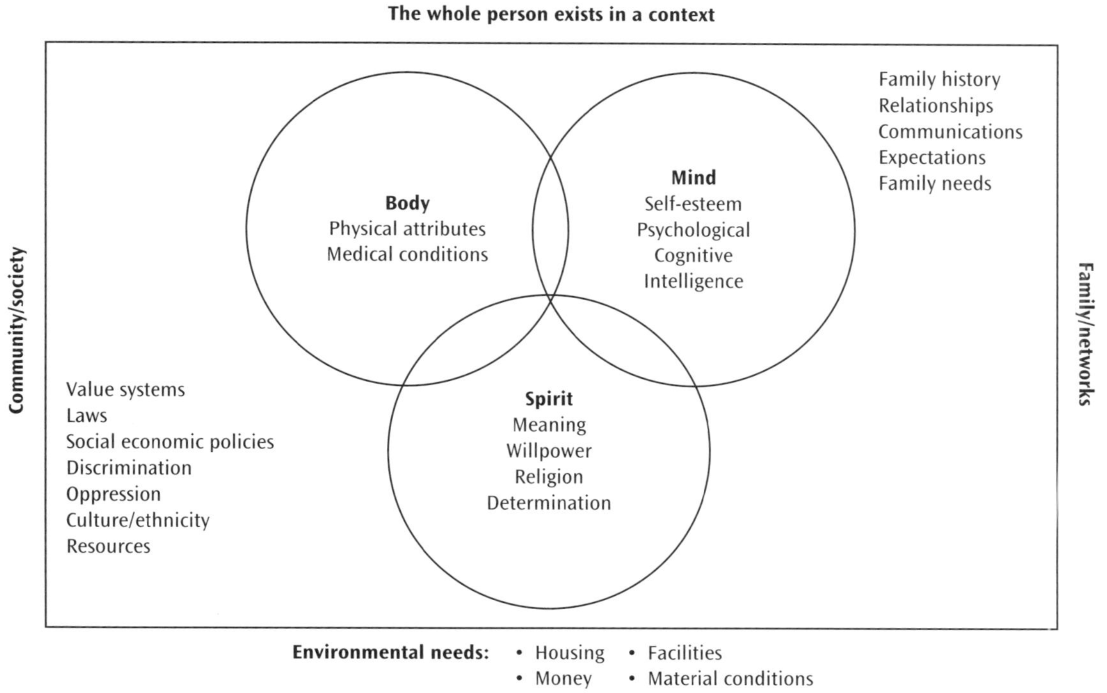

The whole person exists in a context
Family history
Relationships
Communications
Expectations
Family needs
Body
Physical attributes
Medical conditions
Mind
Self-esteem
Psychological
Cognitive
Intelligence
Community/society
Family/networks
Value systems
Laws
Social economic policies
Discrimination
Oppression
Culture/ethnicity
Resources
Spirit
Meaning
Willpower
Religion
Determination
Environmental needs:
• Housing
• Facilities
• Money
• Material conditions

Figure 5.2 *Framework for holistic assessment (from Oliviere* et al.*[38] with permission).*

effective intervention, which will be aimed at reducing the impact of existing losses, preventing further losses, promoting coping, and providing a sense of control and engagement in the decision-making process. Options will be maximized if individuals are given an adequate flow of information at the pace of their choosing and an opportunity to express and, where possible, share their feelings and help to preserve relationships.[38] Assessment is not a one-off process.[32] Assessments should be made early and often. People change their minds and circumstances alter. It is often part of an indistinguishable cycle with intervention; indeed, the assessment process itself will often be therapeutic. The aim is to create a partnership between the patient and those close to him or her and the health care team.

Randall and Downie[39] have emphasized the moral and ethical issues evident in questioning individuals and those close to them about personal and sensitive information. It is important to agree with the ill person and the family the reason for enquiries, to obtain consent, and to check on it at regular intervals: "Please let me know if there is something I ask that you would rather not discuss." Patients should always be asked if they would like to be seen alone or with someone else and, if so, with whom. It is also important to discuss confidentiality and with whom information may be shared, both within the patient's family and friendship network and within the professional team. Good professional recording and communication are vital if effective care is to be achieved and duplication of enquiry avoided. The use of genograms and ecomaps can assist health care professionals to record information in a clear, easily updated manner that leaves the patient in control of the material disclosed.[38,40] Such pictorial mapping generates additional information about roles, patterns of communication, and losses and gaps in care.[41,42]

Assessments may be informal or follow predetermined formats, including the use of questionnaires such as the Hospital Anxiety and Depression Scale. It may be helpful to think of psychological risk assessment divided into

- predisposing factors, such as previous unresolved losses;
- perpetuating factors, such as long-standing marital difficulties;
- psychodynamic factors, such as family disruption caused by shifting roles.[43]

Whatever the format, assessments will contain four main perspectives: the individual, the family and those close to the individual, physical resources, and social resources.[44]

The individual

A psychosocial assessment aims to discover what changes the patient thinks the illness has brought, who or what currently provides support, any gaps in the support network, and the patient's reaction to the illness and its implications for his or her values, beliefs, and aims.

Helpful questions include: What worries you most about your illness? What is helping most at the moment? What has kept you going at other difficult times? Has being ill made any difference to what you believe in? What is the worst thing at the moment? Is there anyone you are especially worried about?

Family, friends, and carers

An assessment will cover:

- the effect of the illness on family roles and relationships;
- personal histories of family members and any likely impact on caring capacity;
- life cycle issues for the family, e.g. births, children leaving home, retirement;
- previous crises and how they were handled and additional concurrent crises, e.g. job loss;
- the presence of other vulnerable individuals in the family, e.g. someone with learning difficulties, a dependent elderly relative.

Physical resources

Assumptions must not be made about the physical resources available to individuals. Housing, money, employment, and unmet physical needs, such as the lack of a commode, can become the most important concerns of the patient or family. They will often not be disclosed unless specifically enquired about by the professional as patients may assume that they are not appropriate subject matter. Patients threatened with eviction for rent arrears because they can no longer work will find it difficult to approach symptom control and treatment compliance in a straightforward way. The prompt provision of a telephone for a patient who lives alone may more helpful in reducing anxiety than any psychological intervention.

Social resources

The patient and family must be set within a context of their community and social network, which may include:

- informal and formal caring resources, e.g. neighbors, churches, social and health care agencies;
- culture and ethnicity – there may be specific requirements or difficulties based on religious or cultural expectations;[45,46]
- potential discrimination – some groups in society are less able than others to voice their needs, e.g. the very poor, the profoundly deaf, the poorly educated.

All of the above will be set within the laws and value systems of the particular society.

THE IMPORTANCE OF EFFECTIVE COMMUNICATION SKILLS

Effective assessments and intervention depend on effective communication. Respect and a nonjudgmental attitude are the key to establishing trust. Patients are clear about what they want from health care professionals: respect, approachability, to be listened to, an unhurried attitude, prompt appointments, repeated explanations of treatments and their side-effects, continuity of care, honesty, referrals to other specialists, and sensitivity to psychological issues.[47] Despite Randall and Downie's[39] rather sanguine view of communication skills in health care professionals – "Genuine professional concern for the patient's welfare will naturally lead to effective communication" – numerous studies have demonstrated deficits in their assessment and communication skills.[48–50] Effective communication is a repeated process that returns control to the patient and helps the family to regain confidence.[51] Unhelpful communication can imply that the truth is too dangerous to share or confronts people with a truth for which they are unprepared or which they are unwilling to receive. Information should be offered in a variety of forms (verbal, written, taped) and interpreters provided where appropriate.[52] It must always be remembered that patients have the right not to know information.

Attention to the beginning and ending of meetings can increase the efficacy of assessment and intervention. It is important, for example, to consider who should attend – patient, family, friends, relevant professionals – and to make proper introductions. On closure there should be a time warning and a "catchall." "We've got about five minutes left, is there anything else that's important for you to mention?" Decisions and agreements should be clearly summarized and the time and date of the next meeting confirmed.

THE IMPORTANCE OF THE FAMILY

Family and friends are important as informal carers for patients with cancer. Increasing numbers of patients are receiving the majority of their care at home. Regarded as a resource to the patient and as potential co-workers with the professional team, it is important that friends and family are supported if they are to continue with their task. Furthermore, depression and anxiety in the family are linked to patient difficulties. The burden of caring has been described in many studies, and there are reports of increased risk of physical and psychological morbidity among carers.[53,54] Caregivers face conflicting demands and conflicting advice; they often have to put their own lives on hold.[55]

A study that examined the concerns of informal carers during the palliative care phase found that 84% reported above normal levels of psychological distress and 41% experienced high levels of strain related to caregiving.[56] Life restrictions, emotional distress, and limited support were among the reported causes of strain. Unmet practical needs are also cited as a source of stress in many studies, along with the failure of health care professionals to meet carers' learning needs adequately.[57,58] It is also clear that, if their educational needs about patient care remain unmet, family members can become a barrier to effective symptom management rather than means of supporting patient compliance.[59]

The family and those close to the patient may also be viewed as co-clients.[60] Care for the family has an important preventive health component as family members will live on into a future shaped in part by their experience of the patient's illness and perhaps death. As Parkes[61] memorably reminds us, "Cancer can affect a family in much the same way as it invades the body, causing it to deteriorate if left untreated." The family is a complex system that changes over time. It has a past and a future that exert pressures on the present. Patients will also belong to other networks of relationships, some of which may be more significant than those with biological links. Unless a clear assessment is undertaken, help for the family can get lost in anxiety for the patient. Family life deteriorates along with the patient, but patient and family members will have different needs at different times. Family members may require different types of support and sometimes have conflicting agendas. Internal and external cultural expectations about the roles, rights, and responsibilities of individual family members will also have an impact.[62] Changes in family structure, e.g. divorce, separation, step-families, geographic distance, which are increasingly common, may add to the burden of informal carers. The literature[63–65] is clear about their needs:

- Adequate nursing support and confident, committed family doctors providing coordinated care.
- Access to specialist care where appropriate.
- The assurance that good symptom control is being given to the patient.
- Knowledge of available support and advocacy to obtain it in time; including practical help with household tasks, personal care and equipment and financial support where necessary.
- Access, where appropriate, to respite care, either as an inpatient or as a home sitting service. Many will be struggling with rapid and frightening changes in the physical needs and capacities of the ill person and the consequent physical caring tasks.
- Knowledge about the illness and training in skills to enhance patient comfort.
- Emotional support directed specifically at the carer.

Ideally, individual time for an assessment and response to carers' needs should be negotiated at the start of the relationship between the professional and patient and family so that it is accepted as a normal part of the contract. If separate meetings are offered only when difficulties arise, they may cause suspicion and guilt.

There are no formal models to predict family psychological status during a cancer trajectory, and relatively little information has been published regarding the psychological state of families of a terminally ill patient, although Kristjanson[66] has produced a useful review. Most studies have examined morbidity after bereavement,[67] although in an important study of families affected by cancer Kissane *et al.*[68] demonstrated a relationship between family functioning during the illness and adaptive grief outcome. The study found spouses' perception of overall family coping as being poor to be correlated with greater grief intensity and depression and poorer social adjustment. Family coping that was perceived as adaptive was linked with a good outcome. This research indicates both the need for an assessment of family functioning as part of good clinical care in order to identify families at risk and the importance of collaborative partnership. What counts is individuals' own view of whether or not they are coping as a family. Professionals must therefore find out from the family how they view themselves and their difficulties.

Significant factors which seem to predispose a family to emotional risk include:[69]

- recent diagnosis of advanced illness;
- anger about delays in diagnosis or treatment;
- close dependent relationship with the ill person;
- other dependants in the family, e.g. children, elderly parents;
- carer isolated with little perceived support;
- carer unable to be realistic about the patient's prognosis;
- previous or current mental health problems or previous losses, especially if recent;
- evidence of dependency on drugs or alcohol;
- practical difficulties such as housing or finance;
- estranged family members or significant conflict within the family;
- history of abuse or trauma.

FAMILY ASSESSMENT – PRACTICAL STEPS

A family assessment should include the following steps:

- Find out how everyone defines the problem, but be neutral. Every individual will need to feel that the professional understands their point of view.
- Consider the impact of the illness on roles and tasks and any care gaps.
- Does the illness challenge the belief structure of the family? Has it brought unfinished business to the fore?
- Anticipate and acknowledge differences and conflicts of need. "You are both feeling lonely and resentful. You want to help your mother but you are worried about giving up your job. You would like to go home to your daughter but you are anxious about the burden this might place on her."
- Help people negotiate and compromise, which often means assisting them to find a dignified way to retreat from fixed positions.
- Facilitate the sharing of emotional pain and anxiety. Generalization may help. "Many families tell us … What is it like for you?"
- Be realistic and encourage a focus on concrete and achievable goals.
- Recognize and respect family coping mechanisms.
- Outline clearly the resources available to the family and find out which they would like to use. Do not coerce them.

CHILDREN

Many research studies have made clear the cost of inadequate support and involvement for children facing serious illness in someone close to them.[70–73] Children may respond with emotional and behavioral disturbance at the time, throughout childhood, and on into adulthood. When the likely outcome of the illness is death, studies confirm the importance of children's pre-death experiences in mediating and influencing the course and outcome of bereavement.[74] Significant factors include the openness of communication in the family, the relationship of the child with the ill person, the availability of community support, and the extent to which the child's parenting needs have continued to be met. When someone in the family is very ill everyone is affected, including children. However, adults' desires to protect children often leave children confused and alone with their fears and fantasies, which may be much worse than the reality. Children are always aware when something significant is happening in the family; they overhear conversations, are aware of body language and practical changes, and often pick up adult gossip from school friends. They also sense adult anxiety. However, they do not always ask unprompted questions, sometimes keeping their worries to themselves out of a desire to protect the adults and family life.

Children need:

- respect and acknowledgement;
- information that is clear, simple, truthful, and repeated about what is happening and why and what might happen next;
- reassurance about practical issues and about their own care;

- reassurance that nothing they did or said made the illness happen;
- a chance to talk about feelings with adults who are prepared to share theirs;
- appropriate involvement in helping the patient.

Parents have good reasons for feeling anxious about talking to their children, and these are often shared by professionals. They are often struggling to maintain their own control in the midst of uncertainty and strong emotion. They may underestimate what a child understands or worry that saying the wrong thing may make matters worse. It is often important to support parents with their own emotional needs before they can contemplate addressing those of their children. The aim should always be to help parents to talk to their own children themselves, to give them the confidence and skills to begin to assess and meet their own children's needs.

Helping parents to talk to children[75]

The following guidance should be given to parents:

- Acknowledge that it will feel uncomfortable and distressing.
- Reassure them that information does not need to be given all at one time, but step by step, using age-appropriate vocabulary and not being afraid to say "I don't know." Offer suggestions about possible explanations.
- Warn parents not to be surprised if children change the subject or focus on the practical. "What's for tea?"
- Help them to understand and respond to their children's emotions and sometimes changed behavior. For example, children may be angry at having their routines upset. They may become more clingy or more naughty.
- Help parents to involve other people in their child's network: friends, relatives, teachers.
- Offer parents resources such as booklets to read themselves and books to read with their children.

Parents need to think about:

- What their children know already. It often helps to start with children's own observations so that any misapprehensions can be corrected. For example, "What have you noticed that's different about mummy? Why do you think mummy is ill?"
- What they want their children to know, e.g. what the doctors have said, what the treatment is, and what the side-effects might be.
- What the children want to know, remembering that they may not ask, e.g. "Is it my fault? Is cancer catching? Will daddy die?"
- Always work with what seems manageable and comfortable to parents themselves. There is no one right way, only the way that is right for them and their family.

SEXUALITY AND INTIMACY

Studies have documented the importance of sexuality as a quality of life issue for patients and their partners.[76] There is a large body of evidence confirming that sexual behaviors, self concepts, and relationships are deeply affected in many adults with life-threatening disease.[77] Studies also confirm the efficacy of sexual counseling programs[78] alongside a conviction among health care professionals that sexuality is an integral part of their responsibility toward patients and those close to them.[79,80] Yet research also demonstrates that professionals seldom address the issue.[81,82] There remains a gap between theory and practice. It is clearly inappropriate to expect every health care professional to be a specialist in sexual counseling. However, the responsibility for making an assessment of whether or not this is an important area for the individual belongs to all.[83]

Potential sexual problems relating to illness fall into two linked categories: mechanical problems that are the direct physical consequences of illness or treatment and the emotional consequences of the illness, including changes in the way people feel about themselves and each other and their body image. Professionals need to be able to initiate dialog and discussion, to identify and assess need, and to offer first-line help with the offer of referral on for specialist support if appropriate. It is important to avoid assumptions, for example that sex is less important to older people or to someone not currently in a relationship. Individuals and those close to them need time to come to terms with their illness and its implications. Anticipation and honest discussion can reduce anxiety, so information should be given in advance, wherever possible in both verbal and written form.

Most people will not ask for help spontaneously. Learning to ask is the professional's responsibility.

Taking a sexual history

The following approach may be helpful:

- See people separately and together.
- Use questions that move from the general to the specific. "How has your illness/treatment affected your work/home/sex life?"
- Use questions that give permission. "Do you have any worries about the sexual side of things?"
- Use phrasing that implies that most people experience these kinds of doubts. "People often have questions they'd like to ask about the sexual side of life."
- Find an appropriate and understandable vocabulary for the individual.
- "In what ways has your illness changed the way you feel about yourself as a man/woman/partner?"
- "How long have you been together? Has the physical

side of your relationship been important to you/your partner?"

- "In what ways has your illness changed the way you can get close to your partner?"
- "What do you want most from your partner at the moment? What do you think your partner's reaction would be?"

Professionals should always be alert to the possibility of violent or abusive relationships.

ASSESSMENT AND COPING MECHANISMS

Denial

Some patients or those close to them may deny the diagnosis or the implications of the disease. Denial is a phase of the coping process that revises or reinterprets a portion of a painful reality. Professionals should tackle denial carefully and consider whose problem it is. People are only at risk when their denial of their symptoms or issues around their illness is so persistent that it jeopardizes aspects of their physical well-being and ultimate prognosis, or the well-being of those close to them.[34]

Questions to ask include:

- Is denial affecting help-seeking behavior and compliance?
- Is denial reducing emotional distress?
- Is denial leaving the patient in immediate, persistent, or extreme anxiety?
- Is the denial temporary or persistent? Many people move in and out of denial.
- Has the information about the diagnosis or treatment been given in way that is clearly understandable?
- Have any underlying major psychiatric disorders or organic mental disorders been excluded?

"What if?" questions may help those in denial as they allow the maintenance of some distance from the painful truth. "Imagine for a moment that you weren't around to look after your children. In those circumstances who would you want to be involved?" Other approaches might include image work, art or music therapy, or very gentle probing. "I know you like to look on the bright side of things but are there ever moments when you find yourself thinking less positive thoughts?"

Anger

Extreme anger can make it hard to assess what is important for the patient or what might be potentially helpful interventions. Strategies to manage anger include:[84]

- Remember that anger is an energy that can be positively harnessed.
- Invite people to sit down in a quiet place. Speak calmly. "Can you explain to me why you are feeling like this?"
- Avoid becoming defensive or patronizing.
- Acknowledge the anger, legitimizing it where appropriate. Be honest if a mistake has been made.
- Recognize the feelings that may be underneath anger: loneliness, fear, a sense of injustice.
- Encourage expression. "Just how angry have you been?"
- Try to suggest a coping strategy, e.g. registering a complaint, talking to a relative.
- Assess the danger to yourself and stop the interview if there is a risk of physical aggression.

RISK ASSESSMENT FOR DEPRESSION, SUICIDE, AND ANXIETY

Depression

Depression is a common symptom among cancer patients, although reports of its prevalence vary enormously.[28,85] There are strong links between poor functional capacity and depression and between depression and chronic pain.[86] Failure to recognize depression can enormously increase physical and psychological suffering for both patients and those close to them. Severe depression can make symptom management more difficult, reduce compliance, and lead to death wishes or a desire for euthanasia. It is important to distinguish between depressed mood, which is often present as part of a natural adjustment reaction, and depressive illness, which is a clinical entity and severely disabling condition that may be potentially life-threatening because of the associated risk of suicide[87] and which benefits from antidepressant therapy and psychological support. It is always important to rule out depression due to a medical condition, e.g. hypercalcemia, hypothyroidism.

A major depressive episode, as widely accepted and encapsulated in the DSM-IV,[88] can be described as the presence of depressed mood or loss of interest or pleasure lasting most of the day, for at least 2 weeks, in the presence of four or more of the following:

- significant loss or increase of appetite/weight;
- psychomotor retardation or agitation almost every day;
- loss of energy or fatigue nearly every day;
- feelings of worthlessness or excessive or inappropriate guilt nearly every day;
- impaired concentration or memory nearly every day;
- recurrent thoughts of death;
- recurrent suicidal ideation.

In the case of patients with severe depression it is important to start drug treatment and then to provide other supportive interventions such as cognitive therapy, relaxation therapy, and personal counseling. One of the difficulties with the quoted criteria is that several of them are somatic in nature and can be confused with the symptoms of cancer itself, such as loss of weight and energy. It is therefore important to consider them within the context of the physical illness. Various writers have suggested distinctive features of depression in cancer patients, such as social withdrawal, complete failure to respond to good news or funny situations, persistent tearfulness, a feeling of being a burden when this is obviously not the case, chronic pain resistant to treatment, and perceiving the illness as a punishment.[89,90]

Health care workers assessing depression should not make assumptions. The patient must be asked directly: "Do you feel depressed?" Several studies have demonstrated that, although medical personnel are good at picking up pain and physical problems, they are much less effective in detecting psychosocial problems.[24] In one study, 58% of patients identified problems not mentioned by professionals, and 52% of these were psychosocial.[91] It therefore follows that a careful history from both patient and close family or friends is essential, including whether the symptoms represent a change from previous functioning. Predisposing factors are:

- a past personal or family history of depressive illness;
- a previous suicide attempt;
- lack of social support;
- recent stressful events;
- alcohol or other substance abuse.

Diagnostic instruments such as the Present State Examination and structured clinical interviews are designed to aid differential diagnosis, but they are time-consuming to administer and require special training. Screening instruments such as the Goldberg Health Questionnaire are also available, but these, too, take time to administer. Another possibility is the use of a self-rating instrument such as the Hospital Anxiety and Depression Scale (HADS). Moorey *et al.*[92] tested the HADS in 560 patients with cancer and concluded that it "seemed to be the best instrument for rapid evaluation of psychological interventions in patients with physical illness." Although the instrument was originally designed to measure severity of anxiety and depression, studies to validate its use as a screening instrument for depression in cancer patients have been carried out.[93] These studies have highlighted some of the drawbacks such as the false-positive and -negative results that emerge with self-screening and the ambiguity of several of the items in patients with poor performance status. General screening questions can play an important role: "How is your morale these days considering what has happened? What can you tell me about how discouraged you ordinarily get?"[34]

Suicide

Cancer patients are at an increased risk of suicide relative to the general population, particularly in the final stage of illness.[94,95] Screening for depressive illness is vital as depression is a factor in 50% of all suicides.[96] Uncontrolled pain is also a very important risk factor.[97,98] Hopelessness is the key variable that links suicide and depression in the general population. In the face of cancer, loss of control and a sense of helplessness are significant factors in suicide vulnerability, as is fatigue.

Evaluation of suicide risk

The following guidelines may be helpful:

- Never be afraid to ask. "How low have you been? Have you ever thought of ending your life? How? When did you think of doing it? What has stopped you?"
- Take threats seriously. Offer appropriate follow-up and avoid prohibiting statements such as "You shouldn't talk like that."
- Recognize despair. This gives people a sense of relief and lets them know they are being taken seriously.
- Check for consistency over time. Some episodes are brief and do not reflect a sustained and committed desire to die.
- Discussing suicide openly can acknowledge the individual's need to retain a sense of control over aspects of his or her death and also allow a fuller discussion about preventable fears and anxieties such as "How will I die? "How might my symptoms be managed?"
- Patients may also need to discuss existential anxieties such as fears of punishment. "What will happen to me after death?"
- Clinicians should also be aware of the danger of the first few weeks on antidepressants, which can lift retardation before improving mood, so that people have the energy to act while remaining very low in spirit.

If suicidal risk is present it is important to refer the patient to a psychiatrist for a professional consultation. However, it is rarely appropriate to refer patients to specialist psychiatric units. According to Breitbart and Krivo[99] "The goal of the intervention should not be to prevent suicide at all costs, but to prevent suicide that is driven by desperation," reminding professionals that the vast majority of cancer patients who express suicidal ideation do so while suffering unrecognized and untreated psychiatric disturbances and poorly controlled physical symptoms, especially pain.

Anxiety

Anxiety is a common response to a fear-provoking diagnosis and an uncertain future. However, if present at a clinical level, it can be disabling and is potentially responsive to an active drug regimen. At any level anxiety can reduce the threshold to physical suffering, especially pain, and make the disclosure and resolution of significant practical and emotional concerns much more difficult.[100] Anxiety and depression often occur together, and both will need to be attended to in many situations with cancer patients.[34,101,102] A clinical anxiety state may include phobic disorders such as claustrophobia, and panic attacks may occur in stressful situations.

Predisposing factors include:

- a past or family history of an anxiety disorder;
- poor social support;
- recent receipt of bad news;
- previous alcohol or substance abuse;
- unstable environment in childhood/early experience of separation;
- overprotection by family or partner;
- previous experience of a distressing death.

A clinical anxiety state is often indicated when the patient reports feeling extremely apprehensive or tense and sometimes tormented and unable to make decisions. It is dominating and intrusive in quality and will often be self-described as significantly different from normal mood. This mood will have persisted for more than 2 weeks for more than 50% of the time. It will be accompanied by the presence of other anxiety-related symptoms, which can be considered to fall into in four categories:

1 psychological apprehension: feelings of dread, threat, fear, worries over trivia, irritability;
2 somatic and autonomic: tremor, diarrhea, sweating, nausea;
3 vigilance and scanning: poor concentration, insomnia, fatigue on waking, distractability;
4 motor tension and behavioral symptoms: shakiness, trembling, muscle aches, fatigue, restlessness, angry outbursts, demands for attention, clinging.

It is always important to exclude organic causes such as endocrine and metabolic disorders, alcohol withdrawal, chronic dementing illness, acute confusional state, and drug-induced motor restlessness.

Upon diagnosis of a clinical anxiety state, appropriate pharmacology is essential, with psychotherapeutic support such as cognitive–behavioral therapy, aromatherapy, and relaxation techniques, as well as general emotional support for patient and family.

CONCLUSION

Psychological distress is key in the patient and family's experience of cancer and interacts with physical distress. Good pain relief is multidimensional and demands a careful, multifaceted, often multiprofessional, approach that does not need to be hugely sophisticated but knows when to call in specialists. The husband of a woman who died of breast cancer declared that in his opinion: "The great deficits in cancer care lie in communication and the psychological care of patient and family."[103] Skills in psychological evaluation are vital if these deficits are to be remedied. Excellent pharmacology, appropriate information, and emotional support are equally important in our efforts to help those with cancer.

REFERENCES

● 1. Gamsa A. The role of psychological factors in chronic pain. II. A critical appraisal. *Pain* 1994; **57:** 17–29.

● 2. Flor H, Fydrich T, Turk DC. Efficacy of multidisciplinary pain treatment centres: a meta-analytic review. *Pain* 1992; **49:** 221–30.

◆ 3. Fallowfield L. Psychosocial interventions in cancer. *Br Med J* 1995; **311:** 1316–17.

● 4. Fawzy FI, Fawzy NW, Arndt LA, Pasnau RO. Critical review of psychosocial interventions in cancer care. *Archiv Gen Psychiatry* 1995; **52:** 100–13.

5. Fawzy FI, Fawzy NW, Canada AL. Psychosocial treatment of cancer: an update. *Curr Opin Psychiatry* 1998; **52:** 601–5.

◆ 6. Vachon M, Kristjanson L, Higginson I. Psychosocial issues in palliative care: the patient, the family and the process and outcome of care. *J Pain Symptom Manage* 1995; **10:** 142–50.

7. Spiegel D, Bloom J, Kraemer HC, Gotheil E. Effect of psychosocial treatment on survival of patients with metastatic cancer. *Lancet* 1989; **2:** 888–91.

8. Fawzy FI, Fawzy NW, Hyun CS, *et al.* Effects of an early structured psychiatric intervention. *Archiv Gen Psychiatry* 1993; **50:** 681–9.

9. Levin DN, Cleeland CS, Dar R. Public attitudes toward cancer pain. *Cancer* 1985; **56:** 2337–9.

10. Daut RL, Cleeland CS. The prevalence and severity of pain in cancer. *Cancer* 1982; **50:** 1913–18.

11. Spiegel D, Bloom JR. Pain in metastatic breast cancer. *Cancer* 1983; **52:** 341–5.

12. Turk DC, Sist TC, Okifuji A, *et al.* Adaptation to metastatic cancer pain, regional/local cancer pain and noncancer pain: role of psychological and behavioural factors. *Pain* 1998; **74:** 247–56.

13. Barkwell DP. Ascribed meaning: a critical factor in coping and pain attenuation in patients with cancer-related pain. *J Palliative Care* 1991; **7:** 5–14.

◆ 14. Herth K. Fostering hope in terminally-ill people. *J Advanced Nursing* 1990; **15:** 1250–9.

● 15. Jensen MP, Turner JA, Romano JM, Karoly P. Coping with chronic pain: a critical review of the literature. *Pain* 1991; **47:** 249–83.

16. Goodwin JS, Hunt WC, Key CR, Samet JM. The effect of marital status on stage, treatment and survival of cancer patients. *JAMA* 1987; **258:** 3125–30.

◆ 17. Redd WH, Silberfarb PM, Andersen BL. Physiologic and psychobehavioural research in oncology. *Cancer* 1991; **67** (Suppl.): 813–22.

18. Strang P. Existential consequences of unrelieved cancer pain. *Palliative Med* 1997; **11:** 299–305.

19. Hodgson C, Higginson I, McDonnell M, Butters E. Family anxiety in advanced cancer: a multicentre prospective study in Ireland. *Br J Cancer* 1997; **76:** 1211–14.

20. Kurtz ME, Kurtz JC, Given CW, Given B. Relationship of caregiver reactions and depression to cancer patients' symptoms, functional states and depression – a longitudinal view. *Social Sci Med* 1995; **40:** 837–46.

21. Parle M, Jones B, Maguire P. Maladaptive coping and affective disorders among cancer patients. *Psychol Med* 1996; **26:** 735–44.

22. Heaven CM, Maguire P. The relationship between patients' concerns and psychological distress in a hospice setting. *Psycho-oncology* 1998; **7:** 502–7.

23. Higginson IJ, McCarthy M. Measuring symptoms in terminal cancer: are pain and dyspnoea controlled? *J Roy Soc Med* 1989; **82:** 264–7.

24. Heaven CM, Maguire P. Disclosure of concerns by hospice patients and their identification by nurses. *Palliative Med* 1997; **11:** 283–90.

25. Miettinen T, Tilvis R, Karppi P, Arve S. Why is the pain relief of dying patients often unsuccessful? The relatives perspectives. *Palliative Med* 1998; **12:** 429–35.

26. Dobratz MC. Analysis of variables that impact psychological adaptation in home hospice patients. *Hospice J* 1995; **10:** 75–88.

27. Davidson P. Facilitating coping with cancer pain. *Palliative Med* 1988; **2:** 107–14.

28. Bukberg J, Penman D, Holland JC. Depression in hospitalised cancer patients. *Psychosomatic Med* 1984; **46:** 199–211.

29. Northouse PG, Northouse LL. Communication and cancer: issues confronting patients, health professionals and family members. *J Psychosoc Oncol* 1987; **5:** 17–46.

30. Saunders C. Introduction – history and challenge. In: Saunders C, Sykes N eds. *The Management of Terminal Malignant Disease,* 3rd edn. London: Edward Arnold, 1993: 1–14.

31. World Health Organization. *Cancer Pain Relief and Palliative Care.* Report of a WHO Expert Committee. WHO Technical Report Series 804. Geneva: World Health Organization, 1990: 21.

32. Lazarus RS, Folkman S. Coping and adaptation. In: Gentry WD ed. *The Handbook of Behavioural Medicine.* New York: Guilford, 1984**:** 282–325.

◆ 33. Vachon M. The emotional problems of the patient. In: Doyle D, Hanks G, MacDonald N eds. *Oxford Textbook of Palliative Medicine*, 2nd edn. Oxford: Oxford University Press, 1998: 883–900.

34. Weisman A. *The Coping Capacity.* New York, NY: Human Sciences Press, 1986.

35. Field D, Hockey J, Small N eds. *Death, Gender and Ethnicity.* London: Routledge, 1997.

36. National Council for Hospice and Specialist Palliative Care Services. *Feeling Better: Psychosocial Care in Specialist Palliative Care.* A discussion paper. Occasional paper 13. London: NCHSPCS, 1997.

37. Monroe B. Psychosocial dimension of palliation. In: Saunders C, Sykes N eds. *The Management of Terminal Malignant Disease,* 3rd edn. London: Edward Arnold, 1993: 174–201.

38. Oliviere D, Hargreaves R, Monroe B. Assessment. In: *Good Practices in Palliative Care: a Psychosocial Perspective.* Aldershot: Ashgate, 1997: 25–48.

39. Randall F, Downie RS. *Palliative Care Ethics. A Companion for all Specialties*, 2nd edn. Oxford: Oxford University Press, 1999.

40. Sheldon F. Mapping the support networks. In: *Psychosocial Palliative Care: Good Practice in the Care of the Dying and Bereaved.* Cheltenham: Stanley Thornes, 1997: 79–80.

41. Kirschling JM ed. *Family Based Palliative Care.* New York, NY: Howarth Press, 1990.

42. McGoldrick M, Gerson R. *Genograms in Family Assessment.* New York, NY: Norton, 1985.

43. Hodgson G. Depression, sadness and anxiety. In: Saunders C, Sykes N eds. *The Management of Terminal Malignant Disease,* 3rd edn. London: Edward Arnold, 1993: 102–30.

◆ 44. Monroe B. Social work in palliative care. In: Doyle D, Hanks G, MacDonald N eds. *Oxford Textbook of Palliative Medicine,* 2nd edn. Oxford: Oxford University Press, 1998: 867–82.

45. Oliviere D. Culture and ethnicity. *Eur J Palliative Care* 1999; **6:** 53–56.

46. Sheldon F. The cultural and spiritual context of death and bereavement. In: *Psychosocial Palliative Care – Good Practice in the Care of the Dying and Bereaved.* Cheltenham: Stanley Thornes, 1997: 17–34.

47. National Cancer Alliance. *Patient-centred Cancer Services? What Patients Say.* Oxford: National Cancer Alliance, 1996.

48. Stedeford A. Couples facing death. II. Unsatisfactory communication. *Br Med J* 1981; **283:** 1098–101.

49. Maguire P. Barriers to psychological care of the dying. *Br Med J* 1985; **291:** 1711–13.

50. Chan A, Woodruff RK. Communicating with patients with advanced cancer. *J Palliative Care* 1997; **13:** 29–33.

◆ 51. Buckman R. Communication in palliative care: a practical guide. In: Doyle D, Hanks G, MacDonald N eds. *Oxford Textbook of Palliative Medicine,* 2nd edn. Oxford: Oxford University Press, 1998: 141–56.

52. Hogbin B, Fallowfield L. Getting it taped – the bad news consultation with cancer patients in a general surgical outpatients department. *Br J Hosp Med* 1989, **41:** 330–3.

● 53. Kinsella G, Cooper B, Picton C. A review of the measurement of caregiver and family burden in palliative care. *J Palliative Care* 1998; **14:** 37–45.

54. Hinton J. Can home care maintain an acceptable quality of life for patients with terminal cancer and their relatives? *Palliative Med* 1994; **8:** 83–96.
55. Hull M. Sources of stress for hospice care-giving families. In: J Kirschling ed. *Family Based Palliative Care.* New York: Howarth, 1990.
56. Payne S, Smith P, Dean S. Identifying the concerns of informal carers in palliative care. *Palliative Med* 1999; **13:** 37–44.
57. Hudson P. The educational needs of lay carers. *Eur J Palliative Care* 1998; **5:** 183–6.
58. Kristjanson L, Leis A, Koop P, *et al.* Family members' care expectations, care perceptions, and satisfaction with advanced cancer care. *J Palliative Care* 1997; **1:** 5–13.
59. Ferrell B. The family. In: Doyle D, Hanks G, MacDonald N eds. *Oxford Textbook of Palliative Medicine,* 2nd edn. Oxford: Oxford University Press, 1998: 909–17.
60. Twigg J. Models of carers: how do social care agencies conceptualise their relationship with informal carers? *J Soc Policy* 1989; **18:** 53–66.
61. Parkes CM. The emotional impact of cancer on patients and their families. *J Oncol Laryngol* 1975; **89:** 1271–9.
62. Die-Trill M. The patient from a different culture. In: Holland JC ed. *Psycho-oncology*. Oxford: Oxford University Press, 1998: 857–66.
63. Sykes N, Pearson S, Chell S. Quality of care: the carer's perspective. *Palliative Med* 1992; **6:** 227–36.
64. Thorpe G. Enabling more dying people to remain at home. *Br Med J* 1993; **307:** 915–18.
65. ● Neale B. *Informal Palliative Care: a Review of Research on Needs, Standards and Service Evaluation*. Occasional Paper No. 3. Sheffield: Trent Palliative Care Centre, 1991.
66. ● Kristjanson LJ. The family's cancer journey: a literature review. *Cancer Nursing* 1994; **17:** 1–17.
67. ● Kissane D, Bloch S. Family grief. *Br J Psychiatry* 1994; **164:** 728–740.
68. ◆ Kissane D, Bloch S, McKenzie D. Family coping and bereavement outcome. *Palliative Med* 1997; **11:** 191–201.
69. Oliviere D, Hargreaves R, Monroe B. Working with families. In: *Good Practices in Palliative Care: a Psychosocial Perspective*. Aldershot: Ashgate, 1998: 54.
70. Black D. Childhood bereavement: distress and long term sequelae can be lessened by early intervention. *Br Med J* 1996; **312:** 1496.
71. Christ GH. *Healing Children's Grief: Surviving a Parent's Death from Cancer*. Oxford: Oxford University Press, 2000.
72. Weller RA, Weller EB, Fristad MA, Bowes BM. Depression in recently bereaved prepubertal children. *Am J Psychiatry* 1991; **148:** 1536–40.
73. Silverman PR. *Never too Young to Know. Death in Children's Lives.* Oxford: Oxford University Press, 2000.
74. ◆ Worden WJ. *Children and Grief. When a Parent Dies*. New York, NY: Guilford Press, 1996.
75. Monroe B. It is impossible not to communicate – helping the grieving family. In: Smith S, Pennells M eds. *Interventions with Bereaved Children.* London: Jessica Kingsley, 1995: 87–106.
76. ◆ Fallowfield L. The quality of life: sexual function and body image following cancer therapy. *Cancer Topics* 1992; **9:** 20–1.
77. Schover LR. Sexual dysfunction. In: Holland JC ed. *Psycho-oncology.* Oxford: Oxford University Press, 1998: 494–9.
78. Capone MA, Good RS, Westie KS, Jacobsen AF. Psychosocial rehabilitation of gynaecologic oncology patients. *Arch Phys Med Rehabil* 1980; **61:** 12–32
79. Jenkins B. Oncology patients' reports of sexual changes after treatment for gynaecological cancer. *Nursing Forum* 1988; **15:** 349–354
80. Gamel C, Davis BD, Hengeveld M. Nurses' provision of teaching and counselling on sexuality: a review of the literature. *J Advanced Nursing* 1993; **18:** 1219–27.
81. Vincent CE, Vincent B, Greiss FC, Linton EB. Some marital concomitants of carcinoma of the cervix. *South Med J* 1975; **68:** 552–8.
82. Wright P. Psychosexual dysfunction in women with gynaecological cancer receiving radiotherapy and their management by healthcare professionals. Unpublished MSc dissertation. University of Southampton, 1996.
83. Monroe B. A sexual-sensitive approach to palliative care. In: Oliviere D, Hargreaves R, Monroe B eds. *Good Practices in Palliative Care: a Psychosocial Perspective.* Aldershot: Ashgate, 1997: 96–111.
84. Faulkner A, Maguire P, Regnard C. The angry person. In: Regnard C,, Hockley J eds. *Flow Diagrams in Advanced Cancer and Other Diseases.* London: Edward Arnold, 1995: 81–5.
85. Lansky SB, List MA, Hermann CA, *et al.* Absence of major depressive disorder in female cancer patients. *J Clin Oncol* 1985; **3:** 1553–60.
86. Foley KM. The treatment of cancer pain. *N Engl J Med* 1985; **313:** 84–95.
87. Brugha TS. Depression in the terminally ill. *Br J Hosp Med* 1993; **50:** 175–81.
88. American Psychiatric Association. *DSM-IV Casebook: a Learning Companion to the Diagnostic and Statistical Manual of the American Psychiatric Association.* Washington, DC: American Psychiatric Association, 1994.
89. Endicott J. Measurement of depression in patients with cancer. *Cancer* 1984; **53** (Suppl.): 2243–9.
90. Casey P. Depression in the dying – disorder or distress? *Prog Palliative Care*1994; **2:** 1–3.
91. Rathbone GV, Horsley S, Goacher J. A self evaluated assessment suitable for seriously ill hospice patients. *Palliative Med* 1994; **8:** 29–34.
92. Moorey S, Greer S, Watson M, *et al.* The factor structure and factor stability of the hospital anxiety and depres-

sion scale in patients with cancer. *Br J Psychiatry* 1991; **158:** 255–9.

93. Robaye E. Screening for adjustment disorders and major depressive disorders in cancer in-patients. *Br J Psychiatry* 1990; **156:** 79–83.
94. Breitbart W. Cancer pain and suicide. In: Foley K, Bonica JJ, Ventafridda V, *et al.* eds. *Advances in Pain Research and Therapy,* vol. 16. New York, NY: Raven Press, 1990: 399–412.
95. Bolund C. Suicide and cancer. *J Psychosocial Oncol* 1985; **3:** 31–52.
96. Fox BH, Stanek EJ, Boyd SC, Flannery JT. Suicide rates among cancer patients in Connecticut. *J Chronic Dis* 1982; **35:** 85–100.
97. Cutler F, Reynolds D. An eight year survey of hospital suicides. *Suicide, Life Threatening Behaviour* 1971; **1:** 184–201.
98. Guze S, Robins E. Suicide and primary affective disorders. *Br J Psychiatry* 1970; **117:** 437–8.
99. Breitbart W, Krivo S. Suicide. In: Holland JC ed. *Psycho-oncology.* Oxford: Oxford University Press, 1998: 541–7.
100. Maguire P, Faulkner A, Regnard C. The anxious person. In: Regnard C, Hockley J eds. *Flow Diagrams in Advanced Cancer and Other Diseases.* London: Edward Arnold, 1995: 73–6.
101. McCartney CF, Cahill P, Larson DB, *et al.* Effect of psychiatric liaison program on consultation rates and on detection of minor psychiatric disorders in cancer patients. *Am J Psychiatry* 1989; **7:** 898–901.
102. Carroll BT, Kathol RG, Noyes R, *et al.* Screening for depression and anxiety in cancer patients using the hospital anxiety and depression scale. *Gen Hosp Psychiatry* 1993; **15:** 69–74.
103. Sinclair S. *Bereavement Services: a Service User's Perspective.* Paper presented at the European Association of Palliative Care Congress. London, September 1997.

6

The role of nursing in pain management

BETTY R FERRELL

Cancer-related pain is multidimensional in that it consists of physiologic, psychologic, social, and spiritual experiences.[1–4] Pain is not restricted to the physical aspect of a person's life, but rather infiltrates every aspect of one's being. The American Pain Society (APS)[5] states that failure to use routine pain assessment and pain relief methods is the most common reason for unrelieved pain. Many patients will not approach the subject of pain unless asked. Patients also frequently underuse medications that have been provided to them. Nurses are in a key position to bridge the gap between possible pain relief and the reality of how pain is generally treated. This chapter reviews nursing roles in providing effective pain management in the areas of eliminating barriers, pain assessment, pharmacological management, nondrug interventions, and education for both patient and family. Also included is discussion of the role of nurses in quality improvement activities in order to improve systems of care.

THE MULTIDIMENSIONAL APPROACH TO NURSING CARE OF CANCER PAIN

Treatment of pain is multidisciplinary, and nurses are recognized as a vital component of the multidisciplinary team. The role of the nurse as a member of the team is also multidimensional. Figure 6.1 illustrates this concept. Nurses work collaboratively with other disciplines to meet the quality of life (QOL) concerns of patients in pain. The QOL of patients in pain includes dimensions of physical, psychological, social, and spiritual well-being. Figure 6.2 provides a more detailed illustration of the aspects of QOL most influenced by pain. Exploring the roles of nursing in contributing to pain relief and QOL may help individual practitioners to examine opportunities to increase their own effectiveness, and may offer institutions a means of evaluating optimum use of nursing pain relief efforts.

ROLES OF NURSING IN CANCER PAIN MANAGEMENT

Elimination of barriers to pain relief

Nurses have played a vital role in eliminating barriers to pain relief. The Agency for Health Care Policy and Research (AHCPR) guidelines for cancer pain management synthesized the literature regarding obstacles to pain relief and provided a succinct table of such barriers.[3] Table 6.1 presents a summary of the barriers, which can be categorized as professional barriers, patient barriers, and system barriers. A tremendous amount of nursing attention has been focused on the category of professional barriers. Although education alone is not sufficient to improve pain relief, most experts have recognized that health care professionals cannot practice what they do not know and that, unfortunately, most professionals are poorly prepared in their formal education programs to assess or to treat pain. Thus, major efforts over the past decade have focused on pain education. It is interesting to note that efforts focused on individuals attending one-off, continuing education programs have now evolved into more formal structures for preparing professionals.[6–10] Several novel educational programs in the USA

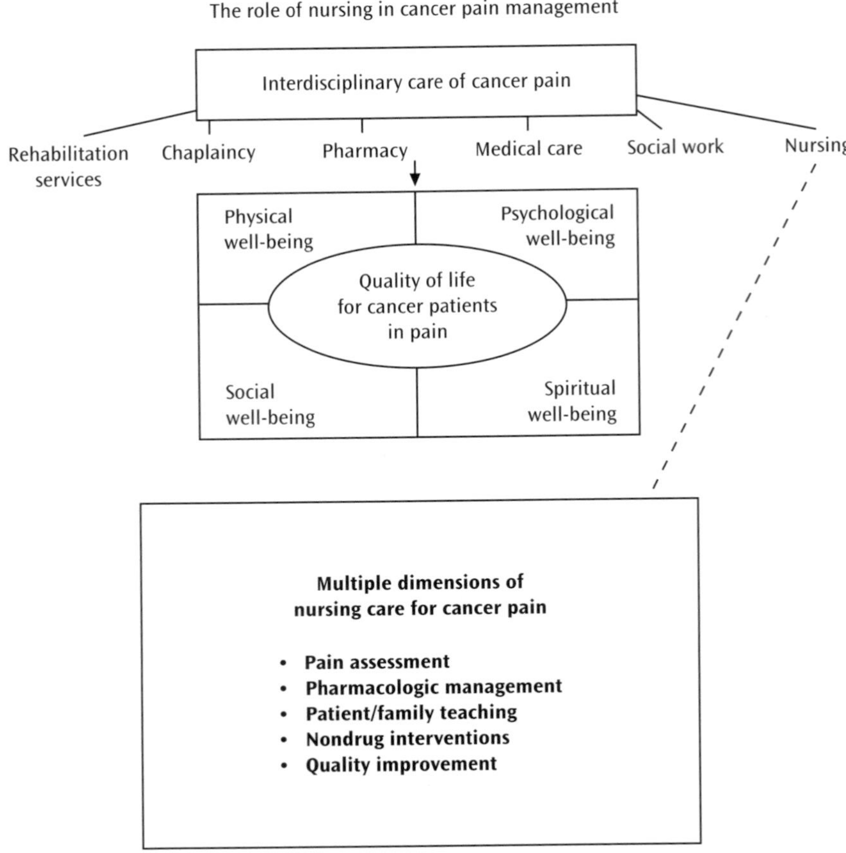

Figure 6.1 *The role of nursing in cancer pain management.*

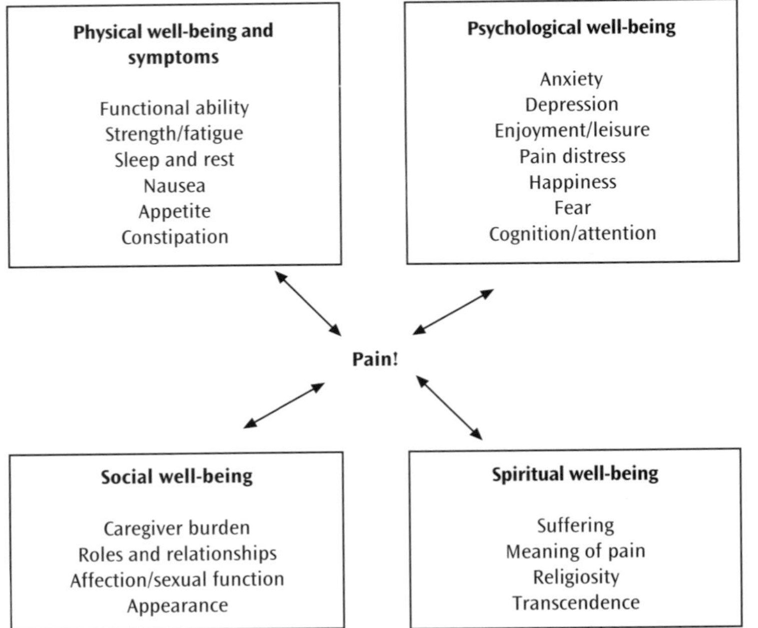

Figure 6.2 *Pain impacts on the dimensions of quality of life.*

Table 6.1 *Barriers to cancer pain management*[3]

Problems related to health care professionals
Inadequate knowledge of pain management
Poor assessment of pain
Concern about regulation of controlled substances
Fear of patient addiction
Concern about side-effects of analgesics
Concern about patients becoming tolerant to analgesics
Problems related to patients
Reluctance to report pain
Concern about distracting physicians from treatment of underlying disease
Fear that pain means disease is worse
Concern about not being a good patient
Reluctance to take pain medications
Fear of addiction or of being thought of as an addict
Worries about unmanageable side-effects
Concern about becoming tolerant to pain medications
Problems related to the health care system
Low priority given to cancer pain treatment
Inadequate reimbursement
The most appropriate treatment may not be reimbursed or may be too costly for patients and families
Restrictive regulation of controlled substances
Problems of availability of treatment or access to it

have demonstrated the value of a comprehensive educational approach, with attendees at such meetings also receiving resources for implementation of their knowledge and supporting structures to guide their efforts. Preparing professionals with knowledge is only one aspect of changing professional practice.[6,10]

One professional education model that has shown some success has been the Pain Resource Nurse (PRN) Program.[11] This program was instituted at the City of Hope, California, in 1992. The PRN Program recognized that, during the 1980s, pain education for many began with one of the numerous continuing education programs across the country. This education usually consisted of a 1-day lecture that individuals attended for their own educational needs, or because they were sent by their institution. However, in the 1990s there came a great awareness that isolated education activities had a minimal impact on changing practice. In the 1990s there began to emerge new models of professional education that incorporated usual education with other key components of institutional change. The PRN program is based on the idea that, within an institution, education of a single individual, such as a pain nurse or member of a pain team, is not sufficient to impact care throughout an entire institution. Through this program at the City of Hope National Medical Center, nurses on every shift and in every unit of the hospital were trained to create an awareness of pain and to provide commitment and expertise in every patient care area.

This program has been widely replicated in more than 25 programs across the USA.[8] Although most programs still struggle to be successful amidst the many challenges of the current health care environment, some common characteristics of success have been demonstrated. For example, most programs have found that a strong institutional commitment from administrators, managers, and organizational structures is essential to maximize the benefit of professional education about pain. It is also evident that nurses need support to realize the potential of increased knowledge. Programs that have also included the education of pharmacists and physicians to work in harmony with nurses toward the common institutional goal of better pain management have been most successful. These programs have often found the need to provide ongoing education to nurses who have been initially prepared in pain management and have recognized the value of rewarding and recognizing commitment to pain management.

Nurses also play a vital role in overcoming barriers to pain relief. Previous studies[12–14] have demonstrated that, even in institutions that offer the highest possible level of pain assessment and management, active patient participation is an essential foundation to effective pain relief. Until patients feel confident in articulating their pain and overcoming major fears of using pain medications, even the best professional efforts are to no avail. Nurses are the largest group of health care providers and work intimately with patients across all settings. Thus, their involvement in reducing patient barriers is essential.[9]

Nurses are also active participants in overcoming system obstacles by addressing regulatory and legislative barriers to pain management. The regulatory barriers have become recognized as a major interference with adequate prescribing and dispensing of pain medications.[3] Many national and international efforts are under way to deal with the regulatory and legal impediments to good pain relief.[15,16] Although, in most areas, nurses do not prescribe opioids, their involvement with patients in pharmacologic management of pain is significant. Nurses have often provided leadership in state cancer pain initiatives and other organizations to bring awareness of the problem of unrelieved pain due to obstacles to obtaining pain medications. Currently, in a project funded by the Robert Wood Johnson Foundation, investigators are working closely with state boards of nursing in the USA in the areas of policy related to pain and also to coordinate nursing reform with that directed at medical and pharmacy boards.[17]

PAIN ASSESSMENT

The recognition of pain as the "fifth vital sign" emerged through efforts of the American Pain Society's Quality Assurance Initiative and has now been echoed through many organizations.[5] It is nurses at the bedside who routinely take "vital signs" and thus are the key professionals to implement routine assessment of pain. Nursing efforts to improve pain assessment have best been accomplished at the institutional level. Nurses have been actively involved in pushing the organization to select a standard pain intensity scale and to make its use routine. Other strategies that have been most effective have included establishing standard documentation on patient records and reinforcing the need for communicating pain problems during change of shift reports or staff meetings in home care settings. Although comprehensive pain assessment tools provide valuable information, the clinical reality is that nurses have minimal time for assessment or documentation. Use of instruments such as the Brief Pain Inventory[18] or similar abbreviated tools are necessary in order to balance the need for comprehensive pain assessment with limited time.

Nurses have also begun to recognize that pain ratings are only one aspect of a good pain assessment, and are starting to place much more emphasis on pain assessment components such as physical examination, patient interview, assessment of neuropathic pain and other pain syndromes, and the importance of constantly assessing for new or treatable sources of pain.[19] Another innovation that holds promise has been the integration of pain assessment in computerized medical records. Some institutions have found ways to incorporate pain assessment in the electronic chart, thus enabling units to have a daily printout of any patient whose pain is above a certain level, i.e. a pain greater than 4. This is one additional way of making pain visible and of focusing the attention of specialty services such as pain teams or clinical nurse specialists on patients who have pain that is out of control. The new recommendation by the Joint Commission on Accreditation of Healthcare Organizations (JCAHO)[20] will certainly increase the emphasis on pain assessment as the cornerstone of all pain treatment.

PHARMACOLOGIC MANAGEMENT OF PAIN

Pharmacologic approaches to pain management have been recognized as the foundation of pain relief.[3] Advances in pain management over the past decade have been considerable, including new routes of analgesic administration, use of combined classes of drugs, increased focus on long-acting analgesics, emphasis on breakthrough pain, and considerable attention given to the use of adjuvant drugs. While these advances are welcome and important to advancing pain relief, they have created a rather complex situation with regards to pain management. It is important to recognize that cancer patients require multiple medications, given by more than one route of administration, on varied time schedules as routine or as p.r.n. dosing schedules. It is this complexity of pharmacologic pain management that necessitates the active involvement of nurses.[21–23]

Studies have previously documented that patients being cared for by skilled physicians prescribing state-of-the-art pain management often fail to achieve pain relief.[24–26] There are many reasons for this, including patients' fears and concerns about medication use, such as fear of addiction, family caregivers' reluctance to give medications which have been prescribed, and untreated side-effects such as nausea or constipation that prevent the patient from using available analgesics. Thus, nurses' involvement in pharmacologic management of pain is critical.[27]

PATIENT EDUCATION

Nurses play a vital role in patient and family education to insure that the optimal pain prescription is a realistic and understandable pain relief regimen. Table 6.2 presents a summary of major teaching points for patient education in cancer pain relief. This content has been developed and tested over the past 10 years in research by the City of Hope National Medical Center.[24,28] This content divides patient education into three components of pain assessment, pharmacologic treatments, and nondrug interventions.

Table 6.2 emphasizes that pain assessment is the first education component, as nurses must first address patient barriers and concerns before medications will be used optimally. Unless patients are willing to communicate their pain, they are unlikely to take medications. Studies involving this teaching plan have demonstrated a

Table 6.2 *Pain education program content*

Part I. General overview of pain
- A. Defining pain
- B. Understanding the causes of pain
- C. Pain assessment and use of pain rating scales to communicate pain
- D. Using a preventive approach to controlling pain
- E. Involvement of the family in pain management

Part II. Pharmacologic management of pain
- A. Overview of drug management of pain
- B. Overcoming fears of addiction
- C. Fear of drug dependence
- D. Understanding tolerance
- E. Understanding respiratory depression
- F. Talking to the doctor about pain
- G. Controlling other symptoms, such as nausea and constipation

Part III. Nondrug management of pain
- A. Importance of nondrug interventions
- B. Use of nondrug modalities as an adjunct to medications
- C. Review of previous experiences with nondrug methods
- D. Demonstration of heat, cold, massage, relaxation/distraction, and imagery

significant increase in the amount of analgesics taken and a reduction in pain intensity.[29,30]

Attention to side-effects must occur concurrently. Uncontrolled side-effects such as nausea, constipation, and sedation make it impossible to achieve optimum pain relief from analgesics. Recent advances in the field of pain relief have demonstrated the value of using written protocols and algorithms. It is also important to note that patient education and detailed attention to pain relief occur in a very constrained environment. Nurses in hospital settings have to deal with many acutely ill patients, and nurses in home care face a caseload of five to seven patients a day, with limited amount of time for patient teaching. Opportunities to use existing protocols, related teaching materials, and novel patient education programs, such as those involving audiotapes or other forms of instruction, are important. Table 6.3 summarizes key teaching points in patient education.

NONDRUG PAIN MANAGEMENT

It has long been recognized that the relief of pain is best accomplished through a combination of pharmacologic and nonpharmacologic interventions. The involvement of nursing and nondrug pain relief methods can be described in two components. The first is the nurse's own involvement in nondrug pain relief methods. In our research at the City of Hope since 1991, we have attempted to include nondrug pain relief as the third aspect of patient teaching following pain assessment and pharmacologic management information.[29,31] We have introduced simple techniques, such as the use of heat, cold, massage, relaxation/distraction, and imagery as methods that nurses can teach to patients in a very inexpensive and simple format. Although virtually all nurses believe in the importance of nondrug interventions, our research has demonstrated that actual use is limited. We believe that this is often because nurses receive little education about the use of these treatments, although the most influential factor is time and resource constraints. In the future, we will need to continue to evolve teaching for nurses so that they are prepared in these treatments and thus can transfer them to patients. We also will need to continue to strive to incorporate nondrug interventions in our patient education.[32] Innovative strategies, such as using volunteers to help implement these interventions, will also be necessary, as nursing time is limited.

The second issue affecting use of nondrug pain interventions is nurses awareness of the role of other colleagues and their willingness to make use of them. Although reimbursement often determines actual clinical use, many beneficial modalities are often available to patients, such as physiotherapy, occupational therapy or psychology. In our PRN training programs, we have attempted to address both of these issues by devoting a major section of our pain education to nondrug interventions. For example, the program includes a laboratory component in which nurses can demonstrate the use of nondrug modalities. This also provides an opportunity

Table 6.3 *Teaching principles for pain education*

Information provided must be accurate and current. Content should be reviewed by experts in the area and pilot tested in a sample of patients
Teaching should be preceded by establishing what the patient already knows about his/her condition/pain management
Establish goals and objectives with the patient/family to enhance cooperation and compliance with the recommended plan of treatment. Information should be immediately useful when teaching adults
Teach the smallest amount possible rather than overload patients who are already burdened by illness and pain. The patient must know enough about his/her condition to understand the rationale behind the regimen and be able to carry out the desired behavior
Use a combination of education methods, such as written materials, lecture, discussion, and audiovisual tools
Keep the teaching session brief, with breaks as needed by the patient
Present the most important material first. For example, it may be necessary to first overcome the patient's overwhelming fear of addiction before he/she will be at all open to drug management of pain
The appropriate materials must be selected to convey the message/information to be taught. Can existing materials be used or is it necessary to produce new materials?
Readability of written materials should be appropriate for the cognitive level of the patient. In general, no higher than a sixth grade reading level is recommended. A readability index should be performed on all written information
Written materials should be in a larger print for elderly patients
Reinforce written information with an audiocassette tape that can be replayed as often as necessary
Illustrations and written materials should be clear and concise. Avoid medical jargon
Repetition is necessary. Encourage questions. Ask questions. Have the patient/family state what they have learned in their own words
Whenever possible, involve family and supportive friends in the educational program
Choose an environment that is quiet with a temperature that is comfortable for the patient and family. The patient should be physically comfortable to learn
Education must be individualized with consideration of cultural influences

Table 6.4 *Select organizations and websites of interest to nurses in pain management*

Organizations

Hospice and Palliative Nurses Association (HPNA)
Medical Center E, Suite 375
211 N. Whitfield
Pittsburgh, PA 15206-3031
USA
Tel: (+1) 412 361 2425
E-mail: HPNA@hpna.org

Oncology Nursing Society (ONS)
501 Holiday Drive
Pittsburgh, PA 15220-2749
USA
Tel: (+1) 412 921 7373
Fax: (+1) 412 921 6565
E-mail: member@ons.org

American Pain Society (APS)
4700 W. Lake Avenue
Glenview, IL 60025
USA
Tel: (+1) 847 375 4715
Fax: (+1) 847 375 4777
E-mail: infor@ampainsoc.org

American Society of Pain Management Nurses (ASPMN)
7794 Grow Drive
Pensacola, FL 32514
USA
Tel: (+1) 888 342 7766
Fax: (+1) 850 484 8762
E-mail: ASPMN@pwetzamc.com

International Association for the Study of Pain (IASP)
IASP Secretariat
909 NE 43rd St., Suite 306
Seattle, WA 98105
USA
Tel: (+1) 206 547 6409
Fax: (+1) 206 547 1703
E-mail: iaspdesk@juno.com

Websites/Internet resources	
Agency for Health Care Policy and Research	www.ahcpr.gov/
American Academy of Hospice and Palliative Medicine	www.aahpm.org
ABCD Americans for Better Care of the Dying	www.abcd-caring.com
American Pain Society	www.ampainsoc.org
Hospice Association of America	www.hospice-america.org
Hospice and Palliative Nurses Association	www.HPNA.org
Hospice Foundation of America	www.hospicefoundation.org
International Association for the Study of Pain	www.pain.org/iasp
Last Acts	www.lastacts.org
National Hospice Association	www.nho.org
Open Society Institute Project on Death in America	www.soros.org/death.html
Oncology Nursing Society	www.ons.org
Resource Center of the American Alliance of Cancer Pain Initiatives	www.wiscinfo.doit.wisc.edu/tnc
UW Pain and Policy Studies Group	www.medsch.wis.edu/painpolicy
International websites	
The Edmonton Palliative Care Program	www.palliative.org
European Association for Palliative Care	www.eapcnet.org
International Institute of Hospice Studies	www.som.fmc.flinders.edu.au/FUSA/PalliativeCare/links/links.htm
Centre for Bioethics/*Journal of Palliative Care*	www.ircm.qc.ca/bioethique/english/publications/journal_of_palliative_care.html
The International Work Group on Death, Dying, and Bereavement	www.wwdc.com/death/iwg/iwg.html
World Health Organization	www.who.int/nce/cancer/
International Psycho-Oncology Society	www.ipos-aspboa.org/iposnews.htm
International Abstracts Palliative Care and Pain Management	www.bestmdsite.com/abstracts-pcpm-home.html

to introduce nurses to the many interventions available through other disciplines.

An additional important benefit of nondrug pain relief methods is that they afford an opportunity to involve family caregivers. Nurses can instruct family members in these methods, which adds to the patient's comfort while also reducing family members' feelings of helplessness when caring for a loved one in pain.[33]

QUALITY IMPROVEMENT IN PAIN MANAGEMENT

In recent years, the focus of nurses has shifted from management of individual patients' pain to a broader institutional perspective. Nurses have come to recognize that influencing institutional policy and reforming systems of care is a more efficient approach than focusing on individual patients' pain problems.[34,35] The ultimate goal of such efforts is to create policies, procedures, staff knowledge, and an environment in which pain relief is expected and uncontrolled pain is viewed as an emergency. The quality assurance mechanism offers many advantages to pain improvement efforts. Most institutions are required to have in place ongoing processes for quality improvement (QI). Many nurses have found that their own efforts are aided tremendously by teaming with quality assurance coordinators in order to take a systems approach to better pain relief. Several model institutions have demonstrated that a systematic QI approach can result in a significant improvement in long-standing pain management practices.[6,7,9,10]

Some of the strategies that have been found most useful for QI efforts are chart audits, patient and family caregiver interviews, and assessment of staff knowledge and belief in order to document the current status of pain management. Nurses have become aware that, unless professionals are aware of the need for improvement, few will be motivated to participate in change. The QI process entails recognition of current strengths and weaknesses in the environments and use of an organized plan to reach goals.[36,37] The QI process also generally emphasizes the importance of an interdisciplinary approach to the system change. Activities often involve coordination of nursing efforts with other key departments such as pharmacy, medicine, and social work. An important aspect of most QI programs is a strong emphasis on evaluation.[38] Mechanisms of ongoing monitoring of pain management practices can provide solid evidence of improvement in types of medications prescribed, use of algorithms, use of protocols for side-effect management, overall pain intensity, patient satisfaction, and can also help to benchmark the institution against a growing body of institutional data related to pain. Certainly, the emphasis by the JCAHO and other regulatory and certifying bodies helps to give credence to pain management as a priority topic for QI topics.[20]

SUMMARY

In summary, as the largest group of health care providers and those most intimately involved in patients' and family caregivers' experiences of pain, nurses have always played a primary role in the treatment of pain. Within the many demands of a constrained health care system, nurses will continue to lead efforts to improve pain management. This requires nurses to become more knowledgeable themselves to stay abreast of the many advances in pain management and to work with interdisciplinary teams to change institutional practice. Table 6.4 provides a list of organizations and websites that are available to support nurses in pain management activities. More detailed listing of resources can be found through the City of Hope Pain Resource Center website at http://prc.coh.org.

The key roles of nurses as described above include pain assessment, pharmacologic and nonpharmacologic interventions, and involvement in the quality improvement efforts. The relief of pain is the essence of nursing care. Nurses assist patients with achieving optimal quality of life despite chronic illness or in the face of terminal illness. Pain relief is a professional mandate for every individual nurse and a challenge to the nursing profession.

REFERENCES

1. McGuire DB. The multiple dimensions of cancer pain: a framework for assessment and management. In: McGuire DB, Henke Yarbro C, Ferrell BR eds. *Cancer Pain Management*. Boston, MA: Jones and Barlett, 1995: 1–18.
2. ● Ferrell BR. The quality of lives: 1,525 voices of cancer. *Oncology Nursing Forum* 1996, **23:** 907–16.
3. ◆ Jacox A, Carr DB, Payne R, *et al. Manage of Cancer Pain.* Agency for Health Care Policy and Research (AHCPR) Clinical Practice Guideline No. 9. Rockville, MD: US Department of Health and Human Services, Public Health Services.
4. Fink R, Gates R. Pain assessment. In: Ferrell BR, Coyle N eds. *Textbook of Palliative Care*. New York, NY: Oxford University Press, 2001: 53–71.
5. American Pain Society. *Principles of Analgesic Use in the Treatment of Acute Pain and Cancer Pain*, 4th edn. Glenview, IL: American Pain Society, 1999.
6. Bookbinder M. Improving the quality of care across all settings. In: Ferrell BR, Coyle N eds. *Textbook of Palliative Care*. New York, NY: Oxford University Press, 2001: 503–30.
7. Breitbart W, Rosenfeld B, Passik SD. The network project: a multidisciplinary cancer education and training program in pain management, rehabilitation, and psychosocial issues. *J Pain Symptom Manage* 1998; **15:** 18–26.
8. Grant M, Rivera LM, Alisangco J, Francisco L. Improv-

ing cancer pain management using a performance improvement framework. *J Nursing Care Quality* 1999; **13(4):** 60–72.

◆ 9. Ferrell BR, Whedon M, Rollins B. Pain and quality assessment/improvement. *J Nursing Care Quality* 1995; **9:** 69–85.

◆ 10. Gordon DB. Critical pathways: a road to institutionalizing pain management. *J Pain Symptom Manage* 1996; **11:** 252–9.

11. Ferrell BR, Grant M, Ritchey KJ, *et al*. The Pain Resource Nursing Training Program: a unique approach to pain management. *J Pain Symptom Manage* 1993; **8:** 549–56.

12. Ward S, Emery Berry P, Misiewicz H. Caregiver and patient concerns about analgesics: a comparison of dyads in a hospice setting. *Res Nursing Hlth* 1996; **19:** 205–11.

13. Ward S, Gatwood J. Concerns about reporting pain and using analgesics: a comparison of persons with and without cancer. *Cancer Nursing* 1995; **17:** 200–6.

◆ 14. Paice JA, Fine PG. Pain at the end of life. In: Ferrell BR, Coyle N eds. *Textbook of Palliative Care*. New York, NY: Oxford University Press, 2001: 76–90.

15. Joranson D, Gilbson AM. Controlled substances and pain management: a new focus for state medical boards. *Fed Bull* 1998; **18(2):** 78–83.

16. Joransen DE, Gilson AM, Ryan KM, *et al. Achieving Balance in Federal and State Pain Policy: a Guide to Evaluation*. Madison, WI: The Pain and Policy Studies Group, University of Wisconsin Comprehensive Cancer Center, 2000.

17. Ferrell BR, Grant M, Virani R. Strengthening nursing education to improve end of life care. *Nursing Outlook* 1999; **47(6):** 252–6.

18. Cleeland CS, Ryan KM. Pain assessment: global use of the brief pain inventory. *Ann Acad Med* 1994; **23:** 129–38.

19. Cleeland CS, Syrjala KL. How to assess cancer pain. In: Turk DC, Melzack R eds. *Handbook of Pain Assessment*. New York, NY: Guilford Press, 1992: 362–87.

20. Joint Commission on Accreditation of Health Care Organizations 2001. Available on-line at http://www.jcaho.org.

◆ 21. McCaffery M, Portenoy RR. Overview of three groups of analgesics. In: McCaffery M, Pasero C eds. *Pain Clinical Manual*. St Louis, MO: Mosby, 1999: 103–28.

22. Deglin JH, Vallerand AH. *Davis Drug Guide for Nurses*, 7th edn. Philadelphia, PA: FA Davis, 2000.

◆ 23. Pasero C, Portenoy RK, McCaffery M. Opioid analgesics. In: McCaffery M, Pasero C eds. *Pain Clinical Manual*. St Louis, MO: Mosby, 1999: 161–299.

◆ 24. Ferrell BR, Rhiner M, Ferrell BA. Development and implementation of a pain education program. *Cancer* 1993; **72:** 3426–32.

◆ 25. Chapman CR. Compliance with pain medication: A hidden problem? *Am Pain Soc Bull* 1996; **6:** 11.

● 26. Levy MH. Pharmacologic treatment of cancer pain. *N Engl J Med* 1996; **335:** 1124–32.

27. Ferrell BR, McCaffery M. Nurses' knowledge about equianalgesia and opioid dosing. *Cancer Nursing* 1997; **20:** 201–12.

28. Ferrell BR, Ferrell BA, Ahn C, Tran K. Pain management for elderly patients with cancer at home. *Cancer* 1994; **74:** 213–146.

29. Ferrell BR, Grant M, Chan J, *et al*. The impact of cancer pain education on family caregivers of elderly cancer patients. *Oncology Nursing Forum* 1995; **22:** 1211–18.

30. Ferrell BR, Borneman T, Juarez, G. Integration of pain education in home care. *J Palliative Care* 1998; **14:** 62–8.

31. Rhiner M, Ferrell BR, Ferrell BA, Grant M. A structured nondrug intervention program for cancer pain. *Cancer Practice* 1993; **1:** 137–43.

◆ 32. McCaffery M, Pasero C. Practical nondrug approaches to pain. In: McCaffery M, Pasero C eds. *Pain Clinical Manual*. St Louis, MO: Mosby, 1999: 399–427.

33. Ferrell BR. Pain observed: the experience of pain from the family caregivers' perspective. *Clin Geriat Med* 2001; **17:** 595–609.

34. Ferrell BR, Dean GE, Grant M, Coluzzi P. An institutional commitment to pain management. *J Clin Oncol* 1995; **13:** 2158–65.

35. Ferrell BR, Jacox A, Miaskowski C, *et al*. Cancer guidelines: now that we have them, what do we do? *Oncology Nursing Forum* 1994; **21:** 1229–38.

36. Weissman DE, Griffie J, Gordon DB, *et al*. A role model program to promote institutional changes for pain management of acute and cancer pain. *J Pain Symptom Manage* 1997; **14:** 274–9.

37. Weissman DE, Dahl JL, Gordon DB, *et al*. The cancer pain role model program of the Wisconsin Cancer Pain Initiative. *J Pain Symptom Manage* 1993; **8:** 29–35.

◆ 38. McCaffery M, Pasero C. Continuous quality improvement. In: McCaffery M, Pasero C eds. *Pain Clinical Manual*. St Louis, MO: Mosby, 1999: 713–15.

7

Teamworking

VICKY ROBINSON AND ROB GEORGE

> No man is an Island, entire of it self; every man is a piece of the Continent, a part of the main; if a clod be washed away by the sea, Europe is the less, as well as if a promontory were, as well as if a manor of thy friends or of thine own were; any man's death diminishes me, because I am involved in Mankind; and therefore never send to know for whom the bell tolls; it tolls for thee.
>
> John Donne
> *Devotions upon Emergent Occasions* (1624)
> "Meditation XVII"

SETTING THE SCENE

Two views of teamwork

Teamworking and interdisciplinary practice are modern mantras. One may therefore be forgiven for viewing this chapter as a sop to political correctness. However, to be ignorant of the elements of effective teamwork is perilous in such a complex area as pain management. Read on!

In order to maintain accessibility and relevance for clinicians, our exploration begins with two slightly stereotypical examples of teams in action. We then use them to:

- contextualize and examine some theories of teamwork;
- offer a framework for those with a strategic role in the formation and development of clinical teams; and
- give readers who have responsibility for leading and managing teams the confidence to influence change processes where their team is weak or dysfunctional.

James's team

It is Friday afternoon in the breast clinic of a large teaching hospital. Dr James Moss, the consultant oncologist, is proud of this clinic. It was his idea to draw counseling, nursing, and medicine together in one place. After all, no-one can be all things to all people, and he had fought hard for the space and staffing necessary. Still, here they all are: a multidisciplinary team in action. In the department each Friday afternoon, apart from James, are a cancer counselor (Linda), a breast care nurse (Julie), and, when requested, a specialist palliative nurse.

Soon it will be 4 p.m. He simply *must* leave by then. The boys are so looking forward to one of their few weekends away sailing. If he is late, they will not get to the coast by seven. Work takes enough of his life as it is. He simply can't break his promise this time.

At 3.40 p.m. Janet Cooper walks in with her husband, Colin. She looks awful. Janet was diagnosed with breast cancer just after her fortieth birthday 2 years ago and has done very well given the aggressiveness of her disease, although she now has widespread liver and bone metastases. She has just had radiotherapy to her hip and chemotherapy starts on Monday. Colin has taken the day off work to come to the hospital with her. James greets them at the door smiling. "Twenty minutes, plenty of time," he thinks.

Janet sits down and bursts into tears. The pain in her side is not responding to simple analgesia. Could she have something stronger? James glances at Colin, and feels a flood of sorrow as he thinks. "I can't take away their hope, but she is unlikely to see Christmas. I'll have to start some morphine too, just whilst we're waiting for the radiotherapy to work." He still couldn't prescribe morphine without feeling he'd lost – irrational, but there it is.

"I'll get Linda to see them. They need to talk. Linda's

such a brick, a real expert at this stuff. I just don't know how she copes with all these tales of woe. Still, that's what a team's for – horses for courses."

James Moss writes the prescription and reassures Janet and Colin that the radiotherapy and chemotherapy really will help and that he is going to ask the cancer counselor to see them both. Three-fifty p.m. Perfect. James knocks on Linda's door on his way out.

"Linda, can you talk to Janet and Colin Cooper for me. Two-year history, nasty disease, bone and liver mets. I've just started her on morphine for pain control. She's taking the whole thing quite badly. I think they both suspect that this could be the beginning of the end, although I've reassured them that this course of radiotherapy and chemo' will make her much better.

"I've arranged to see them both again in 6 weeks' time after the chemo' has finished. Can you keep an eye on her and do your stuff for me until then. My secretary's got the notes – all the information you need is there."

Linda makes to say something, but James is already out of the door. He shakes off a strange feeling of melancholy as he hurries down the corridor. However, he quickly reassures himself

"That's what I like. Someone to pick up the psychological bit. Good teamwork. It really is excellent to have a holistic service."

Linda fumes. "Here we go again: another shot in the dark. Why do I always feel that I have to pick up all the pieces? I'll talk to Julie first to see if she knows the patient." Linda sails into Julie's office and slumps in the chair.

"Can I talk to you? He's done it again: a typical Friday afternoon catastrophe on my doorstep. I don't know them, I haven't been introduced, and I didn't hear what he said. I'm not clairvoyant you know. How many times do I have to tell him? We're going to have to sit him down and pin his ears back." Julie just nods and shrugs at the right moments as there is no point in trying to interrupt Linda when she is in full flood, but it does seem she has a point. What neither knows is that, although he would never admit it, James Moss finds Linda very intimidating when she is in the room with him and a patient – she makes him feel so inadequate that he stumbles over simple interactions and he doesn't quite know how to deal with it. Subconsciously he will do almost anything to avoid joint consultations.

James's team is coming up to its first anniversary – it is still very young. Referring on to another professional is not teamwork, it is only the beginning of teamwork – James doesn't know that, and he is also saddled with his inhibitions with Linda – this will come out sooner or later. Equally, Linda does not make his task easy or her difficulties clear. James will probably be mortified when he hears of the tension he is causing. Teams only form once there is open communication. We will come back to this.

The experienced team

This second scenario highlights something else: the need for a breadth of experience and the professional affiliations and backgrounds required to help a young man who is dying from disseminated malignancy.

Steve is a 28-year-old artist, engaged to Jenny. He was referred to the local interdisciplinary† specialist palliative care team (PCT) by his general practitioner (GP) following a left below-knee amputation for an aggressive osteosarcoma. Six weeks after surgery, Steve was diagnosed with liver metastases. His GP is asking for advice on how to manage Steve's phantom limb pain, and for some general support for Jenny and for Steve's parents. The team discusses the case at referral and decides on a joint assessment by one of the more experienced clinical nurse specialists (CNS) and a team doctor.

Steve's phantom limb pain is well controlled with appropriate neuropathic agents and he says that this isn't the issue. He wants a second opinion on treatment for his cancer.

"You are not here to discuss my death. I was told that you were coming to advise on treating my pain. It's obvious that you should do this by treating my cancer." It is also clear to the CNS that there is a lot of tension in the family.

Over the next few weeks and several hours of tirades against doctors, the CNS learns several things. Jenny is 4 months pregnant, and Steve's own parents had lost a child, Jason, at the age of 9. This was before Steve was born and was never spoken of. Steve was therefore feeling guilty and very angry at the prospect of "deserting" his family so soon.

"I simply refuse to give in to this." He sobs.

The case is clearly complex and operates at several levels beyond Steve's pain. It is also affecting the clinicians who are involved and threatens to draw them into the family's vortex of fear and anxiety. Here, the strength of teamwork should offer a check and a protection for the CNS and GP as well as a framework for managing the case. Here is what happens.

The referral by the GP for assistance with Steve's phantom limb pain also legitimizes his need for some personal support in managing the case. On feeding back, this is brought up with the GP (who is used to working with specialist palliative care). He is quite open about the distress that the case is causing the practice. He has known the family for 30 years and was involved at the time of Jason's death. "I've been looking for an excuse to get you guys involved – there is too much going on for me to handle on my own and I feel part of it."

The CNS presents Steve and his family at the large interdisciplinary team meeting and the GP attends too. She too confesses to feeling helpless and asks for assis-

†Inter- and multidisciplinary are usually used interchangeably, although there is a subtle difference.

tance in deciding the most effective strategy now that the complexity of the family dynamic has emerged. After half an hour's discussion, there is a clear game-plan and contingent approaches should one or more of the family fail to cope or should the disease progress unexpectedly.

It is self-evident that this case is beyond one practitioner, and both clinicians, who are familiar with teamwork, know it. The human problems associated with managing pain and uncertainty are "up front" with Steve: denial, fear of addressing the meaning of pain and symptoms, unresolved matters from the past, etc. Complex problems require more than one brain and more than one discipline. In this mature team, however, although mechanisms are in place for calm and controlled management of this type of case, it has taken 9 years to get there.

The need for teamworking in cancer

Issues for the patient

People with malignant disease perceive pain as telling them that the cancer is alive and well, and they are not. It is a powerful message, a reminder of mortality, the prospect of suffering, and of a future lost. The experience may well precipitate a crisis or be a watershed. It raises questions of mortality, existence, priorities, and relationship that need emotional or psychological support ranging from an effective listening ear through to a psychologist in difficult cases.

Pain also raises practical questions: "how am I going to manage if I have to give up work, or how do I get out of bed, up and down stairs, to and from hospital appointments, etc.?" These may need occupational therapy, physiotherapy, or social support.

Issues for the clinician

Donne was right that "No man is an island," especially when we are working with people facing crisis. Pain does something to us. It's not hard to imagine the pain and suffering being experienced by our two patients. The experience of pain signals that something is happening inside. For doctors in particular, whose imperative so often is to cure a patient, acknowledging the feelings of helplessness and sadness that accompany progressive disease can be a very hard thing to do.

To benefit fully from team life, one must come to acknowledge that we need not only each other's professional expertise but also each other for professional companionship. This enables us to share the burden of often impossibly difficult and sometimes tragic situations – situations that at times challenge us as people as well as professionals.

Our overriding obligation to such patients must be to ensure that we provide a caring environment in which the diverse facets of a patient's pain can be managed. We must ensure appropriate information, choice, and therapeutic diversity for all our patients through involving individuals from different professional backgrounds who each take a different approach to pain management.

Both our cameos demonstrate the need for more than one professional to be involved in caring for a patient and family. We can also say that both scenarios demonstrate a team approach. But what are the key differences between James's team and the experienced team? The following section will take us through some of the theories of teamwork and look at some of the problems and pitfalls that must be overcome to become a successful team. Having visited the theories, we shall return to our cameos.

SOME THEORY

So what is a team?

We all know what a team is. It is a group of people who work together to achieve a common goal that cannot be achieved alone. Every member usually has a specific role and brings a unique talent, while being able to "turn their hand" to another skill. Sports such as football demonstrate this.

The equivalent in clinical practice is *interdisciplinary care*. A doctor is not a counselor and vice versa. Nor is a nurse a psychologist. Each has skills specific to their professions, but some are transferable. Good team players, while knowing their own area and general limitations, should be able to perform the basics of their colleagues' areas. Functioning together, their effectiveness far exceeds that of an individual provided they understand each other's personal and professional skills and help each other to recognize and develop their strengths and abilities within the group. However, it needs more than just a collection of well-meaning professionals to deliver interdisciplinary care effectively. What else is necessary?

The diverse needs of patients with pain need to be addressed seamlessly and effectively, and it is far easier for a team to achieve this. This is one of the foundations on which specialist palliative care and hospice services are built, and is now required in all cancer centers across the UK. However, much of the evidence in support of teamworking in cancer pain and palliative care still remains anecdotal,[1,2] despite some objective evidence that bereaved carers perceive pain and symptom management, as well as financial information and information on local services, to be better when a specialist interdisciplinary team is involved.[3]

From research we find two essential groups of ingredients aside from the people: one to do with the job in hand (the task) and the other to do with managing the problems that arise when people work together (the relationships). Both areas must be understood, developed, and fostered. This takes both time and effort. We now come onto this.

What makes a team succeed?

Factors contributing to the effectiveness of a team are listed in Table 7.1.

Clarity

The overarching theme around tasks and operations is the need for clarity and consistency. The majority of research relevant to us has been undertaken in primary care and mental health. Basically, the themes are common and there are no real surprises, perhaps with the exception of evaluation and accountability, as emphasized by Field and West.[6] This is perhaps because they refer to mature teams and demonstrate the endpoints of a time-consuming growth process.

Variety

Equally, it is not surprising that teams comprising people with identical characteristics do not work well. In fact, having the brightest people in a team in no way guarantees that it will be the best team.[7] This is because the most effective teams have members who express characteristics that fulfill a variety of roles and behaviors necessary for balance. Within reason, the presence of these is as important to a good team as the caliber of its members. The most comprehensive study in this area was conducted by Belbin[7] and its findings are summarized in Table 7.2.

Belbin's work is essential reading for anyone interested in increasing effectiveness and understanding the essential ingredients of a successful team.[7] It is one of the few pieces of organizational development research of this kind that has stood the test of time and proved to be both valid and reliable.

In short, there are eight roles necessary to a team performing at its peak. This does not mean that an effective team has to have eight members, as one person can assume two and occasionally three roles. Note also that a person may fulfill different roles in different groups or circumstances. According to Belbin, roles are sometimes "clustered" and can be filled by one person and, although people tend to have one or two "natural roles," these are not fixed. For example, one person may function in one group principally as the shaper, but in another as the resource investigator if a more effective shaper is present or if there is no resource investigator in the second group.

So, teams need different types of people with clearly defined roles, not just technically but also within the organic world of that team.

Support and peer supervision

Everyone acknowledges that cancer and palliative care are stressful areas of work and clinicians need peer support and supervision.[8] Not surprisingly, these are much valued characteristics of a good working environment.[6] We see this between the lines in the experienced team and explicitly in Linda's support from her colleague Julie. Social support at work has also been identified as a crucial stress-reducing factor.[9,10] However, this is a two-edged sword, as those working in hospice environments have identified. Vachon[8] found that over 70% of stress in hospice staff was attributed to organizational or role issues rather than relationships with patients and families or working with death and dying.

West[11] has helpfully described four types of social support in the team environment:

1 *Emotional support* – the provision of a "shoulder to cry on."
2 *Informational support* – being pointed in the right direction.
3 *Instrumental support* – practical help in times of heavy workload or simply "helping each other out."
4 *Appraisal support* – different perspectives on a given problem, not necessarily solution-generating.

A useful note here is that it is often these types of support that cross the barriers of role suspicion, historical hierarchies, and "ownership" of patients to forge a team in which loyalty and affiliation are balanced properly between the team and one's profession. We see this, for example, with the CNS and GP in the experienced team.

Time

It is common sense that a group of people who know what they are doing and why, and who can manage the aggravations and pressures of working together and still develop and keep the principal goal in view, will be a good team.The time investment to get to this point is considerable. It is our experience that it takes 5 years from inception to reach this stage. Furthermore, it does not stop there: teams go through cycles of function and dysfunction as members leave, as new ones join, and as the tasks and goals change over time. In short, a team is never static and the building process is never over!

The downside of teamwork and how it may fail

Time

On the one hand, time is essential to building teams, but on the other it is often at a premium, both overall (above) and as part of daily practice. In this regard, teamworking is inefficient. Interdisciplinary teamwork is slower than working alone, but, although decision-making can take longer, the quality of a decision made by a team is likely to be higher than that of one made alone by an average team member.[11]

Conflict and communication breakdown

Furthermore, team members do not always agree. Indeed, performing teams need a degree of conflict/tension (overt

Table 7.1 *Factors contributing to an effective team*

	Firth-Cozens[4]	McGrath[5] (mental health)	Field and West[6] (primary care)
Staff	Staff with diverse skills and knowledge	Competent and committed staff Agreed definitions of members' roles Open communication systems and shared information	Individuals' contributions should be identifiable
Tasks	A common goal	Goals and priorities must be agreed Open communication systems and shared information There should be a task-centered, problem-solving approach	Group goals must be clear The team's task is interesting in itself Individual tasks should be intrinsically rewarding
Relationships	Staff who accept and manage conflict Staff who work towards unity Support for team members Opportunities for individuals to develop	Staff who are self-critical, self-managing, and able to cope with conflict Participative management An environment that is supportive, informal, and member-orientated, creative and stimulating	Individuals who feel that their own work is essential to the success of the team An environment that is supportive, informal, and member-orientated, creative and stimulating Individuals who are subject to evaluation Inbuilt performance feedback as part of goals setting

Table 7.2 *Summary of Belbin's classification of team roles*[7]

Chairman/coordinator	Coordinating role, focusing and balancing the group and its judgments. This person is not necessarily the brightest in a group or, oddly, the leader. Doctors are often forced into this role but frequently do it badly
Company person	A practical person, good at administration and implementing decisions
Teamworker	The engine room of the team, someone who is loyal, committed, and noncompetitive and who is good at resolving conflicts and disputes
Completer–finisher	The person who makes sure that projects are completed and kept on schedule. A very important role and often seen in administrators
Monitor–evaluator	The team analyst, who always solves the problems, is bright and can stand one step back
Shaper	The natural leader, who drives ahead with an idea and can be quite ruthless but is inclined to take umbrage
Plant	Another intellectual who often works alone but comes up with ideas
Resource investigator	The charismatic member, entrepreneurial and popular, who knows where to get what is needed but is poor on follow-through

and covert) to maintain creativity and momentum. Without it there is no force for change. If this tension is not managed well or communication is allowed to deteriorate, people will polarize to their profession, form cliques, or withdraw. In any event, trouble comes when we stop communicating and healthy tensions turn into civil war. It is here that the social links will work to maintain team integrity and where good management is necessary.

At such times in a team's developmental cycles, it does seem easier to go it alone, but so often poor communication lies at the root of team tensions or poor service delivery. In reality, problems such as these are occupational hazards and a function of historical barriers between primary, secondary, and tertiary care, between professions, and between professionals, patients, and families. This leads us to an important warning.

Problems with power, status, and communication

Among colleagues

It would be naive and irresponsible were we not to say that effective teamwork usually requires professional or organizational status to be set aside. Much has been written over the years about the power-based relationships between caring professions. For example, the stereotypical doctor–nurse relationship portrays the nurse as subservient handmaiden to the doctor's masculine authority and sacred medical knowledge.[12] Anyone who enters the worlds of cancer, pain management, or palliative care and adheres to these stereotypes will be not only a bad team member, but also a real obstruction to good patient care and partnership. We see shades of this in James Moss.

With our patients

From first presentation to discharge home it is quite usual for a patient to come into contact with at least 13 different professionals. It may seem unbelievable that so many people are involved in a cancer journey. However, the various professionals in the community [family doctor, community nurses(s)], the cancer center (consultant junior doctors; clinic, ward, and specialist nurses; and allied health professionals), not to mention the multidisclinary care service if it is necessary, comes easily to double figures in a short time. As an exercise, count the professionals involved in a patient's journey in relation to your own practice. The deluge of information with which they are provided can be confusing and distressing if different sources conflict or are inconsistent. This is a major risk with uncoordinated teamwork. The best solution is to ensure that patients feel that they too are part of the team. However, reasonable differences in professional opinion around optimum treatments may be the last thing a patient needs to experience. It is at times like this that the quality and maturity of teamworking will find the necessary balance between disclosure and paternalism and the team will be comfortable with the need on occasions to plan behind closed doors in order to reach consensus, free from individual interests, and to present clear choices to the patient.

Absent planning and maintenance

One of the major obstacles to the formation and functioning of teams, within acute settings in particular, is lack of strategic planning and investment in the new team development. A documented, though little discussed, example of this was the Charing Cross Hospital experience.[13]

Briefly, the palliative care support services at the hospital had a short and dysfunctional life and were disbanded. Charing Cross Hospital was ill-designed architecturally, medically, or socially, for a team approach to care. Additional areas of difficulty that led to their team's collapse were:

- an amorphous team;
- understaffing, with only one full-time member (a nurse);
- no designated leader or role clarity;
- no clear referral criteria;
- lack of common office space;
- poor communication; and
- underfunding from senior management with other priorities.

The Charing Cross Hospital experience gives us a very clear message: without planning and development a team will fail, and because the structure and constituency of teams differ between organizations there can be no shortcut or "off-the-shelf solution." We now come to this.

Planning and developing a team

In these days of outcome measures there is little room for throwing resources at organizations and leaving them to get on with it. Any service development strategy must be justifiable, evidence based, and take into account the need for in-built team development strategies that promote the development of good characteristics.

Planning

Øvretveit[14] suggests a useful model to assist those responsible for designing multidisciplinary services. Although developed around community care, the model can easily be transferred to any sector of health care. Øvretveit stresses that teams should not be set up before a survey of local need. He emphasizes that such an approach will not only focus development on local need but will also foster genuine long-term commitment from senior managers and consultants.

Table 7.3 describes the approach. The left-hand column defines and analyzes each element of need from various perspectives, and the right-hand column lists the mechanisms that are necessary to make sense of the analysis in a coherent and doable organizational mechanism that demands accurate information, clear communication, and care planning. This next section offers some clues as to how to achieve this.

Processes: organizational development (OD)

> We trained very hard, but it seemed that every time we were beginning to form up into teams, we would be reorganized. I was to learn in later life that we tend to meet any new situation by reorganizing and a wonderful method it can be for creating the illusion of progress, while producing confusion, inefficiency and demoralization.
>
> Caius Petronius (AD 66)

Petronius is highlighting the time and opportunity that must be given to allow teams to pass through their developmental phase and stabilize. This is the value of organizational development (OD).

OD refers to those efforts intended to improve an organization's culture and processes as a group and between individuals in the group. Essentially, this means that one needs to use techniques and skills that foster relationships that will help people work well together.[15]

Table 7.3 *Øvretveit's[14] "needs–response" dynamic showing the essential elements in creating an effective and responsive team infrastructure*

Elements to be analyzed separately	The means to bring coherence
Assessment of need and the services to meet the need	Care plans
Level of need of individuals, communities, and populations	Information systems
The different types of need	Organizational structures
The various perspectives as to need, e.g. those of the patient, carers, and various professionals	Representatives operating in relationships of trust and understanding

Team-building is the best-known aspect of OD. Some consider it to be the single most important element.[16] Its aim is to improve team effectiveness by enabling teams to analyze how they work together and improve their skills and effectiveness. However, for those readers who go cold at the prospect of playing silly games with colleagues, take heart! Guzzo and Shea[17] found that team-building has a positive effect on team members' attitudes to and perceptions of each other but does not increase team performance. Despite this, there are some essential elements of organizational development strategy which must exist if the team is to develop in a healthy way (Table 7.4). However, what managers will find is that, once again, time is the key, combined with objectives and, in extreme circumstances, external help from an expert. Table 7.4 lists the type of OD technique that may be of value, using Tuckman's[18] natural stages of team development. We refer interested readers to the literature.[16]

Summary

The theory so far has told us that there is more to a team than a group of professionals.

First, it should be clear, not just from this chapter, that patients with cancer need care from more than one discipline and that this is best delivered by a team. Studies in palliative care and of bereaved relatives seem to confirm this.[19]

Second, although elements of good teamwork are common sense, clarity about roles and tasks, and the development of stable, flexible, and accountable team life needs time, skilled management, and hard work.[20]

Third, the task never ends and, regardless of the ingredients, teams will cycle through phases of internal conflict, consolidation, and performance (the so-called processes of forming, storming, norming, and performing[18]). With these data, we can now return to our two examples of teams at work.

REVIEWING OUR SCENARIOS

James's team

We have just a small snapshot of James's team, but let us assume that it is representative of many groups of clinicians working together. From these we can take one of two views: this is a team in its early stages of development or this is a group of professionals working in the same place at the same time, rather than a team.

Table 7.4 *The natural stages of team development and behaviors*

Stage of development	Associated member behavior	Objective	Process and developmental need
Forming	Polite, enquiring, avoiding conflict	Agree on team's mission statement and setting of initial objectives	Strong internal leadership through meetings, brainstorming, and objective setting. An emphasis on unity and desire to be part of the group
Storming	Emotions begin to emerge as underlying conflicts begin to surface; some withdraw	Agree on rules of engagement, e.g. operational policy within the team, decision-making process, and establish leadership	Emerging differences of opinion among members, sometimes involving a challenge to leadership, when external help may be needed
Norming	Mutual respect, shared responsibilities	Improve relationships and test relationships with others outside the team	Personal and group evaluation, recognizing the strength of diversity while maintaining core values. The values rather than the wish to be part of the group begin to maintain unity
Performing	Maturity and mutual acceptance (warts and all!)	Productive and seeking to better	Understanding that none of us is as good as all of us. Celebrating the achievements of the team rather than the individuals. Striving together to improve

Either way, the outcome falls short of teamwork. The patient and her husband left with a prescription for a very strong pain-killer and were told that they needed to see a counselor. Communication between doctor and nurse is at best poor; there seems to be little understanding of each other's roles; there are no clear rules/protocols for case review or management; and it appears that there is no agreed time or format to discuss difficulties.

James's perception was that he had given plenty of his time to the patient, that he had nothing more to offer as a doctor, and that he needed to hand over the psychological and emotional care to the counselor. Linda's view was that he was yet again shirking his responsibilities as a team member in communicating with her and his patient the real truth about what was happening. Both, of course, are right. What went wrong was in the area of communication and an agreed *modus operandi* (an operational policy to use management-speak). What is encouraging is that these problems are soluble using basic approaches with open discussion, negotiation, and an agreed framework of accountability within the team. With some candid discussion, both Linda and James will realize that both of them needs to change. What they need is help to do this.

Let us look at an alternative scenario.

Janet walks in to the consulting room, sits down, and bursts into tears, saying that the pain in her side is not responding to the pain-killers. James glances at Colin, thinking to himself, "I can't take away their hope. Her chances of surviving more than 6 months are less than 10%. I'm going to need some help with this one." Addressing them together, he might say:

"We all know that the success of treatment is uncertain in the long term, but we do need to wait to see how well the radiotherapy controls the pain. In the meantime we can try stronger pain-killers.

"This is a very difficult time and I can see how terribly anxious you and Colin are this afternoon. I think there are other strategies we need to look at to help you both to cope with this situation, but I cannot do this on my own. Fortunately, I am part of a team and, with your permission, I'd like to take some advice from Linda, our counselor. May I ask her in to introduce you? You can then have an initial chat with her and we will all meet for a full discussion next week.

"Can I suggest that over the next few days you sit down together and write down all the questions you have for us and then, when you come back next Friday, we can sit down together with Linda to answer them all to the best of our ability."

In taking this approach, James has fulfilled his medical role in addressing the physical pain. Second, he is beginning to introduce other team members and their skills to help this couple cope with advancing disease and the pain of loss, change, and uncertainty. However, he has given some very important signals to Janet and Colin:

1 He understands that they are in crisis, he is taking things seriously, and he wants to keep a close eye on things.
2 They do not have to wait another month until the next appointment.
3 He does not know everything.
4 He works as part of a team.

"On your way out, make sure that you tell reception that you want a long appointment with Linda and I. That will ensure that we have sufficient time together to come up with a game-plan."

James then calls Linda in and makes the introductions. This takes a few moments longer, though he is still able to leave at 4 p.m., but this time everyone is clear about what is going on.

A long appointment is a 30-min one as opposed to a 10-min one. As part of their team development strategy, James and Linda had already agreed on criteria for joint consultations and their mutual roles for such interactions. This has resulted in a highly effective working relationship that provides a safer environment in which patients can ask difficult questions of the doctor. The team counselor is then able to arrange a further 30-min appointment with the patient if necessary, at which time more specific psychoemotional issues can be addressed. Mutual cases are then discussed at the regular interdisciplinary team meetings, which provide an environment for peer support and supervision.

By now we hope that you have concluded that, on the one hand, James's team demonstrates poor teamwork but, on the other hand, for there to be improvement does not require a completely different approach or group therapy, just common sense and communication. This is a young team about to enter the storming stage. Figure 7.1, adapted from Cummings,[21] illustrates the conflict management and strategies that the team may need.

The experienced team

Scenario 2 encapsulates the work of a team that has been in existence for more than 5 years. The apparent ease of assessment and the inclusion of the GP (and later the district nurses and hospital consultant) are only possible because of the structures that surround clinical practice. The team has clear referral criteria and goals, a mission statement, minimum standards of communication, clinical practice, notekeeping, a strong sense of corporate identity, and a clearly negotiated relationship between team members and those outside the team.

This does not mean that this kind of team is perfect, but the existence of checks and balances to engage complex problems minimizes the risk of patient or staff morbidity from poor communication. Needless to say, this has developed over the years and will have needed hard work and more than a little give and take. It is, however,

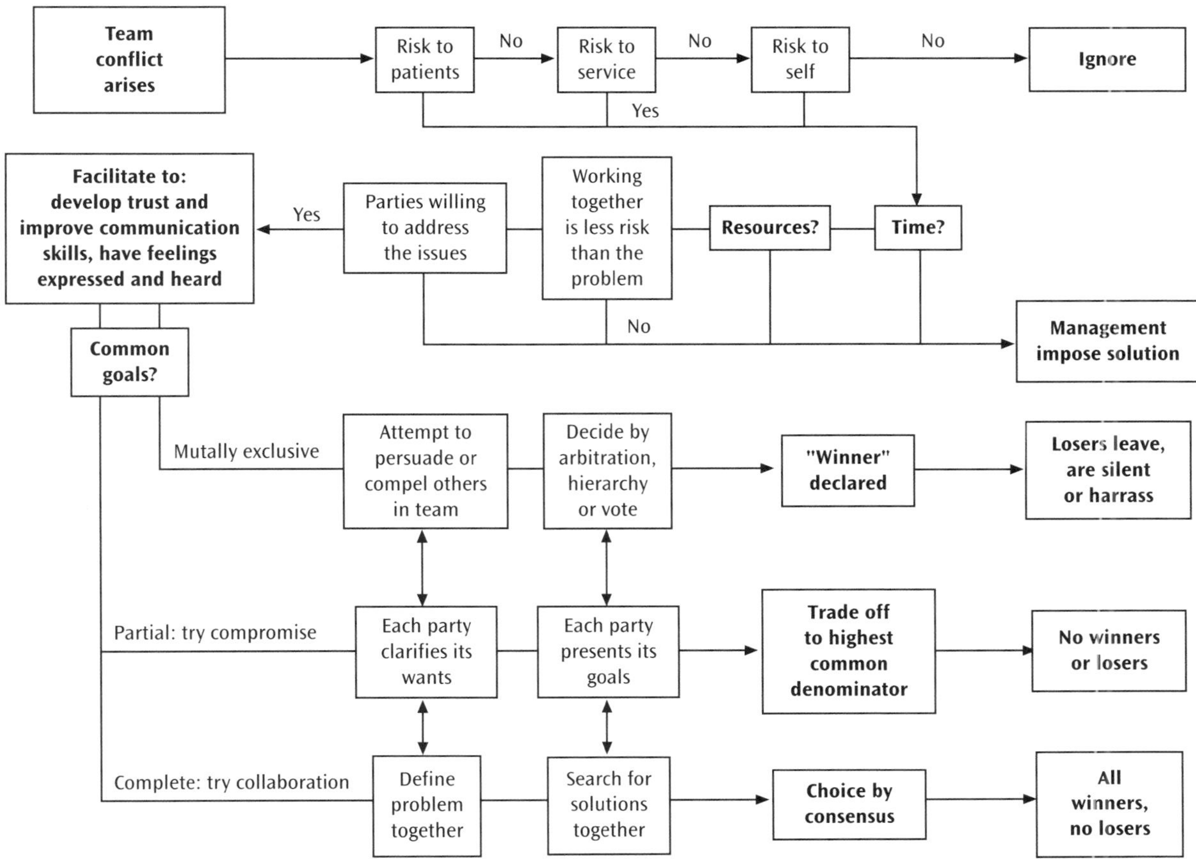

Figure 7.1 *An algorithm adapted from Cummings[21] suggesting means to resolve conflicts within teams.*

as a highly functional team, at risk of complacency and unthinking routine based in the belief that their way is the right way simply because it is the way that they do things.

Sooner or later, this team will begin to dysfunction and the arrival of a new member may well expose it (Fig. 7.1).

CONCLUSION

In this chapter we have attempted to illustrate how teamworking can make a difference to our patient care and our own working lives. Our cameos represent the two poles of teamwork. One extreme claims to be a team because they are in the same place at the same time once a week and make referrals to each other. The other is a team because they are so interdependent that they cannot function without each other. Each has strengths and weaknesses, and there are infinite shades between one and the other. It is also worth saying that any one team can operate along the spectrum according to the problem in hand, and in fact the most experienced teams are those in which the *modus operandi* is fluid and adaptable both to the environment and to the problems in hand. Only you will know at which point to balance your team.

REFERENCES

● 1. Dunlop R, Hockley J. In: Saunders C ed. *Hospice and Palliative Care. An Interdisciplinary Approach*. Sevenoaks: Edward Arnold, 1990: 14.
● 2. Sheldon F. Teamwork and palliative care: is it effective? In: Sheldon F ed. *Psychosocial Palliative Care*. Cheltenham: Stanley Thornes, 1997: 112.
3. Jones RVH. Teams and terminal cancer at home: do patients and carers benefit? *J Interprofessional Care* 1993; **7:** 239–44.
4. Firth-Cozens J. Building teams for effective audit. *Quality Hlth Care* 1992; **1:** 252–5.
● 5. McGrath M. *Multidisciplinary Teams*. Aldershot: Gower, 1991.
6. Field R, West M. Teamwork in primary health care. 1. Perspectives from practices. *J Interprofessional Care* 1995; **9:** 122–30.
◆ 7. Belbin M. *Management Teams: Why They Succeed or Fail*. Oxford: Butterworth-Heinemann, 1994.
◆ 8. Vachon MLS. Staff stress in hospice/palliative care: a review. *Palliative Med* **9:** 91–122.
9. Cooper CL, Mitchell S. Nursing the critically ill and dying. *Human Relations* 1990; **43:** 297–311.

10. Mallett K, Price JH, Jurs SG, Slenker S. Relationships amongst burnout, death anxiety and social support in hospice and critical care nurses. *Psychol Rep* 1991; **68:** 1347–59.

● 11. West M. *Effective Teamwork*. Leicester: BPS Books, 1994: 66.

12. Pietroni PC. Towards reflective practice: the languages of health and social care. *J Interprofessional Care* 1992; **6:** 7–16.

◆ 13. Herxheimer I, Begent R, Maclean D, *et al*. The short life of a terminal care support team: the experience at Charing Cross Hospital. *Br Med J* 1985; **290:** 1877–9.

14. Øvretveit J. *Co-ordinating Community Care*. Buckingham: Open University Press, 1993: 26–7.

15. Iles P, Auluck R. From organizational to interorganizational development in nursing practice: improving the effectiveness of interdisciplinary teamwork and collaboration. *J Advanced Nursing* 1990, **15:** 50–8.

● 16. Moxon P. *Building a Better Team*. Aldershot: Gower, 1993.

17. Guzzo RA, Shea GP. In: Dunnette MD, Hough LM eds. *Handbook of Industrial and Organizational Psychology*, Consulting Psychologists Press: Palo Alto, CA, 1992.

● 18. Tuckman BW Development Sequence in Small Groups. *Psychol Bull* 1965; **63:** 284–499.

19. Hearn J, Higginson IJ. Do specialist palliative care teams improve outcomes for cancer patients? A systematic literature review. *Palliative Med* 1998; **12:** 317–32.

20. Smeenk FWJM, van Haastegt JCM, de Witte LP, Crebolder HFJM. Effectiveness of homecare programmes for patients with incurable cancer on their quality of life and time spent in hospital: a systematic review. *Br Med J* 1998; **316:** 1939–44.

◆ 21. Cummings I. Interdisciplinary teamworking. In: Doyle D, Hanks G, MacDonald N eds. *Oxford Textbook of Palliative Medicine*. Oxford: Oxford University Press, 1999: 28.

8

Palliative care – care for the dying, home care, the last days of life

MALGORZATA KRAJNIK AND ZBIGNIEW ZYLICZ

This chapter deals with the characteristics of palliative care, its definition, and its aims. It will focus on the needs of dying patients and the likelihood of these needs being met at home, in hospital, and in other institutions specifically designed for the care of the terminally ill. The preventive and proactive potential of palliative care will be highlighted. In addition, ethical problems and the increasing pressure from patients and the family to end the patient's life will be discussed.

DEFINITION

Palliative care is usually defined as total and continuous care for patients and/or their families when the patient's disease does not respond to curative treatment and death becomes inevitable. Control of pain and other symptoms, including psychological, social, and spiritual problems, is paramount. The goal of palliative care is to achieve the best possible quality of life for patients and their families.[1]

ANTICIPATION OF PATIENTS' NEEDS

From the above definition it is clear that care for the terminally ill is primarily based on recognizing the needs of patients and their families. Carers need to be ready to listen to and look out for the real needs of their clients. Not all patients' needs are obvious, and some may not be communicated to the carers. Understanding the patient requires considerable communication skills.

When analyzing and classifying the needs of terminally ill patients, one should recognize that some needs are hidden in the subconscious. Patients often do not communicate with their carers about their needs because they do not realize how important these needs are. For example, as long as a particular bodily function works properly, patients do not realize how important it is for their quality of life. They take it for granted until things deteriorate. At this time, patients feel very stongly that unnecessary loss of bodily functions should be prevented or delayed. To do this properly, carers need to know more about the hidden needs of the patient, e.g. coping style and culture, but they also need to anticipate the losses by understanding the natural history of the disease. A breast cancer patient with bone metastases may remark to her physician that her left leg is "slower" than the right one. For a healthy person this would be a vague sign not necessitating any action and justifying a wait and see policy. For a cancer patient with vertebral metastases, the same symptom may herald spinal cord compression. Not anticipating this may delay and compromise treatment. These unrecognized needs may be seen as the foundations of a house. The whole house of needs stands on them although the patient does not realize how important they are. So, here at this level, prevention of unnecessary loss is the major task of professional carers.

The second level of the house of needs is the living

room. These are the needs that are easy to see and to discuss: "Control my pain, my discomfort or anxiety." Most of the symptoms have a physical, measurable dimension. At this physical level, it is easy for patients to communicate with their carers. Proper diagnosis should lead to adequate treatment. However, this approach has its own limitations.

Some patients will take their carers to the third level of the house. This is the top floor, hidden under the roof. It is a private and intimate bedroom, full of emotions, memories, good and bad experiences, shame, and unresolved losses – sometimes from the past. These experiences, for example the death of a partner, however long ago, may have an important influence on patients' current behavior. If a lost partner suffered severe, uncontrolled dyspnea before death, then patients may be afraid that breathlessness, even if it is unlikely, will complicate their terminal illness. In the past, physicians believed this third level, necessitating spiritual care, to be the domain of priests and psychologists. The third level, however, contains valuable information about patients' behavior and understanding of their disease. The problem is that not every carer and not every physician is allowed to visit this level. Carers need to earn their patients' trust. Palliative care depends on the integration of all three levels of need: prevention of loss, symptom control, and spiritual care.

THE AIMS OF PALLIATIVE CARE

The main purpose of curative treatment is to restore health by eradicating disease. In patients with terminal disease, restoration of health is not possible and the physician must accept death as the inevitable and natural consequence of disease. The issue here is to bring the patient into the best possible balance – physically as well as emotionally and spiritually. This balance will facilitate adaptation, making losses easier to communicate and to tolerate. Questions raised by patients about death include not only why and when, but also how. In this respect carers may provide a great deal of comfort by patiently explaining the symptoms and processes of dying, making the inevitable less frightening for the patient. Carers should provide comfort and a feeling of security. In hospices these two aims are paramount. The processes of adaptation to dying are not forced but facilitated.

Another aim of palliative care is to maintain the best possible quality of life. This is achieved by trying to make the patient as independent as possible. Meeting this aim starts with pain therapy. For example, morphine may provide sufficient pain relief to allow the patient to be more active and able to visit the toilet. However, in toxic doses morphine may result in the patient being less active, somnolent, and confused. The more specific the pain treatment strategy, the better the effect on activity. For instance, treating pain that is poorly responsive to opioids with morphine alone necessitates higher morphine doses, which increase the chance of toxic effects. The patient suffers now not from pain but from limitations on activity.

Patients' goals may be different from those of the healthy professional carer, who may presume that pain relief is the patient's top priority. A terminally ill patient may prefer to tolerate pain in order to be able to drive a car and visit a daughter who has just given birth to the patient's first grandchild. The recognition of the patient's agenda must be included in the whole strategy of pain and symptom control. Professionals in palliative care should therefore be very creative in their choices of therapies. Pain should be viewed not separately but in the context of the whole person and his or her needs.

ACCEPTANCE OF DEATH

Palliative care accepts that death and dying are natural elements of life, like birth. However, this acceptance does not imply that palliative care is a passive activity. Palliative care is active and total care in which anticipation and prevention of unnecessary losses play an important role. Acceptance of death causes a change in the priorities of the care. Some drugs and treatments useful in the earlier stages of disease have no value when death is approaching. Other therapies rarely used in the early stages of disease become valuable in the terminal phase. However, some patients, families, and carers never reach an acceptance of death. As a result, there is a real risk of loss of dignity and frustrations that may complicate grieving and bereavement.

Failure to accept death and dying may increase the distress around the patient and make proper recognition of the patient's needs more difficult. However, the healing role of acceptance in the hospice environment should not be overemphasized. According to Higginson *et al.*,[2] the main problems identified at referrals to hospital palliative care units are family anxiety, symptom control, and communication between patient and family. In the same study, 15 of the 17 key indicators of STAS (support team assessment schedule) were found to improve significantly between referral and the last week of life; there was no improvement in family anxiety or spiritual needs. Patient anxiety, family anxiety, pain control, and symptom control continued until death.

THE CONCEPT OF TOTAL PAIN

Total pain is experienced by the whole person and consists of physical, psychological, social, or spiritual dimensions. The suffering caused by physical pain is worsened when the patient does not believe that it can be relieved and when the meaning of the pain is directly related to approaching death.[3] Therefore, it is important to control symptoms properly, and to make the cause of pain known and understandable for the patient. A sense of loss of meaning and purpose, helplessness, hopelessness, and endlessness are other elements of total pain.[4,5] It is important to remember that hope may be increased by showing that the patient is valued, which reinforces the patient as a person; meaningful relationships with the proper dose of humor; and good symptom control. Giving realistic goals to patient and family can ease helplessness and endlessness. Broken relationships may also cause psychological pain; many patients need to forgive and be forgiven.[6] The patient must also be sustained spiritually as everybody has spiritual needs, even those without a formal faith. Common existential issues include hopelessness, disappointment, remorse, death anxiety, disruption of personal identity, and the meaninglessness of continued life.[5] The spiritual pain should be addressed, and dying patients and their families face questions of purpose and the need to understand the story of their lives.[7] The physician may suggest to the patient that it would be helpful to bring spiritual issues to the attention of a spiritual leader. The release from anxiety and feelings of guilt, which may be observed, for example, after confession or sacramental rituals among Roman Catholics and other Christians, often produces physical relaxation with relief of pain and makes dying easier.[8] However, it should be remembered that spiritual distress is related not only to a deity or religious beliefs but also to how comfortable an individual is with himself and those around him. The relief of total pain may allow a patient to regain a sense of integration by discovering a renewed sense of meaning and purpose within his or her own personal experience of discomfort and dying.[9,10]

PLACE OF DYING

Dying at home or in the hospital?

For centuries, many cultures have embraced the notion that people should remain at home to die,[11] and even in the early twentieth century most people died at home. However, the number of people dying at home has fallen progressively, and more patients are now admitted to hospital. The reasons for this phenomenon include an increase in the number of elderly people living in residential and nursing homes and in the number of people living alone or in small families; so there are fewer people to share the burden of looking after the terminally ill.[11] Despite the introduction and growth of the palliative care movement in the UK and USA, more than 60% of deaths occur in hospitals.[12,13] By contrast, the demand for home care in many countries has grown rapidly in the past decade. In the USA between 1980 and 1996, the number of patients in home health care increased by more than 400%.[14] For home hospice care this growth is even more significant. Patients and families are choosing the option of home care more frequently for many reasons, including:[15]

- an aging population;
- the increasing prevalence of chronic incurable diseases;
- increased hospital costs due to high-technology services;
- earlier discharge from hospitals to homes;
- in some countries the desire of patients or their families to avoid prolonged expensive care at the end of life;
- patients' choice to receive care at home;
- preference for autonomy.

It has been shown that home care is a viable option for both patient and carers provided they are given the support they require. Factors significantly associated with dying at home are the patient's preference for this and the availability of a family member other than the spouse to be involved in the patient's care.[16] When good support services are available, most patients who express a preference for dying at home have their wish fulfilled: some patients who initially would prefer to be admitted to hospital change their mind when they find out how well they can be supported at home. A hospital environment is not ideal for attending to the needs of the terminally ill and their families, and both families and staff feel the frustration of the situation. Home care for the terminally ill is increasing in popularity as a result of three important factors:[17]

- Death at home is a more cost-effective option than death in an institutionalized setting.[18,19]
- In the hospital system, social, psychological, and spiritual needs are often ignored; difficulties in communication between hospital staff and the patient and family have been linked to fragmentation of care and to marginalization or exclusion of both the patient and family.[20]
- Death at home contributes to an overall higher quality of life for patients and family, giving a sense of normality.[21]

In addition, many patients and families equate care at home with freedom and control.[22]

However, home care is very demanding. Studies show that the proportion of patients admitted to institutions from home care services increases with the length of the care period.[23] The principal reasons for the discontinuance of home care have been identified as poor pain control, unrelieved emotional distress, and family strain for a multitude of reasons.[24] When choosing home care, it is important to recognize the increased demands that will be placed on family members or other caregivers assisting the patient. Home care requires family members or the patient to be capable of learning the necessary skills such as wound care or drug administration. Although costs are reduced compared with hospitalization, home care may only be achieved at the expense of increased personal cost to family members' emotional, social, physical, and financial well-being. Home care until death requires a fit relative who can cope with serious illness, nurses who can visit the patient at least once daily, an available capable physician, a team that can respond quickly to a new problem, and a guarantee of rapid admission in the event of a major crisis.

In general, the public regards hospitals rather than home as the best place to cope with patients with pain and other symptoms. However, most studies have found that a better level of pain control is achieved at home and in hospices than in hospitals. In addition, patients' satisfaction with home care is significantly higher than satisfaction with conventional care.[25] This supports the view that a less interventionist approach and a caring atmosphere are appreciated. Generally, hospice patients are more likely to die at home, and families are satisfied with that outcome.[26] Interestingly, even in a study in which the quality of life of cancer patients nursed at home was assessed as not very high, only 3% of relatives of patients who died at home subsequently wished that death had occurred in hospital.[27] Sometimes the patients, family, and staff know that symptom relief could be improved by inpatient admission, but the patient prefers to tolerate pain or other symptoms in order to stay at home. One of the reasons why patients and their families might avoid inpatient admission for pain control may be the way the patient was treated in the hospital in the past. Return to hospital may recall the disappointment the patient experienced when tumor recurrence had been diagnosed. The way this was communicated to the patient may also be critical. At the beginning of the disease patients are frequently encouraged to accept unpleasant treatments.

Whatever the patient's choices, one should remember that 90% of days in the last year before death are spent at home and that the general practitioner is the main person responsible for the well-being of patients at any stage in their illness, but particularly in the terminal phase.[28]

Home care by general practitioners

McWhinney[29] identified two attitudes assumed by general practitioners in dealing with patients and their needs: proactive and reactive. Reactive physicians wait for the symptom, then diagnose and prescribe treatment: the principle of action and reaction. Proactive physicians, especially when dealing with patients at home, will plan the care and anticipate many problems of the terminally ill. They will try to avoid critical situations and unnecessary losses.[30] At least half of palliative care is anticipatory and preventive. However, this type of care can be very complex. At any one time, terminally ill patients have, on average, 10 problems requiring attention. Only 50% of these problems will be reported as symptoms; the others, although equally important to the patient, are not reported because the patient believes that they are too trivial to be worthy of the doctor's attention.[31] Experience of such problems as well as knowledge about the natural course of the disease is paramount.

General practitioners see few terminal cancer patients dying at home and may therefore have insufficient knowledge and experience to anticipate all problems. This may be an important determinant of reactive practice.

In The Netherlands the desire for autonomy and the wish to die at home may be a reason for the increase in the number of requests for euthanasia.[32] Most euthanasia is carried out by general practitioners at home. These practitioners need to make life and death decisions about their patients alone, without the support of a multidisciplinary team. As patients who prefer to die at home will not want to be readmitted to hospital, even when they have complex problems, their general practitioners may run short of ideas as to how to treat their patients' symptoms. As the suffering increases, both general practitioner and the patient may reach the conclusion that all options have been exhausted and euthanasia is the most logical and humane solution. Bedside consultations by experienced palliative care physicians or specialist nurses may dramatically change this situation.

Hospice or palliative care unit? Is this the solution?

A great deal has been written about palliative care units and hospices, which in the last 30 years have flourished throughout the world.[33] Hospices may be divided into two types with different aims and responsibilities. Low-care hospices provide 24-h care with a minimal staff (including general practitioner, district nurses, and volunteers), especially to those who are alone. High-care hospitals and palliative care units are usually larger institutions that specialize in palliative care for the terminally ill patient. They may have their own admission capacity, but may also provide support to general practitioners, low-care hospices, and residents of nursing homes. One of our patients with multiple sclerosis and brain tumor, when asked what she thought of hospice care, told us "It's the best choice in a situation where there is no choice."

EUTHANASIA REQUESTS: HOW TO DEAL WITH THEM?

In recent years, it has been increasingly common for patients to want to discuss euthanasia. In The Netherlands, about 25% of patients referred to hospice care requested assisted death, usually before admission.[32] Some patients may refuse to be admitted to hospice because it does not provide euthanasia. Different reasons underlie requests for euthanasia.

Group A (afraid)

Patients in this group, who account for 80% of requests for euthanasia, are afraid of something. Their fears may be real or imagined, but are very often exacerbated by the feelings of hopelessness and lack of purpose associated with suffering. In many cases, the unhealed "soul wounds" of the patient can be recognized and treated.[34] The request in these cases can be interpreted as a cry for help and for recognition of real, if sometimes hidden, needs. Continuous professional care and a safe environment provide the best means of comfort. Most patients in this group will never mention assisted death again.

Group B (burn-out)

Group B consists of a small proportion of patients (approximately 5%) who wish to die early because they are "burnt out." If the terminal phase of disease is prolonged, burn-out may become a real threat, affecting both patient and carers. In the case of "burn-out syndrome," it is better to concentrate on its prevention. Making the right decision at the right moment is as important as treating symptoms. Withdrawal of treatment aimed at prolonging life may also be important in the prevention of critical situations that may lead to burn-out. As such patients are not depressed, but exhausted, treatment with antidepressants is pointless.

Group C (control-oriented)

Patients who fall into group C (less than 1%) are "control-oriented." They rarely seek help from a hospice. They have an intrinsic drive to control every single minute of their life and they are very much self-oriented. They do not always see the suffering that their decision causes their family. The risk of pathological bereavement for the family may be increased.

Group D (depressed)

Patients in D group (approximately 10%) are "depressed." Most cases of depression are treatable with psychotherapy, together with the prescription of antidepressants. The important issue is early diagnosis.

Group E (extreme)

The patients from E group suffer "extreme" pain or other intractable symptoms. It is not unknown for patients to refuse treatment so that symptoms become intractable, their subsequent suffering being used to justify their wish to die sooner. More frequently, these situations are similar to the case of patients with unrelieved total pain.[5] In these cases, when everything possible has been done, sedation may be increased. There should be a clear difference between this treatment and euthanasia.

Through the accurate assessment of each group of patients different interventions may be designed. These interventions may be successful in allowing patients to die a peaceful death and families to undergo, as far as possible, an uncomplicated bereavement.

INTERVENTIONS AT THE END OF LIFE

Simplifying treatment

When death is very near some treatments may become irrelevant. Their aims may be unrealistic and their toxicity increased. In addition, these treatments may interfere with the drugs that are necessary to control pain or other symptoms. Patients may be psychologically dependent on the treatment they have received in the past, and it may be difficult to accept that these measures are now unnecessary or even toxic. Discontinuing all of these treatments on the first day of admission to the palliative care unit may reflect badly on the care provided by the general practitioner or medical specialist before admission. It is not unusual for a patient's condition to improve after discontinuation of some treatments, which may challenge the relationship between the patient and the previous prescriber.

Terminal cancer syndrome

Many patients with different types of malignancies go through a common clinical pathway that has been defined as "terminal cancer syndrome."[35] Despite differences in tumor types, patients present similarly with declining performance and nutritional status, fatigue, anorexia, lack of feeling of well-being, pain, and insomnia. How people die remains in the memories of those who live on, and for them, as for the patient, one should be aware of the nature and management of terminal pain and distress.

Symptom control when death is near

Symptom relief in the last days of a patient's life is a continuation of what is already being done. However, new problems may emerge in the terminal phase. Symptom management and patient comfort have been identified by the family members as their primary concerns in caring for patients with cancer at home.[36] Even when pain is controlled optimally, about one-quarter of patients experience no relief of other symptoms, such as nausea, vomiting, dyspnea, dysphagia, and confusion.[37] So pain must not be seen as the only and most important symptom, and its absence does not equal good quality of life or dying. Pain should always be seen in the context of the whole person and other symptoms. Pain, paradoxically, may also be the easiest symptom to control.

In a small percentage of patients, death at home or in a hospice is not peaceful (Tables 8.1 and 8.2),[38] but good control of symptoms and a peaceful death (as perceived by the doctors) can be achieved by most patients, in contrast to public expectations and fears.

The control of symptoms other than pain is discussed in detail in Chapter Ca22.

CARE FOR THE FAMILY

The family needs to be prepared not only psychologically but also practically for what to do in case of different eventualities. A syringe driver should be available, and a supply of essential drugs in suppository or parenteral form should be kept in the home. Early decisions of what, in an emergency, may be done by the family and what by the nurse should be clear. Contrary to what many believe, most patients and relatives do want to know what to expect and what is not likely to happen. Lack of such planning often precipitates unnecessary stress.

As death approaches the family members need to be aware of what might happen and should be made aware that the patient's means of communication may be impaired. Based on observations during patients' final 24 h, it has been reported that about 67% of patients are drowsy or semiconscious, 23% are unconscious or unresponsive, and 10% are alert.[38] Lightening or a lucid interval before death may be seen occasionally, but occurs less often if extra medication is given.

Relatives often feel a strong need to be present at the moment when their loved one dies, and this is much more likely to be the case if the patient dies at home. The loss of a loved one is a very distressing experience, but there is evidence that being present at the death can help relatives and friends to cope better with their loss and grief.[39] Sometimes patients "choose" to die during the only short period when the family has left the room. In such cases, family members may feel that they let down their loved one and it is essential to stress that some patients need their final solitary space. Telling the family that they can speak normally, move, and even laugh sometimes is all part of the mental preparation for death. When the final stage of illness lasts for days, emotional pain may cause exhaustion among family members. They might wonder why the loved one has not died yet. Sometimes the answer is that the patient has not had a chance to say goodbye to everybody, but sometimes the family will beg the patient not to die. In such a situation, discussion about "letting go" and learning to say goodbye may be helpful. Making the final communication by sharing thoughts and feelings can help the relatives cope with the separation. The loss of the loved one always leaves a mark on those who survive. Studies confirm that encouraging families to focus on the actual death and being present for it make the process of bereavement easier.

Table 8.1 *Frequency of symptoms in the last 48 h of life (from Lichter and Hunt[38] with permission)*

Symptom	%
Noisy and moist breathing	56
Urinary dysfunction	53
Incontinence	32
Retention	21
Pain	51
Restlessness and agitation	42
Dyspnea	22
Nausea and vomiting	14
Sweating	14
Jerking, twitching, plucking	12
Confusion	9

Table 8.2 *Causes of nonpeaceful death (from Lichter and Hunt[38] with permission)*

Symptoms	%
Hemorrhage and hemoptysis	2
Respiratory distress	2
Restlessness	1.5
Pain	1
Myocardial infarction	1
Regurgitation	1
Total	8.5

CONCLUSION

The goals of palliative care have been summarized by Roy[40] as:

- to help those who need not die to live, and to live with a maximum of freedom from constraints on their quality of life arising from acute and chronic conditions of the body;
- to help those who can no longer live to die on time – not too early and not too late;
- to help the dying, whether in hospital, nursing home, hospice, or at home, to die with dignity and in peace.

REFERENCES

◆ 1. World Health Organization. *Cancer Pain Relief and Palliative Care.* Report of a WHO Expert Committee.

Technical Report Series 804, Geneva: World Health Organization, 1990: 11–12.

2. Higginson I, Wade A, McCarthy M. Effectiveness of two palliative care support teams. *J Publ Hlth Med* 1992; **14:** 50–6.

● 3. Twycross R, Lichter I. The terminal phase. In: Doyle D, Hanks, G, MacDonald N eds. *Oxford Textbook of Palliative Medicine*. Oxford, Oxford University Press, 1998: 977–92.

4. Chapman CR, Gavrin J. Suffering and its relation to pain. *J Palliative Care* 1993; **9:** 5–13.

5. Cherny NI, Coyle N, Foley KM. Suffering in the advanced cancer patient: a definition and taxonomy. *J Palliative Care* 1994; **10:** 57–70.

6. Clark R. Forgiveness in the hospice setting. *Palliative Med* 1990; **4:** 305–10.

7. McGee EM. Can suicide intervention in hospice be ethical? *J Palliative Care* 1997; **13:** 27–33.

8. Saunders C. The care of the dying patient and his family. *Contact* 1972; Suppl. 38, 12–18.

● 9. Saunders C, Baines M. *Living with Dying*. Oxford: Oxford University Press, 1984.

10. Byock I. When suffering persists. *J Palliative Care* 1994; **10:** 8–13.

11. Thorpe G. Enabling more dying people to remain at home. *Br Med J* 1993; **307:** 915–18.

12. O'Henley A, Curzio J, Hunt J. Palliative care services and settings: comparing care. *Int J Palliative Nursing* 1997; **3:** 161–7.

◆ 13. Foley KM. Competent care for the dying instead of physician-assisted suicide. *N Engl J Med* 1997; **336:** 54–7.

14. Vladeck BC. From the health care financing administration. *JAMA* 1996; **274**: 449.

15. Montauk SL. Home health care. *Am Family Phys* 1998; **57:** 1608–14.

16. McWhinney MD, Bass MJ, Orr V. Factors associated with location of death (home or hospital) of patients referred to a palliative care team. *Can Med Assoc J* 1995; **152:** 361–7.

17. Osuna E, Perz-Carceles MD, Esteban MA, Luna A. The right to information for the terminally ill patient. *J Med Ethics* 1998; **24:** 106–9.

18. Chochinov HM, Kristjanson L. Dying to pay: the cost of end-of-life care. *J Palliative Care* 1998; **14:** 5–15.

19. Aiken LH. Evaluation research and public policy: lessons learned from the National Hospice Study. *J Chron Dis* 1986; **39:** 1–4.

● 20. Field D, James N. Where and how people die. In: Clark D ed. *The Future of Palliative Care: Issues of Policy and Practice*. Philadelphia, PA: Open University Press, 1993: 43–61.

21. Roe DJ. Palliative care 2000 – home care. *J Palliative Care* 1992; **8:** 28–32.

22. Davies B, Reimer JC, Brown P, Martens N. *Fading away: The Experience of Transition in Families with Terminal Illness*. New York, NY: Baywood, 1995.

◆ 23. Hinton J. Can home care maintain an acceptable quality of life for patients with terminal cancer and their relatives? *Palliative Med* 1994; **8:** 183–96.

24. Parkes CM. Home or hospital? Terminal care as seen by surviving spouses. *J R Coll Gen Pract* 1978; **28:** 19–30.

25. Seale C. A comparison of hospice and conventional care. *Soc Sci Med* 1991; **32:** 147–52.

26. Greer DS, Mor V, Morris JN, *et al*. An alternative in terminal care: results of the National Hospice Study. *J Chron Dis* 1986; **39:** 9–26.

◆ 27. Wilkes E. Occasional survey: dying now. *Lancet* 1984; **323:** 950–2.

28. Levy B, Searle AB. Fatal illness in general practice. *J R Coll Gen Pract* 1976; 26, 303–7.

29. McWhinney IR. *Textbook of Family Medicine*. London: Oxford University Press, 1989.

● 30. Doyle D. Domiciliary palliative care. In: Doyle D, Hanks G, MacDonald N eds. *Oxford Textbook of Palliative Medicine*. Oxford: Oxford University Press, 1998: 957–73.

31. Cartwright A, Hockey L, Anderson R. *Life before Death*. London: Kegan Paul, 1973.

◆ 32. Zylicz Z, Janssens MJPA. Options in palliative care: dealing with those who want to die. *Baillière's Clin Anaesthesiol* 1998; **12:** 121–31.

33. Saunders C, Kastenbaum R eds. *Hospice Care on the International Scene*. New York, NY: Springer, 1997.

◆ 34. Kearney M. *Mortally Wounded. Stories of Soul Pain, Death and Healing*. Dublin: Mercier Press, 1996.

35. Vigano A, Bruera E, Suarez-Almaroz ME. Terminal cancer syndrome: myth or reality, 12th International Congress on care of the terminally ill. *J Palliative Care* 1998; **14:** 127.

36. Kristjanson LJ. Quality of terminal care: salient indicators identified by families. *J Palliative Care* 1989; **5:** 21–28.

37. Jones RVH, Hansford J, Fiske J. Death from cancer at home: the carers' perspective. *Br Med J* 1993; **306:** 249–51.

◆ 38. Lichter I, Hunt E. The last 48 h of life. *J Palliative Care* 1990; **6:** 7–15.

39. Legrand M, Gomas JM. Being present at the last moments of life. *Eur J Palliative Care* 1998; **5:** 191–4.

40. Roy DJ. The relief of pain and suffering: ethical principles and imperatives. *J Palliative Care* 1998; **14:** 3–5.

9

Ethical issues

FIONA RANDALL

The relief of suffering and the prolongation of life are the essential aims of health care. As the relief of pain, a major component of suffering, is an aim of health care, it follows that attempting to relieve pain is a *moral obligation* in health care, and must be an intrinsic part of the professional's role.

We should also note that, as the prolongation of life is an aim of health care, there must be an underlying assumption that there is a moral obligation not to cause the patient's death.

Pain control is not one of those areas normally associated with major moral dilemmas, but it does give rise to important moral issues that tend to be overlooked amidst the more dramatic ethical problems in health care.

PAIN CONTROL AS A MORAL OBLIGATION

As pain control is an intrinsic part of the health care professional role, and is a moral obligation within that role, the importance accorded by professionals to pain relief is a moral issue in itself. It is strange and morally questionable that, in general, a low priority is given to education about pain relief in undergraduate and postgraduate medical education, especially when compared with the priority given to life-prolonging measures. The low priority given to pain control in education is reflected in doctors' attitudes to the importance of pain relief.

For example, all physicians would consider that they should have a good basic knowledge of the management of common life-threatening disorders such as diabetes. They consider that they should be able to commence a simple insulin regimen, giving the correct sort of insulin at the appropriate intervals, in such a way as to balance the blood sugar. Yet relatively few consider that they should be able to commence a comparable simple opiate regimen, giving the morphine at the appropriate intervals, in such a way as to balance the pain. Thus, all hospital physicians could manage diabetes adequately if not well, but many would have great difficulty with pain control because it is not accorded sufficient importance in education.

Doctors should be competent in basic pain control, which should be accorded the same importance in education as basic life-prolonging treatment. They should also be sufficiently motivated to ensure that good pain control is provided as a priority for every patient.

It is likely that the standard of pain relief we offer patients will not improve until we manage to remind doctors that pain relief is a moral obligation in health care, not an optional extra. It follows from this that doctors have an obligation to be *competent* at a basic level in pain control, and that they have an obligation to *provide the treatment* that achieves pain control. Doctors with specialist knowledge and experience should take every opportunity to pass that knowledge on to others, and should also to try to encourage others to strive continuously to achieve the best possible pain control in all patients.

INFORMED CONSENT AND HONESTY IN PAIN CONTROL

The second issue that we tend to forget is that pain control is most likely to be successful when patients understand their illness and the ways in which the medication is intended to alleviate pain. Informed consent is, of course, a basic tenet of health care. Yet much more than a minimum standard of consent is required before patients are able to work in partnership with their doctors to control pain. We know that patients usually require understanding of their illness and the medications in order to ensure compliance and safety with drug regimens.

For example, patients with advanced malignant disease are often afraid to take morphine at all, let alone take it regularly, unless they understand both the nature of their disease and the ways in which morphine works best. Where knowledge of their diagnosis has been withheld from patients, sometimes at the instigation of well-meaning relatives, patients are not in a position to comprehend the importance and advantages of having good pain control. They often suffer unnecessarily because this lack of understanding leads to a reluctance to take analgesics. Explanation is required to reassure them that addiction to morphine will not occur, and that if taken early in the illness it will not become ineffective in the later stages. Patients who are unaware of the nature of their illness may decline to take adequate analgesia as they always expect to get better and so hope not to require it.

Thus, seeking informed consent to treatment with appropriate analgesic regimens usually entails a discussion about the clinical circumstances in general – it is not just a matter of asking the patient to take morphine. Of course, patients may decline analgesia, or may occasionally want to retain a degree of pain as a yardstick of how the illness is going, but doctors should make sure that a refusal of analgesia is made only after the patient has had the opportunity to comprehend the medical facts of the situation. In other words, by offering information doctors should endeavor to ensure that refusal of consent is informed.

Seeking informed consent from patients includes informing them about the harms and risks of treatment, and this includes the side-effects of medications. It is easy to become so overwhelmed by a desire to relieve the patient's pain that we lose sight of the parallel obligation to inform patients of the significant side-effects of the drugs or procedures. This happens particularly when it seems to the professionals that the benefit of pain relief far outweighs the harm of a particular side-effect, such as constipation or sedation. Some drugs, for instance non-steroidal anti-inflammatory agents, are associated with a multitude of side-effects, some of which are serious and not uncommon, especially in the context of advanced malignancy. In particular, gastrointestinal hemorrhage may be precipitated by their use. It is easy in our enthusiasm to try to control pain, and because we consider that the benefits of the drugs outweigh their harms in the circumstances, to fail to mention serious and relatively common side-effects that present harms or risks.

There is an objective medical view of the importance of these harms and risks in the circumstances, and this view is based on value judgments as well as factual information. However, we know that patients place different values on various harms and benefits, so that what may seem to the doctor to be an acceptable harm or risk may not be acceptable to the patient. Therefore, even if the doctor considers that the benefits of an analgesic outweigh the side-effects, it can be argued that the doctor should mention the side-effects to the patient, because the latter may consider certain adverse effects as particularly undesirable.

For example, whereas some patients would rather be completely pain free, even if this means being drowsy, others would rather accept some pain, for instance on movement, rather than feel sedated by the analgesics. Patients need to be offered the chance to participate fully in decision-making regarding analgesia, because full participation increases the chance of establishing the best regimen for them. Therefore, doctors have a moral obligation to try to enable patients to have a basic *understanding* of their illness and pain-killers so that they can work together with their doctors to overcome the pain.

On the other hand, the right to give informed consent and to be fully involved in decision-making regarding pain control should not be transformed into a duty. In other words, giving fully informed consent should not become a condition of receiving adequate pain control. It seems intuitively wrong that patients who do not want much information should have to have it forced upon them and thus be forced to give fully informed consent before pain control is provided. Some patients, especially those who are terminally ill and exhausted, do not wish to be fully informed or involved in decision-making, and it seems reasonable to respect their choice in this regard. They may state that they do not want to discuss all the details of their illness or to receive a list of side-effects of medications. Instead, they may want professionals to offer what they consider is the best option and then they choose to accept that option on less information than would be regarded as adequate for fully informed consent. It seems reasonable that such patients should be able to choose the extent of their involvement in decision-making. They are responsible then for that choice.

CONTROL OF PSYCHOSOCIAL ASPECTS OF PAIN

The multifactorial etiology of pain has become appreciated, and the concept of "total pain" has been generally accepted. Total pain is a concept relating to distress that includes emotional, social, and spiritual components as well as the purely physical pain aspect of the pathology. In terminally ill patients and those suffering chronic pain, professionals are increasingly encouraged to consider that the aim is to alleviate total pain, which, of course, entails addressing emotional, social, and spiritual sources of distress. This goes way beyond the traditional remit of health care, and it raises some moral issues. For example, is it realistic to imply that professionals can alleviate non-physical sources of distress? How cost-effective in terms of resources (especially professional time) is it to attempt to do this? Has the patient given any form of consent to interventions designed to alleviate emotional, social or spiritual distress?

In particular, in the context of palliative care it is generally considered that professionals should try to alleviate emotional and social pain, and that doing so entails knowing how the patient and family are adjusting to the whole illness scenario and how it is affecting their relationships with each other. All of this entails questioning the patient and family about intimate relationships. Such questioning is unjustifiably intrusive if the patient has not requested such assistance, or at least given consent freely to discussions about his or her very private affairs. It is all too easy, especially if buoyed up by an almost missionary zeal to alleviate total pain, for professionals to intrude into people's private affairs under the (probably misguided) impression that we can alleviate emotional, social, and spiritual distress. Our motivation to alleviate these components of total pain should not drive us to intervene without the patient's consent, just as our motivation to alleviate the physical component of pain with analgesics does not justify treating the patient without his or her consent.

THE OBLIGATION NOT TO HARM PATIENTS

Health care professionals have a clear obligation not to harm patients in terms of increasing suffering or causing threat to life, and so should not provide treatments whose associated harms and risks in these respects outweigh their benefits in the clinical circumstances. At the same time, we have already acknowledged that the patient's subjective assessment of the importance of those harms and risks is of crucial relevance in the decision. For example, a nerve block may alleviate pain but at the cost of rendering a limb numb, and there may be other risks of loss of function through misadventure. The patient may or may not consider a numb and possibly weak limb to be better than a painful one, whereas the physician, from experience, may know that other patients often find a numb and useless limb more distressing than a painful one. Patient and doctor between them need to weigh up the harms, risks, and benefits. If agreement is not reached then, in the final analysis, the doctor can and should decline to provide a treatment requested by the patient if the doctor considers that the harms and risks outweigh any possible benefits. The moral basis of pain control is summarized in Table 9.1.

MORAL BALANCES IN PAIN CONTROL

Health care professionals must achieve a delicate moral balance between their obligations:

- We have an obligation to strive to alleviate pain yet we are obliged not to impose treatment without consent.
- We should not offer or provide treatments that will confer overall harm yet there is usually a subjective element to assessment of harm and benefit.
- We are obliged to seek consent but yet must not force unwanted information on patients in the process, nor deny pain control to those who do not wish to be fully informed.

Even if all of these obligations are accepted in the conscious minds of doctors and the delicate moral balances required are achieved, there will still remain those moral problems that occur when there is a conflict between our two main aims in health care and their corresponding obligations. The most common conflict in the area of pain control is that which is perceived to occur between the obligation to relieve suffering and the obligation to prolong life.

CONFLICT BETWEEN OUR OBLIGATION TO RELIEVE SUFFERING AND OUR OBLIGATION TO PROLONG LIFE

We will all be familiar with the scenario, often reported dramatically in the media, in which a patient with a terminal illness has pain and distress that has been difficult to control and it is found that drug regimens that effectively alleviate the pain also inevitably result in sedation with possible shortening of life. Unfortunately, one would be led to believe by the media, certainly in the UK, that such situations are the norm, if indeed pain can be controlled at all. Those reading this book will be aware that with good pain control such situations are not common, but they do still occur and treatment decisions have to be made.

The legal and moral prohibition against causing the death of another

We are all bound by the laws of our communities and countries. The vast majority of communities and countries have laws that prohibit one person from intentionally causing the death of another. Intentionally causing the death of another person, i.e. killing another person, is a major offence and is punishable by law. This law quite rightly applies to doctors, and indeed it could be argued that it must apply particularly to doctors, who are entrusted with the care of their patients and who are normally considered to have an obligation to try

Table 9.1 *The moral basis of pain control*

- Relief of suffering is an essential aim of health care but, as in all other areas of medicine, is accompanied by an obligation not to cause harm
- There is an obligation upon doctors to attain competence in pain control
- There is a requirement for honest discussion with patients about the risks and benefits of proposed pain therapies
- There should be acceptance of patients' control over therapies and the level of information they desire for decision-making
- An understanding of the multifactorial nature of the pain experienced should be balanced by a parallel understanding of the need for consent to intrusive personal enquiry

to prolong life. So, although doctors have a moral obligation to alleviate pain, they also have moral and legal obligations not *intentionally to cause* the deaths of their patients. The legal prohibition is to do with both intention and causation and it reflects the consensus that there is a moral prohibition against intentionally causing the death of another. Thus, in most countries, there are legal and moral prohibitions against health care professionals intentionally causing the deaths of their patients.

The need to alleviate pain even at the cost of shortening life

To return to our problem scenario. We have said that occasionally it happens when a patient is terminally ill that the drug regimen required to alleviate distress will have other effects, such as sedation or respiratory depression, which in the context of the patient's grave illness will possibly hasten death. But doctors are morally and legally prohibited from intentionally causing the patient's death. At the same time they have an obligation to relieve suffering. Two main approaches are commonly used to justify the use of a drug regimen given to alleviate distress in those terminally ill when it may result in hastening death.

The balance of benefit to harm and risk in the dying patient

The first or "common-sense" approach is to argue that on the basis of a relatively simple balance of benefits to harms and risks the analgesic regimen is morally justified. One might say that the benefit of freedom from pain in the context of a terminal illness outweighs the harms of sedation and the risk of shortening life. Of course, the patient's views are essential in quantifying the benefit of pain relief, the harm of sedation, and the risk of death. Some dying patients like and want a degree of sedation; others do not like it and do not want it. Some want to live as long as possible, and to take advantage of life-prolonging treatments; others do not.

It is generally accepted that when a patient who is terminally ill wants to be free of pain, even at the cost of sedation and possible shortening of life, then the necessary drug regimen should be provided, even if it may result in death slightly earlier. When the patient is unable to take part in decision-making doctors may take this view and implement the drug regimen on the basis of the patient's overall benefit. Patients, doctors, and the law in the UK accept this practice and consider it to be morally as well as legally justified in the circumstances. It is also reasonable to conclude that the analgesic regimen was not the fundamental cause of the patient's death – the illness is usually considered the primary or fundamental cause of the patient's death, although it is acknowledged that death may occur slightly earlier as a result of the side-effects of sedation.

The doctrine or rule of double effect

The second is a philosophical approach called the rule or doctrine of "double effect". It is invoked to justify claims that a single act that has two anticipated effects, one good (such as pain relief) and one bad (such as death), may be morally justifiable if the bad effect is not intended although it is foreseen. This rule or doctrine is sometimes used to justify the use of drug regimens to prevent distress, which is considered the good effect, even if that may entail a risk of shortening life, which is considered a bad effect. The doctrine of double effect relies upon the distinction between intending the good effect of treatment and foreseeing but not intending the bad or adverse effect.

The intended and good effect of the drug regimen is the relief of suffering in a patient who is dying. The professional must intend only this good effect. The effect that is considered harmful but which is unintended is the risk of shortening life; the professional may foresee this effect but must not intend it. The harmful effect, i.e. the possible earlier death of the patient, is not the means of achieving the good effect, which is the relief of suffering. Relief of suffering is achieved through the use of the drug regimen. It is considered in this clinical situation that the benefit of the *intended* good effect of alleviating distress in a dying patient outweighs the harm of the *foreseen* effect of possibly hastening death.

The doctrine of double effect has four conditions which must be satisfied if the doctrine is to justify the action. These conditions have been illustrated in the scenario of the dying patient just described. They are as follows:

1 The act itself must be good. Pain control is a good act.
2 The agent must intend only the good effect, i.e. pain relief.
3 The bad effect (shortening life) must not be the means to the good effect (relief of suffering).
4 The good effect must outweigh the bad effect.

The distinction between intended and foreseen effects

The moral distinction between intended and foreseen effects of treatment is accepted in general medical practice. Virtually all treatments have foreseen harms and risks. Although doctors intend the benefits from treatments, the fact that they foresee side-effects and risks does not mean that they intend those harms and risks in the sense of wanting, seeking, or aiming at those harms and risks. For example, surgeons do not intend the discomfort and anxiety that accompany an operation, although they foresee them. Similarly, oncologists do not intend the adverse effects of chemotherapy, such as nausea, although they foresee them. In both cases, it is generally accepted that the doctors intend only the benefits, and that they foresee but do not intend the harms and risks.

Intention is itself a highly complex psychological concept in moral philosophy. Intention has to do with planning toward the consequence, or wanting, desiring, or willing that consequence, or seeking a consequence as an aim. This is how it is understood in ordinary usage, when its meaning is distinguished from the concept of foreseeing but not aiming at, willing, or planning a consequence or effect. Complex philosophical arguments can be constructed to defend or refute the existence of a distinction between intending and foreseeing a consequence of an action, but they are not really relevant to the ordinary clinical situation in which health care professionals and the public accept the distinction at face value. Almost every treatment has side-effects, but it is generally accepted that health care professionals intend only the beneficial effects of treatment and not the side-effects, although the latter may be foreseen.

The importance of clear thinking and integrity

The public acceptance of the moral distinction between intending and foreseeing effects of treatment is based on trust in the integrity of doctors. In return, doctors have to be worthy of that trust. This entails being clear in our thinking and being honest with ourselves and others about our intentions. In health care, the aim of a treatment is the effect which is intended. We cannot be clear and honest about our intentions unless we have thought clearly and been honest with ourselves about the aim of the treatment.

At the beginning I stated that the prolongation of life is an essential aim of health care. If doctors were permitted to intend to cause or hasten their patients' deaths, then the aim of prolonging life in health care would be irretrievably undermined, and patients would no longer be able to trust that doctors would not intentionally cause or hasten their deaths for whatever reason.

The problem of what causes death

The issue of what actually causes death must also be discussed. It is argued, quite appropriately, that in the situation described the cause of death is the terminal illness, and not the drug regimen given to alleviate distress or even the absence of more life-prolonging technology. This is certainly the case if the same drug regimen given to a fitter person would not cause death. In the same way it is argued that the cause of death of a patient who dies of renal failure is in fact renal failure and not the absence of a renal transplant or dialysis. Issues around causality are very complex philosophically, but for the public, the law, and health care professionals a more common-sense approach is needed and is accepted.

We have said that the essential aims of health care are the relief of suffering and the prolongation of life. I have stressed that there is *always* a moral obligation for health care professionals to minimize suffering. In contrast, the aim of prolonging life must be seen in the light of the inevitability of human death, so that for all people there comes a time when further attempts to prolong or sustain life by means of health care will fail. Thus, there is *not always* a moral obligation to strive to prolong or sustain life. On the other hand, doctors must not intentionally shorten the life of their patients or cause their deaths, because the prohibition against killing to which the vast majority of societies subscribe must be upheld, especially where vulnerable people such as patients are concerned.

The use of the doctrine of double effect

It is obvious that very fine moral lines exist in all these matters. Harms and risks of treatment must be carefully weighed against benefits, and distinctions are sometimes finely drawn. Yet this must be so. For moral decision-making in medicine is very complex, and cannot be simplified by any theory into a simple formula that will give the answer when applied to the particular situation. So communities and health care professionals agree some basic legal rules and moral rules (such as the doctrine of double effect). Within the necessary constraints of those rules it is for patients and their doctors to work out the best course of action in each particular clinical situation.

Praiseworthy and blameworthy actions

One may be held blameworthy in health care for what one has not done as well as for what one has done. Thus, doctors might be considered blameworthy for not relieving the patient's pain. The fact that the doctor did not do something does not mean that no blame may be attributed to that decision. Similarly, one may be praised for making a correct decision to withhold an inappropriate treatment, just as one may be praised for giving an appropriate treatment. So the issue of rightness or wrongness of a treatment decision, and the corresponding attribution of praise or blame, cannot be simplified into a distinction between doing and not doing something.

The doctrine of double effect cannot justify euthanasia

Euthanasia, defined as an intentional act that brings about the death of the patient in order to alleviate suffering, cannot be justified by the doctrine of double effect. The doctrine will not justify an intentional act of killing, which euthanasia is. Moreover, where euthanasia is concerned, the good effect (relief of suffering) is brought about by means of the bad effect (the death of the patient). Thus, the conditions of the doctrine of double effect are not satisfied by euthanasia. So the doctrine cannot be used to justify euthanasia.

Conflicts between the obligations to relieve suffering and prolong life are summarized in Table 9.2.

THE ROLE OF RELATIVES IN DECISION-MAKING FOR COMPETENT PATIENTS

In Western society the wishes of the patient are currently considered to be more important than those of their relatives as far as treatment decisions are concerned. Thus, the patient is entitled to give informed consent to treatment or to refuse treatment (but the patient cannot demand treatment that the health care team considers to be clinically inappropriate).

In contrast, in some other cultures, the relatives' views are considered to be as important as, or sometimes more important than, those of the patient, and in these cultures knowledge of the diagnosis may be given to the relatives and withheld from the patient. Of course, in these cultures the patient will be aware that this is occurring as he or she will be familiar with the culture. Where the views of relatives are given priority in this way, the relatives may make decisions on behalf of the patient. This means that they may consent to or refuse an analgesic regimen on behalf of the patient (but they cannot demand a treatment that the health care team considers to be clinically inappropriate).

DECISION-MAKING FOR INCOMPETENT PATIENTS

At the end of life many patients will be unable to make decisions for themselves, by reason of confusion or diminished consciousness. When it is clear that the illness will result in death and that some life-prolonging treatments are no longer appropriate, the moral obligation to relieve pain logically supersedes any obligation to continue to strive to prolong life. Health care professionals should then make the patient's comfort their first priority. They will then wish to provide an analgesic regimen that will enable the patient to be comfortable but without causing more sedation than is necessary to achieve this. However, the question as to who should make health care decisions for patients who cannot make them for themselves inevitably arises.

In Western society, when the patient's wishes are not known and cannot be ascertained, relatives may or may not be given decision-making authority on behalf of the patient, depending on the law of the country concerned. For example, in the UK relatives do not have decision-making authority, and so cannot consent to or refuse treatment on behalf of the patient. On the other hand, in some other countries, including the USA, relatives can consent to or refuse treatment on behalf of the patient, and may be expected to take this responsibility.

However, it should be noted that relatives cannot force the health care team to give treatment that the professionals consider is inappropriate because of an adverse balance of harms and risks to benefits. In other words, relatives cannot insist that the patient be given a treatment (for example excessive sedation) that has very little chance of benefit, or very small benefit, in comparison with more major and/or more certain harms and risks.

The differences between the laws of various countries reflect the fact that there are moral arguments both for and against giving relatives decision-making authority for incompetent patients. Such decision-making authority enables and perhaps requires relatives to consent to or refuse an analgesic regimen on behalf of the patient. The policy regarding decision-making for incompetent patients is generally decided on the basis of two issues: firstly, who is likely to make decisions that most accord with what is best for the patient; and, secondly, who can be said to have some sort of entitlement to make decisions for the patient.

It can be argued that the health care professionals are better placed, on the grounds of professional knowledge and experience, to know what is the best analgesic regimen for the patient. On the other hand, relatives are likely to have a better knowledge of the patient's previously expressed wishes and values. Ideally, health care professionals and relatives should work together to formulate the analgesic regimen that best accords with attaining comfort without going against the patient's known val-

Table 9.2 *Conflicts between the obligations to relieve suffering and prolong life*

- As death is inevitable, the obligation to relieve suffering must ultimately outweigh the obligation to prolong life
- With competent use of pain therapies, the risk of shortening life in order to relieve suffering arises occasionally, not frequently
- Where it is foreseen that adequate pain relief might shorten life, it may legitimately be considered that this risk is outweighed by the benefit of comfort, but this decision belongs to the patient, not the doctor
- Ill-effects of treatment can be foreseen without being intended
- The cause of death remains the disease which has given rise to the situation necessitating the treatment, not the treatment itself
- For the doctrine of double effect to be invoked legitimately, the shortening of life must not be the *means* to relieve pain. The doctrine cannot justify euthanasia
- Moral culpability applies equally to the failure to provide a necessary treatment and to the giving of an inappropriate treatment

ues. Disagreement about an analgesic regimen is very rare, but if relatives refuse the analgesic regimen considered most appropriate by the health care team the consequences for the patient may be very serious. Therefore, in some countries, such as the UK, decision-making authority for incompetent patients lies with the health care team and not with the relatives.

However, in other countries decision-making authority lies with the relatives, who can therefore refuse the analgesic regimen on behalf of the patient. They might do this if they believed it would or might shorten life. Decision-making authority may be granted to relatives because of a view that they are entitled in some way to make decisions for the patient. Such an entitlement may be based on the idea of an ownership or property right, but this idea is intuitively unattractive. It is more plausible to base an entitlement for relatives to make decisions on behalf of incompetent patients on the idea that such a policy affirms and fosters intimate relationships between family members. Alternatively, it may be thought that relatives may be most likely to decide in the patient's best interests, but where pain control is concerned it must be admitted that the experience of the health care professionals makes them more likely to know what regimen is most likely to be effective.

Regardless of whether the health care team or the relatives are granted legal decision-making authority for incompetent patients, there is a moral duty for both parties to work together to try to achieve the analgesic regimen that will enable the patient to be comfortable while at the same time respecting as far as possible the patient's previously stated values.

Some patients make oral or written statements while mentally competent in order to influence treatment decisions that may arise when they are incompetent to make those decisions. Such statements are called "advance statements", or may be referred to as "living wills." A doctor presented with an advance statement has to decide (as far as is possible) whether it was competently made and whether it was intended to apply to the circumstances that have actually arisen. The legal status of advance statements varies in different countries. Concerns may arise that patients should not be able to refuse adequate pain control in advance; for this reason the British Law Commission has suggested that a patient should not be able to refuse measures *essential* for pain relief via an advance statement.[1] It would be extraordinarily rare for patients to state that they did not want to be pain free at the end of their lives, or for them to want their relatives and carers to see them distressed at this time. Fortunately, when adequate explanation is given to relatives, agreement about treatment is normally reached without conflict, and patients at the end of life can and should be as free of distress as current medical knowledge allows.

REFERENCE

1. Lord Chancellor's Department. *Who Decides?* London: Lord Chancellor's Department, 1997: 30.

PART II

Clinical management – therapies

10

Principles of oral analgesic therapy in cancer pain

STEPHAN A SCHUG AND JO E RITCHIE

Pain is the most common symptom of cancer; it is estimated that up to 30% of cancer patients have pain as the presenting complaint. This incidence increases with progress of the disease, so that up to 70% of all patients with advanced cancer report significant pain.[1] There are also data suggesting that the impact on daily living and enjoyment of life is greater in patients with cancer pain than in those with other chronic pain.[2]

In the past, cancer pain had a low priority for treatment, and until the early 1980s was a largely neglected problem.[3,4] It has been estimated that over 25% of all cancer patients worldwide died without any relief from pain.[5] Now, as it was then, this is quite unacceptable, but over the last two decades there have been major advances in the management of cancer pain.

After the laudable initial efforts and successes of the hospice movement,[6] management guidelines were drafted in 1982 by the World Health Organization (WHO), and were then finalized as treatment guidelines and published in the booklet *Cancer Pain Relief* in 1986.[3,4,7] This booklet was revised and updated in a second edition in 1996.[8]

These guidelines have become the internationally accepted standard for the principles governing treatment of cancer pain, focusing on oral analgesic use as the mainstay of therapy. Their use has been studied in over 30,000 patients, proving their usefulness and efficacy.[3,9]

Even so, cancer pain often remains a poorly treated problem. The reasons for this continued undertreatment of cancer pain include:[10–15]

- a lack of understanding of the nature of pain due to inadequate training of health care professionals;
- failure to assess pain fully;
- poor communication between patients and physicians;
- difficulties in communicating the subjective feeling of pain;
- a lack of understanding of or misconceptions about the actions of various analgesics, in particular opioids;
- underdosage of drugs;
- inadequate intake schedule (p.r.n. or irregular dosing);
- failure to tailor the regimen to the individual;
- poor coordination of care as patients move from one health care professional to another;
- barriers to opioid availability or reluctance to use opioids (by government and/or society).

To combat this, the World Health Organization has instigated pain relief programs on a worldwide basis through establishment of governmental policies and education of physicians, the public, and policy-makers, with the aim of increasing the availability of strong analgesics such as morphine.[3,4,13] Improvement in cancer pain management and in attitudes toward opioid use has been reflected in a worldwide increase in morphine use.[13] However, although there have been well-documented improvements in the attitudes and knowledge of medical practitioners regarding cancer pain and its treatment, there are still deficiencies in problem areas such as overconcern with the development of tolerance, instituting high-dose therapy on the basis of prognosis rather than pain intensity, and a persistence of the idea that it is possible to overmedicate.[14]

PRINCIPLES OF CANCER PAIN TREATMENT

The goal of cancer pain treatment is to provide pain relief and thereby to enable patients to continue to have a good quality of life, to function at an acceptable level, to be able to tolerate diagnostic and therapeutic procedures, and to die relatively free of pain while maintaining freedom of choice and minimizing adverse effects.[12,15]

However, cancer pain is not a homogeneous problem, and many patients will have more than one type and more than one localization of pain. "Cancer pain" is therefore an insufficient diagnosis on which to base a targeted therapy. The term describes a variety of acute and chronic pain states in a group of patients who have little in common other than malignant disease as the underlying cause of pain. Only in some specific conditions is the primary diagnosis of malignant disease relevant to successful treatment of the resulting pain.[16]

There are numerous ways of classifying cancer pain depending on the cause, pathophysiology, temporal pattern, and effect on the life and well-being of a patient.[17] In an attempt to classify pain from a causal point of view, a system distinguishing between tumor-related pain, therapy-related pain, disability-related pain, and pain unrelated to cancer has been suggested (Table 10.1).[5] In up to 80% of patients, pain will be related to the tumor itself and depend on the localization of the primary or its metastases. In this scenario, the tissue mass itself (of the tumor or its metastases) will cause either distension or compression of other tissues, leading to either nociceptor stimulation or nerve irritation. However, pain may also be due to treatment (e.g. postsurgical or postchemotherapy pain syndromes) or debility caused by the cancer, such as herpes zoster or pressure sores. In addition, patients with cancer may experience pain unrelated to the cancer, such as migraines and back pain.

From a therapeutic point of view, it is particularly important to identify the type of pain, i.e. to determine if a specific pain is nociceptive or neurogenic (often also called neuropathic). Nociceptive pain can be further classified according to the source of the pain as somatic or visceral (Table 10.2).

Neurogenic pain results not from nociceptor irritation, but from damage to parts of the peripheral and/or central nervous system. In general, neurogenic pain is more difficult to manage with analgesics than nociceptive pain.[18] In addition, both of these types of pain can occur at the same location.

With regard to temporal patterns a useful distinction is between acute, chronic, and breakthrough pain. Although breakthrough pain can be caused by low plasma levels of analgesics, it can also be caused by precipitating factors such as movement or pressure, in which case it is termed incident pain.[19]

Last but not least, cancer disrupts many aspects of normal life, such as social support, financial independence, and family relationships, all of which are likely to lead to a reduction in coping skills and pain tolerance. These factors and the multidimensional nature of pain have appropriately been described by Saunders[6] as "total pain."

A holistic approach to the complex patterns of cancer pain requires that all the above issues be addressed.

Successful pain therapy begins with a comprehensive pain assessment and diagnosis, including functional limitations caused by pain, while taking into account the individual patient's goals and priorities and their definition of pain and suffering.[15,20] A treatment plan should then

Table 10.1 *Etiology of cancer pain (examples)*

Pain caused by cancer
Bone metastases
Primary bone cancer
Infiltration of peripheral nerves or spinal cord by cancer
Compression of peripheral nerves or spinal cord by cancer
Cancer of abdominal or thoracic organs
Soft-tissue infiltration by cancer
Infiltration or compression of blood vessels by cancer
Pain related to treatment of cancer
Surgical intervention
Stump pain
Phantom limb pain
Post-thoracotomy pain
Pain after radical neck dissection
Chemotherapy
Polyneuropathy
Mucositis
Radiotherapy
Fibrosis of nerve plexus caused by radiation
Mucositis
Pain associated with disability of cancer
Acute pain of shingles
Postherpetic neuralgia
Pressure sores
Pain unrelated to cancer or cancer therapy
Migraine
Osteoporosis
Degenerative musculoskeletal pain

Table 10.2 *Types of cancer pain (examples)*

Nociceptive pain
Somatic pain
Bone pain
Soft-tissue pain
Muscle pain
Visceral pain
Pancreatic pain
Liver capsule tension pain
Neuropathic pain
Brachial plexopathy
Spinal cord compression
Intercostal neuralgia
Phantom limb pain

be formulated. Treatment should be viewed as a dynamic process, changing in response to the underlying progressive disease and perhaps involving multiple treatment interventions over time. The treatment plan should consider the following approaches to the pain problem:

- explanation;
- treatment of the underlying cause (e.g. tumor ablation, reduction of tumor size);
- elevation of pain threshold;
- interruption, destruction, or stimulation of pathways;
- change of lifestyle.

The WHO guidelines stress that, although systemic pharmacotherapy is the mainstay of the control of cancer pain, it is not only the only solution.[8]

Treatment should always begin with a straightforward explanation of the cause of the pain and the various options available to the patient.[21*] This not only reinforces patient autonomy but also helps to increase pain tolerance and to encourage improved coping skills. Very often, it helps also to allay misconceptions that patients have about their pain, its cause and mechanism, and its consequences (e.g. patient beliefs about pain as a cause of death). Such thoughts can be a major obstacle to successful pain therapy, and to overcome them often takes time and involves careful questioning and objective, understandable conversation with the patients and significant others.[22,23] In addition, identifying and relieving stress, anxieties, and depression, often through counseling, is of paramount importance, as these problems may prevent optimal pain relief. Ignoring the multidimensional components of cancer pain and focusing exclusively on the use of drugs can lead to situations of "intractable" pain that could be avoidable by a more careful approach.[24] Another useful term in this context is "opioid-irrelevant pain," which reflects the social, spiritual, and/or psychological circumstances of the patient more than the nociception caused by cancer.

Many pains are treated with a number of drug and nondrug combinations. Although systemic analgesic pharmacotherapy has the advantages of being noninvasive, readily available, and acceptable to most patients,[25**] the modification of the pathological process with radiotherapy,[26] chemotherapy,[27] or surgery[28,29] may provide an important and often more appropriate method of pain treatment. As such therapy is usually aimed more at the cause than the symptoms, it is useful to consider these options early and re-evaluate this decision repeatedly.

However, in contrast to most other areas of medicine, in palliative care, therapy aimed at the tumor should not necessarily be given the highest priority; often, a symptomatic approach needs to be chosen. Elevation of the pain threshold by means of analgesics and coanalgesics is the topic of this chapter. Some pain responds well to an opioid and nonopioid combination; other types of pain, such as neurogenic pain, may require coanalgesics such as corticosteroids, tricyclic antidepressants, anticonvulsants, or antiarrhythmics. Recognizing that not all pain responds to opioids in a similar way is an important step in the optimal management of cancer pain.

When a pharmacologic approach fails to relieve pain, multiple neurosurgical and anesthesiological approaches to treatment are available, aimed at interrupting, destroying, and stimulating pain pathways. However, as improved pharmacologic options are continually being introduced, the indications for such interventions are becoming increasingly limited.

In rare cases, some pain states, in particular pain on movement in patients with pathological fractures of vertebral structures, are not amenable to any of the above interventions. In such situations, modification of lifestyle (e.g. limited periods of bed rest, reduced mobility, or spinal braces) might be the only option available.[30*] This approach might sometimes be superior to desperate attempts to control these situations with increasing doses of analgesics, often leading to severe side-effects without sufficient analgesia and then even more reduced quality of life.

PRINCIPLES OF ANALGESIC THERAPY OF CANCER PAIN

The WHO guidelines can be summarized in five key points:[8]

- by the mouth;
- by the clock;
- by the ladder;
- for the individual;
- attention to detail.

By mouth – the oral route

Most analgesics, including opioids, have reasonably good oral bioavailability.The oral route is preferred as it is simple, acceptable, and relatively cheap.[15***] It requires little medical intervention and therefore makes the patient independent of infrastructure and medical personnel. Further, there are no needles or syringes to dispose of nor risks of needlestick injury for the administrator. In addition, the delayed absorption that occurs after oral administration prolongs the duration of action of most drugs, giving further benefits. However, a slower onset of action is accompanied by a delayed peak time, thereby conveying disadvantages in the management of acute (e.g. incident) pain.

Unfortunately, the oral route is not always suitable, and indications to abandon the oral route include emesis, dysphagia, gastrointestinal obstruction, malabsorption, and coma.[31*] However, simple failure of the oral therapy used is an indication not to change route of administration, but to re-evaluate the pain diagnosis and thereafter the treatment plan.[32]

By the clock – regular around-the-clock medication

Chronic pain requires preventive therapy on a regular basis, thus avoiding repeated recurrence of pain with unnecessary suffering and subsequently the potential development of chronic pain behavior.[33*,34*]

Thus, analgesic drugs should be given regularly in doses that are high enough to suppress pain continuously.[10*] The timing of the repetitions should be guided by the pharmacokinetics of the drugs utilized; each successive dose should be given before the previous dose has worn off. This allows the plasma concentration to reach a relative steady state without unnecessary troughs. It is clear that slow- or sustained-release preparations should be used whenever they are available, as their use extends dosing intervals and stabilizes plasma concentrations. Regular dosing also increases the efficacy of a regimen, providing continuous pain relief. Not surprisingly, it has been found that demands for rescue analgesia are reduced and analgesia is improved, even in patients with pain of nonmalignant origin, when analgesia is administered at timed intervals rather than on demand.[35**]

The timing of analgesic administration should suit the patient's daily activities and schedule and should consider the day–night rhythm of the patient.[36*] It is useful to provide a medication plan including the timing in writing to avoid confusion for the patient and caregivers.

By the ladder – sequential use of analgesic medication

One basic principle of pain management in cancer patients is to begin treatment with less potent analgesics and to progress in response to more severe or increasing pain intensity with the use of more potent agents, making use of adjuvant and coanalgesic agents as appropriate. The WHO has suggested the successful model of an "analgesic ladder" to provide a framework for this approach to oral pharmacotherapy of cancer pain (Fig. 10.1). Drugs are selected according to increasing pain intensity in a sequential approach; inadequate pain relief at one level results in a step up to the next level instead of changing to a drug on the same level.[8*]

This WHO ladder of analgesic drug therapy thus presents a simple method to introduce increasingly potent drugs sequentially. In addition, it encourages the combined use of nonopioid and opioid analgesics and so-called coanalgesics, which are defined as drugs that are not usually regarded as analgesics but which have analgesic properties in certain defined conditions (i.e. steroids in liver capsule distension).[5*] The ladder concept is useful in titrating initial therapy as well as in adapting an established therapy to take account of progression of the malignant disease.[11]

The base of the analgesic ladder (step 1) is the use of simple nonopioids. These are recommended to control pain of mild to moderate intensity. They are used in established standard doses and frequency. Nonopioids exhibit a ceiling effect, i.e., in contrast to opioids, a further increase in dose beyond an established maximum effective dose will not result in improved analgesia. Thus, if pain is not adequately controlled by the maximum dose of nonopioid analgesics, and if appropriate coanalgesic therapy is already in use and cannot be improved, it is necessary to climb the analgesic ladder.[37*]

The next step (step 2) is the addition of a weak opioid without discontinuation of the nonopioid. This step is necessary when the maximum effective doses of nonopioids fail to relieve pain because of its intensity or because of further progression of the malignant disease. However, the use of weak opioids here is currently the subject of a wide-ranging controversy, having being described as a "didactic instrument"[38] or an "educational substitute for morphine."[39] A more detailed analysis of this issue follows later.

When the combination of a nonopioid and a weak opioid fails despite the use of appropriate doses, the weak opioid is replaced by a strong opioid (step 3), again without abandoning the nonopioid if possible. Any further increase in pain is then treated by an increase in dose.

It is recommended that only one agent from each group be used at a time. When one drug fails to provide pain relief, a drug from those recommended for the next step should be used rather than switching within a group of drugs with similar efficacy and potency.[8*] However, if one drug results in unacceptable side-effects, then clearly it should be replaced by another agent from the same group, as opioid rotation is useful to minimize side-effects.[40–42] This is particularly useful if morphine causes neuroexcitatory effects, presumably by retention of the metabolite morphine 3-glucuronide.[43] The same applies to morphine-induced hyperalgesia.[44]

At any step, additional coanalgesics should be added as appropriate for the individual patient and the pain diagnosis.[33*]

Obviously, patients presenting with moderate or severe pain should be started on step 2 or even step 3 immediately, rather than working slowly up the ladder. This decision may sometimes take experience but is clearly useful as long as the individual patient is taken into account.[9**,11**]

For the individual

Pain is, by definition, "a sensory and emotional experience" and "always subjective."[45] Any analgesic regimen must therefore be adapted to the individual patient, the nature of the disease, and the intensity and cause of the pain. Although the analgesic ladder gives the impression of a schematic, standardized approach to the problem of

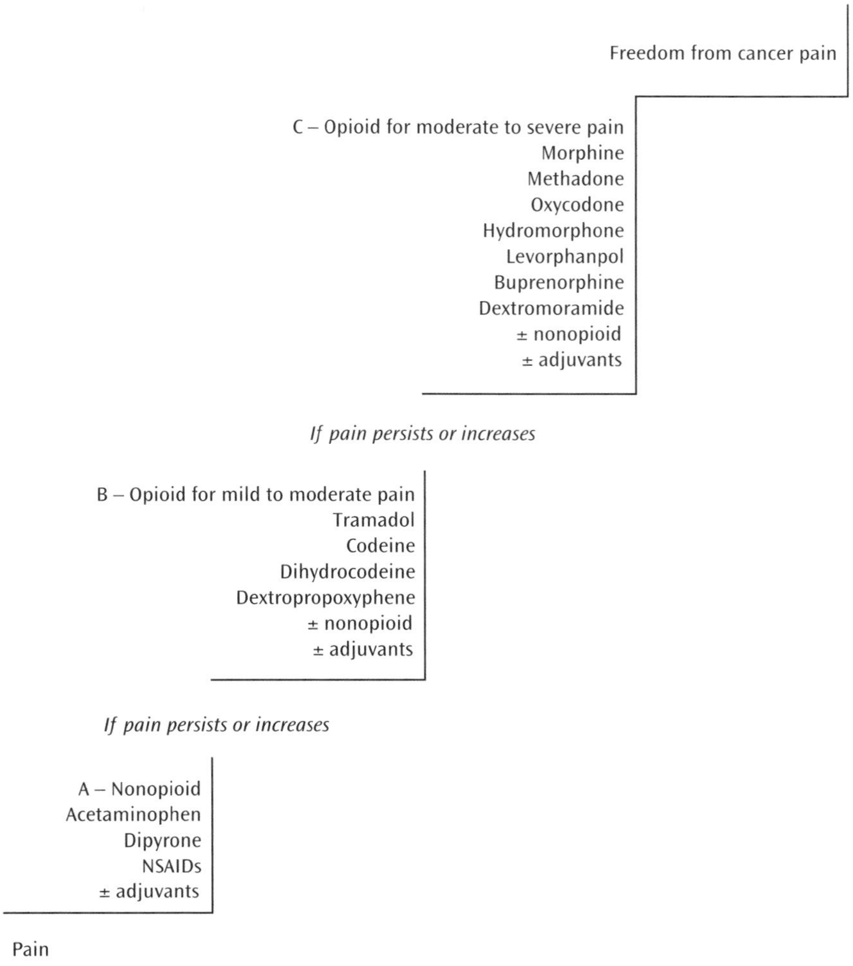

Freedom from cancer pain

C – Opioid for moderate to severe pain
Morphine
Methadone
Oxycodone
Hydromorphone
Levorphanpol
Buprenorphine
Dextromoramide
± nonopioid
± adjuvants

If pain persists or increases

B – Opioid for mild to moderate pain
Tramadol
Codeine
Dihydrocodeine
Dextropropoxyphene
± nonopioid
± adjuvants

If pain persists or increases

A – Nonopioid
Acetaminophen
Dipyrone
NSAIDs
± adjuvants

Pain

Figure 10.1 *The WHO analgesic ladder. For adjuvants, see Coanalgesics.*

cancer pain, it should be seen more as a guideline to the development of an individualized treatment plan.

There is no "right" medication and/or dose for every patient: the correct dose of an opioid is the one that treats the patient's pain. It is best found by individual dose titration until a patient is comfortable. As an example of the individual variability of opioid response, the commonly quoted dose range for oral morphine is 5–1,000 mg every 4 h.[8] Such a wide dose range is confirmed by a recent publication.[46]

Aiming for realistic obtainable goals helps to improve this titration process. It is important to be aware of and to take into account the patient's own priorities and goals. Improving sleep patterns and obtaining a reasonable night's sleep without pain would be a good place to start. Subsequently, most patients may also be able to become pain free at rest, while many ultimately may even achieve pain-free activity.[47]* Aiming for too high a goal immediately can result in early failure, thereby frustrating the patient and possibly undermining his or her trust in the treating physician.

The starting doses of strong opioids recommended for the titration process depend on a number of patient factors: age, disease, concurrent disease, and previous exposure to opioids. However, experience of the treating physician is another relevant factor. In general, titration should be performed only with immediate-release and not with slow- or sustained-release preparations, the long half-life of which makes titration more difficult and protracted.[48–50] During titration to establish the correct level of background analgesia, patients must have free access to additional rescue medication. The pattern of use of rescue medication is a good indicator of the adequacy of the background analgesia and of the need for changes in the analgesic regimen.

A rule of thumb states that, if a starting dose provides good analgesia, but with excessive sedation, then the next dose should be 50% lower. If pain relief with the starting dose is inadequate after 24 h, then doses should be increased, based on the rescue drug used, but a typical increase would be 50%, with frequent re-evaluation at intervals of least at 48 or 72 h.

Medication must be continued throughout the night, and doses may need to be increased to cover the period of sleep, unless a longer acting drug such as slow-release morphine or methadone is used.

Attention to detail

The regimen should be written out in full, listing each drug and the reason for its use as well as outlining possible side-effects and relevant treatments.[33] Patients should be encouraged to maintain a diary of analgesia, pain intensity, and adverse events; thus, daily fluctuations in pain can be monitored and treated accordingly.

Frequent reassessment ensures that correct diagnoses are made and that goals are being reached. If treatment is not providing adequate pain relief then the analgesic regimen or the original diagnoses should be reviewed, remembering that any patient may have more than one source of pain.

Patient review must be sufficiently frequent to detect and treat side-effects while continuing to tailor the analgesic regimen.[51*] In a recent study, modification of the analgesic prescription was required, on average, every 2 weeks.[25]

EVALUATION OF THE EFFICACY OF ORAL ANALGESIC THERAPY

It has been found that using the principles of the WHO ladder in managing oral medication provides adequate analgesia in 70–90% of patients.[11*,20*,52*] Hence, it is now the internationally accepted standard for treatment of cancer pain.[8] In treatment programs involving a large number of patients with previously severe, intractable pain followed for a long period of time, following the WHO guidelines has been shown to reduce pain intensity to none to moderate for 80–90% of the treatment period.[11,25] Improvement in pain relief is rapid:* use of the WHO guidelines in patients with previously difficult to treat pain can provide adequate pain relief within a week.[11,37]

Enteral treatment is possible in approximately 95% of patients.[25*] In other cases, more invasive routes of administration or procedures may be required.[53] These invasive procedures, such as neurolytic and non-neurolytic blocks, should be undertaken only after systemic analgesics have failed; about 10% of patients with severe pain will require such measures.[11,25,51,52,54*] Oral treatment continues to be effective even in the last days of life:[51,52] at the time of death up to 50–70% of patients may be pain free, with less than 5% suffering severe pain.[51,55] In contrast, it is estimated that worldwide 25% of patients suffer severe pain at the time of death. In addition, up to 80% of patients may be able to maintain communication, orientation, and consciousness during the last 24 h of life.[51]

The judicious use of coanalgesics and other adjuvant drugs, which is the case in about 90% of patients, means that serious side-effects are rare. Overall, side-effects are unlikely to lead to a change of regimen, with the WHO guidelines providing a safe and effective means for treatment of cancer pain.[9,11,25,51]

OTHER ROUTES OF ADMINISTRATION

The oral route is the most common and preferred route of drug administration for treatment of cancer pain.[56*] Unfortunately, its use is not always possible because a number of absorption or swallowing problems, such as emesis or gastrointestinal obstruction. In this case, the rectal[57] or subcutaneous[58] routes are preferred for reasons of ease, comfort, acceptability, and availability.

Morphine is well absorbed rectally, and most others opioids and nonopioids can be given per rectum.[59**] Morphine is available as both immediate-release and controlled-release preparations, as suppositories or enemas. Alternatively, controlled-release morphine tablets may be administered as suppositories.[60] Doses should be equivalent to oral dosage but show greater variation of bioavailability owing to differing first-pass effects depending on site of absorption. Recently, a study found that the onset of action of rectal morphine in producing pain relief may be more rapid than that of oral morphine (10 min compared with 60 min[57]), suggesting that this route could be especially useful for rescue analgesia.

Other routes of administration of morphine, such as sublingual and buccal administration, have also been assessed.[61*]

The availability of simple portable syringe pumps has made continuous subcutaneous morphine administration easy and acceptable for the patient who is unable to take oral medication.[62*] This method avoids repeated injections and is relatively cheap, requiring little medical input for administration.[63] Changing the route of administration of morphine from enteral to parenteral should result in a dose reduction of at least a half, and more commonly two-thirds, and frequent reassessment is necessary to take into account bioavailability differences resulting from the absence of a first-pass effect.[64]

Sublingual administration is possible with buprenorphine[65*] or fentanyl. However, the pharmacology of these drugs makes them second to morphine as the drug of choice. Sublingual transmucosal fentanyl may be useful as rescue analgesia, with a rapid onset of action within 5 min.[66]

Fentanyl is also available in patch form for transdermal administration. The patches are applied for 72 h to provide doses between 25 and 100 μg/h, depending on patch size. They are not yet universally available because they are expensive, but they have been found to be similar, if not superior, to controlled-release morphine in analgesic efficacy and safety.[67**,68**] Fentanyl transdermal patches are an easy and acceptable alternative to morphine in those patients unable to tolerate oral medication.[67*]

Other forms of analgesia include epidural or intrathecal opioid administration or neurolytic blocks. Each has its own advantages and disadvantages. However, they require expertise and specialized equipment and are invasive. These forms of treatment should only be necessary for 5–10% of patients when following the WHO analgesic guidelines.

SPECIFIC PHARMACOLOGICAL MANAGEMENT

Nonopioids (step 1)

Nonopioids provide the basis of nearly all regimens of cancer pain management, commonly not as the only medication but in combination with opioids.[37]* However, nonopioids used alone in step 1 of the analgesic ladder are useful for the treatment of mild to moderate pain.[8] Nonopioid analgesics are readily available, widely acceptable to physicians, patients, and relatives, and easy to prescribe.

In a supervised program, up to 25% of patients referred for management of cancer pain could initially be treated effectively with nonopioids alone.[37]* Calculated on the basis of total treatment time, cancer pain can be managed with nonopioids alone for 15–20% of the time.[37,69] However, the number of patients that can be treated with nonopioids decreases with disease progression, until in final stages of the disease only 5% of patients can be managed with nonopioids alone.[11,70]

Even in patients with far advanced disease, problems with pain management have often been due to failure to use nonopioids, and to recognize their importance in combination with opioids.[25]* Combining a nonopioid analgesic with an opioid treats pain at both central and peripheral sites.[37] This increases the efficacy of treatment while decreasing opioid requirements,[51,71,72] thus possibly decreasing the incidence and severity of opioid side-effects, such as nausea, constipation, and dizziness.[37,51]

The WHO lists acetaminophen (paracetamol), dipyrone, and nonsteroidal anti-inflammatory drugs (NSAIDs) as nonopioids suitable for use on step 1 of the analgesic ladder. Only the first two of these agents are true nonopioid analgesics, while NSAIDs in addition have a profound anti-inflammatory effect. This is linked to a significantly worse side-effect profile of these drugs. It is therefore the opinion of the authors that only acetaminophen and dipyrone should be used routinely as nonopioids, as limited data suggest that no improvement of analgesia in this setting is achieved by the use of NSAIDs.[73]** The nonopioid nefopam is not recommended for the treatment of cancer pain, as its analgesic effect is no better than that of acetaminophen but it is associated with significantly more side-effects.[74–76]

The use of NSAIDs should be limited to clear indications for this group of drugs. They might therefore be regarded as coanalgesics for defined pain states rather than representatives of nonopioids for all pain states. Conditions in which, after a careful risk–benefit analysis, their use is justified include bone and soft-tissue pain, in particular if linked to swelling with resulting distension or compression. There is limited empirical evidence that combination of an NSAID with a simple nonopioid might be helpful.

The recent arrival of specific COX-2 antagonists might change this attitude, although there is as yet insufficient information on their use in the relief of cancer pain.

Acetaminophen

Acetaminophen is very commonly used.It provides very safe and effective pain relief.[73]* It has high oral and rectal bioavailability as it is well absorbed, with a low first-pass metabolism.[77] Several oral and rectal preparations are available either alone or in combination with other analgesics such as weak opioids. However, it may only be given enterally, limiting its use in some situations; propacetamol, a prodrug for parenteral administration, is registered in only a small number of countries (e.g. France).[78] Acetaminophen has a low to negligible incidence of side-effects and it has no effect on platelet function or the gastrointestinal mucosa. Hepatotoxicity in overdose is the most feared problem but is most unlikely to occur in the recommended dosages of 1 g every 4 h to a maximum of 6 g/day.[8]

Dipyrone

Dipyrone, 3–6 g/day, may be another useful alternative to other nonopioid analgesics.[79] It has a higher efficacy than acetaminophen,[80] and has mild spasmolytic properties, making dipyrone especially useful for the treatment of visceral pain.[81] With a low side-effect profile,[82] it has also been found to be effective in combination with a weak opioid such as codeine, and it may be useful instead of an NSAID when a corticosteroid is used as adjuvant or coanalgesic treatment. The usefulness of this drug is also enhanced by the availability of a parental preparation.

Nonsteroidal anti-inflammatory drugs

WHO guidelines recommend acetylsalicylic acid (ASA) as the nonopioid of choice because of its worldwide availability but, as mentioned above, acetaminophen has been found to be equianalgesic to ASA with a lower side-effect profile.[73]** Newer NSAIDs have also been found to have more favorable side-effect profiles than ASA.[83]

The standard dose of ASA is 500–1,000 mg every 4 –6 h. To decrease the incidence of gastric irritation, it should be taken with food and or an antacid medication. ASA may also be given as a suppository and has been found to be useful in the treatment of postpelvic radiation diarrhea, particularly in prostate cancer patients.

NSAIDs have been found to be effective and relatively well tolerated in the treatment of cancer pain.[84]** In most situations, there may be no proven benefits of NSAIDs over acetaminophen except in selected patients with an inflammatory response to a tumor. Therefore, NSAIDs offer a treatment advantage in bone pain due to periosteal distension or soft-tissue tumors associated with distension of tendon, muscle, or subcutaneous tissue. In these scenarios, a high concentration of prostaglandins is often produced by tumor cells; inhibition of synthesis of these by NSAIDs provides effective analgesia.[8] In these cases, NSAIDs are used as specific coanalgesics, rather than simple nonopioids. Combining paracetamol with NSAIDs increases the efficacy in these situations.[85]

The major problem with NSAIDs is their significant side-effect profile. Side-effects include gastric erosions, peptic ulcer disease, inhibition of platelet function, renal impairment, exacerbation of asthma in susceptible patients, and a number of idiosyncratic reactions. Although the analgesic effect of NSAIDs displays a ceiling effect, this is not the case for their side-effects, and these continue to increase with dose and over time with multiple dosing.[86]

Because of the high incidence of gastrointestinal mucosal damage, it is recommended that NSAIDs are administered concomitantly with a mucoprotective agent such as an H_2 receptor antagonist, a prostaglandin analog, or a proton pump inhibitor. Misoprostol, a prostaglandin analog, has been found to be significantly superior to ranitidine in reducing the incidence of upper gastrointestinal lesions in cancer patients on diclofenac.[87]** Proton pump inhibitors such as omeprazole are another, possibly superior, protective option.[88]

The choice of NSAID may be individual and dictated by local availability and cost, as there are no significant differences in efficacy at appropriate doses.[86] For reasons of convenience, a long-acting agent such as tenoxicam in a single daily dose of 20 mg or slow-release diclofenac, 100 mg every 8–12 h, may be preferable. Other alternatives include naproxen, 500 mg 8- to 12-hourly, or flurbiprofen up to 50 mg every 4 h. When one agent is used as indicated, but still fails, it may be of use to try a second NSAID in place of the first.[33]

In the future, use of the COX-2-specific antagonists celecoxib and rofecoxib might be the safest option here, although specific data on efficacy and adverse effects in cancer pain patients are lacking.[89]

NSAIDs in combination with a strong opioid, with or without acetaminophen, have been found to enhance analgesia and decrease opioid use without an increase in side-effects while increasing patient satisfaction.[90–92]*** However, adding an NSAID to weak opioids produces little increase in analgesia over NSAIDs alone but is associated with an increase in the incidence of side-effects.[86,93]

Weak opioids (step 2)

As outlined above, the sequential approach of the WHO guidelines suggests that failure of a monotherapy with a nonopioid should lead to addition of a weak opioid to the treatment regimen. However, in view of the limited efficacy and the considerable difficulties with the drugs available in this group, there is an increasing debate about the usefulness of this step in principle.[38,39]

The strongest arguments in this discussion are the findings of the above-quoted recent meta-analysis on the use of NSAIDs in cancer pain, which also analyzed the effects of a combination of these drugs with weak opioids in a step 2 approach. The quite surprising main findings were an increase in side-effects without an improvement in analgesia in this setting.[86]***

In most countries, weak opioids are nonscheduled drugs, making them convenient and easy to prescribe for the physician, and at the same time more readily available and more acceptable to patients, the general public, and government authorities. The above finding, and others, have led to the increasing doubt as to the value and usefulness of step 2 of the analgesic ladder. It is increasingly believed that there are only be two reasons why a treatment on step 2 might be superior to the introduction of low doses of strong opioids. One is the stigma attached to the word "morphine" in many societies and the resulting reluctance of patients to accept a suggested strong opioid therapy.[94] In such cases, introduction of a weak opioid might facilitate patient acceptance and compliance, as drugs such as codeine are commonly not stigmatized. Further, combination preparations of nonopioids with weak opioids are widely utilized for everyday pain problems and are not usually thought of as containing "drugs of addiction." The second reason is the reluctance of medical practitioners to use strong opioids at an early stage or even at all (so called "opiophobia").[95] Thus, there is often a much lower barrier to the use of weak opioids, which are usually not subject to specific drug control measures and therefore much easier to prescribe. It is important to realize that neither of these reasons is of a pharmacologic nature but rather the result of inappropriate education and societal pressures.[96]

The increasing worldwide availability of tramadol will reopen the discussion of these issues.[97] The analgesic efficacy of this compound and its superior side-effect profile in comparison with conventional opioids adds a new and useful drug to our armamentarium. Its dual mode of action should result in a revival of the concept of step 2 of the WHO ladder, as it provides a real step between the nonopioids and the strong opioids.

The benefits of the second step of the analgesic ladder are unclear. The weak opioids such as codeine have been described as no more efficacious than standard dosages of acetaminophen or aspirin,[98] with higher side-effects. Adding a weak opioid to NSAIDs has been found to produce no increase in efficacy over NSAID alone with an increase in incidence of side-effects.[86]

Codeine phosphate is the classic weak opioid analgesic, given in doses of 30–120 mg every 4 h, with additive effects from retaining the nonopioid medication in the regimen.[8]

It is well absorbed from the gastrointestinal tract with a low first-pass metabolism. It has about 10% of the potency of morphine, with most, if not all, of the analgesic effect from metabolism of codeine to morphine and its subsequent metabolites.[99]

Its efficacy is limited by side-effects such as constipation, nausea and vomiting, and confusion, in particular in higher doses; therefore doses should ideally be limited to those mentioned above.[100]

Dextropropoxyphene, a derivative of methadone, has been seen as a useful agent by WHO. However, it has poor and unpredictable oral bioavailability due to a high, but saturable, first-pass effect.[101**] Despite these disadvantages, it compared well with low-dose morphine in a cancer pain population.[102***] However, a meta-analysis found little benefit in adding dextropropoxyphene to acetaminophen for postoperative pain.[103]

Dextropropoxyphene is relatively long acting and may be given every 6 h in dosages of 50–100 mg. Again, possible side-effects include nausea, vomiting, and constipation. It may cause central nervous system disturbances such as confusion or hallucinations, especially in high doses and in the elderly.

Dihydrocodeine is a semisynthetic derivative of codeine with a slightly greater potency. Its effect seems to be independent of metabolization to dihydromorphine.[104] An advantage over codeine is the availability of a slow-release preparation for use every 12 h.[105]

Tramadol is probably the most useful step 2 drug available. It has been found to be safe and effective in the treatment of cancer pain, when used in conjunction with the WHO guidelines and in combination with a nonopioid.[69,97] A relatively recent alternative to conventional opioids in many countries, tramadol has been used extensively in Germany, but also in many Asian countries, with good effects. Tramadol is a dual-acting analgesic agent with weak opioid actions that also activates descending pain pathways by inhibition of reuptake of serotonin and norepinephrine (noradrenaline) at nerve endings.[106] Thus, it has potency similar to that of parenteral meperidine (pethidine), but is associated with a low incidence and severity of the traditional opioid side-effects, in particular constipation and sedation. Unfortunately, nausea and vomiting still occur with this drug, and these are the most frequently reported side-effects.[97] However, another advantage is the low dependency potential of tramadol; as a result it is either a noncontrolled drug or a drug of a lower schedule than morphine in all countries.[107]

Tramadol is available in both parenteral and enteral preparations with a good oral bioavailability of about 70%. It is used in dosages of 50–100 mg every 4 h.

In some patients, tramadol may even be effective in the treatment of severe pain with fewer side-effects than morphine.[106**,108**] It may also be of use in neurogenic pain. However, it might not have the efficacy of morphine in severe pain and patients with progressive disease will require change to morphine as pain increases.[97]

Strong opioids (step 3)

Over 50% of patients with pain and advanced cancer will require treatment with strong opioids (i.e. morphine) at some stage of their disease.[72] According to the WHO guidelines, strong opioids are used to treat pain of high intensity that is not responsive to nonopioid or a nonopioid–weak opioid combination. This substitution process is safe and effective.[49]

Fears of side-effects such as respiratory depression, tolerance, and physical and psychological dependence have led to the worldwide underutilization of this very important group of drugs in the management of cancer pain.[109,110]

Pain acts as a stimulant to counteract any initial respiratory center depression, while the respiratory center rapidly becomes tolerant to the effect of opioids over time. Thus, respiratory depression due to opioid treatment of cancer pain almost never occurs; fear of this side-effect is not a good reason for failing to make use of opioids[111] except in patients in whom pain has been treated by other procedures (e.g. neurolysis or spinal cord compression); in such patients, high doses of opioids in the absence of pain can lead to respiratory depression.[111,112]

Drug tolerance is characterized by decreased efficacy of a drug with repeated use over time. Patients with chronic pain rarely develop tolerance, and cancer pain patients with stable disease remain on stable doses of strong opioids for long periods of time. An increased pain in association with stable opioid dosage indicates progressive disease and not tolerance.[72]

Physical dependence causes withdrawal symptoms to occur on discontinuation of a drug or with the administration of an antagonist. The terminal nature of their disease spares many cancer patients this fear. In a study of opioid withdrawal in cancer pain patients, intolerable pain rather than withdrawal symptoms made withdrawal impossible.[113] However, it has been found that a patient can stop or reduce strong opioids if pain levels are decreased by other means.[72,114] To avoid withdrawal symptoms, however, after a decrease in pain, the opioid dose should be reduced gradually. After an abrupt reduction in pain, for example after a nerve block, the dose should be reduced to 25% of the original dose, then reduced further every 2–3 days, and opioids may be stopped altogether if pain does not recur. Thus, although physical dependence does necessarily occur after opioid intake exceeding 7–10 days, it is not a major practical problem.[72]

Fears of inducing psychological addiction by appropriate pain therapy have been unfounded. Widespread clinical experience in supervised pain management programs shows that when strong opioids are used for the treatment of pain psychological dependence is a very rare occurrence;[115,116] specifically, in cancer pain patients treated with strong opioids, two surveys independently found an incidence of psychological dependence of 0.2%.[72,113]

The risk of drug diversion has also been found to be low. In Wisconsin, a significant increase in the use of opioids to combat a large problem of cancer pain was not associated with any significant increase in drug diversion to illicit users. Thus, provided drug distribution is well regulated, an increase in opioid use is not likely to result in an increase in abuse.[13]

Thus, many fears about the use of strong opioids are unfounded. Despite this, the effective and safe use of opioids still requires the consideration of several factors: previous opioid exposure, the severity and nature of the pain, the age of patient, the extent of disease, and concurrent disease.[8]

Because of the high prevalence of nausea and constipation associated with the use of opioids, it is advisable to start them in combination with a regular antiemetic and laxative.[72,117] Problems with nausea often subside as treatment continues over a few weeks, but treatment for constipation needs to be continued and aggressive.[118,119] Despite this, constipation occurs in approximately 10–12% of patients on morphine.[72]

Other side-effects of morphine are pruritus, urinary retention (3–5%), and sweating.[72]

Sedation is also common with initial and increasing doses of opioids. Sedation, nausea, and vomiting usually subside within a week of achieving a stable dose.[120] However, if sedation or nausea persists, changing opioid may be useful, as cross-tolerance between strong opioids is often incomplete.[41]

Cognitive impairment has been found to occur in patients started on opioid treatment or who undergo a significant increase in opioid dosage. This effect is unlikely to last longer than a week, and patients on stable doses of opioid experience no change in cognitive abilities.[120] However, comparisons of patients on stable doses of opioids and patients not on opioids or healthy volunteers have found small, but statistically significant, differences in cognitive abilities.[121–123]

Psychostimulants can be combined with opioids in cancer pain treatment to reduce sedation and cognitive impairment.

All of these side-effects may be decreased by the addition of a nonopioid drug or a suitable coanalgesic drug, subsequently lowering the dosage of opioid required.[72]

Morphine

Morphine is the gold standard strong opioid of choice; wide experience has been gained in its use, and acceptable analgesia can be achieved over 80% of the time by using morphine in combination with a nonopioid analgesic.[72]

Morphine is available in multiple preparations. Enteral preparations include immediate- and controlled-release tablets, capsules, elixir, or suspension.

Morphine is fully absorbed, but is subject to substantial first-pass metabolism, with an oral bioavailability of between 10% and 45%.[124] However, with chronic use, significant levels of the metabolite morphine 6-glucuronide (M6G) are produced, which has an additive analgesic effect and enhances the practical bioavailability of the drug. The metabolite is excreted via the kidney with a half-life of about 2.5–7.5 h.[64] Thus, it has the potential to accumulate in patients with renal dysfunction, and morphine should be used with care in such patients.

As there is a large inter-patient variability in morphine pharmacokinetics, dosages must be carefully determined on an individual basis by titration to pain relief. Whenever possible, morphine should be given orally, starting with an immediate-release preparation such as elixir or tablets. This ensures flexibility in dose titration. Controlled-release preparations may be started when daily requirements are established.

For such a titration, it is recommended that loading doses in opioid-naive patients start at 2.5–10 mg of an immediate-release preparation, depending on age, coexisting diseases, and pain severity. This dose may be repeated every 30–90 min in a patient-controlled approach after an effect from the previous dose is established.

Additionally, the starting dose of morphine needs to be guided by previous analgesic use. For example, a patient on a 60–100 mg dosage of codeine will normally require 10- to 15-mg doses of morphine for loading dose and titration.[125]

Once an effective analgesic dose has been reached, this dose should be given every 4–6 h. If excessive sedation occurs with adequate analgesia, the dose over 24 h will need to be decreased, usually by 50%. If, after 24 h, pain relief is inadequate, the 24-h dosage will need to be increased, usually by 50%, but by up to 100% if the 24-h dosage is less than 100 mg, and depending on rescue analgesia use.

Immediate-release morphine

Immediate-release morphine is available as 10- or 20-mg tablets as well as an elixir. Compared with the elixir, the tablets have the advantages that they have no bitter taste and are easy to swallow, the dose can be measured accurately, and distribution is easily regulated. Although they are scored for easy division into two, the tablets cannot be divided into very small doses, such as 2.5 mg, as can the elixir. Otherwise, they have the same pharmacokinetic and pharmacodynamic profile of other immediate-release preparations.

Once a 24-h dosing regimen is established, patients

may be switched to a controlled-release preparation of morphine. Dosage should be given every 12–24 h depending on the preparation.

Controlled-release preparations

Controlled-release preparations are available in strengths from 10 to 200 mg. There are two main types of preparation: a film-coated tablet with a matrix of active drug and an inactive core (MS-Contin™) and the more recently introduced capsule containing a large number of polymer-coated pellets, each designed to release morphine at different rates (Kadian, Kapanol™). A controlled-release suspension with similar efficacy to MS-Contin™ when given 12-hourly is also available.[126]

Most studies have been carried out with drugs such as MS-Contin™. It has been found that 12-hourly morphine dosage improves the quality of night-time sleep and daytime functioning as well as overall quality of life when compared with previous regimens.[118,125,127]** However, although simpler and more convenient,[128] overall pain relief and side-effects are similar when comparing 4-hourly regimens with 12-hourly ones.[128–131,132] However, simply by making a regimen easier for patients, the use of controlled-release morphine may increase the efficacy of a regimen as a whole by increasing patient acceptability and therefore compliance.[125,130,131]

Owing to the prolonged activity of these drugs, it is difficult to titrate dosages with controlled-release morphine. Ideally, daily dosage should be established with an immediate-release preparation before switching to equivalent daily dosage with controlled-release morphine, usually after 48 h of stable pain relief on stable doses of an immediate-release preparation.[125] At least 24 h should elapse before changing the dose of controlled-release morphine, to allow steady-state plasma levels of both morphine and M6G to be reached. This period should be increased in patients with renal or hepatic failure. In this case, the daily dose should be increased by at least 50%, or even 100%, if doses less than 100 mg are used.[125]

Comparisons of the two main controlled-release preparations show little difference in efficacy or side-effects,[133,134] although 24-hourly dosage of Kadian has been shown to be associated with less fluctuation in plasma levels than 12-hourly MS-Contin™.[134] However, 24-hourly dosage of Kadian does have advantages over MS-Contin™ in terms of ease of administration and patient acceptability.[133] In addition, the capsule formulation enables the contents to be sprinkled over food or down a feeding tube while retaining its controlled-release properties, whereas crushing a MS-Contin™ tablet will release the active drug from the matrix, converting it to an immediate release preparation.

Controlled-release morphine relies on slowed absorption from the gastrointestinal tract to delay and prolong its effects. In patients with "short bowel" syndrome following surgery, the effect of these preparations is diminished as a result of their rapid transit through the gut. Hence, use of these preparations should be avoided in such patients. Similar problems occur in patients who lose their slow-release tablets due to vomiting soon after intake.

**Rescue medication* must be available for all patients on controlled-release preparations. This should a short-acting opioid (usually immediate-release morphine) used to treat pain not covered by the regular dosage.[135,136]

Incident pain, i.e. increased pain due to activity, is best treated with rescue analgesia prior to the incident. This provides a safety net during periods of inactivity, which are relatively easily treated with the background controlled-release morphine.[137] Increasing controlled-release dosages may only cause excessive sedation during periods of inactivity.[138]

Breakthrough pain, i.e. pain occurring before the next dose of controlled-release morphine, often indicates progressing disease or inadequate regular dosage and needs to be met with reassessment of the pain and, usually, an increase in the dose of controlled-release preparation depending on rescue analgesic use.[19]

Rescue analgesic dosage should be approximately 25% of a 4-hourly dose or a single controlled-release dose.[125]*

For most patients, morphine will be the first-choice drug; however, if patients are in any way intolerant to morphine then alternatives should be tried.

Methadone

Methadone is a very useful and effective potent opioid alternative to morphine in the treatment of cancer pain.[139] It is well absorbed with good oral (60–95%)[124] and rectal bioavailability in both elixir and tablet form.[63] Methadone is a long-acting drug (6–12 h), making it useful for a regular dosing regimen. However, it has a variable and unpredictable half-life,[63] from 8 to 80 h,[8,124] especially in the elderly, in whom it may accumulate, resulting in excessive sedation and delayed toxicity.[140] In addition, it may take several days to weeks to achieve a steady state, which must be taken into account when changing dose. This highlights the need for careful and individual determination of dose and dosing interval.[124] Methadone should be started in doses of up to 5 mg repeated hourly until pain relief is achieved. After 1 week of this type of use, it is possible to introduce a regular dosing pattern.[141]

Recent evidence suggests that methadone is more potent than previously thought, so that rotation from morphine or other strong opioids, especially hydromorphone, to methadone must be undertaken with care, as cross-tolerance is incomplete with these drugs.[40] Rotation may also take into account previous total opioid dose.[40,142] According to tables currently in use, the equipotency ratio of oral morphine to oral methadone is 1:1 to 4:1. Calculated dose ratios for patients on a stable dose of morphine for long-term use are in the range 1:5–1:15.[143] The ratios are highest for patients receiving more than 1,000 mg of morphine per day. This again highlights the great need for care and an individualized approach when prescribing methadone, especially when rotating from other strong opioids to methadone,[143] as this may be accompanied by severe side-effects, such as respiratory depression.[140]

Methadone seems to have an advantage over other opioids in the treatment of neuropathic pain as it has inhibitory effects on serotonin and nonadrenergic uptake[144] and is a noncompetitive *N*-methyl-D-aspartate (NMDA) antagonist, albeit a weak one.[145]

Oxycodone

Oxycodone is another strong opioid alternative with potency similar to morphine.[146] It may be given orally, rectally, or parenterally and has a good oral bioavailability of 50–70%.[8] Oral conversion from morphine can be done on a 1:1 ratio.[146,147**] It has been shown to be as effective as oral morphine for cancer pain,[148,149] and there are no disadvantages associated with its long-term use.[150**] A slow-release preparation with equivalent efficacy to the immediate-release preparation is available.[151]

Hydromorphone

Hydromorphone is a potent alternative to morphine; the usual oral starting dose is 1–2 mg every 3–4 h.[8] The potency ratio to morphine is in the range of 1:3–5.[152**] A slow-release preparation with identical efficacy to the immediate-release preparation is available.[153]

Levorphanol

Like methadone, this drug has a long half-life and a tendency to accumulate and cause excessive sedation with repeated doses. Levorphanol is usually started in oral doses of 2 mg every 6 h.[8]

Meperidine (pethidine)

Long-term treatment with meperidine, especially in patients with renal impairment, may lead to the accumulation of the metabolite, normeperidine. This metabolite can cause central nervous system (CNS) excitability and even seizures in high concentrations.[154] Thus, the drug should be used with care, and avoided in those with renal failure. In addition, meperidine is a relatively short-acting drug, and must be administered every 3 h. Hence, meperidine should not be used to treat chronic cancer pain if alternatives are available.[8]

Buprenorphine

Buprenorphine is a partial opioid agonist; thus, a ceiling effect is seen with the use of this drug.[155] At low doses, 0.2 mg every 8 h, it may be used as an alternative to codeine, and at high doses, 1 mg every 8 h, buprenorphine is equivalent to 30 mg of oral morphine every 4 h.[8,156] Average daily doses of 1.5–1.7 mg provide good long-term analgesia in cancer pain patients.[157,158] However, at 3–5 mg/day a ceiling effect is seen, with any further increase in dose failing to produce any further increase in analgesia. As a partial agonist, buprenorphine may antagonize the effects of other opioid agonists and may induce a withdrawal state in some patients previously on opioid medication. Buprenorphine has a high affinity for μ-opioid receptors; as a result it is difficult to displace it by other antagonists or agonists in patients with respiratory depression or withdrawal induced by buprenorphine.

However, buprenorphine has a relatively rapid onset of 30 min with a long duration of analgesia of 6–9 h. Oral administration is accompanied by a high first-pass metabolism, but the drug can be given and is well absorbed sublingually in those who are unable to swallow.[65,155]

In a comparison with tramadol, buprenorphine was less effective and caused more serious side-effects.[159**,160**]

Dextromoramide

This is a short-acting opioid that may be useful as a rescue analgesic in patients who are intolerant of morphine, but it is unlikely to be of use as a continuous analgesic in those with chronic cancer pain because of its short half-life.[8]

Coanalgesics

On all steps of the analgesic ladder, therapy may be supplemented by the use of coanalgesic drugs.[8] These provide an alternative for patients who cannot be treated with conventional analgesics alone without encountering unacceptable side-effects.[20,161–163] The recognition that not all pain responds to morphine is of paramount importance as coanalgesics may be required by up to 90% of patients at death.[51] However, because of the not insubstantial risk of side-effects, most of these drugs should be reserved until the more conventional methods are failing to treat specific pain types.[33]

Membrane stabilizers

This group of drugs comprises the anticonvulsants and class 1 antiarrhythmics. They are particularly useful in treating neurogenic pain caused by damage to the peripheral or central nervous system. This pain is often difficult to treat as traditional analgesics may often be of little use.

Anticonvulsants

Anticonvulsants have been found to be particularly useful when pain has a stabbing or paroxysmal quality.[8,33***] A meta-analysis of randomized trials found that the number needed to treat (NNT) ranged from 2.1 to 3.8 for the various agents studied.[164] As use of these agents is often associated with sedation, it is recommended that low doses are used to begin with and doses slowly increased until analgesia is reached or side-effects become intolerable.

Clonazepam is a good first choice,[165] starting at 0.5 mg at bedtime (up to 1–4 mg/day).[33] A newer alternative is gabapentin, which has been shown to have good efficacy and a very low rate of adverse effects.[166] Alternatives are carbamazepine or sodium valproate. Carbamazepine should be started at 200 mg at bedtime or 100 mg twice daily, increasing by 200 mg every 2–3 days. Sodium valproate is started at 600 mg daily. However, it can cause significant sedation and the dose should be reduced in elderly patients.

Antiarrhythmic agents

Antiarrhythmic agents are as effective as, or even more effective than, anticonvulsants, particularly mexilitine. The concurrent use of tricyclic antidepressant drugs or other antiarrhythmic agents also enhances the arrhythmogenic potential of these drugs. Mexilitine is used in doses of 150 mg 2–4 times daily. Rapid analgesia may be achieved with an intravenous bolus of lidocaine (lignocaine) 3 mg/kg over 5 min; this may last hours to days and may be followed by oral drugs such as mexiletine.[167] In rare cases, lidocaine needs to be continued subcutaneously.[168]

Tricyclic antidepressants

These may be a useful group of drugs in some types of nerve pain, especially burning dysesthetic pain.[25,33] Doses are usually lower than those required for an antidepressant effect. Amitriptyline and imipramine are the most commonly used drugs at doses of 10–75 mg at bedtime.[33] The dose should be started low, but increased to 30–50 mg as soon as tolerated; after this doses should be increased weekly until pain is relieved or until side-effects prohibit further increases.[8]

Effects should be seen after a few days of doses in the range of 50–100 mg. However, pain may not always be completely relieved. Anticholinergic side-effects limit the usefulness of most of these agents, especially in the elderly; however, the sedative effects may be particularly useful in those experiencing sleep difficulties and depression.

Steroids

Steroids act as anti-inflammatory agents but may also have membrane-stabilizing effects and so are particularly useful in patients with spinal cord compression, intracranial tumors, organ capsule distension, and bone infiltration. High doses are usually required. Dexamethasone is a long-acting drug with no mineralocorticoid actions. Other alternatives include prednisolone (1 mg of dexamethasone is equivalent to 7 mg of prednisolone[8]) and methylprednisone. Depending on the indication, dexamethasone may be used in dosages up to 60–100 mg daily for short periods in patients with spinal cord compression.[8] Otherwise, dosages of 8–16 mg would be appropriate in patients with raised intracranial pressure, or 4–16mg[8,25] for patients with nerve compression syndrome. Administration should continue for at least a week, and be discontinued if there is no response. Otherwise doses should be reduced to the lowest dose that maintains the response seen.

In addition to their analgesic and anti-inflammatory properties, steroids can improve mood and sense of well-being, thus increasing pain tolerance and efficacy of any regimen; they may also help to improve appetite and general strength. Side-effects may include gastric irritation or even ulceration, opportunistic sepsis, myopathies, agitation, hypomania, and Cushing's syndrome. Gastrointestinal side-effects are increased if steroids are combined with NSAIDs.

Calcitonin

Pain due to tumor osteolysis and hypercalcemia has been found to be relieved by parenteral calcitonin.[169]

The usefulness of calcitonin is limited by its slow onset and unreliability, and so its use should, whenever possible, be preceded by NSAIDs in the treatment of bone pain. It is not available in an oral formulation; recent investigations suggest benefit of high-dose subcutaneous infusion.[170]

Bisphosphonates

Members of this relatively new group of synthetic drugs, like calcitonin, decrease bone resorption and increase bone mineralization through inhibition of osteoclasts. Thus, bisphosphonates are particularly useful in patients with osteolytic tumors associated with hypercalcemia. In such cases, analgesic effects have been found to be encouraging.[171]

Other oral medication

Many other groups of drugs may be used to treat the adverse effects of analgesics, to enhance pain relief, and to treat concomitant psychological disturbances, such as insomnia, anxiety, and depression.[8]

Anxiolytics

Benzodiazepines, psychotropic drugs, and major tranquilizers have no specific analgesic effects and they often cause sedation without adding to analgesia. Hence, they should only be used for unrelieved anxiety or identifiable depression; any problems with sleeping should be first addressed by treatment of the cause: analgesia, counseling regarding fears. However, for some patients, pharmacological treatment of these problems may be necessary, with benzodiazepines being of further use in muscle spasm or myofascial pain.

Laxatives

Laxatives are essential to chronic opioid therapy. Coloxyl and senna is a common combination, as this provides both a softener and peristaltic stimulant. The dose is usually given at night and titrated to the patient's needs. An alternative is lactulose, but in 30–50% of patients suppositories or enemas may also need to be used in combination with oral preparations.

Antiemetics

Antiemetics should be prescribed regularly for any patient starting on opioid treatment. Prochlorperazine may be used in 10-mg doses before each morphine dose, or metoclopramide 10–20 mg every 4–6 h. Other drugs that may have better efficacy include droperidol or ondansetron. The need for these depends on tolerability of side-effects and availability of individual drug classes. These can usually be discontinued within a week.

SUMMARY

Cancer pain is a worldwide problem that has only recently been addressed and resolved. The World Health Organization has been fundamental in setting up cancer pain relief programs worldwide.

Treatment of cancer pain involves a multimodal approach, with oral pharmacotherapy being the mainstay. An analgesic ladder has been developed giving a structured method for introducing increasingly potent drugs in a sequential manner to treat increasing pain intensity.

Strong opioids such as morphine have been underutilized in the past for number of reasons, including misconceptions regarding use and side-effects. However, these drugs in combination with nonopioid analgesics form the basis of an effective analgesic regimen.

After full pain assessment, treatment regimens must be tailored to meet individual patients' needs depending on the nature and intensity of their pain and their goals and priorities.

There is no right dose of drugs such as morphine, so doses must be titrated to pain relief for each individual patient. Once this is established, then constant, regular, around the clock, dosage must be used to treat and then to prevent chronic recurring pain.

If the pain is not responding despite high-dosage morphine, or a patient is experiencing excessive sedation without pain relief, then further assessment is required. Not all pain responds fully to opioids. Examples include neurogenic pain, bone pain, and visceral pain; each may require the use of an appropriate coanalgesic drug. Conversely, unrelieved anxiety or depression may prevent adequate analgesia. Thus, recognition and treatment of psychological problems is of paramount importance in cancer pain treatment. Oral drugs may not be fully absorbed in a number of situations such as emesis, short bowel syndrome, or gastrointestinal obstruction. In such situations, other routes of administration are available and acceptable.

Increasing pain almost always reflects disease progression rather than true opioid tolerance. In addition, fear of respiratory depression and psychological dependence is almost universally unfounded, with physiological dependence causing no practical problems to cancer patients with decreased pain if opioid doses are tapered off over a few days.

Used appropriately, the WHO analgesic guidelines for cancer pain relief will significantly improve pain levels and quality of life in up to 80–90% of cancer patients with severe pain even in the last days of life.

REFERENCES

◆ 1. Portenoy R. Cancer pain. Epidemiology and syndromes. *Cancer* 1989; **63:** 2298–307.
2. Daut R, Cleeland C. The prevalence and severity of pain in cancer. *Cancer* 1982; **50:** 1913–18.
3. Stjernsward J, Colleau S, Ventafridda V. The World Health Organization cancer pain and palliative care program. Past, present and future. *J Pain Symptom Manage* 1996; **12:** 65–72.
4. Foley K, Portenoy R. World Health Organization –International Association for the Study of Pain: joint initiatives in cancer pain relief. *J Pain Symptom Manage* 1993; **8:** 335–9.
● 5. Foley K. The treatment of cancer pain. *N Engl J Med* 1985; **313:** 84–95.
6. Saunders C. *The Management of Terminal Illness.* London: Edward Arnold, 1967.
◆ 7. World Health Organization. *Cancer Pain Relief,* 2nd edn. Geneva: WHO, 1986.
◆ 8. World Health Organization. *Cancer Pain Relief and Palliative Care,* 2nd edn. Geneva: WHO, 1996.
◆ 9. Zech D, Grond S, Lynch J, *et al.* Validation of the World Health Organization Guidelines for cancer pain relief: a 10-year prospective study. *Pain* 1995; **63(1):** 65–76.
10. Tuttle C. Drug management of pain in cancer patients. *Can Med Assoc J* 1985; **132:** 121–34.
◆ 11. Schug SA, Zech D, Doerr U. Cancer pain management according to WHO Analgesic Guidelines. *J Pain Symptom Manage* 1990; **5:** 27–32.
12. Skaer T. Management of pain in cancer patients. *Clin Ther* 1993; **15:** 638–49.
13. Joranson D. Availability of opioids for cancer pain: recent trends, assessment of system barriers, new World Health Organization guidelines, and the risk of diversion. *J Pain Symptom Manage* 1993; **8:** 353–60.

14. Fife BL, Irick N, Painter JD. A comparative study of the attitudes of physicians and nurses toward the management of cancer pain. *J Pain Symptom Manage* 1993; **8:** 132–9.
15. Hammack J, Loprinzi C. Use of orally administered opioids for cancer-related pain. *Mayo Clin Proc* 1994; **69:** 384–90.
16. Alastair JJ, Wood MD. Pharmacologic treatment of cancer pain. *N Engl J Med* 1996; **335:** 1124–32.
17. Ventafridda V, Caraceni A. Cancer pain classification: a controversial issue. *Pain* 1991; **46:** 1–2.
18. Payne R, Gonzalez G. Pathophysiology of pain in cancer and other terminal disease. In: Doyle D, Hanks G, MacDonald N eds. *Oxford Textbook of Palliative Medicine.* Oxford: Oxford Medical Publications, 1993: 140–8.
19. Portenoy R, Hagen N. Breakthrough pain: definition, prevalence and characteristics. *Pain* 1990; **41:** 273–81.
● 20. Portenoy R. Pharmacologic management of cancer pain. *Semin Oncol* 1995; **22** (2 Suppl. 3): 112–120.
21. Hillier R. Control of pain in terminal cancer. *Br Med Bull* 1990; **46:** 279–91.
22. Blanchard CG, Ruckdeschel JC. Psychosocial aspects of cancer in adults: implications for teaching medical students. *J Cancer Ed* 1986; **1:** 237–48.
23. Gadow S. An ethical case for patient self-determination. *Semin Oncol Nursing* 1989; **5(2):** 99–101.
24. Levenson BS. A multidimensional approach to the treatment of pain in the oncology patient. *Front Radiat Ther Oncol* 1980; **15:** 138–41.
25. Grond S, Zech D, Lynch J, *et al.* Validation of the World Health Organization guidelines for pain relief in head and neck cancer. A prospective study. *Ann Otol Rhinol Laryngol* 1993; **102:** 342–8.
26. Donato V, Montagna A, Musio D, Cellini N. Radiotherapy in the symptomatic treatment of the oncological patients. *Anticancer Res* 1999; **19(4C):** 3375–82.
27. Ramirez AJ, Towlson KE, Leaning MS, *et al.* Do patients with advanced breast cancer benefit from chemotherapy? *Br J Cancer* 1998; **78:** 1488–94.
28. Fourneau I, Broos P. Pathologic fractures due to metastatic disease. A retrospective study of 160 surgically treated fractures. *Acta Chir Belg* 1998; **98:** 255–60.
29. Weigel B, Maghsudi M, Neumann C, *et al.* Surgical management of symptomatic spinal metastases. Postoperative outcome and quality of life. *Spine* 1999; **24:** 2240–6.
30. Ippolito V, Micheletti E, Saccalani M, *et al.* Radiotherapy and spinal brace: still first-choice treatment for vertebral metastases from breast cancer. *Chir Organi Mov* 1998; **83:** 177–83.
● 31. Mercadante SG. When oral morphine fails in cancer pain: the role of the alternative routes. *Am J Hosp Palliat Care* 1998; **15:** 333–42.
● 32. Glare P. Problems with opiates in cancer pain: parenteral opioids. *Support Care Cancer* 1997; **5:** 445–50.
● 33. Schug SA, Dunlop R, Zech D. Pharmacological management of cancer pain. *Drugs* 1992; **43:** 44–53.
34. Moote C. The prevention of postoperative pain. *Can J Anaesth* 1994; **41:** 527.
35. McCormack J, Warriner C, Levine M, Glick N. A Comparison of regularly dosed oral morphine and on-demand intramuscular morphine in the treatment of postsurgical pain. *Can J Anaesthesiol* 1993; **40:** 819.
36. Goughnour BR, Arkinstall WW, Stewart JH. Analgesic response to single and multiple doses of controlled-release morphine tablets and morphine oral solution in cancer patients. *Cancer* 1989; **63** (11 Suppl.): 2294–7.
37. Grond S, Zech D, Schug SA, *et al.* The importance of non-opioid analgesics for cancer pain relief according to the guidelines of the World Health Organization (WHO). *Int J Clin Pharm Res* 1991; **6:** 253–60.
◆ 38. Freynhagen R, Zenz M, Strumpf M. WHO step II – clinical reality or a didactic instrument? *Der Schmerz* 1994; **8:** 210–15.
◆ 39. Grond S, Meuser T. Weak opioids – an educational substitute for morphine? *Curr Opin Anaesthesiol* 1998; **11:** 559–65.
40. Bruera E, Pereira J, Watanabe S, *et al.* Opioid rotation in patients with cancer pain. A retrospective comparison of dose ratios between methadone, hydromorphone, and morphine. *Cancer* 1996; **78:** 852–7.
41. de Stoutz ND, Bruera E, Suarez-Almazor M. Opioid rotation for toxicity reduction in terminal cancer patients. *J Pain Symptom Manage* 1995; **10:** 378–84.
● 42. Mercadante S. Opioid rotation for cancer pain: rationale and clinical aspects. *Cancer* 1999; **86:** 1856–66.
43. Smith MT. Neuroexcitatory effects of morphine and hydromorphone: evidence implicating the 3-glucuronide metabolites. *Clin Exp Pharmacol Physiol* 2000; **27:** 524–8.
44. Sjogren P, Jensen NH, Jensen TS. Disappearance of morphine-induced hyperalgesia after discontinuing or substituting morphine with other opioid agonists. *Pain* 1994; **59:** 313–16.
45. IASP. Pain terms. *Pain* 1979; **6:** 249.
46. Boisvert M, Cohen SR. Opioid use in advanced malignant disease: why do different centers use vastly different doses? A plea for standardized reporting. *J Pain Symptom Manage* 1995; **10:** 632–8.
47. Twycross R. Medical treatment of cancer pain. *Bull Cancer* 1980; **67:** 209–16.
48. Klepstad P, Kaasa S, Borchgrevink PC. Start of oral morphine to cancer patients: effective serum morphine concentrations and contribution from morphine-6-glucuronide to the analgesia produced by morphine. *Eur J Clin Pharmacol* 2000; **55:** 713–19.
49. Klepstad P, Kaasa S, Skauge M, Borchgrevink PC. Pain intensity and side-effects during titration of morphine to cancer patients using a fixed schedule dose escalation. *Acta Anaesthesiol Scand* 2000; **44:** 656–64.
50. Brooks I, De Jager R, Blumenreich M, *et al.* Principles of cancer pain management. Use of long-acting oral morphine. *J Fam Pract* 1989; **28:** 275–80.

◆ 51. Grond S, Zech D, Schug SA, *et al.* Validation of WHO guidelines for cancer pain relief during the last days and hours of life. *J Pain Symptom Manage* 1991; **6:** 411–22.

◆ 52. Ventafridda V, Tamburini M, Caraceni A. A validation study of the WHO method for cancer pain relief. *Cancer* 1987; **59:** 850–6.

53. Portenoy RK. Managing cancer pain poorly responsive to systemic opioid therapy. *Oncology (Huntingt)* 1999; **13** (5 Suppl. 2): 25–9.

◆ 54. Takeda F. Results of field testing in Japan of the WHO Draft Interim Guidelines on relief of cancer pain. *Pain Clin* 1986; **1:** 83–9.

55. Lichter I, Hunt E. The last 48 h of life. *J Palliative Care* 1990; **6(4):** 7–15.

56. Walsh TD. Oral morphine in chronic cancer pain. *Pain* 1984; **18:** 1–11.

57. DeConno F, Ripamonti C, Saita L, *et al.* Role of rectal route in treating cancer pain: a randomised crossover clinical trial of oral versus rectal morphine administration in opioid-naive cancer patients with pain. *J Clin Oncol* 1995; **13:** 1004–8.

58. Moulin DE, Johnson NG, Murray-Parsons N, *et al.* Subcutaneous narcotic infusions for cancer pain: treatment outcome and guidelines for use. *CMAJ* 1992; **146:** 891–7.

59. Breda M, Bianchi M, Ripamonti C, *et al.* Plasma morphine and morphine-6-glucuronide patterns in cancer patients after oral, subcutaneous, sublabial and rectal short-term administration. *Int J Clin Pharmacol Res* 1991; **11:** 93–7.

60. Wilkinson TJ, Robinson BA, Begg EJ, *et al.* Pharmacokinetics and efficacy of rectal versus oral sustained-release morphine in cancer patients. *Cancer Chemother Pharmacol* 1992; **31:** 251–4.

61. Ripamonti C, Bruera E. Rectal, buccal, and sublingual narcotics for the management of cancer pain. *J Palliat Care* 1991; **7:** 30–5.

62. Nelson KA, Glare PA, Walsh D, Groh ES. A prospective, within-patient, crossover study of continuous intravenous and subcutaneous morphine for chronic cancer pain. *J Pain Symptom Manage* 1997; **13:** 262–7.

● 63. Ripamonti C, Zecca E, Bruera E. An update on the clinical use of methadone for cancer pain. *Pain* 1997; **70:** 109–15.

● 64. Glare PA, Walsh TD. Clinical pharmacokinetics of morphine. *Ther Drug Monit* 1991; **13(1):** 1–23.

65. Robbie DS. A trial of sublingual buprenorphine in cancer pain. *Br J Clin Pharmacol* 1979; **7** (Suppl. 3): 315S–17S.

66. Farrar J, Cleary J, Rauck R, *et al.* Oral transmucosal fentanyl citrate: randomised, double-blinded, placebo-controlled trial for treatment of breakthrough pain in cancer patients. *J Natl Cancer Inst* 1998; **90:** 611–16.

67. Wong J, Chiu G, Tsao C, Chang C. Comparison of oral controlled-release morphine with transdermal fentanyl in terminal cancer pain. *Acta Anaesthesiol Sin* 1997; **35:** 25–32.

◆ 68. Ahmedzai S, Brooks D. Transdermal fentanyl versus sustained-release oral morphine in cancer pain: preference, efficacy, and quality of life. *J Pain Symptom Manage* 1997; **13:** 254–61.

69. Grond S, Zech D, Lynch J, Schug S, Lehmann KA. Tramadol – a weak opioid for relief of cancer pain. *Pain Clin* 1992; **5:** 241–7.

70. Grond S, Zech D, Meuser T, *et al.* Cancer pain relief in dying patients. *Pain* 1990; Suppl. 5: 355.

71. Schug S, Zech D, Grond S. Morphine dosages in the treatment of cancer pain. *Pain* 1990; Suppl. 5: 365.

◆ 72. Schug SA, Zech D, Grond S, *et al.* A long-term survey of morphine in cancer pain patients. *J Pain Symptom Manage* 1992; **7:** 259–66.

73. Cooper S. Comparative efficacies of aspirin and acetaminophen. *Archiv Internal Med* 1981; **141:** 282–5.

74. Minotti V, Patoia L, Roila F, *et al.* Double-blind evaluation of analgesic efficacy of orally administered diclofenac, nefopam, and acetylsalicylic acid (ASA) plus codeine in chronic cancer pain. *Pain* 1989; **36:** 177–83.

75. Pillans PI, Woods DJ. Adverse reactions associated with nefopam. *N Z Med J* 1995; **108:** 382–4.

76. Wang RI, Waite EM. The clinical analgesic efficacy of oral nefopam hydrochloride. *J Clin Pharmacol* 1979; **19:** 395–402.

77. Sahajwalla CG, Ayres JW. Multiple-dose acetaminophen pharmacokinetics. *J Pharm Sci* 1991; **80:** 855–60.

78. Viel E, Langlade A, Osman M, *et al.* Propacetamol: from basic action to clinical utilization. *Ann Fr Anesth Reanim* 1999; **18:** 332–40.

79. Rodriguez M, Barutell C, Rull M, *et al.* Efficacy and tolerance of oral dipyrone versus oral morphine for cancer pain. *Eur J Cancer* 1994; **5:** 584–7.

80. Daftary SN, Mehta AC, Nanavati M. A controlled comparison of dipyrone and paracetamol in post-episiotomy pain. *Curr Med Res Opin* 1980; **6:** 614–8.

81. Schmieder G, Stankov G, Zerle G, *et al.* Observer-blind study with metamizole versus tramadol and butylscopolamine in acute biliary colic pain. *Arzneimittelforschung* 1993; **43:** 1216–21.

82. Kewitz H. Rare but serious risks associated with non-narcotic analgesics: clinical experience. *Med Toxicol* 1986; **1** (Suppl. 1): 86–92.

83. Saxena A, Andley M, Gnanasekaran N. Comparison of piroxicam and acetylsalicylic acid for pain in head and neck cancers: a double-blind study. *Palliative Med* 1994; **8:** 223–9.

84. Ventafridda V, Conno FD, Panerai A, *et al.* Non-steroidal anti-inflammatory drugs as the first step in cancer pain therapy: double-blind, within-patient study comparing nine drugs. *J Int Med Res* 1990; **18:** 21–9.

85. Breivik EK, Barkvoll P, Skovlund E. Combining diclofenac with acetaminophen or acetaminophen–codeine

after oral surgery: a randomized, double-blind single-dose study. *Clin Pharmacol Ther* 1999; **66:** 625–35.

● 86. Eisenberg E, Berkey C, Carr D, *et al.* Efficacy and safety of nonsteroidal antiinflammatory drugs for cancer pain: a meta-analysis. *J Clin Oncol* 1994; **12:** 2756–65.

87. Valentini M, Cannizzaro R, Poletti M, *et al.* Nonsteroidal antiinflammatory drugs for cancer pain: comparison between misoprostol and ranitidine in prevention of upper gastrointestinal damage. *J Clin Oncol* 1995; **13:** 2637–42.

88. Lazzaroni M, Bianchi Porro G. Non-steroidal anti-inflammatory drug gastropathy: clinical results with H2 antagonists and proton pump inhibitors. *Ital J Gastroenterol Hepatol* 1999; **31** (Suppl. 1): S73–8.

● 89. Jackson LM, Hawkey CJ. COX-2 selective nonsteroidal anti-Inflammatory drugs: do they really offer any advantages? *Drugs* 2000; **59:** 1207–16.

90. Stambaugh J, Drew J. The combination of ibuprofen and oxycodone/acetaminophen in the management of chronic cancer pain. *Clin Pharmacol Ther* 1988; **44:** 665–9.

91. Weingart W, Sorkness C, Earhart R. Analgesia with oral narcotics and added ibuprofen in cancer patients. *Clin Pharmacy* 1985; **4:** 53–8.

92. Mercadante S, Sapio M, Caligara M, *et al.* Opioid-sparing effect of diclofenac in cancer pain. *J Pain Symptom Manage* 1997; **14:** 15–20.

93. Minotti V, Angelis VD, Righetti E, *et al.* Double-blind evaluation of short-term analgesic efficacy of orally administered diclofenac, diclofenac plus codeine, and diclofenac plus imipramine in chronic cancer pain. *Pain* 1998; **74:** 133–7.

94. Lander J. Fallacies and phobias about addiction and pain. *Br J Addict* 1990; **85:** 803–9.

◆ 95. Morgan JP. American opiophobia: customary underutilization of opioid analgesics. *Adv Alcohol Subst Abuse* 1985; **5:** 163–73.

96. Weinstein SM, Laux LF, Thornby JI, *et al.* Medical students' attitudes toward pain and the use of opioid analgesics: implications for changing medical school curriculum. *South Med J* 2000; **93:** 472–8.

● 97. Radbruch L, Grond S, Lehmann K. A risk–benefit assessment of tramadol in the management of pain. *Drug Safety* 1996; **15:** 8–29.

98. Beaver W. Impact of non-narcotic oral analgesics on pain management. *Am J Med* 1988; **84(5A):** 3–15.

99. Caraco Y, Sheller J, Wood AJJ. Pharmacogenetic determination of the effects of codeine and prediction of drug interactions. *J Pharmacol Exp Ther* 1996; **278:** 1165–74.

100. Jochimsen PR, Noyes R, Jr. Appraisal of codeine as an analgesic in older patients. *J Am Geriatr Soc* 1978; **26:** 521–3.

●101. Collins SL, Edwards JE, Moore RA, McQuay HJ. Single-dose dextropropoxyphene in post-operative pain: a quantitative systematic review. *Eur J Clin Pharmacol* 1998; **54:** 107–12.

102. Mercadante S, Salvaggio L, Dardanoni G, *et al.* Dextropropoxyphene versus morphine in opioid-naive cancer patients with pain. *J Pain Symptom Manage* 1998; **15:** 76–81.

103. Li Wan Po A, Zhang WY. Systematic overview of co-proxamol to assess analgesic effects of addition of dextropropoxyphene to paracetamol. *Br Med J* 1997; **315:** 1565–71.

104. Jurna I, Komen W, Baldauf J, Fleischer W. Analgesia by dihydrocodeine is not due to formation of dihydromorphine: evidence from nociceptive activity in rat thalamus. *J Pharmacol Exp Ther* 1997; **281:** 1164–70.

105. Frazer N, Galloway DB, Quinn K, *et al.* *A Multiple Dose, Randomised, Comparative Pharmacokinetic Study of DHC Continuous 60 mg and Normal Release Dihydrocodeine 30 mg (DF118 Tablets).* Cambridge: Clinical Pharmacology Department, Napp Research Centre Ltd, 1987.

106. Wilder-Smith C, Schimke J, Osterwalder B, Senn H. Oral tramadol, a mu-opioid agonist and monoamine reuptake-blocker, and morphine for strong cancer-related pain. *Ann Oncol* 1994; **5:** 141–6.

◆107. Preston KL, Jasinski DR, Testa M. Abuse potential and pharmacological comparison of tramadol and morphine. *Drug Alcohol Depend* 1991; **27:** 7–17.

108. Grond S, Radbruch L, Meuser T, *et al.* High-dose tramadol in comparison to low-dose morphine for cancer pain relief. *J Pain Symptom Manage* 1999; **18:** 174–9.

109. Venegas G, Ripamonti C, Sbanotto A, Conno FD. Side-effects of morphine administration in cancer pain. *Cancer Nursing* 1998; **21:** 289–97.

●110. Walsh TD. Prevention of opioid side-effects. *J Pain Symptom Manage* 1990; **5:** 362–7.

111. Ravenscroft P, Schneider J. Bedside perspectives on the use of opioids: transferring results of clinical research into practice. *Clin Exp Pharmacol Physiol* 2000; **27:** 529–32.

112. Quevedo F, Walsh D. Morphine-induced ventilatory failure after spinal cord compression. *J Pain Symptom Manage* 1999; **18:** 140–2.

113. Sun WZ, Chen TL, Fan SZ, *et al.* Can cancer pain attenuate the physical dependence on chronic long-term morphine treatment? *J Formos Med Assoc* 1992; **91:** 513–20.

114. Jackson MB, Pounder D, Price C, *et al.* Percutaneous cervical cordotomy for the control of pain in patients with pleural mesothelioma. *Thorax* 1999; **54:** 238–41.

115. Porter J, Jick H. Addiction rate in patients treated with narcotics. *N Engl J Med* 1980; **302:** 123.

◆116. Chapman C, Hill H. Prolonged morphine self-administration and addiction liability. *Cancer* 1989; **63:** 1636–44.

117. Curtis EB, Walsh TD. Prescribing practices of a palliative care service. *J Pain Symptom Manage* 1993; **8:** 312–16.

118. Lazarus H, Fitzmartin R, Goldenheim P. A multi-investigator clinical evaluation of oral controlled-release

morphine (MS Contin tablets) administered to cancer patients. *Hospice J* 1990; **6:** 1–15.

◆119. Mancini I, Bruera E. Constipation in advanced cancer patients. *Support Care Cancer* 1998; **6:** 356–64.

●120. Bruera E, Macmillan K, Hanson J, MacDonald R. The cognitive effects of the administration of narcotic analgesics in patients with cancer pain. *Pain* 1989; **39:** 13–16.

121. Vainio A, Ollila J, Matikainen E, *et al.* Driving ability in cancer patients receiving long-term morphine analgesia. *Lancet* 1995; **346:** 667–70.

122. Banning A, Sjogren P. Cerebral effects of long-term oral opioids in cancer patients measured by continuous reaction time. *Clin J Pain* 1990; **6:** 91–5.

123. Banning A, Sjogren P, Kaiser F. Reaction time in cancer patients receiving peripherally acting analgesics alone or in combination with opioids. *Acta Anaesthesiol Scand* 1992; **36:** 480–2.

◆124. Gourlay GK, Cherry DA, Cousins MJ. A comparative study of the efficacy and pharmacokinetics of oral methadone and morphine in the treatment of severe pain in patients with cancer. *Pain* 1986; **25:** 297–312.

125. Lapin J, Portenoy R, Coyle N, *et al.* Guidelines for the use of controlled-release oral morphine in cancer pain management. *Cancer Nursing* 1989; **12:** 202–8.

126. Boureau F, Saudubray F, d'Arnoux C, *et al.* A comparative study of controlled-release morphine (CRM) suspension and CRM tablets in chronic cancer pain. *J Pain Symptom Manage* 1992; **7:** 393–9.

127. Meed S, Kleinman P, Kantor T, *et al.* Management of cancer pain with oral controlled-release morphine sulphate. *J Clin Pharmacol* 1987; **27:** 155–61.

128. Hanks G, Twycross R, Bliss J. Controlled release morphine tablets: a double-blind trial in patients with advanced cancer. *Anaesthesia* 1987; **42:** 840–4.

129. Cundiff D, McCarthy K, Savarese J, *et al.* Evaluation of a cancer pain model for the testing of long acting analgesics. The effect of MS Contin in a double-blind, randomised crossover design. *Cancer* 1989; **63** (11 Suppl.): 2355–9.

130. Portenoy R, Maldonado M, Fitzmartin R, *et al.* Oral controlled-release morphine sulphate. Analgesic efficacy and side-effects of a 100-mg tablet in cancer patients. *Cancer* 1989; **63** (11 Suppl.): 2284–8.

131. Goughnour B, Arkinstall W, Stewart J. Analgesic response to single and multiple doses of controlled-release morphine tablets and morphine oral solution in cancer patients. *Cancer* 1989; **63:** 2294–7.

132. Warfield C. Controlled-release morphine tablets in patients with chronic cancer pain: a narrative review of controlled clinical trials. *Cancer* 1998; **82:** 2299–306.

133. Broomhead A, Kerr R, Tester W, *et al.* Comparison of once-a-day sustained-release morphine formulation with standard oral morphine treatment for cancer pain. *J Pain Symptom Manage* 1997; **14:** 63–76.

134. Gourlay GK, Cherry DA, Onley MM, *et al.* Pharmacokinetics and pharmacodynamics of twenty-four-hourly kapanol compared to twelve-hourly MS Contin in the treatment of severe cancer pain. *Pain* 1997; **69:** 295–302.

135. Simmonds MA. Management of breakthrough pain due to cancer. *Oncology (Huntingt)* 1999; **13:** 1103–8.

136. Patt RB, Ellison NM. Breakthrough pain in cancer patients: characteristics, prevalence, and treatment. *Oncology (Huntingt)* 1998; **12:** 1035–46.

137. Rogers AG. How to manage incident pain. *J Pain Symptom Manage* 1987; **2:** 99.

●138. McQuay HJ, Jadad AR. Incident pain. *Cancer Surveys* 1994; **21:** 17–24.

139. DeConno F, Groff L, Brunelli C, *et al.* Clinical experience with oral methadone administration in the treatment of pain in 196 advanced cancer patients. *J Clin Oncol* 1996; **14:** 2836–42.

140. Hunt G, Bruera E. Respiratory depression in a patient receiving oral methadone for cancer pain. *J Pain Symptom Manage* 1995; **10:** 401–4.

◆141. Sawe J, Hansen J, Ginman C, *et al.* Patient-controlled dose regimen of methadone for chronic cancer pain. *Br Med J* 1981; **282:** 771–3.

142. Ripamonto C, Conno FD, Groff L, *et al.* Equianalgesic dose/ratio between methadone and other opioid agonists in cancer pain: comparison of two clinical experiences. *Ann Oncol* 1998; **9:** 79–83.

◆143. Lawler P, Turner K, Hanson J, Bruera E. Dose ratio between morphine and methadone in patients with cancer pain: a retrospective study. *Cancer* 1998; **82:** 1167–73.

144. Codd EE, Shank RP, Schupsky JJ, Raffa RB. Serotonin and norepinephrine uptake inhibiting activity of centrally acting analgesics: structural determinants and role in antinociception. *J Pharmacol Exp Ther* **274:** 1263–70.

145. Ebert B, Andersen S, Korgsgaard-Larsen P. Ketobemidone, methadone and pethidine are non-competitive *N*-methyl-D-aspartate (NMDA) antagonists in the rat cortex and spinal cord. *Neurosci Lett* **187:** 165–8.

146. Glare PA, Walsh TD. Dose-ranging study of oxycodone for chronic pain in advanced cancer. *J Clin Oncol* 1993; **11:** 973–8.

147. Zhukovsky DS, Walsh D, Doona M. The relative potency between high dose oral oxycodone and intravenous morphine: a case illustration. *J Pain Symptom Manage* 1999; **18:** 53–5.

148. Mucci-LoRusso P, Berman BS, Silberstein PT, *et al.* Controlled-release oxycodone compared with controlled-release morphine in the treatment of cancer pain: a randomized, double-blind, parallel-group study. *Eur J Pain* 1998; **2:** 239–49.

149. Bruera E, Belzile M, Pituskin E, *et al.* Randomized, double-blind, cross-over trial comparing safety and efficacy of oral controlled-release oxycodone with controlled-release morphine in patients with cancer pain. *J Clin Oncol* 1998; **16:** 3222–9.

150. Citron ML, Kaplan R, Parris WC, *et al.* Long-term administration of controlled-release oxycodone tablets for

the treatment of cancer pain. *Cancer Invest* 1998; **16:** 562–71.

151. Parris WC, Johnson BW, Jr, Croghan MK, *et al.* The use of controlled-release oxycodone for the treatment of chronic cancer pain: a randomized, double-blind study. *J Pain Symptom Manage* 1998; **16:** 205–11.
152. Lawlor P, Turner K, Hanson J, Bruera E. Dose ratio between morphine and hydromorphone in patients with cancer pain: a retrospective study. *Pain* 1997; **72(1–2):** 79–85.
153. Hays H, Hagen N, Thirlwell M, *et al.* Comparative clinical efficacy and safety of immediate release and controlled release hydromorphone for chronic severe cancer pain. *Cancer* 1994; **74:** 1808–16.
154. Armstrong PJ, Bersten A. Normeperidine toxicity. *Anesth Analg* 1986; **65:** 536–8.
155. Hanks GW. The clinical usefulness of agonist–antagonistic opioid analgesics in chronic pain. *Drug Alcohol Depend* 1987; **20:** 339–46.
156. Wallenstein SL, Kaiko RF, Rogers AG, Houde RW. Crossover trials in clinical analgesic assays: studies of buprenorphine and morphine. *Pharmacotherapy* 1986; **6:** 228–35.
157. Zenz M, Piepenbrock S, Tryba M, *et al.* Long-term therapy of cancer pain. A controlled study on buprenorphine. *Dtsch Med Wochenschr* 1985; **110:** 448–53.
158. Zenz M, Piepenbrock S, Tryba M, *et al.* Sublingual buprenorphine tablets: initial clinical experiences in long-term therapy of cancer pain. *Fortschr Med* 1983; **101:** 191–4.
159. Brema F, Pastorino G, Martini MC, *et al.* Oral tramadol and buprenorphine in tumour pain. An Italian multicentre trial. *Int J Clin Pharmacol Res* 1996; **16(4–5):** 109–16.
160. Bono AV, Cuffari S. Effectiveness and tolerance of tramadol in cancer pain. A comparative study with respect to buprenorphine. *Drugs* 1997; **53** (Suppl. 2): 40–9.
161. Kopf A. Co-analgesics in the treatment of chronic pain. *Ther Umsch* 1999; **56:** 441–5.
162. Mancini I, Body JJ. Treatment of cancer pain: the role of co-analgesics. *Rev Med Brux* 1998; **19:** A319–22.
163. Rouveix B, Bauwens MC, Giroud JP. Treatment of different types of pain. *Bull Acad Natl Med* 1999; **183:** 889–901.
164. Wiffen P, Collins S, McQuay H, Carroll D, *et al.* Anticonvulsant drugs for acute and chronic pain (Cochrane review). *The Cochrane Library* 2002; **2.**

◆165. Swerdlow M, Cundill JG. Anticonvulsant drugs used in the treatment of lancinating pain. A comparison. *Anaesthesia* 1981; **36:** 1129–32.

●166. Nicholson B. Gabapentin use in neuropathic pain syndromes. *Acta Neurol Scand* 2000; **101:** 359–71.

◆167. Boas R, Covino B, Shahnarian A. Analgesic responses to IV lignocaine. *Br J Anaesth* 1982; **54:** 501–5.

168. Devulder JE, Ghys L, Dhondt W, Rolly G. Neuropathic pain in a cancer patient responding to subcutaneously administered lignocaine. *Clin J Pain* 1993; **9:** 220–3.
169. Schiraldi GF, Soresi E, Locicero S, *et al.* Salmon calcitonin in cancer pain: comparison between two different treatment schedules. *Int J Clin Pharmacol Ther Toxicol* 1987; **25:** 229–32.
170. Mystakidou K, Befon S, Hondros K, *et al.* Continuous subcutaneous administration of high-dose salmon calcitonin in bone metastasis: pain control and beta-endorphin plasma levels. *J Pain Symptom Manage* 1999; **18:** 323–30.
171. Fulfaro F, Casuccio A, Ticozzi C, Ripamonti C. The role of bisphosphonates in the treatment of painful metastatic bone disease: a review of phase III trials. *Pain* 1998; **78:** 157–69.

11

When the WHO ladder appears to be failing: approaches to refractory or unstable cancer pain

MICHAEL ASHBY AND KATE JACKSON

The World Health Organization (WHO)'s analgesic "ladder" has been the internationally recommended approach to the pharmacological management of cancer pain for the last two decades.[1] In essence, this approach (hereafter referred to as the "WHO ladder") describes a three-step progression from nonopioid to opioid drugs, depending on an assessment of pain intensity. It also emphasizes the preferential use of the oral route of administration wherever possible. This simplicity and clarity has been the secret of its widely attested success in improving pain control in palliative care practice. However, nothing in clinical medicine can be that simple, and any approach has its flaws and omissions. Although the ladder appears to be an effective strategy for the majority of patients, all practitioners will be aware of situations in which the interventions that it describes "fail" to achieve acceptable pain control. This ladder "failure" cannot be conceptualized as a homogeneous set of clinical circumstances, and there is no one identifiable underpinning biological mechanism at play. In this chapter, the history and background to the present-day ladder will be briefly considered as a prelude to an examination of its underlying pharmacological principles. It will be shown that the ladder is not a static concept, and that a more complex clinical and biological understanding of pain mechanisms is emerging. The principles of a mechanistic approach to individual patient management will be described.[2]

BACKGROUND

The WHO analgesic ladder approach to cancer pain management (Fig. 11.1) is one of the tablets of stone of the hospice and palliative care movement, being the bedrock of three successive WHO technical reports on cancer pain and palliative care and the principal international textbook on the subject.[3–6] An editorial in 1986 by Robert Twycross sums up the initial WHO policy thrust,[7] and Stjernsward and Teoh[8] summarized the history of the ladder approach, also in an editorial, in 1989. It originated from the WHO consultation in Milan in 1982, which resulted in draft guidelines, and the first official appearance in the influential 1986 WHO report entitled *Cancer Pain Relief*.[3]

The three key elements of the ladder approach are that analgesic drugs are administered "by the mouth," "by the clock," and "by the ladder," to which, in 1990, were added, "for the individual" and "attention to detail." Drug class choice is determined in a sequence (or additive sequence, an important distinction; see below), going from nonopioid, to "weak" opioid, and then "strong" opioid, depending on the severity of the pain (placed in three categories: mild, moderate or severe). The drugs are given regularly, respecting their pharmacokinetic characteristics, with the aim of achieving steady-state plasma drug concentrations. The oral route is preferred, wherever possible, as, traditionally, nonoral routes of administration seem to have been (wrongly) felt to be more effective, and, in particular, the hitherto not uncommon practice of the administration of multiple intramuscular injections is to be avoided.

Overall, these principles are sound and applicable with considerable success to the majority of patients with can-

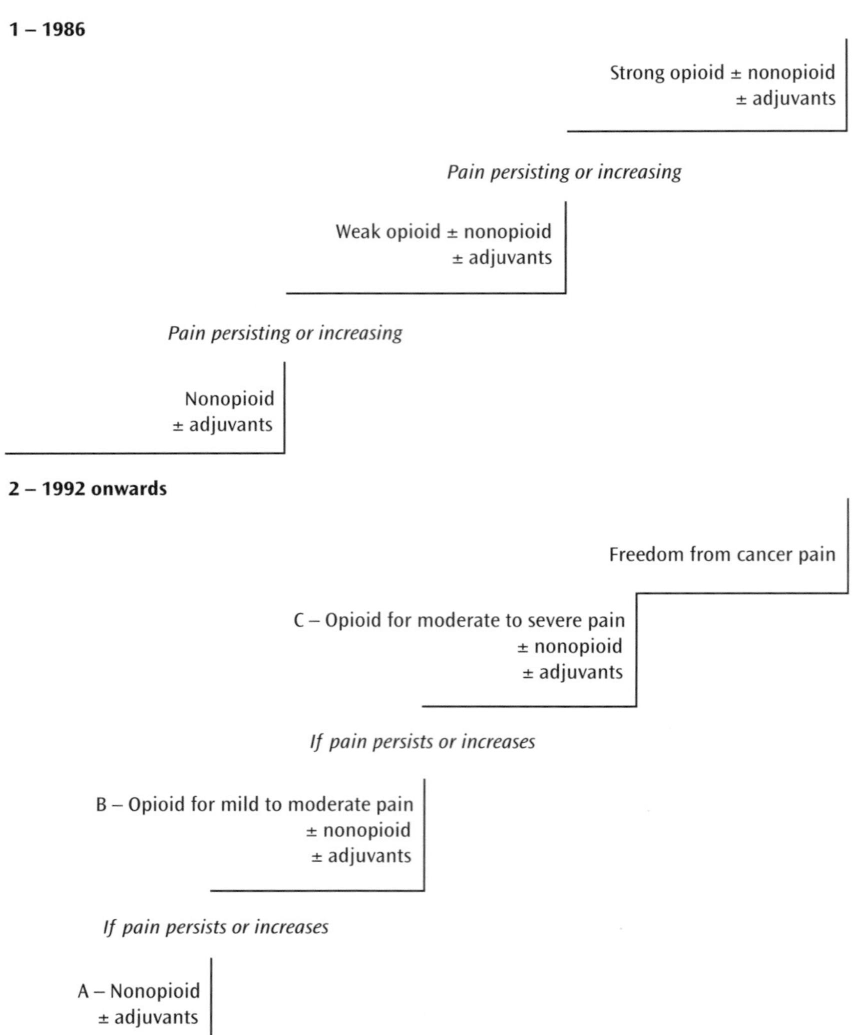

Figure 11.1 *WHO analgesic ladder for cancer pain management.*

cer pain, as the major validation studies appear to confirm.[9,10*,11,12] The WHO ladder has stood the test of time as a succinct practical system for cancer pain relief that started well before practice guidelines became fashionable. However, as all clinicians know, no guidelines fit all clinical circumstances and deviation from the simple three-step ladder approach is often necessary, particularly now that the subject of palliative medicine has continued to develop and a greater degree of clinical and scientific detail is being applied to pain management.

LIMITATIONS OF THE LADDER CONCEPT

Political and social acceptance of morphine

It is clear that the ladder was firmly focused on gaining clinical, social, and political acceptance for the use of oral morphine in cancer pain management. The magnitude of this hurdle over the last 30 years cannot be understated, and there seems little doubt that the ladder has been very effective in bringing about substantial change in most countries of the world, although varying degrees of resistance persist.[13] Although morphine clearly remains the most important and widely used opioid in palliative care practice, the role of other opioids and drug classes is now being actively explored as biological knowledge and clinical experience expand, resulting in a more mechanistic approach to pain relief as well as a greater focus on the minimization of adverse effects (see below).

The opioid drug class

The distinction between strong and weak opioids, on which the middle step of the first ladder was based, has not proven to be very helpful, except in settings when morphine is not available. The standard drug in this category is codeine. However, the administration of codeine is a somewhat inefficient way to give a low dose of an opioid, and the upper limit of the dose range in most patients is tightly limited by the incidence of adverse effects such as cognitive impairment and constipation. It is a prodrug, being converted to morphine by an O-demethylation step in the liver, for which some people lack the enzyme CYP 2D6.[14] It is of note that in the second ladder (1990), the wording changed from "weak opioid" to "opioid for moderate pain" (compare 1986 and 1990 ladders in Fig. 11.1). There seems to be little if any remaining justification for the use of codeine in countries where morphine is available for cancer pain management. If an opioid is indicated for mild or moderate pain, it is now increasingly common for morphine to be used as the first-line drug, with other members of the class being reserved for those who experience unacceptable adverse effects with morphine (opioid substitution)[15*] or develop renal failure, or to exploit putative mechanistic advantages [e.g. methadone and *N*-methyl-D-aspartate (NMDA) receptor antagonism] or incomplete cross-tolerance (opioid rotation) (see Chapter Ca12).

Opioid "substitution" or "switching" is the practice of changing from one member of the opioid class to another in an attempt to improve the adverse effect profile for patients who experience unacceptable and refractory adverse effects (e.g. confusion, drowsiness, nausea, and vomiting).[15*,16*] It is no longer a tenable assumption that all opioids, in currently accepted equianalgesic doses,[17] are similar in efficacy and side-effect profiles. It is increasingly apparent that individual patients tolerate one opioid better than another and that significant reductions in the frequency of opioid-induced adverse effects can be achieved by opioid substitution. Two prospective audits from inpatient palliative care units found an improvement in the leading symptom in more than 70% of patients. The major substitutions were hydromorphone for morphine in 55/80 patients[16] and fentanyl for morphine in 31/55 substitutions.[15] It is now clear that some opioids are associated with lower incidences of specific adverse effects than others, for instance constipation caused by fentanyl is less severe than that caused by morphine. It is also possible that, by virtue of their broader receptor-binding capacity, some opioids have the potential to provide better analgesia than others. Methadone, for example, has been shown in animal studies to bind to the NMDA receptor, and there are anecdotal reports of improved control of neuropathic pain when patients are switched to methadone from other opioids.[18] There is also growing interest in the ability of some opioid drugs, especially oxycodone, to bind to the κ subtype of opioid receptors.

The term "opioid rotation" is better reserved for its original use, i.e. the practice of the sequential use (or rotation) of the different available opioids to maintain pain control that is thought to be compromised by the development of tolerance to a particular opioid (however, documented clinical or scientific evidence in favor of this practice appears to be lacking).

Pain mechanism

When the ladder model was first promulgated, pain mechanisms, and consequently analgesic drug actions, were widely held to be either peripherally or centrally mediated. This is an oversimplification of a much more complicated situation. It is now known that the nervous system is "plastic," that drugs act both centrally and peripherally, and that several major receptor systems are in play (and no doubt further new ones will be described). It also seems probable that spatial cooperation (i.e. reduction in pain by blockade of two or more sites of action) could be important. Therefore, instead of moving serially in a set sequence from one drug class to another as the pain intensity worsens (serial sequential approach), where there is evidence of partial response to one drug class, the addition of one or several drugs from other classes may improve control (additive or synergistic approach). The mechanistic hypothesis here is that enhanced pain control is achieved by the combined use of agents blocking different sites and receptors in the pain pathways, resulting in the possibility of additive or synergistic analgesia.

The terms "adjuvant" and "coanalgesic" drug require further examination as some drugs may be analgesic in their own right at known and unknown sites of action, and others may be truly synergistic with drugs on the ladder. It has been proposed that analgesic drugs be reclassified as primary analgesics, if their the main pharmacodynamic property is pain relief [e.g. opioids, nonsteroidal anti-inflammatory drugs (NSAIDs), local anesthetics], and secondary analgesics, if the drug or class has another major dynamic property (e.g. antidepressants, membrane-stabilizing agents) but also displays analgesic properties through mechanisms understood or not.[2] A better mechanistic understanding of the various drugs used in cancer pain management may lead to improved therapeutic practices and results.

Assessing and categorizing pain intensity and response

Despite its widespread use in palliative care, the practice of categorization of pain into mild, moderate, and severe is arbitrary and subjective.[19] Although pain scores are useful for evaluating intensity trends for individual patients, they do not provide a reliable and valid basis for comparison between patients, and the possibility exists of a delay in the initiation of appropriate drugs or drug combinations because the pain is underestimated and/or wrongly categorized.

It is also necessary to consider how response to therapeutic interventions in pain management is described. Analgesic response is a clinical observation of pain abolition (complete response) or amelioration (partial response, for which a consensus is emerging for a definition of reduction in pain score of 50%),[20,21] or no response at all. If pain fails to respond at all to a given drug class, this may be termed primary resistance, and if initial response occurs but the pain subsequently returns or worsens then this might be referred to as secondary or acquired resistance. If pain control with an opioid is restored by dose escalation, then either the pain signal intensity or mechanism has changed, or tolerance has developed. Such response can only really be properly assessed when plasma morphine concentrations are steady (steady state) and after several dose escalation steps.

Although pain improvement that is initially short of a complete response will usually be disappointing for patients and their carers, this should not necessarily lead to premature cessation of the drug. Further dose escalation (where possible), or the addition of a member of another drug class, may lead to substantial improvements in pain control.

Other interventions

The ladder was never intended to encapsulate all that might be done for cancer pain. Knowledge about the role of oncological interventions, neurolytic procedures, nonoral drug delivery systems, together with novel pathophysiological insights, and hence pharmacological approaches, have developed rapidly over the last few years. Increasing knowledge and sophistication in pain management, together with earlier and more complex referrals, make it ever more important for practitioners to have a broader view of pain mechanisms and treatment options than the ladder permits.

Advances in the understanding of pain pathophysiology

Recent developments in pain research (see Chapters A1, A2, and Ch14) have shown the importance of central nervous system plasticity, i.e. that sensory (pain) processing is not "hard wired" but "plastic," with changes in structure, function, and connections occurring in response to not only prior pain experience and a patient's reaction to current pain, but also the nature of the incoming sensory (pain) information. The dorsal horn is not merely a passive relay station, but is the major site at which nociceptive input is modified. This modification may be inhibitory or stimulatory, with descending inhibitory input releasing enkephalin (Enk), norepinephrine (NE) (noradrenaline), γ-aminobutyric acid (GABA), or serotonin (5-HT). This is the rationale for the spinal administration of opioids[22,23] and other drugs, e.g. midazolam[24] and clonidine,[25] and probably the site of action of the tricyclic antidepressants as analgesics. More recently, it has been recognized that with ongoing nociceptive input, for example major surgery, fractures or malignancy, dorsal horn function undergoes changes known as central sensitization. This results in clinical features such as persistent and escalating pain, hyperalgesia, and allodynia. Some of these patients will develop chronic pain states, although the mechanism(s) whereby these are maintained remain uncertain. They may or may not be mechanistically related to the initial central sensitization process.

The NMDA receptor is implicated in these changes.[26,27] It is usually inactive in the initial acute phase; however, with ongoing and repetitive nociceptive input and/or nerve section/damage it may be activated. NMDA activation results in further changes which set up a vicious cycle of reactivation. This phenomenon is known experimentally as "windup" or central sensitization,[25–27] and it correlates clinically with excessive responsiveness persisting after the stimulus has ceased.[25–27]

Theoretically there are a number of ways of preventing or reducing "windup:"

1 reduction in the inflammatory response (mainly by the use of steroidal or nonsteroidal anti-inflammatory drugs);
2 preventing nociceptive input to the spinal cord by local anesthetic blocks;
3 using the presynaptic action of opioids to reduce glutamate release to a level lower than that required for NMDA receptor activation;
4 use of NMDA receptor antagonists.

Once central sensitization has occurred, the dose of an opioid required for presynaptic block is often associated with unacceptable adverse effects. The combined use of an opioid, an NSAID, and a NMDA receptor antagonist may inhibit the "windup" response,[27] and may restore opioid sensitivity in patients with neuropathic pain (including pain associated with nerve invasion) or ongoing nociceptive input such as refractory incident-related bone pain, mucositis, skin ulceration, or poorly controlled pain of whatever cause. The most readily currently commercially available NMDA antagonist is ketamine. Although ketamine in subanesthetic doses, given by continuous subcutaneous infusion, is used for refractory cancer pain limited data are available. A prospective audit of continuous subcutaneous infusion (CSCI) ketamine for refractory cancer-associated pain has shown an overall efficacy of 67% for mucositis, incident bone pain, and tumor-associated neuropathic pain.[28–30*] Other potential mechanisms for apparent opioid-refractory pain are opioid tolerance, disease progression (particularly if this results in a change of pain mechanism),[31] drug interactions, and other (perhaps unidentified) pharmacokinetic characteristics. It is also clear that almost any other feature of an individual's environment may have an impact on his or her pain experience, most notably spiritual concerns, premorbid personality characteristics, drug and alcohol behaviors, anxiety and depression,[32] changing social or family factors, alteration in the location of care, feelings of insecurity, and changing expectations or levels of physical activity. Although it is not fashionable to say so (pain, after all, is what the patient says it is), there may also be occasions when a chronic illness behavior pattern[33] becomes established in a palliative care setting, and the pain–drug therapeutic feedback loop may lead to both a failure to improve the pain and the generation of unacceptable adverse effects.

LADDER "FAILURE"

For the purposes of this exercise, optimal "ladder" management will be considered to be the concomitant use of a nonsteroidal anti-inflammatory and oral morphine with appropriate dose escalation (the "top" of the ladder). Clinically, the situations that most frequently generate management difficulties are intrinsic damage to the nervous system (neurogenic or neuropathic pain), incident pain, e.g. movement-related exacerbations due to bone metastases, skin or mucosal inflammation, and nerve compression. These circumstances will be addressed in the mechanistic approach outlined below.

It seems inappropriate to view situations in which the oral route is not effective or possible as ladder "failure." Oral drug administration has no intrinsic benefit for *per se*, apart from the avoidance of more invasive routes when they are unnecessary or inappropriate. The more important question is to ascertain when route changes are indicated, and how effective they are.

NONORAL ROUTES OF DRUG ADMINISTRATION

It is widely agreed that the oral route is the preferred route of drug administration in palliative care practice. In particular, it is important to bury the myth that the parenteral routes of opioid administration are more effective than the oral route. This appears to have been largely achieved. The simplicity and cost-effectiveness of the oral route generally enables good analgesia in all settings, including, most importantly, at home. However, frequently oral administration is either undesirable or impossible (Table 11.1). In terminally ill patients who are drowsy or comatose, agitated and uncooperative, or whose memory is poor or in whom compliance is a problem, the oral route is not reliable.

There is, to date, no conclusive evidence that changing the route of opioid administration alone improves pain control. No route of administration in clinical practice, with the possible exception of spinal delivery, has been demonstrated to produce a consistently superior therapeutic ratio than any other. Such changes are also rarely undertaken alone, in controlled conditions, and substantial environmental factors and placebo effect may be operating.

Table 11.1 *Indications for changing from oral to parenteral analgesics*

Obstruction of gastrointestinal tract
Nausea and vomiting
Inability to cooperate and swallow medication (e.g. acute organic brain syndrome)
Impaired conscious state or coma
Agent not absorbed satisfactorily from gastrointestinal tract
Unstable pain for which pharmacokinetics may be responsible (e.g. unreliable absorption)
Erratic compliance
Patient preference (e.g. elderly person who finds tablets hard to swallow)
Ease of drug administration, especially where several agents may be given in one subcutaneous infusion

Subcutaneous route

The use of the subcutaneous route is widespread in palliative care practice worldwide, taking the form either of intermittent injection or, where available, infusion with a syringe driver. It has proved to be a viable and reliable alternative to the oral route for most of the key drugs that are commonly used by palliative care services. It is placed on the second rung of the intervention/complexity ladders outlined later, for each pain mechanism, because it is a second-line intervention that requires specialist expertise (although it is now common for these to be regarded as core skills by many general practitioners and community nurses in countries where palliative care is well established). Subcutaneous route changes are commonly undertaken in order to improve pain control or to reduce the severity of adverse effects. In part, any favorable responses that result from such a change may be due to the achievement of smoother pharmacokinetics with infusions or better absorption in some patients. The widespread availability and use of sustained-release opioid formulations may have reduced the need for a route change for this indication, at least as a first-line step.

Transdermal route

The availability of multilayer transdermal therapeutic system (TTS) fentanyl has allowed the widespread use of fentanyl for cancer pain, a use that was previously restricted by drug delivery system limitations. The TTS patches release the drug at a constant rate over 72 h, achieving therapeutic serum levels after a mean of approximately 13 h due to depot accumulation within the skin.[34] The main advantage over morphine may be in adverse effect profile, but this has not yet been conclusively demonstrated. Effective analgesia and patient preference have been demonstrated, with a reduction in severe constipation in patients in one study with good follow-up.[35*]

Spinal opioids

Spinal opioids (either epidural or intrathecal[36**]) are indicated for refractory cancer pain below the head and neck when other drugs, including opioids, have been ineffective or accompanied by adverse effects not reversed by opioid substitution.[15]

Spinally administered opioids gain access to the cerebrospinal fluid and hence the substantia gelatinosa cells of the dorsal horn. Because drugs are applied directly close to the site of action, low doses are used, for example initial morphine doses of 0.5–2 mg intrathecally, or 5–10 mg epidurally, are effective, and adverse effects, particularly nausea and vomiting, drowsiness, or confusion, are often minimal.

Morphine is generally the drug of choice for spinal administration in cancer pain management because of its high water solubility, and hence long duration of action (12–24 h), and extensive dermatomal spread.[25] However, spinal opioids are not always effective, particularly when nerve compression or invasion has occurred and/or when pain has a significant incident element. Other drugs may be added, including low-dose local anesthetics,[25,37] midazolam,[24] or clonidine.[25] Combinations of drugs may be both more effective and associated with less adverse effects as a result of a synergistic rather than additive action.[38]

Catheters may be inserted either epidurally or intrathecally. The catheters are generally tunneled subcutaneously and attached to a percutaneous filter system or an implanted reservoir. They can be accessed for either intermittent bolus dosing (once or twice per day) or continuous infusion. Often, local factors, including available expertise and resources, determine what system is chosen. When a spinal opioid and low-dose local anesthetic are used, an infusion system is preferable to intermittent boluses in order to minimize motor paralysis and hemodynamic instability.[39]

Recent trends in practice have favored the intrathecal over the epidural route. Factors influencing this choice are a lower incidence of technical complications, particularly catheter occlusion, usually about 3 weeks after insertion,[40] efficacy in the presence of suspected or proven presence of epidural tumor deposits,[25] lower doses and volumes,[41] and, in the unlikely event of infection occurring despite scrupulous insertion and top-up techniques, the easier management of meningitis as opposed to an epidural abscess (see Chapters P23 and P24).

A MECHANISTIC APPROACH TO CANCER PAIN MANAGEMENT

Modern pain management approaches usually attempt to match the type of pain mechanism to the most effective treatment.[2] A pain experience may be described in the following three categories, somatic, visceral, and neuropathic, these categories being determined by which embryologically defined part of the body the nociceptive stimulus emerges in and hence which part of the nervous system mediates the message. Somatic pain is, in addition, subdivided into superficial and deep, as the nonpharmacological management of the two categories is very different. Neuropathic pain is divided into two further categories: tumor associated (or "mixed" nociceptive/neuropathic pain) and nontumor associated (or "pure" neuropathic pain), because the pharmacological and nonpharmacological management is also substantially different.

The diagnostic and therapeutic characteristics of these categories are summarized in Table 11.2. The principal features are as follows. Firstly, somatic pain responds well to anti-inflammatory agents, and it is usual (as per the ladder) to start treatment with a trial of such an agent alone, although if pain is severe and acute concomitant commencement of an opioid may be indicated. Secondly, visceral pain responds well to opioids alone (unless colicky smooth muscle spasm is responsible, in which case anti-inflammatory and muscle relaxant drugs are usually considered). Thirdly, neuropathic pain requires the use of drug classes that are specific to this mechanism (antidepressants and membrane stabilizers of various types). Lastly, involvement of nervous and visceral structures may coexist in the same patient because of tumor extension or metastatic spread, and several mechanisms may be operative for a patient at the same time.[2]

The principles of a three-level approach to cancer pain management, according to the level of complexity of interventions, and hence severity and responsiveness of the pain, are summarized in Fig. 11.2, and set out for somatic (deep and superficial), visceral and neuropathic pain in Figs 11.3, 11.4, and 11.5. Interventions are allocated to one of the three steps as a rough indication of sequence of use. Position on this "ladder" is therefore proportional to pain severity and difficulty in achieving pain control, and the interventions tend to become more complex, specialized, and/or experimental, and therefore more likely to be undertaken with specialist involvement, although the categories are not intended to be rigid.

The first level describes interventions that may reasonably be undertaken in a primary care and general hospital setting, usually without the need for any specialist input. This would correspond to the three steps of the WHO ladder. At the second level are interventions that require some form of specialist input because the ladder approach has failed to produce acceptable and enduring pain control, and in these circumstances shared care arrangements are usually required. On the third level are located highly specialized (and often incompletely evaluated) interventions for refractory and unstable pain. Naturally, the degree of complexity undertaken by practitioners and teams will depend on individual experience and access to the techniques in question. Collaborative

Table 11.2 *Mechanistic classification of cancer pain (adapted from Ashby et al.)*

	Superficial somatic	Deep somatic	Visceral	Neuropathic
Origin of stimulus	1 Skin, subcutaneous tissue 2 Mucosa of mouth, nose, sinuses, urethra, anus	1 Bone, joints, muscles, tendons, ligaments 2 Superficial lymph nodes 3 Organ capsules and mesothelial membranes (pleura and peritoneum)	1 Solid or hollow organs 2 Deep tumor masses 3 Deep lymph nodes	1 Mixed: nociceptive element present due to tumor invasion or compression of nerve pathway 2 Pure (deafferentation): nociceptive element absent
Examples	Malignant ulcers, chemotherapy/ radiotherapy mucositis	Bone metastases, liver capsule distension, or inflammation	Deep abdominal or chest masses Intestinal, biliary, and ureteric colic	Mixed: brachial, lumbosacral plexus, or chest wall invasion, spinal cord compression Pure: postherpetic neuralgia, post-thoracotomy syndrome, phantom pain
Description	Burning, stinging	Dull, aching	Dull, deep	1 Dysesthesia,[a] e.g. pins and needles, tingling, burning or lancinating/shooting 2 Allodynia[b] 3 Phantom pain 4 Pain in a numb area
Localization (to site of stimulus)	Very well defined	Well defined	Poorly defined	Nerve or dermatome distribution
Movement	No effect	Worsening pain (patient prefers to be still)	Movement may improve pain	Nerve traction provokes pain (e.g. sciatic stretch test)
Referral	No	Yes	Yes	Yes
Local tenderness	Yes	Yes	May be	No
Autonomic effects	No	No	Nausea, vomiting, sweating, blood pressure and heart rate changes	Autonomic instability: warmth, sweating, pallor, cold, cyanosis (dermatomal localization)
First-choice drug class	AI	AI	O	Mixed: AI Pure: AD or AC[c]
Second-choice drug class	LA	O	AS if colicky	Mixed: O Pure: AC or AD
Third-choice drug class	O	Ketamine	?AI	Mixed: S Pure: O
Fourth-choice drug class	Ketamine		–	Mixed: AD, AC, or ketamine Pure: ketamine
Other measures	Radiotherapy Irrigation Heat or cold	Radiotherapy Heat Immobilization	Radiotherapy Pressure Heat	Epidural LA Neurolytic procedure or block Radiotherapy[d] TENS

a. Dysesthesia: an unpleasant abnormal sensation whether spontaneous or evoked (IASP). b. Allodynia: pain due to a stimulus which does not normally provoke pain (IASP).
c. AC first if lancinating features. d. Only if nociceptive tumor invasion and/or compression are present.
AC, anticonvulsant; AD, antidepressant; AI, anti-inflammatory; AS, antispasmodic; LA, local anesthetic; O, opioid; S, steroid; TENS, transcutaneous electrical nerve stimulation.

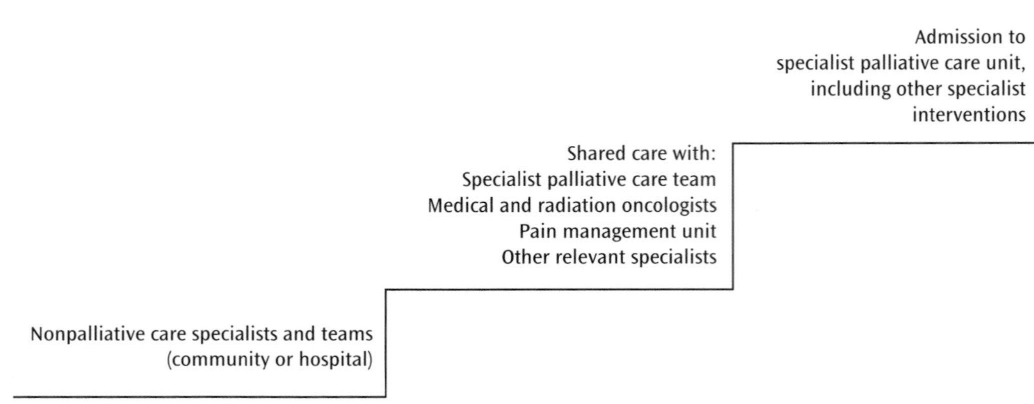

Figure 11.2 *The three levels of cancer pain management.*

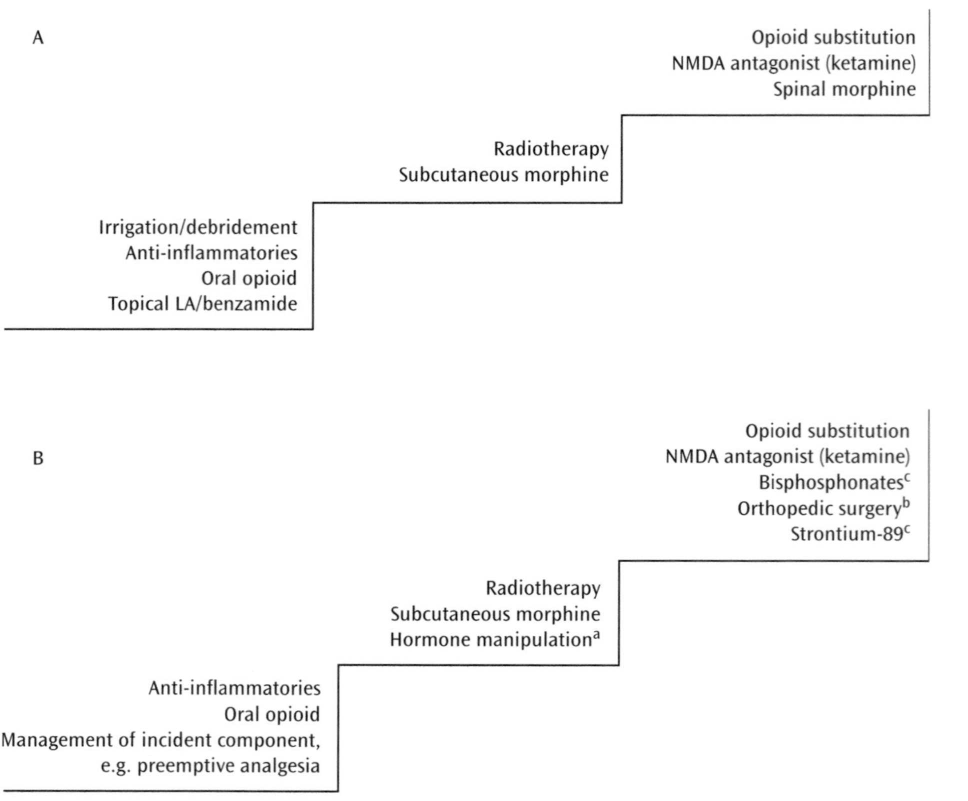

Figure 11.3 *Somatic pain interventions. (A) Superficial. (B) Deep.*
a, In hormone-responsive diseases, e.g. breast and prostate cancer; b, internal fixation for a fracture, or to prevent imminent fracture; c, widespread bone pain where focal external beam irradiation has failed or is not indicated and pharmacological response has been poor.

management and teamwork are therefore essential to an optimal outcome.

Somatic pain

Somatic pain (Fig. 11.3) arises from structures that are embryologically derived from ectoderm. These mainly constitute the surface covering of the body (skin and subcutaneous tissues), the lining of the upper aerodigestive tract and the final part of the digestive and urogenital tracts (urethra, anus, vagina), the musculoskeletal system (bone, joints, muscles, tendons, ligaments), and the outer layers of mesothelial membranes (somatic pleura and peritoneum). Its clinical characteristics are set out in Table 11.2, it tends to be well localized, and the pain is of a "bright" quality. Management is divided into that of superficial and deep somatic pain, mainly because of the local measures which are possible for pain arising from superficial (and accessible) lesions. The pharmacological principles are similar for both groups. See also Chapters Ca18 and Ca21.

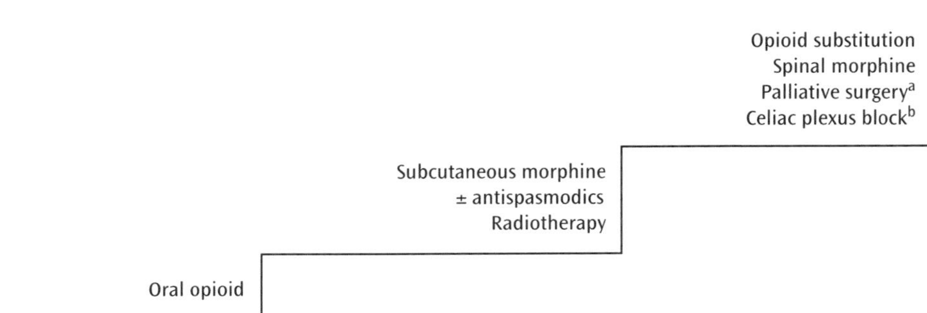

Figure 11.4 *Visceral pain interventions.*
a, Where indicated, e.g. surgical relief of bowel obstruction; b, where anatomically appropriate, e.g. carcinoma of the pancreas.

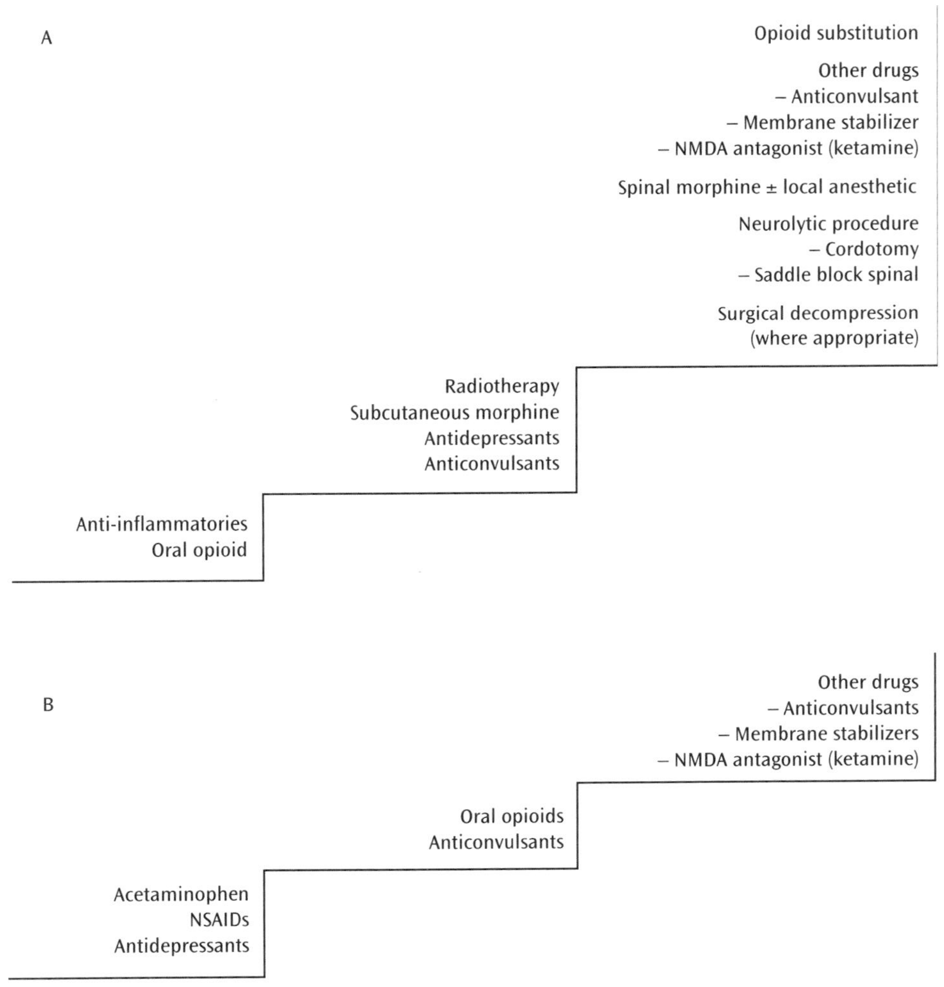

Figure 11.5 *Neuropathic pain.*
(A) Mixed – tumor associated. (B) Pure – nontumor associated (e.g. postmastectomy, peripheral neuropathy, postherpetic neuralgia).

Superficial

Superficial tumors and ulcers are often tender to touch, and there is frequent evidence of accompanying inflammation, with surrounding erythema and tissue irritation. As mediators of the inflammatory response are clearly at play here, it is usual to use anti-inflammatory agents and to pay attention to local measures for ulcer surfaces and cavities, by irrigation and dressings. By maintaining good wound care, the build-up of chemical mediators of inflammatory pain is presumably reduced. Application of topical analgesics, usually a local anesthetic agent, may be helpful, although clear efficacy data are lacking.

There is experimental and limited clinical evidence of the role of peripheral opioid receptors in inflammation.[42] There is also increasing interest in the possible role of topical opioids for malignant and nonmalignant ulcers, with the aim of pain control without systemic adverse effects such as drowsiness, confusion, or constipation. There are substantial data to support the efficacy of intra-articular morphine in arthroscopic surgery.[43] The potential usefulness of peripherally acting opioids, which do not cross the blood–brain barrier, needs to be explored.

The application of heat and cold may also be soothing in some acute situations, and palliative irradiation has a good track record of reducing or even healing malignant ulcers.[47] It is usual to assess response to a nonsteroidal agent first, followed by the addition of morphine if this fails to give adequate relief.

Deep

This is the commonest mechanism of cancer pain generation because of the high incidence of bone metastases with the common malignancies (especially breast, lung, and prostate primaries). It is characterized by a close relationship to movement, giving rise to so-called incident pain.[44*] In particular, titrating the opioid dose up to the level required to relieve the incident pain peaks can lead to unacceptable adverse effects at rest. The standard management of incident and other so-called "breakthrough" pain is the administration of oral or subcutaneous bolus doses. Ideally, such boluses should consist of a drug and route that has a rapid onset, early peak effect, and short duration of action. Transmucosal (sublingual and intranasal) administration of the fentanyl series of drugs is being explored for this role. This route avoids first-pass metabolism, allows for rapid absorption in an area with a rich blood supply, and is not painful. It requires limited equipment and expertise compared with conventional patient-controlled analgesic (PCA) regimens.[45**,46*] As with superficial somatic pain, inflammation appears to be the dominant nociceptive mechanism and, therefore, a trial of an anti-inflammatory agent is the first step in pain management, often in combination with morphine as there does appear to be a "ceiling" effect with anti-inflammatory drugs in terms of pain response and adverse effects. A trial of steroids can often have significant short-term impact on pain, mobility, and well-being in patients with advanced skeletal disease. In the case of bone disease, oncological interventions such as hormonal therapy, chemotherapy, and radiotherapy are important tools in pain management throughout the disease's natural history. The use of bisphosphonates and, in specialist centers, the systemic administration of radioisotopes (e.g. strontium-89) are now common for both pain prevention (prophylaxis) and treatment of resistant diffuse skeletal pain (see Chapters Ca18 and Ca21).

Visceral

Visceral pain arises from deep body structures that are embryologically derived from endoderm and are innervated by the autonomic nervous system. Relay is via the slow C-fibers, with extensive connections in the primitive rhinencephalon, often leading to accompanying autonomic effects. Pain tends to be deep, dull, diffuse, and referred to the midline in the appropriate segment. With the exception of smooth muscle spasm, which responds to antispasmodics, most visceral cancer pain is very sensitive to opioids. Morphine as the sole agent will often provide enduring relief. The absence of an incident component usually makes management easier. Sometimes palliative surgical or oncological interventions may be helpful.

Celiac plexus block should always be considered for refractory pancreatic cancer pain. It can produce complete pain relief or a significant reduction in opioid requirements. In a review of 15 studies, 418 out of 480 (87%) patients obtained good relief, with the best results in patients with pancreatic cancer.[48] Efficacy is highest early in the disease as with advanced disease local tumor or scar tissue may prevent good spread of the neurolytic agent. In addition, in patients with advanced disease there is frequently a mixed pain picture with metastatic disease or local extension to adjacent structures such as retroperitoneal nodes or thoracic wall, i.e. tissues not innervated by the celiac plexus. The standard procedure is a posterior approach, as outlined by Cousins and Bridenbaugh.[25] However, an anterior computed tomography (CT)-guided approach[49] is also possible; this is quicker and easier and is associated with a reduced risk of neurological complications. The supine position also offers less discomfort to the patient and increased safety and ease of sedation (to mask the pain of the alcohol injection).

Neuropathic

Neuropathic pain arises as a result of damage to nervous system structures, and subsequent neurophysiological changes, such as "windup." It is the hardest mechanism to treat, and accounts for the majority of difficult pain management situations in palliative care practice. Diagnosis is usually straightforward, with specific clinical features and dermatome or specific neurological referral distribution (see Table 11.2). Management differs according to whether the damage is due to the direct effect of tumor deposits (tumor associated or "mixed" nociceptive/neuropathic) or not (nontumor associated or "pure" neuropathic pain).

Mixed – tumor associated

If the pain is caused either by tumor growing adjacent to, or actually invading, nervous tissue, then management consists of the usual interventions for somatic nociceptive pain, i.e. anti-inflammatory drugs (steroidal and nonsteroidal), opioids,and oncological interventions plus consideration of secondary analgesics. Despite negative prior reports of the use of opioids in neuropathic pain, it is clear that opioids do have a role in the management of neuropathic cancer pain, although results tend to be inferior to those achieved in somatic and visceral pain. Some patients report that the pain is still present but that they are better able to tolerate it. Surgical decompression and both chemical and surgical neurolysis are all used. The techniques include laminectomy, chemical or surgical rhizotomy, cordotomy, and saddle block spinal. The choice of technique depends on local expertise and resources, and results are variable, with few large series reported.

Cordotomy, that is spinothalamic tractotomy, has a limited place in refractory cancer pain, and is undergoing re-examination. It is indicated for unilateral pain below the C5 dermatome, classically for tumor invasion of the lumbosacral plexus in patients with a reasonable respiratory reserve.[25] Cordotomy may be performed by an open approach, i.e. mini-laminectomy, usually at T1–2, or by a C1 percutaneous CT-guide radiofrequency approach. Although respiratory complications are the major risk, the technique has been reported by Stuart and Cramond[50*] as safe and effective in controlling refractory chest wall pain (39% of their 230 patients had mesotheliomia or lung cancer). Expertise in percutaneous cordotomy has waned subsequent to the widespread use of subcutaneous and spinal opioid administration, but there may be a resurgence of its use in well-defined and audited circumstances.

A saddle block spinal consists of the administration of anesthesia/analgesia confined to the perineal area. This achieved by the injection of hyperbaric phenol (5–15% phenol in glycerine) with the patient seated and tipped backwards to 45°, with this maintained at least 15 min after injection.[25] In our unit it is restricted to patients with a colostomy or ileostomy and some form of urinary diversion (or who are prepared to accept a permanent indwelling catheter) and who have intractable perineal pain, usually due to tumor invasion of the nerves of the sacral plexus. It may be preceded by a diagnostic block with "heavy" xylocaine or bupivacaine to assess likely efficacy, reassure patients, and to determine a safe volume of neurolytic solution.

More studies of most of these techniques are required to determine both criteria for patient selection and results.

It is also for this group of patients that spinally administered opioids, local anesthetics, and other receptor blockers (e.g. $GABA_A$ receptor blockers, i.e. midazolam, and noradrenergic blockers, e.g. clonidine) have been used most frequently (see Spinal opioids). It is usually necessary to try a number of agents and interventions in a serial manner to achieve optimal results.

Pure – nontumor associated

In patients with nontumor-associated pain, it is common to delay the use of opioids until secondary analgesics, such as tricyclic antidepressants, anticonvulsants (e.g. carbemazepine, gabapentin or sodium valproate), or membrane stabilizers, (e.g. mexiletine or flecainide), have been tried.

Responses are more uncertain. Oncological interventions are not indicated, but occasionally opioid substitution/rotation and/or NMDA antagonists are tried; however, so far, as for all types of neuropathic pain, conclusive outcome data are not available (see Chapter Ca15).

CONCLUSIONS

The WHO ladder is a well-established and effective initial general approach to cancer pain management. A wide range of additional interventions and strategies can be tried when pain has not been adequately controlled by a combination of escalating doses of opioids and a nonsteroidal anti-inflammatory drug (the "top" of the ladder). As the level of sophistication in pain management continues to rise, and earlier referrals are made to pain and palliative care services, it seems likely that a more complex and individualized mechanistic approach will be adopted, with involvement of generalists as well as palliative care, pain, and other relevant specialists, and the various oncological disciplines. This requires a high level of effective interaction between these specialties and the other health service professions, especially nursing. It is important that palliative care practitioners are aware of the general pain and anesthetic literature, particularly the basic sciences, as these are the areas from which new knowledge of relevance to clinical practice is most likely to emerge.

It seems fairly clear that all practitioners find that neuropathic and incident pain are most resistant to standard treatments. Research over the next few years will continue to address the area of basic pharmacology and pathophysiology (especially with regard to the "windup" phenomenon, receptor systems, and novel drugs and novel routes of administration), indications for, and results of, neurolytic and spinal drug delivery techniques, opioid substitution and rotation, and pain behavior. The location of this knowledge and practice within a framework of the total oncological management of patients is also an ongoing imperative. Finally, it should be emphasized that, although there is a considerable body of clinical experience with interventions for refractory and unstable pain, few have been subjected to clinical trials to validate their widespread use, and many should be regarded as experimental at this stage.

REFERENCES

1. Expert Working Group of the European Association for Palliative Care. Morphine in cancer pain: modes of administration. *Br Med J* 1996; **312:** 823–6.
2. Ashby M, Fleming BG, Brooksbank M, *et al.* Description of a mechanistic approach to pain management in advanced cancer. Preliminary report. *Pain* 1992; **51:** 153–61.
3. World Health Organization. *Cancer Pain Relief*. Geneva: World Health Organization, 1986.
4. World Health Organization. *Cancer Pain Relief and Palliative Care*. Report of a WHO Expert Committee. Geneva: World Health Organization, 1990.
5. ◆ World Health Organization. *Cancer Pain Relief, With a Guide to Opioid Availability*, 2nd edn. Geneva: World Health Organization,1996.
6. Hanks G, Cherny N. Opioid analgesic therapy. In: Doyle D, Hanks G, MacDonald N eds. *Oxford Textbook of Palliative Medicine*, 2nd edn. Oxford: Oxford University Press, 1998: 331–55.
7. Twycross RJ. Easing the pain of cancer. *Pain Clinic* 1986; **1(2):** 75–6.
8. Stjernsward J, Teoh N. The cancer pain relief programme of the World Health Organization. *Palliative Med* 1989; **4:** 1–3.
9. Walker V, Hoskin P, Hanks GW, White ID. Evaluation of WHO analgesic guidelines in a hospital based palliative care unit. *J Pain Symptom Manage* 1988; **3:** 145–9.
10. Zech DF, Grond S, Lynch J, *et al.* Validation of World Health Organization Guidelines for cancer pain relief: a 10-year prospective study. *Pain* 1995; **63:** 65–76.
11. Takeda F. Results of field-testing in Japan of the WHO Draft Interim Guidelines on relief of cancer pain. *Pain Clinic* 1986; **1(2):** 83–9.
12. Ventafridda V, Tamburini M, Caraceni A, *et al.* A validation of the WHO method of cancer pain relief. *Cancer* 1987; **59:** 850–6.
13. Zenz M, Willweber-Strumpf A. Opiophobia and cancer pain in Europe. *Lancet* 1993; **341:** 1075–6.
14. Chen ZR, Bochner F, Somogyi A. Polymorphic O-demethylation of codeine. *Lancet* 1988; **2:** 914–15.
15. Ashby M, Martin P, Jackson K. Opioid substitution to reduce adverse effects in cancer pain management. *Med J Aust* 1999; **170:** 68–71.
16. de Stoutz ND, Bruera E, Suarez-Almazor M. Opioid rotation for toxicity reduction in terminal cancer patients. *J Pain Symptom Manage* 1995; **10:** 378–84.
17. Anderson R, Saiers JH, Abram S, Schlicht C. Accuracy in equianalgesics dosing: conversion dilemmas. *J Pain Symptom Manage* 2001; **21:** 397–406.
18. Twycross R. Opioid rotation: does it have a role? *Palliative Med* 1998; **12:** 60–1.
19. Serlin RC, Mendoza TR, Nakamura Y, *et al.* When is cancer pain mild, moderate or severe? Grading pain severity by its interference with function. *Pain* 1995; **61:** 277–84.
20. Campbell WL, Paterson CC. Quantifying meaningful changes in pain. *Anaesthesia* 1998; **53:** 121–5.
21. Keefe FJ, Gil KM, Rose SC. Behavioral approaches in the multidisciplinary management of chronic pain: programs and issues. *Clin Psychol Rev* 1986; **6:** 87–113.
22. ◆ Yaksh TL, Rudy TA. Analgesia mediated by a direct spinal action of narcotics. *Science* 1976; **192:** 1357–8.
23. ◆ Wang JK. Analgesic effect of intrathecally administered morphine. *Reg Anesth* 1977; **2:** 8.
24. ◆ Goodchild CS. Nonopioid spinal analgesics: animal experimentation and implications for clinical developments. *Pain Rev* 1997; **4:** 33–58.
25. Cousins MJ, Bridenbaugh PO eds. *Neural Blockade in Clinical Anesthesia and Management of Pain*, 3rd edn. New York, NY: Lippincott-Raven Publishers, 1998.
26. ◆ Woolf CJ. Somatic pain: pathogenesis and prevention. *Br J Anesth* 1995; **75:** 169–76.
27. ◆ Dickenson AH. Spinal cord pharmacology of pain. *Br J Anaesth* 1995; **75:** 193–200.
28. Jackson K, Ashby M, Martin P, White M. Can "burst" ketamine wind down wind up: a prospective audit. 9th World Congress on Pain, Vienna, 1999.
29. Ashby M, Jackson K, Martin P, White M. The incidence of adverse effects with the use of "burst" ketamine: a prospective audit. 9th World Congress on Pain, Vienna, 1999.
30. Jackson K, Ashby M, Martin P, *et al.* "Burst" ketamine for refractory cancer pain: an open-label audit of 39 patients. *J Pain Symptom Manage* 2001; **22:** 834–42.
31. Collin E, Poulain P, Gauvain-Piquard A, *et al.* Is disease progression the major factor in morphine "tolerance" in cancer pain treatment? *Pain* 1993; **55:** 319–26.
32. Bruera E, MacMillan K, Hanson J, MacDonald RN. The Edmonton staging system for cancer pain: preliminary report. Pain 1989; **37:** 203–9.
33. Pilowsky I. *Abnormal illness Behaviour*. London: John Wiley, 1997.
34. Gourlay GK, Kowolski FR, Plummer J, *et al.* The transdermal administration of fentanyl in the treatment of postoperative pain: pharmacokinetic and pharmacodynamic effects. *Pain* 1989; **37:** 193–292.
35. Nugent MD. Long term observations of patients receiving transdermal fentanyl after a randomized trial. *J Pain Symptom Manage* 2001; **21:** 385–91.
36. ● Mercadante S. Problems of long-term spinal opioid treatment in advanced cancer patients. *Pain* 1999; **79:** 1–13.
37. Akerman B, Arwestrom E. Local anesthetics potentiate spinal morphine antinociception. *Anesth Analg* 1988; **67:** 943–8.
38. Barnes RK, Rosenfeld JV, Fennessy SS, Goodchild CS. Continuous subarachnoid infusion to control severe cancer pain in an ambulant patient. *Med J Aust* 1994; **161:** 549.

39. Sjoberg M, Nitescu P, Appelgren L, Curelaru I. Long-term intrathecal morphine and bupivacaine in patients with refractory cancer pain. *Anesthesiology* 1994; **80:** 284–97.
40. Crul BJ, Delhaas EM. Technical complications during long-term subarachnoid or epidural administration of morphine in terminally ill cancer patients: a review of 140 cases. *Reg Anesth* 1991; **16:** 209–13.
41. Nitescu P, Appelgren L, Linder LE, *et al*. Epidural versus intrathecal morphine-bupivacaine: assessment of consecutive treatments in advanced cancer pain. *J Pain Symptom Manage* 1990; **5:** 18–26.
● 42. Gupta ABL, Holmstrom B, Berggen L. A systematic review of the peripheral analgesic effects of intra-articular morphine. *Anesth Analg* 2001; **93:** 761–70.
● 43. Stein C, Haimerl E, Yassouridis A, *et al*. Analgesic effect of intra-articular morphine after arthroscopic knee surgery. *N Engl J Med* 1991; **325:** 1123–6.
◆ 44. Portenoy RK, Hagen NA. Breakthrough pain: definition, prevalence and characteristics. *Pain* 1990; **41:** 273–82.
45. Porteny RK, Payne R, Coluzzi P, *et al*. Oral transmucosal fentanyl citrate (OTFC) for the treatment of breakthrough pain in cancer patients: a controlled dose titration study. *Pain* 1999; **79:** 303–12.
46. Jackson K, Ashby MA, Keech J. Pilot dose finding study of intranasal sufentanil for breakthrough and incident cancer-associated pain. *J Pain Sympton Manage* 2002; **23:** 450–2.
47. Ashby M. The role of radiotherapy in management of cancer related pain. In: Arbit E ed. *Management of Cancer-Related Pain*. Mount Kisko, NY: Futura, 1993.
● 48. Sharfman WH, Walsh TD. Has the analgesic efficacy of neurolytic coeliac plexus block been demonstrated in pancreatic cancer pain? *Pain* 1990; **41:** 267–71.
49. Romanelli DF, Beckmann CF, Heiss FW. Celiac plexus block: efficacy and safety of the anterior approach. *Am J Roentgenol* 1993; **160:** 497–500.
50. Stuart G, Cramond T. Role of percutaneous cervical cordotomy for pain of malignant origin. *Med J Aust* 1993; **158:** 667–70.

12

Opioid switching and rotation

MARIE FALLON

Opioid-based pharmacotherapy is the mainstay approach to the management of cancer pain. An extraordinary success rate justifies the widely held view that long-term opioid therapy is the first-line approach for moderate or severe cancer pain.[1] Morphine remains the most commonly used opioid.[2] However, some patients are sensitive to the side-effects of morphine, particularly the central effects, even at very low doses. There has been an increase in the use of alternative opioids to morphine, partly because of increased availability and partly because of clinical observation that individual patients respond differently to different opioids.[3–6] Numerous reports exist of an improved balance between analgesia and side-effects after an opioid switch or even sequential trials of opioids.[7–23]

BASIC CONCEPTS IN OPIOID PHARMACOLOGY OF RELEVANCE TO OPIOID SWITCHING

All opioid drugs produce analgesia and other effects by mimicking the actions of endogenous opioid compounds (endorphins) at multiple subtypes of the three major opioid receptors (mu, kappa, and delta)† in the spinal cord, brainstem, and peripheral tissues. The opioid drugs most commonly used in clinical practice bind selectively to the mu receptor, and morphine is the prototype of this class. In the central nervous system these drugs act both presynaptically and postsynaptically to inhibit the release of transmitters and the firing of neurons in pain pathways. Binding of opioids to receptors in peripheral tissues could contribute a peripheral mechanism that may be most appropriate in pain associated with inflammatory conditions.[24]

Opioid analgesics can be classified as pure agonists or agonist/antagonists based on their interactions with opioid receptors. The agonist/antagonist drugs can be divided into a mixed agonist/antagonist subclass and a partial agonist subclass. The mixed agonist/antagonist drugs are weak antagonists at the mu receptor and agonists at the kappa receptor. The partial agonist drugs are selective agonists at the mu receptor but have a limited intrinsic efficacy at the site.

The agonist/antagonist subclasses are not preferred for the treatment of cancer pain because they have a pharmacological ceiling effect for analgesia and can reverse the effects of pure agonists in patients who are physically dependent. Some produce psychotomimetic side-effects more readily than the pure agonist opioids.

In clinical practice in cancer pain management the pure mu agonists are the opioids most commonly used.

A further concept in clinical pharmacology is the difference between efficacy and potency. For practical purposes, one can think of the potency of a drug as being irrelevant so long as it can reach adequate efficacy without unacceptable side-effects. Thus, efficacy refers to the effect of a given dose of the drug or the maximal effect that can be produced, and potency refers to the dose required to produce a specified effect. However, potency becomes an important issue when opioid drugs or routes of opioid administration are changed. Some understanding of the relative potency of the different drugs or routes of drug administration must be known to avoid overdos-

†Mu, delta, and kappa are used because of clinician familiarity. However, a revised IUPHAR nomenclature for these receptors can be found in the *IUPHAR Compendium of Receptor Characterization and Classification* 2000.

ing or underdosing when treatment with a new drug or route is instigated. Clearly, factors other than the drug potency and efficacy are also of relevance, such as duration of treatment with the current drug and dose, which may affect tolerance to side-effects when switching opioids.[17,25]

OPIOID RESPONSIVENESS

In many ways, the degree of opioid responsiveness of moderate or severe cancer pain is the keystone to further decisions about pharmacological and other management. There is a large degree of variability in opioid responsiveness, and this is not a phenomenon that can be predicted in any given situation. However, we do know that some clinical situations are likely to be less responsive to opioids than others, for example neuropathic pain.[26*] In addition, patients with sudden onset of severe pain, for example related to voluntary actions, patients with a high level of psychological distress, and those who need a rapid dose escalation after initiation of therapy are all likely to have a less favorable balance between wanted and unwanted effects of opioids and hence opioid responsiveness. In addition, elderly patients and patients with renal dysfunction are more likely to have a less favorable balance between wanted and unwanted opioid effects.

It is clear that the factors which determine the degree of opioid responsiveness are often not the opioid, or even the pain syndrome, but are other patient-centered factors.

None of the factors mentioned above represents an inherent unresponsiveness to opioid analgesia, except psychological distress, with some patients mistakenly using an opioid as an anxiolytic. There is evidence that neuropathic pain will respond to opioid analgesia; however, the doses required are higher than the doses required for non-neuropathic pain, with an associated increased likelihood of side-effects, and it is this that is the dose-limiting effect, leading to a less favorable outcome of opioid responsiveness.[26***]

In summary, opioid responsiveness is essentially a retrospective diagnosis. However, more vigilance is required in some clinical situations, such as in elderly patients, patients with impaired renal function, neuropathic pain, or incident pain, psychologically distressed patients, and any situation in which opioid dose is titrated rapidly. In practice, the limiting side-effect is sedation associated with varying degrees of opioid toxicity: hallucinations, vivid dreams, agitation, confusion, myoclonic jerks, and paradoxical complaints of increased pain with increased analgesia in the agitated/confused patient. The other common side-effects of opioid administration are dry mouth, constipation, nausea and vomiting, and although these can be very troublesome for individual patients they are rarely the dose-limiting factor.

The subject of this chapter is opioid switching and rotation; however, from what has been said above, it will be clear that there are a number of pharmacological and nonpharmacological strategies that need to be part of routine practice at the initiation of any opioid treatment, to give the best possible balance between wanted and unwanted opioid effects and hence maximum opioid responsiveness. It is essential to conduct a thorough patient assessment, both physical and nonphysical, to identify the most likely cause of the pain and therefore facilitate the choice of optimum analgesia, including adjuvant analgesics. The complete patient assessment should help to distinguish between pain distress and pain severity, i.e. some patients have pain but are generally more distressed by that pain because of exacerbating nonphysical factors such as anxiety, fear, or depression. In addition, at initiation of opioid prescribing it is good practice to prescribe a laxative, unless the patient has diarrhea, to give advice about regular mouth care using a mouthwash such as chlorhexidine, and the use of iced water and artificial saliva and oral gels as appropriate, and to prescribe an antiemetic, usually metoclopramide or haloperidol. Somewhere between 30% and 60% of patients experience nausea and/or vomiting on initiation of opioid treatment, and the availability of an antiemetic is clearly important. In addition to the prescription of an adjuvant analgesic, depending on the pain syndrome, there is evidence that nonsteroidal anti-inflammatory drugs (NSAIDs) or acetaminophen (paracetamol) in combination with opioids provide improved analgesia over opioids alone.[27***] The prescription of an NSAID will depend very much on the individual patient and the risk–benefit analysis.

RATIONALE FOR THE PRESCRIPTION OF AN ALTERNATIVE OPIOID

The rationale for switching opioid in a patient who has not achieved opioid responsiveness with the first opioid is to achieve a better balance between analgesia and unwanted effects and is based on a combination of:

1 knowledge of the different pharmacology of opioid analgesics;
2 preclinical evidence of genetic variability in response to opioids;
3 clinical experience of the use of alternative opioids in patients who encounter difficulty with the opioid analgesia and side-effect balance.*

PHARMACOLOGY OF DIFFERENT OPIOID ANALGESICS

Different opioid drugs have different receptor-binding profiles, half-lives, toxic metabolites, and side-effect profiles and also vary in the time of onset of analgesia and duration of analgesia. In addition, pharmacokinetic profiles in patients with renal dysfunction and, to some degree, hepatic dysfunction, will lead to a different balance in the outcome of wanted and unwanted effects with different drugs in any individual patient. Table 12.1 summarizes the opioid drugs available, although not all are available in every country.

PRECLINICAL EVIDENCE FOR A DIFFERENT OPIOID RESPONSE WITH DIFFERENT OPIOID ANALGESICS

It is known, from molecular approaches to the study of pain-differential gene expression, that different genes are involved in alteration of pain pathways. Working on the hypothesis that changes in the expression of individual genes are responsible for many of the functional sequelae of nerve damage and inflammation, a challenge then is to define the nature of the changes that occur in the known genes as well as to identify and investigate unknown genes whose regulation may contribute to the pathophysiological processes that occur, such as the generation of neuropathic or inflammatory pain. In addition to this, however, there is now a fascinating body of work looking at the genetic profile of opioid receptors. Work by Pasternak's group using mice lacking morphine receptors (mor-knockout mice) has nicely demonstrated the effect of different opioids. These studies have shown that mice which have no morphine receptors will still in fact respond to other opioids, such as fentanyl and diacetyl morphine.[28]

The preclinical evidence goes some way to explaining the phenomenon, commonly encountered in clinical practice, of patients preferring and doing better on one analgesic over another.[29–40]

CLINICAL EVIDENCE FOR A BENEFIT IN OPIOID SWITCH*

The idea of switching from one opioid to another, sometimes more than once (so-called opioid rotation), was first reported in a small case series by Galer *et al.* in 1992.[41] Since then, larger case series, many also retrospective but some providing prospective data, support the finding of clinical improvement when patients are switched to a second opioid.* Many of these studies report cases of patients suffering from opioid-induced neurotoxicity, and one could argue that, in such cases, the first step should be to reduce the dose of the first opioid and review the clinical situation rather than automatically switching to a second opioid.[42] However, the case series reported have raised the interesting issue that a lower than expected equianalgesic dose of the second opioid is frequently successful in achieving analgesia. This phenomenon can be explained by any combination of the following:

1 The dose of the first opioid was simply too high in relation to the patient's true analgesic requirement or degree of opioid responsiveness.
2 A degree of pharmacological tolerance developed to the first opioid, with the result that a lower dose of the second opioid could be introduced.
3 The effect was the result of the phenomenon of incomplete cross-tolerance at receptor level. This means that the second opioid works in a different way to the first either at the receptor site or at the secondary messenger level. The degree of incomplete cross-tolerance is unpredictable within and between patients.
4 The genetic make-up of the patient resulted in a differential response to different opioids.
5 Neuroplasticity of the nervous system in chronic pain may have resulted in a different response to different opioids. Methadone is interesting in this respect, being up to 14 times as potent as morphine, possibly because of its *N*-methyl-D-aspartate (NMDA) antagonist activity, although the mechanisms underlying its increased potency and efficacy are not fully understood.[17*,25] For this reason, great clinical care is needed when switching to methadone.

Randomized controlled trials have been conducted with the aim of determining the effects of different opioids in cancer pain. However, there has been only one double-blind randomized controlled trial and that examined the effects of oxycodone and morphine (small numbers).[43***] This study found the two drugs to be equally as effective as analgesics, although oxycodone seemed to be associated with fewer hallucinations and less sleep disturbance.

EVIDENCE FOR SELECTION OF A PARTICULAR ALTERNATIVE OPIOID TO MORPHINE

There is little justification for the administration of another opioid as an alternative to morphine. However, from a combination of first principles drawn from the known pharmacology of different opioids, the nature of cancer pain, and published work on different opioids, it is possible to come to some logical conclusions.

Patients with very severe pain, who require rapid dose titration, are generally best treated with drugs that reach steady state soon after treatment is initiated or the dose is changed. Controlled-release drugs, including long-acting morphine, hydromorphone, and oxycodone preparations, and the transdermal fentanyl system, can require up to several days to approach steady-state concentrations and are not the preferred approach in patients with severe, uncontrolled cancer pain. In addition, drugs such as methadone and levorphanol, which have long half-lives, can cause problems in situations of rapid dose adjustments. Normal-release morphine, oxycodone, or hydromorphone would be appropriate if rapid dose titration is required.

Methadone has a uniquely long and highly variable half-life, and presents special considerations in drug

Table 12.1 *Opioid analgesics (pure mu agonists) used for the treatment of chronic pain*

Morphine-like agonists	Equianalgesic doses[a]	Half-life (h)	Peak effect (h)	Duration (h)	Toxicity	Comments
Morphine	10 s.c.	2–3	0.5–1	3–6	Constipation, nausea, sedation most common; respiratory depression rare in cancer patients	Standard comparison for opioids; multiple routes available
	20–60 p.o.[b]	2–3	1.5–2	4–7		
Controlled-release morphine	20–60 p.o.[b]	2–3	3–4	8–12		
Sustained-release morphine	20–60 p.o.[b]	2–3	4–6	24		Once-a-day morphine approved in some countries
Hydromorphone	1.5 s.c. 7.5 p.o.	2–3 2–3	0.5–1 1–2	3–4 3–4	Same as morphine	Used for multiple routes
Oxycodone	20–30	2–3	1	3–6	Same as morphine	Combined with aspirin or acetaminophen for moderate pain in USA; available orally without co-analgesic for severe pain
Controlled-release oxycodone	20–30	2–3	3–4	8–12		
Oxymorphone	1 s.c.	–	0.5–1	3–6	Same as morphine	No oral formulation
	10 p.r.	–	1.5–3	4–6		
Meperidine (pethidine)	75 s.c.	2–3	0.5–1	3–4	Same as morphine + CNS excitation; contraindicated in patients on monoamine oxidase inhibitors	Not used for cancer pain because of toxicity in higher doses and short half-life
Diamorphine	5 s.c.	0.5	0.5–1	4–5	Same as morphine	Analgesic action due to metabolites, predominantly morphine; only available in some countries
Levorphanol	2 s.c.	12–15	0.5–1	3–6	Same as morphine	With long half-life, accumulation occurs after beginning or increasing dose
	4 p.o.					
Methadone[c]	10 s.c.	12 to >150	0.5–1.5	4–8	Same as morphine	Risk of delayed toxicity due to accumulation; useful to start dosing on p.r.n.
	20 p.o. (see text)					
Codeine	130 s.c. 200 p.o.	2–3	1.5–2	3–6	Same as morphine	Usually combined with nonopioid
Propoxyphene HCl (dextropropoxyphene)	–	12	1.5–2	3–6	Same as morphine plus seizures with overdose	Toxic metabolite accumulates but not significant at doses used clinically; usually combined with nonopioid

Propoxyphene napsylate (dextropropoxyphene)	–	12	1.5–2	3–6	Same as hydrochloride	Same as hydrochloride
Hydrocodone	–	2–4	0.5–1	3–4	Same as morphine	Only available combined with acetaminophen; only available in some countries
Dihydrocodone	–	2–4	0.5–1	3–4	Same as morphine	Only available combined with aspirin or acetaminophen
Fentanyl	–	7–12	–	–	Same as morphine	Can be administered as a continuous i.v. or s.c. infusion; based on clinical experience, 100 μg/h is roughly equianalgesic to morphine 4 mg/h
Fentanyl transdermal system	–	6–24	–	48–72		Based on clinical experience 100 μg/h is roughly equianalgesic to morphine 4 mg/h; recent study indicates a ratio of oral morphine to transdermal fentanyl of 100:1

a. Dose that provides analgesia equivalent to 10 mg i.m. morphine. These ratios are useful guidelines when switching drugs or routes of administration.
b. Extensive survey data suggest that the relative potency of i.m. to p.o. or s.c. to p.o. morphine changes from 1:6 to 1:2–3 with chronic dosing.
c. When switching from another opioid to methadone, the potency of methadone is much greater than indicated in this table.

selection. The half-life of this opioid is usually about 1 day, but ranges from 12 h to more than 150 h.[44] This variability implies that the four to five half-lives required to approach steady state after treatment begins or is changed can be as brief as several days or as long as 2 weeks. If the dose is rapidly increased to an effective level, the plasma concentration continues to rise toward steady-state levels and late toxicity can occur. For this reason, careful monitoring is required for a prolonged period after methadone dosing is initiated or the dose is increased. These characteristics suggest that methadone should be considered a second-line drug for patients who are difficult to monitor (e.g. noncompliant patients or those who live alone or at a distance) and those predisposed to opioid side-effects (e.g. the elderly and those with encephalopathy or other major organ dysfunction). As mentioned already, the equianalgesic dose of methadone can be as little as 1/14 that of morphine.

TRANSDERMAL FENTANYL

The transdermal route of administration is available for the highly lipophilic opioid fentanyl.[8] This formulation, which offers a 48–72 h dosing interval, may be most useful for the patient who is unable to swallow or absorb an orally administered opioid, particularly if the pain syndrome is relatively stable. Pains that are rapidly fluctuating and require multiple supplemental doses may be more easily managed using an ambulatory infusion device with a patient-controlled analgesia option or another opioid until a stable situation is achieved.

Based on clinical observation, there may be other indications for a trial of transdermal fentanyl. This formulation easily permits a trial of fentanyl after other opioids have failed. If patient compliance has been a problem, the longer dosing interval associated with the transdermal system may be helpful. The observation in open-label studies that transdermal fentanyl produces less constipation than oral morphine suggests that severe constipation may be another indication for a trial. Finally, some patients prefer the transdermal route over oral medication. If a patient expresses such a preference, or it is perceived independently by the clinician, this, too, may be an indication for a trial of the transdermal system.

The pharmacokinetics of the transdermal system are complex and vary between patients.[45] The formulation produces a subcutaneous depot, which results in a slow onset of effects following a dose change and a prolonged apparent elimination half-life (usually 24 h) after the patch is removed. Steady-state concentrations are not approached for 1–3 days, and sometimes longer. Absorption from the patch can be accelerated when fever occurs.

These kinetics reinforce the importance of dose titration, the need to have an alternative means of analgesia available during the potentially prolonged period before stable analgesia is attained, and the need for prolonged monitoring after the transdermal system is removed. Even when stable, patients usually require access to an opioid by an alternative route to treat intermittent breakthrough pains. Patients who develop toxicity and require discontinuation of therapy must be observed for a day or more after the patch is removed.

OPIOID SWITCHING – DRUG AND/OR ROUTE?

The level of evidence for switching between opioid drugs to achieve an improved balance between analgesia and side-effects is poor.* Clearly, it can be very difficult to conduct randomized controlled trials in patients with advanced, uncontrolled cancer pain. It can be disappointing when a maneuver that is undoubtedly clinically useful in the palliative care of patients cannot be given a higher level of evidence. It is important to remember that lack of evidence does not make a particular maneuver less important, although it can make it more of a challenge. It is likely that the enthusiasm for preclinical evidence will encourage future well-conducted prospective controlled trials looking at the role of alternative opioids. Currently, all that can be said with certainty is that adherence to a proper patient assessment and dosing guidelines, as outlined by the World Health Organization (WHO) and others, is a greater determinant of analgesic success than choice of a particular opioid or route of administration.

Switch of route*

Opioid route switching is an everyday practice in basic palliative care, e.g. oral → subcutaneous or oral → rectal (when the patient is unable to swallow or has nausea and vomiting). Generally, this type of maneuver simply involves administering the same drug in an appropriate equianalgesic dose by a different route.*

A more complicated maneuver involves a switch to the epidural or intrathecal route.* This is sometimes necessary if systemic opioid therapy is limited by side-effects and all appropriate adjuvants have been tried. Usually the pain has to be below mid-chest level. Opioids are usually combined with local anesthetic and/or clonidine and given by continuous infusion in chronic cancer pain management (Table 12.2).

SUMMARY

Although morphine is often the first-line drug, based on extensive clinical experience, relative ease of oral titration, and availability of numerous formulations, variability in the response to different opioids is very substantial, and morphine may or may not be preferred by any indi-

Table 12.2 *Routes of opioid administration used for chronic pain*

Route	Comment
Oral	Preferred in cancer pain management
Sublingual	Buprenorphine effective but not available in all countries. Efficacy of highly lipid-soluble drugs, such as fentanyl, is likely, but no studies and very little clinical experience. Efficacy of morphine controversial
Rectal	Available for morphine, oxymorphone, and hydromorphone. Methadone has been compounded and used successfully. Customarily used as if dose is equianalgesic to oral dose. Absorption is variable, however, and relative potency may be higher or lower than expected
Transdermal	Available for fentanyl. Dosing interval is 2–3 days. Empirical indications include difficulty with swallowing or gastrointestinal absorption, desire for fentanyl trial, compliance problems with oral dosing, possibly severe constipation, and possibly desire to offer an alternative that the patient perceives may improve quality of life
Oral transmucosal	Formulation using fentanyl for breakthrough pain
Subcutaneous Repetitive bolus Continuous infusion Continuous infusion with patient-controlled analgesia	Ambulatory infusion pumps can provide continuous infusion with any parenteral opioid formulation. More advanced pumps can also provide patient-controlled analgesia. Clearest indication is inability to tolerate oral route
Intravenous	Continuous infusion possible if permanent venous access device available – sometimes the nonoral route of choice in children
Repetitive bolus	
Continuous infusion	
Continuous infusion with patient-controlled analgesia	
Epidural	Clearest indication is pain below mid-chest and treatment-limiting side-effects from systemic opioid. Often co-administered with local anesthetic
Repetitive bolus	
Continuous infusion using percutaneous or implanted system	
Intrathecal	Sometimes administered via a totally implanted infusion pump. May be cost-effective for those patients with clear indication for intraspinal therapy and long life expectancy
Intracerebroventricular	Rarely indicated. Experience is limited

vidual patient. Sequential trials of different opioid drugs may be needed to identify the opioid that yields the most favorable balance between analgesia and side-effects.[46]* In addition, a change in the route of administration may be the solution in some situations.* The most important factors to remember in any switching of drugs are the basic principles of cancer pain control. Switching opioids will never be the right solution in patients who are generally distressed or in those in whom a proper pain assessment has not been carried out and appropriate treatment modalities instituted, such as adjuvant analgesics, radiotherapy, physiotherapy, and many more treatment options.

Great care should be taken in patients who experience opioid toxicity, with a general review, appropriate hydration, and reduction in dose in the first instance.

Future preclinical studies should add to our understanding of this complex clinical area.

REFERENCES

1. World Health Organization. *Cancer Pain Relief*, 2nd edn. Geneva: World Health Organization, 1996.
2. European Association for Palliative Care. Morphine in cancer pain: modes of administration – Expert working group of the European Association for Palliative Care. *Br Med J* 1996; **312:** 823–6.
3. Pulsen L, Brosen K, Arendt-Nielsen L, *et al.* Codeine and morphine in extensive and poor metabolizers of sparteine: pharmacokinetics, analgesic effect and side-effects. *Eur J Clin Pharmacol* 1996; **51:** 289–95.
4. Sindrup SH, Brosen K. The pharmacogenetics of codeine hypoalgesia. *Pharmacogenetics* 1995; **5:** 335–46.
5. Fromm MF, Hofmann U, Griese EU, *et al.* Dihydrocodeine: a new opioid substrate for the polymorphic

CYP2D6 in humans. *Clin Pharmacol Ther* 1995; **58:** 374–82.

6. Lurcott G. The effects of the genetic absence and inhibition of CYP2D6 on the metabolism of codeine and its derivatives, hydrocodone and oxycodone. *Anesth Prog* 1998; **45:** 154–6.
7. Ahmedzai S, Brooks D. Transdermal fentanyl versus sustained-release oral morphine in cancer pain: Preference, efficacy, and quality of life – The TTS Fentanyl Comparative Trial Group. *J Pain Symptom Manage* 1997; **13:** 254–61.
8. Donner B, Zenz M, Tryba M, *et al.* Direct conversion from oral morphine to transdermal fentanyl: a multicenter study in patients with cancer pain. *Pain* 1996; **64:** 527–34.
9. Payne R, Mathias SD, Pasta DJ, *et al.* Quality of life and cancer pain: satisfaction and side-effects with transdermal fentanyl versus oral morphine. *J Clin Oncol* 1998; **16:** 1588–93.
10. Lawlor P, Turner K, Hanson J, *et al.* Dose ratio between morphine and hydromorphone in patients with cancer pain: a retrospective study. *Pain* 1997; **72:** 79–85.
11. ◆ Bruera E, Pereira J, Watanabe S, *et al.* Opioid rotation in patients with cancer pain: a retrospective comparison of dose ratios between methadone, hydromorphone, and morphine. *Cancer* 1996; **78:** 852–7.
12. Bruera E, Franco JJ, Maltoni M, *et al.* Changing pattern of agitated impaired mental status in patients with advanced cancer: association with cognitive monitoring, hydration, and opioid rotation. *J Pain Symptom Manage* 1995; **10:** 287–91.
13. De Stoutz ND, Bruera E, Suarez-Almazor M. Opioid rotation for toxicity reduction in terminal cancer patients. *J Pain Symptom Manage* 1995; **10:** 378–84.
14. Thomas Z, Bruera E. Use of methadone in a highly tolerant patient receiving parenteral hydromorphone. *J Pain symptom Manage* 1995; **10:** 315–17.
15. Galer BS, Coyle N, Pasternak GW, *et al.* Individual variability in the response to different opioids: report of five cases. *Pain* 1992; **49:** 87–91
16. Fitzgibbon DR, Ready LB. Intravenous high-dose methadone administered by patient controlled analgesia and continuous infusion for the treatment of cancer pain refractory to high-dose morphine. *Pain* 1997; **73:** 259–61.
17. ◆ Ripamonti C, Groff L, Brunelli C, *et al.* Switching from morphine to oral dose methadone in treating cancer pain: what is the equianalgesic dose ratio? *J Clin Oncol* 1998; **16:** 3216–21.
18. Maddocks I, Somogyi A, Abbott F, *et al.* Attenuation of morphine-induced delirium in palliative care by substitution with infusion of oxycodone. *J Pain Symptom Manage* 1996; **12:** 182–9.
19. Vigano Am Fan D, Bruera E. Individualized use of methadone and opioid rotation in the comprehensive management of cancer pain associated with poor prognostic indicators. *Pain* 1996; **67:** 115–19.
20. Paix A, Coleman A, Lees J, *et al.* Subcutaneous fentanyl and sufentanil infusion substitution for morphine intolerance in cancer pain management. *Pain* 1995; **63:** 263–9.
21. ◆ Ashby MA, Martin P, Jackson KA. Opioid substitution to reduce adverse effects in cancer pain management. *Med J Aust* 1999; **170:** 68–71.
22. Makin MK, Ellershaw JE. Substitution of another opioid for morphine: methadone can be used to manage neuropathic pain related to cancer [letter]. *Br Med J* 1998; **317:** 81.
23. Mercadante S. Opioid rotation for cancer pain: rationale and clinical aspects. *Cancer* 1999; **86:** 1856–66.
24. Stein C, Hassan AHS, Lehrberger K, *et al.* Local analgesic effect of endogenous opioid peptides. *Lancet* 1993; **342:** 321–4.
25. Foley KM, Houde RW. Methadone in cancer pain management: individualize dose and titrate to effect [editorial]. *J Clin Oncol* 1998; **16:** 3213–15.
26. Fallon M, Hanks GW. Opioid responsiveness – sense or nonsense? *Pain Clin* 1993; **6:** 205–206.
27. Moore A, McQuay H. *An Evidence-based Resource for Pain Relief*. Oxford: Oxford University Press, 1998: 58–77.
28. Rossi GC, Pan YX, Brown GP, *et al.* Antisense mapping the MOR-1 opioid receptor: Evidence for alternative splicing and a novel morphine-6 beta-glucuronide receptor. *FEBS Lett* 1995; **369:** 192–6.
29. Leventhal L, Stevens LB, Rossi GC, *et al.* Antisense mapping of the MOR-1 opioid receptor clone: modulation of hyperphagia induced by DAMGO. *J Pharmacol Exp Ther* 1997; **282:** 1402–7.
30. Brown GP, Yang K, King MA, *et al.* 3-Methoxynaltrexone, a selective heroin/morphine-6 beta-glucuronide antagonist. *FEBS Lett* 1997; **412:** 35–8.
31. Blake Ad, Bot G, Li S, *et al.* Differential agonist regulation of the human kappa-opioid receptor. *J Neurochem* 1997; **68:** 1846–52.
32. Rossi GC, Brown GP, Leventhal L, *et al.* Novel receptor mechanisms for heroin and morphine-6 beta glucuronide analgesia. *Neurosci Lett* 1996; **216:** 1–4.
33. ◆ Pasternak GW, Standifer KM. Mapping of opioid receptors using antisense oligodeoxynucleotides: correlating their molecular biology and pharmacology. *Trends Pharmacol Sci* 1995; **16:** 334–50.
34. Zadina JE, Kastin AJ, Harrison LM, *et al.* Opiate receptor changes after chronic exposure to agonists and antagonists. *Ann NY Acad Sci* 1995; **757:** 353–61.
35. Pasternak GW. Pharmacological mechanisms of opioid analgesics. *Clin Neuropharmacol* 1993; **16:** 1–18.
36. Moulin DE, Ling GS, Pasternak GW. Unidirectional analgesic cross-tolerance between morphine and levorphanol in the rat. *Pain* 1988; **33:** 233–9.
37. Brosen K, Sindrup SH, Skjelbo E, *et al.* Role of genetic polymorphism in psychopharmacology: an update. *Psychopharmacol Ser* 1993; **10:** 199–211.
38. Heiskanen T, Olkkola KT, Kalso E. Effects of blocking

CYP2D6 on the pharmacokinetics and pharmacodynamics of oxycodone. *Clin Pharmacol Ther* 1998; **64:** 603–11.

39. Kirkwood LC, Nation RL, Somogyi AA. Characterization of the human cytochrome P450 enzymes involved in the metabolism of dihydrocodeine. *Br J Clin Pharmacol* 1997; **44:** 549–55.
40. Sindrup SH, Poulsen L, Brosen K, *et al.* Are poor metabolisers of sparteine/debrisoquine less pain tolerant than extensive metabolisers? *Pain* 1993; **53:** 335–9.
41. Galer BS, Coyle N, Pasternak GW, Portenoy RK. Individual variability in the response to different opioids: report of five cases. *Pain* 1992; **49:** 87–91.
42. Fallon MT, O'Neill B. Substitution of another opioid for morphine: Opioid toxicity should be managed initially by decreasing the opioid dose [letter]. *Br Med J* 1998; **317:** 81.
43. Kalso E, Vainio A. Morphine and oxycodone hydrochloride in the management of cancer pain. *Clin Pharmacol Ther* 1990; **47:** 639–46.
44. Plummer JL, Gourlay GK, Cherry DA, *et al.* Estimation of methadone clearance: application in the management of cancer pain. *Pain* 1988; **33:** 313–22.
45. Portenoy RK, Southam MA, Gupta SK, *et al.* Transdermal fentanyl for cancer pain: repeated dose pharmacokinetics. *Anesthesiology* 1993; **78:** 36–43.
46. ◆ Cherny N, Ripamonti C, Pereira J, *et al.* Strategies to manage the adverse effects of oral morphine: an evidence-based report. *J Clin Oncol* 2001; **19:** 2452–4.

13

Management of side-effects

JUAN M NÚÑEZ OLARTE

Opioid analgesics are certainly the mainstay of cancer pain therapy.[1,2] Skillful use of the World Health Organization (WHO) method for cancer pain relief can achieve success in approximately 80% of patients.[3] Although excessive concern about opioid toxicity (for example addiction) can become an important barrier to adequate pain therapy,[4] improper management of opioid side-effects might result in decreased quality of life for the patients, and even failures in pain control.

This chapter reviews the management of the most important opioid side-effects. It is emphasized that side-effects of opioid therapy cannot be avoided but can and must be minimized. In most cases, a beneficial balance between pain relief and adverse effects can be achieved.

CLASSIFICATION OF IMPORTANT OPIOID SIDE-EFFECTS

See Table 13.1.

GENERAL ETIOLOGY AND PATHOPHYSIOLOGY

The likelihood of opioid toxicity is associated with several factors, such as the patient's age, organ dysfunction, pharmacodynamic considerations, concurrent use of medications with overlapping toxicity, and the patient's prior experience with opioids.[5]

Traditionally, adverse side-effects were considered to be a consequence of the binding of opioids at specific receptors in the encephalon, spinal cord, and periphery to either activate or suppress different nerve populations. In addition to its action on the central nervous system (CNS), opioids are known to have effects on the cardiovascular, pulmonary, gastrointestinal, genitourinary, and immune systems, which account for some of their side-effects.[6] On the other hand, some authors have recently proposed a role for several nonopioid receptors in the potential mechanisms of opioid neurotoxicity either through the binding of the parent drug or its metabolites or, in the case of morphine, via a more specific mechanism.[7–9] The role of morphine metabolites (morphine 6-glucuronide, morphine 3-glucuronide, and normorphine) in the development of morphine neurotoxicity has been the subject of a heated debate.[10–12] There is a growing consensus that these metabolites and their parent drug are important in the development of some opioid side-effects, but their true clinical relevance as regards opioid toxicity merits further investigation.[13–18]

GENERAL EPIDEMIOLOGY

It is difficult to establish overall frequencies of opioid-induced symptoms because of the multifactorial etiology of the symptoms recorded in cancer patients, in whom it can be impossible to attribute any given symptom to an opioid side-effect. Nevertheless, some authors have

Table 13.1 *Classification of important opioid side-effects*

Sedation
Cognitive failure
Organic hallucinosis
Delirium
Myoclonus and seizures
Hyperalgesia
Constipation
Nausea and vomiting
Respiratory depression
Tolerance, physical dependence, and addiction
Other
Urinary retention
Biliary spasm
Pruritus and allergy
Noncardiac pulmonary edema
Amenorrhea
Dry mouth

attempted to study the association of the prevalence of different symptoms with the use of weak or strong opioids within a larger prospective study,[19] or to record prospectively the prevalence of opioid side-effects.[20,21] The results of these studies are summarized in Table 13.2.

OVERALL MANAGEMENT STRATEGIES

Several global strategies that may reduce the incidence of side-effects sometimes associated with opioid therapy have been proposed. Summarizing some of them,[5,21–25] it might be concluded that there is a degree of consensus in the following strategies:

- careful monitoring until tolerance to side-effects develops;
- adding an agent to treat the side-effect;
- switching to a different opioid or to a different route of administration;
- decreasing the opioid dose, mostly by adding nonopioid analgesics and/or adjuvant analgesic medication and/or nonpharmacological treatment.

Some authors have proposed a stepwise approach to the management of opioid-induced CNS side-effects, specially when dealing with sedation and cognitive impairment.[21–23] Two of these authors[22,23] suggest the following stepwise strategy:

- Eliminate nonessential CNS depressant medications and evaluate the patient for concurrent causes (sepsis, metabolic derangement, metastases, etc.).
- If analgesia is satisfactory reduce the opioid dose by 25%.
- If analgesia is unsatisfactory and the patient is somnolent consider the addition of a psychostimulant.
- If the patient is hallucinating and delirious, consider a trial of haloperidol.
- If these problems persist, consider the addition of a nonopioid or adjuvant analgesic (which may allow reduction in the opioid dose), a switch to a different opioid, or an anesthetic or neurolytic drug.

Recently, other authors have advocated a different strategy for the management of opioid-induced neurotoxicity.[7,8,26–28] This approach places maximum emphasis on a routine changing of opioids (opioid rotation), coupled with hydration in order to increase the elimination of water-soluble active metabolites. Other alternative measures proposed are reducing the opioid dose or prescribing other drugs (such as haloperidol to manage agitation). To summarize this new approach, the alternatives would be:

- Try opioid rotation and/or hydration or, alternatively,
- Opioid dose reduction or circadian modulation.
- Try psychostimulants for sedation.
- Try other drugs for specific side-effects such as haloperidol in the setting of agitated delirium.

Table 13.2 *Prevalence of opioid side-effects*

Side-effects (*n*)	Grond *et al.*[18] (289) (%)	Schug *et al.*[19] (550) (%)	Cherny *et al.*[20] (124) (%)
a. Nil			20.1
b. Somnolence	26 (b + c + d + e + f)		35.4
c. Cognitive impairment			33.1
d. Hallucinations			14.5
e. Myoclonus			8.8
f. Seizure			1.6
g. Constipation	42	11.5	21.7
h. Nausea and vomiting	33 + 26	6.5	12.9
i. Respiratory depression			0.8
j. Urinary retention		4.7	0.8
k. Itch	6	3.7	0.8
l. Dizziness			2.4
m. Sweating	0	2.0	

Not only is there a lack of agreement on the sequence of therapies to be implemented when confronting opioid neurotoxicity, with some groups preferring opioid reduction[29–32] and others favoring opioid rotation,[8,27,28,33–36] but other areas are also currently under discussion. The role of adjuvant drugs to help diminish the opioid dose has also been a contentious issue. Although nonsteroidal anti-inflammatory drugs (NSAIDs) and other adjuvant drugs are widely considered to be one of the basic tenets of cancer pain relief,[1,2,37] caution in their use by applying our knowledge of their indications, pharmacology, and potential for additive and new side-effects has long been advocated.[38]

More recently, some authors have raised concerns about the possibility of a "dark side" to adjuvant analgesic drugs, a new concept that might undermine our previous reliance on these drugs to allow for a reduction in the opioid dose.[39] The evidence presented to support this thesis is not new, and relies heavily on studies of adverse effects in different populations. With regard to cancer pain, there is only anecdotal evidence that the risk of opioid toxicity is precipitated by impaired renal function secondary to the administration of NSAIDs in the presence of dehydration.[40,41]

On the other hand, old controlled trials in cancer pain patients have already demonstrated that the addition of a nonopioid can provide analgesia additive to that of opioids,[42,43] and support a role for NSAIDs in the management of malignant bone pain.[44] Newer, well-designed cohort studies and randomized controlled trials have again addressed the impact of NSAIDs and have provided evidence of their analgesic efficacy in cancer pain due not only to somatic but also to visceral mechanisms,[45*] and also evidence of the opioid-sparing effect of diclofenac in cancer pain.[46**,47**] This action is not secondary to a modification of morphine or methadone bioavailability induced by diclofenac.[48,49] Interestingly, ketorolac has been found to be safe for high-dose, long-term use, even in the setting of a frail patient population, with no evidence that it precipitates renal dysfunction. In this same case series, ketorolac was found to be useful in reverting opioid bowel syndrome thanks to its morphine-sparing effect.[50*]

Finally, a recent review of the literature concerning the use of NSAIDs as adjuvant analgesics to opioids found nine studies, all of which reported favorable results for this combination of drugs.[51***] In summary, the broad analgesic effect of NSAIDs seems to be useful in optimizing the balance between analgesia and side-effects in conditions in which increases in opioid dosage cause opioid toxicity. Nevertheless, further research is needed to assess the safety of NSAIDs as adjuvants on a long-term basis, specifically addressing the significant ulcerogenic gastrointestinal effects of NSAIDs.[12,51]

SEDATION

Etiology and pathophysiology

There is some preliminary evidence suggesting that a rapid increase in morphine concentration causes more sedation than increasing concentration more gradually.[52]

Epidemiology

It has been suggested that sedation remains a major problem in 7–10% of patients with advanced cancer treated with opioids in spite of opioid dose titration and opioid switch.[53]

Clinical presentation

Sedation is a common adverse effect either when patients are started on opioid analgesics or after they receive a significant increase in dose. After a few days, tolerance to sedation usually develops. It should be noted that in some cases somnolence may reflect an increase in comfort after the patient has been relieved from severe pain, rather than true sedation. On the other hand, rapidly progressive sedation in the setting of a stable opioid dose should trigger a review of concurrent medications and potential complications (metabolic disturbances, sepsis, CNS metastases, etc.) prior to considering somnolence only as an opioid side-effect.[5,8,27,28]

Evidence-based evaluation of management

There is evidence from well-designed open trials that transdermal fentanyl is less sedating than oral morphine in the setting of cancer pain.[54*,55*,56*] In the first of these three studies, significant improvement in morning vigilance with transdermal fentanyl was associated also with significant improvement in sleep quality.[54] In the second and larger study, fentanyl was associated with significantly less daytime drowsiness but greater sleep disturbance and shorter sleep duration than morphine.[55] On the other hand, a recent randomized controlled trial comparing subcutaneous morphine and fentanyl in stable (nonopioid toxic) hospice patients failed to confirm the range of benefits of fentanyl suggested in other studies.[57**] Possible explanations for these different findings might be differences in number of patients, the stigma associated with oral morphine acting as a bias, and differences in routes of administration.

Oral methadone may also be less sedating than oral morphine, as found in a recent randomized prospective study.[58**] Summarizing the available data, there is not as yet enough evidence to favor any strong opioid or route of administration as being less sedating than another, although clinical evidence is starting to accumulate that points in the direction of the presumed etiology mentioned above.

With regard to the weak opioids commonly used in the WHO guidelines,[1,2] some studies have tried to address the issue of whether the second step "makes any sense," and in doing so have found that dextropropoxyphene[59★★] and tramadol[60★] seem to be less sedating than low-dose morphine. However, tramadol failed to show this profile in a randomized controlled trial.[61★★]

Other strategies that have been advocated for managing opioid-induced sedation include:[2,5]

- discontinuation of nonessential CNS depressant medications;
- reducing the fixed-schedule opioid analgesic dose by 25% (if analgesia is adequate);
- addition of a psychostimulant (if analgesia is inadequate);
- addition of a relatively nonsedating nonopioid or adjuvant (which would allow for a reduction in the opioid dose);
- a trial of intraspinal analgesia, nerve block, or other analgesic technique (which would also allow for a reduction in the opioid dose).

The role of psychostimulants in the management of opioid-induced sedation has been the subject of extensive reviews.[8,27,62] Studies in human subjects have confirmed the enhancement of opioid analgesia by amphetamines shown in animal studies. In addition, clinical studies have demonstrated that psychostimulant drugs produce a decrease in opioid-induced somnolence and an increase in general cognitive abilities. Moreover, the greater alertness allows for the use of larger opioid doses, which can produce a substantial increase in analgesia.[8★★★,27★★★,62★★★]

Nevertheless, the randomized controlled clinical trials that have addressed the impact of amphetamines in opioid-induced sedation in cancer patients show conflicting results,[63,64] although the cumulative evidence of other open studies and retrospective studies, plus studies on different patient populations, strongly supports the positive influence of amphetamines.

Methylphenidate and dextroamphetamine are usually initiated at doses of 2.5–5 mg q.i.d. or b.i.d. (typically in the morning and at noon in order not to disturb sleep). The dose can be escalated as required, and the therapeutic effect is evident within 2 days of starting the treatment. Experience is greater with methylphenidate.

Psychostimulants can produce adverse effects such as paranoid ideation, hallucinations, delirium, anorexia, insomnia, and tremulousness. Tolerance to their positive effects can develop. Amphetamines are contraindicated relatively or even completely in the setting of a previous history of psychiatric disorders, substance abuse, cardiac ischemia, and arrhythmia. Severe extreme manifestations might also include intracranial hemorrhage.

Caffeine also may be useful in the reversal of sedation from opioid analgesics.[5★,65★]

COGNITIVE FAILURE

Introduction and definition

Research has shown that subtle changes in cognitive function in cancer patients can be detected under opioid exposure. On the other hand, cognitive failure in the terminal cancer population usually happens in the setting of the broader syndromic category of delirium. This section will focus only on cognitive dysfunction without delirium.

Clinical presentation

In most cases, the cognitive failure resembles more a generalized slowdown of cognitive function, rather than an increase in the number of errors or major errors in judgment.[8,66,67]

Clinical findings

A 30% increase in the regular opioid dose used for cancer pain relief produces a significant cognitive impairment, measured by specific cognitive tests, that can be detected 45 min after receiving the new increased dose. In some cases, this impairment is still detectable 1 week after the increase in the dose.[68,69]

Cognitive function has been assessed in cancer patients by means of reaction time and compared with other populations.[70–72] Cancer patients on stable opioid doses have also been tested for their driving ability by means of computerized psychomotor tests originally designed for professional motor vehicle drivers,[73] and by driving regularly on a driving simulator.[74] It was concluded that opioids had a slight and selective effect on psychomotor performance, and that long-term stable opioid doses do not necessarily impair driving ability, but with the caveat that each patient requires an individual examination. Other researchers have found reduced awareness and global cognitive function in patients with advanced cancer on a stable opioid dose compared with other populations.[75]

Recently, a small group of patients with very advanced cancer in a hospice setting were tested with a range of instruments for higher cognitive function. The study found the patients to have intellectual functioning below average despite having no clinical evidence of impairment of cognitive function.[16]

Evidence-based evaluation of management

In a randomized controlled trial, methylphenidate significantly improved cognitive function as measured by specific testing in patients receiving high doses of opioids subcutaneously.[76] Other noncontrolled studies have shown similar results.[77]**

The general management suggested for opioid-induced sedation is usually also advocated in the setting of opioid-induced cognitive failure (see above).

ORGANIC HALLUCINOSIS

Introduction and definition

Hallucinations secondary to opioid toxicity are usually part of the wider syndromic category of delirium. On the other hand, the syndrome of "organic hallucinosis," characterized by hallucinations in the setting of clear consciousness and intact intellectual function, is considered a separate entity in the DSM-IV[78] and ISCD-10.[79]

Clinical presentation and findings

Some clinicians have described patients with opioid-induced organic hallucinosis with no evidence of delirium.[80–83] It was observed that in some cases a transition took place from organic hallucinosis to delirium in spite of opioid rotation, and that in most cases the presence of hallucinations was not reported spontaneously by patients but was revealed by a sudden change in mood.[83]

Evidence-based evaluation of management

The limited number of cases described in the literature does not allow for a proper discussion of treatment options, but it seems that haloperidol and opioid switch/rotation might be effective options.[83]

DELIRIUM

Definition

The definition of delirium in DSM-IV is based on clinical characteristics considered to be crucial to the diagnosis:

- disturbance of consciousness/impaired attention;
- change in cognition (such as memory deficit, disorientation, language disturbances) or perception disturbances not due to dementia;
- acute presentation and fluctuation during the course of the day;
- evidence of a general medical condition or drugs or several etiologies judged to be etiologically related to the disturbance.[78]

There are some differences in the diagnostic criteria established for delirium when comparing DSM-IV and ISCD-10, although the general concept is similar. The ISCD-10 system of classification includes also some additional points such as: short-term memory impairment with preservation of long-term memory, disorientation, psychomotor disturbances, and sleep problems.[79]

Etiology and pathophysiology

It is important to emphasize that in the medically ill, and in cancer patients, opioids are seldom the only causal factor implicated in the genesis of delirium.[80] Multiple etiologies and concomitant conditions usually contribute to development of this syndrome, with polypharmacy and toxic metabolic abnormalities affecting a large percentage of cancer patients.[84]

Nevertheless, it is possible that in some cases opioids are the only factor behind the development of delirium.[85] In a recent prospective study, the only factor associated with a higher frequency of delirious symptoms in terminal cancer patients was higher daily opioid dosage (P =0.08).[86] Some researchers have suggested that oxycodone is less likely to induce delirium/hallucinations than morphine,[87] but these claims have not been proven when both drugs were compared in randomized clinical trials.[88,89]

There are several theoretical models that try to explain the pathophysiology of delirium in the setting of advanced cancer, including:

- reduction in cerebral oxidative metabolism;
- imbalance between the neurotransmitters acetylcholine and dopamine;
- stress-induced hypercortisolism;[90]
- neuroanatomical models, changes in endorphin levels.[90]

Epidemiology

Delirium is most prevalent in the advanced cancer population, with several studies suggesting that at least one-third of cancer patients admitted for terminal care may develop delirium before death,[86] although in some studies the proportion of patients experiencing terminal delirium in the last week is as high as 83–88%.[91,92]

Clinical presentation

Delirium, unfortunately, still goes unrecognized or is misdiagnosed as depression or dementia. Delirium can present in three categories: hyperactive or agitated, hypoactive, and mixed. Whereas agitated delirium is easily recognizable, the hypoactive and mixed forms are less easily detectable. Patients' relatives are usually aware of the subtle changes that precede florid delirium.[84]

Delirium is very common in advanced cancer patients and is reversible in 50% of cases. The most common delirium subtype is mixed.[92]

Delirious patients with advanced cancer are an important stressing factor for relatives and the professionals caring for them. Health professionals tend to overestimate the intensity of pain in delirious patients.[93] Without a high index of suspicion, delirium might go undetected and the attending physician my increase the opioid dose in response to the situation, thereby exacerbating the patient's delirious symptoms. If this "analgesic spiral" goes undetected, a serious deterioration in the patient's condition, and even death, can occur.[94]

Examination and diagnostic criteria

The diagnosis of delirium is primarily clinical and relies on precise criteria already described above. The Mini-Mental State Exam (MMSE) is perhaps the most utilized cognitive screening tool,[95] and its use has long been advocated in the setting of advanced cancer.[7,96] Although the MMSE is effective in measuring delirium severity, the determination of impairment in the MMSE is not specific to delirium.

A number of instruments have been developed to help to diagnose delirium accurately, including the Confusion Assessment Method (CAM),[97] which has been frequently selected by clinicians and researchers in the field of advanced cancer because of its simplicity.[96]

Recently, a new tool has been developed, the Memorial Delirium Assessment Scale (MDAS).[98] Although the scale was developed for assessing severity of delirium, it may also be useful to establish a diagnosis of delirium in medically ill patients.

Evidence-based evaluation of management

The management of delirium in advanced/terminal cancer has been summarized in the following points:

- provision of a safe environment;
- treatment of underlying etiology;
- psychological interventions;
- pharmacological interventions;
  - tranquilization
  - sedation
  - anesthesia.[99]

Despite advanced malignancy, and the fact that the precise etiology can be discovered in less than 50% of the cases,[91] managing treatable causes (e.g. hypercalcemia, infection, dehydration) is perhaps the most effective and rapid method of dealing with delirium. In this setting it is quite relevant to remember the overall management strategies for opioid toxicity described in the introductory sections of this chapter. When comparing the relative merits of opioid switching/rotation plus hydration versus opioid reduction in the treatment of delirium, it is clear that the most relevant evidence[32★,100★,101★] supporting each of these treatments is retrospective or prospective nonrandomized in nature, and therefore still weak. Morphine, hydromorphone, methadone,[102] oxycodone,[101] and fentanyl[82] have been successfully used for opioid rotation in this setting.

There are no published studies formally evaluating psychological approaches to the delirious patient such as clocks, calendars, reassuring interjections, etc.[99,103]

Regarding pharmacological interventions, haloperidol is widely considered to be the drug of choice for tranquilization in delirium. Haloperidol is a high-potency, relatively low-toxicity neuroleptic with a wide safety margin and great administration versatility (p.o., p.r., s.c., i.m., i.v.). Adverse effects are rare, except for extrapyramidal reactions. Titration of the dosage against the clinical state is feasible, and oral starting doses are around 0.5–1.5 mg (parenteral doses should be a half to two-thirds of the oral dose). Doses are repeated at regular intervals (2–5 mg at 1 mg/min every 30 min i.v. maximum if rapid tranquilization is necessary), and increased as needed, with most advanced cancer patients settling down with an oral total daily dose of 1.5–20 mg every 12 or 24 h.[96,99] The newer atypical antipsychotics risperidone and olanzapine might be useful in the setting of complicated delirium when extrapyramidal side-effects develop with haloperidol.[104]

Sedation with benzodiazepines should be used cautiously because of the risk of worsening the delirium, but occasionally it is unavoidable. Lorazepam is usually preferred because of its short half-life and lack of active metabolites, although midazolam is becoming very popular because of its very short half-life, water solubility, and ease of administration. The dose range for midazolam is 30–120 mg parenteral (s.c. or i.v.) total daily dose. As a last resort in patients with very advanced cancer, and when everything else has failed, phenobarbitone and propofol can be considered.[96,99]

Prognosis

In prospective studies delirium in advanced cancer is reversible in 44–50% of cases.[86,92] Retrospective studies have shown sustained cognitive impairment to be a poor prognostic indicator for discharge in patients with advanced cancer,[105] with some prospective studies even suggesting an expected survival of less than 4 weeks in the event of delirium not reverting to normal cognition.[106]

MYOCLONUS AND SEIZURES

Definition

Myoclonus is characterized by sudden, brief, shock-like involuntary movements caused by muscular contractions or inhibitions arising from the CNS. There are various patterns. The amplitude of the jerks can range from small contractions that have no effect on a joint to gross contractions that move limbs, head, or trunk.

Single muscles, or a group of muscles, can be involved in a myoclonic jerk, with a frequency that ranges from rare, isolated events to several contractions a minute. The distribution of myoclonus in the body can be focal (involving a single region), segmental (involving two or more contiguous regions), or generalized (involving multiple regions of the body). Myoclonic jerks can occur bilaterally (symmetrical or asymmetrical) or unilaterally.[107]

Both myoclonus and seizures can be a manifestation of opioid-induced neurotoxicity. The sequence of events is usually that of nocturnal myoclonus preceding diurnal myoclonus, which in turn might precede convulsions if the opioids are not removed.[108] There is a theoretical potential of myoclonus to become a specific early marker of opioid-induced neuroexcitation.[109]

Etiology and pathophysiology

As with delirium, it is possible that in advanced cancer patients multiple etiologies might be interacting in order to produce the myoclonic activity. Focal CNS damage, dementias, metabolic encephalopathies, and toxic encephalopathies induced by other drugs other than opioids can contribute with the offending opioid in the genesis of myoclonus.[107] Nevertheless, the role of hypomagnesemia and hypoglycemia in opioid-induced myoclonus has been rejected as a result of two studies,[110,111] and the role of other metabolic abnormalities such as hypermagnesemia, hypocalcemia, hypercalcemia, hyponatremia, hypernatremia, hypokalemia, and hyperkalemia seems to be irrelevant.[107]

Myoclonus as a side-effect of opioid therapy has been described after administration of morphine, hydromorphone, diamorphine, meperidine (pethidine), methadone, and fentanyl.[9,112] High doses of opioids are not strictly a prerequisite for myoclonus,[111] although they seem to be a prerequisite for seizures.[108]

Our understanding of the pathophysiology of opioid-induced myoclonus is greatly limited by the lack of neurophysiological studies.[107] Animal models have provided evidence of the role of *N*-methyl-D-aspartate (NMDA), γ-aminobutyric acid (GABA), opioid, and serotonin receptors in opioid-induced neuroexcitation.[9]

Epidemiology

The incidence of myoclonus as a side-effect of treatment with an opioid in advanced cancer varies widely, ranging from 2.7% to 87%. This wide discrepancy can be explained by the different nature and methodology of the studies, the absence of validated assessment measures for myoclonus, and different perceptions of myoclonus as an alarming symptom in different settings. There is a very real danger of underdiagnosing myoclonus if it is restricted to sleep.[107]

Clinical presentation and findings

Myoclonus associated with systemic opioid therapy is usually described as uncontrollable jerks affecting the arms, legs, or both. The duration of spasms is commonly about 1 s, and spasms are asymmetrical and vary in frequency between patients. Jerking can occur either at night or during the day or both, with nocturnal myoclonus commonly preceding the appearance of diurnal myoclonus for weeks or months. In patients with a low intensity of myoclonus, the phenomenon is frequently not noticed by physicians or nurses but perceived by patients and/or relatives. Some patients associate myoclonus with poor quality of sleep or feelings of clumsiness, but the true impact of myoclonus as one of the possible etiologies of sleep fragmentation in advanced cancer remains to be determined.[107]

Spinal opioid therapy is particularly associated with focal/segmental myoclonus restricted to myoclonic spasms with spinal jerking distal to the segment of the spinal cord where the tip of the catheter is located, although it might also progress to generalized myoclonus. In this setting the patient usually complains of a severe increase in pain with the involuntary jerking of spine and lower limbs. Systemic opioid therapy can also induce this type of segmental myoclonus when there is coexistence of pathologic changes within the spine.[9] The risk of developing myoclonus with spinal opioid therapy is highly associated with neural dysfunction due to pathologic damage within the spine.[113]

Diagnostic criteria

Assessment is perhaps one of the most neglected areas of research in myoclonus, and failure to produce a validated tool greatly limits the conclusions of several investigations. A preliminary severity scale for opioid-induced myoclonus has been produced[107] but still has to undergo appropriate testing to assess its validity. It is presented in Table 13.3.

Table 13.3 *Marañón's Myoclonus Assessment Scale (MMAS)*[107]

Myoclonus absent
Myoclonus restricted to sleep that goes undetected
Myoclonus restricted to sleep that wakens the patient
Myoclonus while awake not appreciable during a short interview
Myoclonus while awake appreciable during a short interview

Evidence-based evaluation of management

Current standard therapeutic approaches to opioid-induced myoclonus include opioid rotation or reduction or discontinuation.[9,112] Unrestricted escalation of the opioid dosage in the setting of significant myoclonus might trigger a convulsive episode,[108] although epileptic seizures have also been reported with intracerebroventricular and intrathecal morphine bolus with no previous myoclonus warning.[114]

Smaller doses may reduce the myoclonus but also result in poor pain control, whereas opioid rotation should not be associated with this problem.[102*] A specific treatment to control myoclonus has the theoretical advantage that it may allow the continuation of opioid escalation when pain is uncontrolled, whereas an alternate opioid therapy may result in a period of poor pain control.[112]

Thus, the role of supplemental drugs is quite promising but very much under discussion. The balance of present evidence, all of it of anecdotal nature, favors the use of either clonazepam or midazolam. Clonazepam appears to be safe in doses ranging from 0.25 to 2.0 mg in a single dose at bedtime or b.i.d., either p.o. or i.v. in a slow push. The role of other drugs such as lorazepam, diazepam, baclofen, bupivacaine, dantrolene, haloperidol, phenytoin, carbamazepine, valproate, phenobarbital, chlomethiazole, and naloxone is either conflicting or difficult to assess in view of the different reports in the literature.[9,112]

Notes on unevaluated treatments

Based on previous treatment anecdotes and animal models, some observational studies have recently been started with ketamine and dextromethorphan with promising preliminary results.[115]

HYPERALGESIA

Introduction and definition

Hyperalgesia and allodynia have occasionally been reported following high doses of morphine administered systemically and intrathecally in humans.[8]

Etiology and pathophysiology

This is presumed to be similar to other manifestations of opioid neurotoxicity with active opioid metabolites playing an important role.[27]

Epidemiology and clinical presentation and diagnostic criteria

Although this a very rare manifestation of opioid neurotoxicity, it is of clinical relevance because of the real risk of physicians misinterpreting this phenomenon. If not recognized as an opioid adverse effect, the clinician may respond by further increasing the opioid dose in an attempt to control pain, thereby aggravating the problem.[28]

A high degree of suspicion should be exerted whenever a patient experiences a sudden aggravation of pain chronologically linked with the administration of an opioid (morphine), and especially if associated with cutaneous hyperalgesia and/or allodynia.[27]

Evidence-based evaluation of management

Opioid switching has been successful in some case series.[116,117]

Notes on unevaluated treatments

In the author's own limited experience (two cases) opioid-induced hyperalgesia can improve dramatically after opioids are discontinued and replaced with an NSAID with no evidence of opioid withdrawal, thereby also suggesting a predominantly nonopioid receptor mechanism involved in the etiology (unpublished results). Our limited knowledge of this phenomenon does not allow for a recommendation on this procedure.

CONSTIPATION

Introduction and definition

Constipation is one of the most frequent and most troublesome side-effects of opioid analgesia, specially with morphine. Constipated patients might become reluctant to accept the morphine doses that they need to control pain.[118]

Constipation is defined as the passage of small hard feces infrequently and with difficulty. Failure to defecate at least three times per week, straining at stool during more than 25% of defecations, and defecation regularly lasting for more than 10 min are usually taken as objective indicators of constipation.[119]

Etiology and pathophysiology

In general, opioids inhibit gastrointestinal motility. Their widespread effects on the gut include:

- delayed gastric emptying associated with constriction of the pyloric sphincter;
- increased tone in ileocecal and anal sphincters;
- impaired transit through small intestine and colon;
- reduced intestinal secretion (in animals);
- impaired defecation reflex.[118,119]

Peripheral opioid receptors on gut smooth muscle presumably mediate these actions.[120] Morphine gastrointestinal effects are preferentially mediated by μ_2-receptors. Central mediation of opioid-induced constipation has been found in animal studies, but its clinical significance in humans remains to be determined.[118,119]

Constipation in advanced cancer is usually multifactorial, but traditionally opioids have been considered an important contributory factor. Dose–response, lack of tolerance to the constipating effect, and large interindividual variability are supposedly common characteristics of opioid-induced constipation.[121] Nevertheless, recent studies have challenged these long-held beliefs and suggest that morphine-induced constipation is not dose dependent, that persistent constipation is related more closely to the patient's condition than to morphine, and that a proportion of patients may become tolerant in the long term to the constipating effects of morphine.[122] In a retrospective study,[123] age, female sex, and abdominal tumor involvement were found to be, along with opioid type, clinical predictors of laxative dose in advanced cancer patients. Opioids seem to account only for about a quarter of the constipation found in terminally ill cancer patients.[120]

The constipation-inducing capacity of different opioids has been the subject of much recent research and will be discussed as a treatment option. There is preclinical evidence from an animal model to support the relatively low incidence of intestinal side-effects observed clinically with transdermal fentanyl in comparison with orally administered morphine.[124]

Epidemiology

It is quite difficult to discriminate in a physically ill population constipation due to opioids from that due to other reasons, as discussed above. Nevertheless, the proportion of patients receiving opioids who suffer from opioid-induced constipation ranges from 11.5% to 42% (Table 13.1).

Clinical presentation and clinical findings

History-taking and an abdominal and rectal examination are essential in the evaluation of constipation but, unfortunately, are easily overlooked.

Diagnostic criteria and critical evaluation of investigations

Investigations are rarely needed in the assessment of constipation. Plain abdominal radiographs may distinguish between constipation and obstruction but are not useful in the systematic assessment of constipation in advanced cancer.[125]

Mean transit time (MMT-S) has been used as a standard to evaluate stool analysis of transit time (SST) and a standardized estimation of stool form as measures of bowel function in advanced cancer.[126] There is presently no widely accepted measurement tool for constipation, and the lack of it may limit the conclusions of the comparative studies.

Evidence-based evaluation of management

The management of opioid-induced constipation is based on a three-step approach:

- choice of opioid;
- prevention;
- pharmacological treatment
  - oral laxatives
  - rectal laxatives
  - prokinetics.

Numerous prospective controlled trials have found transdermal fentanyl to be less constipating than oral morphine.[54**,55**,56,**127,**128,**129,**130**] This conclusion was challenged in one of the studies because of the short-term nature of the study and the possibility that opioid withdrawal syndrome might be playing a role.[131] However, these criticisms have been convincingly rebutted.[132] Fentanyl is also less constipating than morphine when both are administered subcutaneously.[57**] Transdermal fentanyl has become the opioid of choice in our institution in the setting of spinal cord compression.

Oral oxycodone was found to be more constipating than oral morphine in one prospective randomized controlled trial.[88] On the other hand, in a similar study, no significant differences in adverse effects were found.[89**] Anecdotal evidence[133] and retrospective[123*] and prospective randomized studies[58**] all suggest that oral methadone might be less constipating than oral morphine, and perhaps hydromorphone. Finally, tramadol has been found in prospective nonrandomized[60] and randomized[61**] studies to induce less constipation than morphine.

Prevention of opioid-induced constipation relies upon:[119,121]

- encouraging activity;
- increasing fiber and fluid intake if the patient is ambulatory and at no risk of gastrointestinal obstruction;
- altering treatment with constipating drugs if achievable[50] or adding laxatives;
- creating a favorable environment for defecation.

Oral laxatives regularly used in opioid-induced constipation can be classified into:[121]

- prokinetics (metoclopramide,[134] cisapride);
- bulk-forming laxatives;
- lubricants (mineral oil – starting dose 1–2 tablespoons);
- osmotic (saline) cathartics (lactulose – starting dose 10–30 ml);
- agents for colonic lavage (polyethylene glycol – starting low dose 13 g/sachet);
- cathartic drugs
  - docusate (starting dose 300 mg)
  - castor oil
  - anthraquinone derivatives (senna – starting dose 1–2 tablets or 1–2 tablespoons)
  - diphenylmethane derivatives (bisacodyl – starting dose 1–2 tablets or one suppository).

A full discussion of these agents is outside the scope of this chapter. Some studies have attempted to compare laxatives in opioid-induced constipation: lactulose and senna in advanced cancer patients,[135]** an ayurvedic formulation and senna in the same population,[136]** and lactulose, senna, and codanthrusate in a volunteer population.[137]* In addition, polyethylene glycol has been tested against lactulose in patients with chronic constipation.[138]**

Notes on unevaluated treatments

There is increasing interest in the therapeutic possibilities of opioid antagonists in opioid-induced constipation. Several studies have tested naloxone and methylnaltrexone,[139–143] but the potential to precipitate opioid withdrawal is real. Drugs that may have a wider margin of safety are under investigation.[118]

NAUSEA AND VOMITING

Etiology and pathophysiology

It has been suggested that high plasma levels of morphine 3-glucuronide[16] and morphine 6-glucuronide[144] might be associated with chronic nausea in the setting of renal insufficiency.

Although typical analgesic doses of opioids are often emetogenic (stimulation of D_2-receptors in the area postrema), very high doses may not be (stimulation of opioid receptors in brainstem).[145]

Epidemiology

The prevalence of opioid-induced nausea in cancer patients has been found to range between 8.3% and 18.3% and the prevalence of vomiting between 22.7% and 40%.[146] A similar study in medical patients with acute pain has found the prevalence of nausea to be 35.4% and the prevalence of emesis to be 13.6%.[147]

Evidence-based evaluation of management

Opioid-induced nausea and vomiting have been traditionally managed with antiemetics on an as-needed basis. Antiemetics have been selected according to the putative triggering mechanism:

- delayed gastric emptying – metoclopramide;
- stimulation of vestibular apparatus – antihistamine;
- stimulation of the chemoreceptor trigger zone – haloperidol.[5]

Some authors have reported transdermal scopolamine[148] and ondansetron[149] to be effective in this setting. In a randomized prospective trial, tropisetron, as a single agent or in combination, was more effective than chlorpromazine plus dexamethasone in the management of nausea and vomiting in advanced cancer patients on opioids.[150]**

In the event of refractory nausea, a trial of an alternative opioid is usually considered.[5] Until now few studies have been able to show significant differences in the emetogenic capacity of different opioids, but there are some nonetheless. Oxycodone has been found to be either less nausea-inducing than[88]** or similarly nausea-inducing to[89]** morphine in controlled trials. Transdermal fentanyl was found to be less emetogenic than oral morphine in one controlled study[54] but not in another one comparing fentanyl and morphine by the same subcutaneous route.[57]** Finally, both oral tramadol[61]** and dextropropoxyphene[59]** seem to be less emetogenic than oral morphine.

RESPIRATORY DEPRESSION

Opioid-induced respiratory depression in patients treated for cancer pain is a very uncommon circumstance due to the protective nature of pain itself. Experimental pain has been found to stimulate respiration and attenuate morphine-induced respiratory depression in a controlled study in human volunteers.[151] Furthermore, the mechanisms underlying placebo analgesia and placebo respiratory depression seem to be independent of each other and might involve different subpopulations of opioid receptors.[152]

In practical terms, caution is advised in patients receiving high doses of opioids in which a change in disease status (e.g. spinal cord compression[153]) or a pain-relieving intervention (e.g. nerve block[154]) may produce rapid pain relief. Judicious use of naloxone might be life-saving in these rare instances.[5] Delayed respiratory depression is a concern with spinal administration of opioids.[6]

TOLERANCE, PHYSICAL DEPENDENCE, AND ADDICTION

Unfortunately, many health care workers as well as patients still believe that there is a significant risk of addiction when using opioids for cancer pain. Irrational fears of addiction to opioids are bolstered by professionals with misconceptions about the phenomena of tolerance, physical dependence, and addiction.[4]

Tolerance is defined as a physiological state characterized by a decrease in the effects of a drug (e.g. analgesia) with chronic administration. Tolerance can be induced experimentally in animals, and has been considered to be a poor prognostic factor in the management of cancer pain.[155] Nevertheless, its true clinical relevance seems to be very low. The vast majority of patients who need an increase in their opioid dose do so because of disease progression rather than tolerance.[20,156] Analgesic tolerance seldom compromises therapy except perhaps in the setting of previous drug addiction or alcoholism.

Physical dependence is the physiological adaptation of the body to the presence of an opioid. It is defined by the development of withdrawal symptoms when opioids are discontinued or reduced abruptly, or when an antagonist is administered. It is frequently mistakenly equated with addiction. If the source of pain is successfully treated or removed, physical dependence is easily treated by gradually decreasing the opioid dose (e.g. 75% of the previous daily dose).[3,4,20]

Addiction is defined as aberrant changes in behavior, with compulsive use of opioids for nonmedical reasons characterized by a craving for mood-altering effects, not pain relief.[4] Addiction is extremely rare in cancer pain and chronic pain patients.[20,157,158]

DRY MOUTH

Definition

Xerostomia is defined as the subjective sensation of dryness of mouth.[159]

Etiology and pathophysiology

Xerostomia is usually associated with a low unstimulated whole salivary flow rate, but not the other way round, in patients with advanced cancer.[160] There is a positive correlation between low parotid gland salivary flow and severity of symptoms in terminally ill patients.[161]

Epidemiology

Dry mouth is considered to be a very common minor side-effect of opioids. The prevalence of xerostomia has been variously reported to be anywhere between 30% and 77% among patients with advanced cancer.[159]

Evidence-based evaluation of management

Dry mouth seems to be less common with methadone[58]** and dextropropoxyphene[59]** than with morphine. Low-tack chewing gum and pilocarpine hydrochloride have been found to be as effective as artificial saliva in the management of xerostomia in advanced cancer patients in prospective randomized studies.[159**,162**]

OTHER SIDE-EFFECTS

Opioids cause increased bladder and sphincter tone, resulting in urgency and retention, most commonly in elderly men. This side-effect is more likely to occur after spinal administration of opioids.[3,5,6]

Biliary spasm is rarely seen, or rather diagnosed, with chronic opioid therapy. Clinically it mimics gallbladder pain, sometimes associated with an elevation of hepatic and pancreatic enzymes. It can occur with almost every opioid and it has been described with morphine[12] and fentanyl.[6] Both meperidine[12] and tramadol[163] are devoid of this side-effect. Only a high index of suspicion will help to detect this problem in cancer pain management.

Pruritus is a well-known side-effect of epidural opioids and is usually treated with antihistamines or naloxone.[6] Opioids cause histamine release, and this is said to contribute to asthma or urticaria in allergic patients. Some authors consider this to be a rare phenomenon and not true "allergy."[3] Nevertheless, there have been reports of severe opioid-induced itching refractory to antihistamines but responding to transnasal butorphanol.[164] In addition, oral morphine-induced pruritus has been reported to disappear after opioid rotation to hydromorphone.[165] Tramadol has been found to induce significantly less pruritus than morphine in a controlled trial.[60]*

Noncardiogenic pulmonary edema has been reported in severely debilitated patients treated with high opioid doses.[166]

REFERENCES

1. World Health Organization. *Cancer Pain Relief.* Geneva: World Health Organization, 1986.
2. World Health Organization. *Cancer Pain Relief*, 2nd edn. Geneva: World Health Organization, 1996.

● 3. Hanks GWC, Cherny N. Opioid analgesic therapy. In: Doyle D, Hanks GWC, MacDonald N eds. *Oxford Textbook of Palliative Medicine*, 2nd edn. Oxford: Oxford University Press, 1998: 331–55.

● 4. Colleau S, Joranson DE. Fear of addiction: confronting a barrier to cancer pain relief. *Cancer Pain Release* 1998; **113:** 1–3.

● 5. Lyss AP, Portenoy RK. Strategies for limiting the side-effects of cancer pain therapy. *Semin Oncol* 1997; **24** (5 Suppl. 16): s16-28–s16-34.

● 6. Lema MJ. Opioid effects and adverse effects. *Reg Anesth* 1996; **21** (6S): 38–42.

● 7. Centeno C, Bruera E. Uso apropiado de opioides y neurotoxicidad. *Medicina Paliativa* 1999; **61:** 3–12.

● 8. Bruera E, Pereira J. Neuropsychiatric toxicity of opioids. In: Jensen TS, Turner JA, Wiesenfeld-Hallin Z eds. *Progress in Pain Research and Management*, vol. 8. Proceedings of the VIIIth World Congress on Pain. Seattle, WA: IASP Press, 1997: 717–38.

● ◆ 9. Núñez Olarte JM, Benedetti C. Ketamine treatment of opioid-induced myoclonus: clinical and theoretical implications. Submitted to *Pain*.

● 10. Sjogren P. Clinical implications of morphine metabolites. In: Portenoy RK, Bruera E eds. *Topics in Palliative Care,* vol. 1. New York: Oxford University Press, 1997: 163–75.

◆ 11. Hanks G, Portenoy RK, MacDonald N, Forbes K. Difficult pain problems. In: Doyle D, Hanks GWC, MacDonald N eds. *Oxford Textbook of Palliative Medicine*, 2nd edn. Oxford: Oxford University Press, 1998: 454–77.

● 12. Twycross R. *Pain Relief in Advanced Cancer*. Edinburgh: Churchill-Livingstone, 1994.

● 13. Faura CC, Collins SL, Moore RA, McQuay HJ. Systematic review of factors affecting the ratios of morphine and its major metabolites. *Pain* 1998; **74:** 43–53.

14. Collins SL, Faura CC, Moore A, McQuay HJ. Peak plasma concentrations after oral morphine: a systematic review. *J Pain Symptom Manage* 1998; **16:** 388–402.

15. Faura CC, Moore RA, Horga JF, *et al.* Morphine and morphine-6-glucuronide: plasma concentrations and effect in cancer pain. *J Pain Symptom Manage* 1996; **11:** 95–102.

◆ 16. Wood MM, Ashby MA, Somogyi AA, Fleming BG. Neuropsychological and pharmacokinetic assessment of hospice inpatients receiving morphine. *J Pain Symptom Manage* 1998; **16:** 112–20.

◆ 17. Tiseo PJ, Thaler HT, Lapin J, *et al.* Morphine-6-glucuronide concentrations and opioid-related side-effects: a survey in cancer patients. *Pain* 1995; **61:** 47–54.

● 18. Mercadante S. The role of morphine glucuronides in cancer pain. *Palliative Med* 1999; **13:** 95–104.

● 19. Grond S, Zech D, Diefenbach C, Bischoff A. Prevalence and pattern of symptoms in patients with cancer pain: a prospective evaluation of 1635 cancer patients referred to a pain clinic. *J Pain Symptom Manage* 1994; **9:** 372–82.

◆ 20. Schug SA, Zech D, Grond S, *et al.* A long-term survey of morphine in cancer pain patients. *J Pain Symptom Manage* 1992; **7:** 259–66.

◆ 21. Cherny NJ, Chang V, Frager G, *et al.* Opioid pharmacotherapy in the management of cancer pain. *Cancer* 1995; **76:** 1288–93.

22. Cherny NI, Foley KM. Nonopioid and opioid analgesic pharmacotherapy of cancer pain. In: Cherny NI, Foley KM eds. *Pain and Palliative Care. Hematology/Oncology Clinics of North America*. Vol. 10, no. 1. Philadelphia, PA: WB Saunders, 1996: 79–102.

23. Cherny N, Portenoy RK. Cancer pain management. *Cancer* 1993; **72:** 3393–415.

24. Inturrisi CE. Management of cancer pain: pharmacology and principles of management. *Cancer* 1989; **63:** 2308–20.

● 25. Twycross R. Oral morphine. In: Twycross R ed. *Pain Relief in Advanced Cancer*. Edinburgh: Churchill-Livingstone, 1994: 307–22.

26. Bruera E, Neumann CM. Management of specific symptom complexes in patients receiving palliative care. *CMAJ* 1998; **158:** 1717–26.

● 27. Ripamonti C, Bruera E. CNS adverse effects of opioids in cancer patients: guidelines for treatment. *CNS Drugs* 1997; **81:** 21–37.

● 28. Pereira J, Bruera E. Emerging neuropsychiatric toxicities of opioids. *J Pharmaceut Care Pain Symptom Control* 1997; **54:** 3–29.

◆ 29. Fallon M. Opioid rotation: does it have a role? [editorial]. *Palliative Med* 1997; **11:** 177–8.

30. Fallon M. Reply [letter]. *Palliative Med* 1997; **12:** 61–2.

31. Fallon MT, O'Neill B. Opioid toxicity should be managed initially by decreasing the opioid dose (letter). *Br Med J* 1998; **317:** 81.

◆ 32. Hawley P, Forbes K, Hanks GW. Opioids, confusion and opioid rotation [letter]. *Palliative Med* 1997; **12:** 63–4.

33. Fainsinger R, Toro R. Opioids, confusion and opioid rotation [letter]. *Palliative Med* 1998; **12:** 463–4.

34. Morley JS. Opioid rotation: does it have a role [letter]. *Palliative Med* 1998; **12:** 464–5.

35. Murray P. Substitution of another opioid for morphine may be useful for pain control [letter]. *Br Med J* 1998; **316:** 702–3.

36. Twycross R. Opioid rotation: does it have a role? [letter]. *Palliative Med* 1997; **12:** 60–1.

37. O'Neill B, Fallon M. Principles of palliative care and pain control. *Br Med J* 1997; **315:** 801–4.

38. Portenoy RK, Waldman SA. Preface. Adjuvant analgesics in pain management: part I. *J Pain Symptom Manage* 1994; **9:** 390–1.

◆ 39. Oneschuk D, Bruera E. The 'dark side' of adjuvant analgesic drugs. *Progr Palliative Care* 1997; **51:** 5–13.

40. Stiefel F, Movant R. Case report: morphine intoxication during acute reversible renal insufficiency. *J Palliative Care* 1991; **7:** 45–7.
41. Fainsinger RL, Miller MJ, Bruera E. Morphine intoxication during acute reversible renal insufficiency. *J Palliative Care* 1992; **8:** 52–3.
42. Stambaugh JE, Drew J. The combination of ibuprofen and oxycodone/acetaminophen in the management of chronic cancer pain. *Clin Pharmacol Ther* 1988; **44:** 665–9.
43. Ferrer-Brechner T, Ganz P. Combination therapy with ibuprofen and methadone for chronic cancer pain. *Am J Med* 1984; **77:** 78–83.
44. Levick S, Jacobs C, Loukas DF, *et al.* Naproxen sodium in treatment of bone pain due to metastatic cancer. *Pain* 1988; **35:** 253–8.
◆ 45. Mercadante S, Cassuccio A, Agnello A, *et al.* Analgesic effects of nonsteroidal anti-inflammatory drugs in cancer pain due to somatic or visceral mechanisms. *J Pain Symptom Manage* 1999; **17:** 351–6.
◆ 46. Bjorkman R, Ullman A, Hedner J. Morphine-sparing effect of diclofenac in cancer pain. *Eur J Clin Pharmacol* 1993; **44:** 1–5.
◆ 47. Mercadante S, Sapio M, Caligara M, *et al.* Opioid sparing effect of diclofenac in cancer pain. *J Pain Symptom Manage* 1997; **14:** 15–20.
48. DeConno F, Ripamonti C, Bianchi M, *et al.* Diclofenac does not modify morphine bioavailability in cancer patients. *Pain* 1992; **48:** 401–2.
49. Bianchi M, Clavenna A, Groff L, *et al.* Diclofenac does not modify methadone bioavailability in cancer patients. *J Pain Symptom Manage* 1999; **17:** 227–8.
● ◆ 50. Joishy SK, Walsh D. The opioid-sparing effect of intravenous ketorolac as an adjuvant analgesic in cancer pain: application in bone metastases and the opioid bowel syndrome. *J Pain Symptom Manage* 1998; **16:** 334–9.
● 51. Jenkins CA, Bruera E. Non-steroidal anti-inflammatory drugs as adjuvant analgesics in cancer patients. *Palliative Med* 1999; **13:** 183–96.
52. Christrup LL, Sjogren P, Jensen NH, *et al.* Steady-state kinetics and dynamics of morphine in cancer patients: is sedation related to the absorption rate of morphine? *J Pain Symptom Manage* 1999; **18:** 164–73.
53. Bruera E, Brenneis C, Paterson AHG, *et al.* Use of methylphenidate as an adjuvant to narcotic analgesics in patients with advanced cancer. *J Pain Symptom Manage* 1989; **4:** 3–6.
54. The TTS Fentanyl Multicentre Study Group. Transdermal fentanyl in cancer pain. *J Drug Development* 1994; **63:** 93–7.
◆ 55. Ahmedzai S, Brooks D on behalf of the TTS-Fentanyl Comparative Trial Group. Transdermal fentanyl versus sustained-release oral morphine in cancer pain: preference, efficacy and quality of life. *J Pain Symptom Manage* 1997; **13:** 254–61.
56. Payne R, Mathias SD, Pasta DJ, *et al.* Quality of life and cancer pain: satisfaction and side-effects with transdermal fentanyl versus oral morphine. *J Clin Oncol* 1998; **16:** 1588–93.
◆ 57. Hunt R, Fazekas B, Thorne D, Brooksbank M. A comparison of subcutaneous morphine and fentanyl in hospice cancer patients. *J Pain Symptom Manage* 1999; **18:** 111–19.
58. Mercadante S, Cassuccio A, Agnello A, *et al.* Morphine versus methadone in the pain treatment of advanced cancer patients followed up at home. *J Clin Oncol* 1998; **16:** 3656–61.
◆ 59. Mercadante S, Salvaggio L, Dardanoni G, *et al.* Dextropropoxyphene versus morphine in opioid-naive cancer patients with pain. *J Pain Symptom Manage* 1998; **15:** 76–81.
◆ 60. Grond S, Radbruch L, Meuser T, *et al.* High-dose tramadol in comparison to low-dose morphine for cancer pain relief. *J Pain Symptom Manage* 1999; **18:** 174–9.
◆ 61. Wilder-Smith CH, Schimke J, Osterwalder B, Senn HJ. Tramadol oral, un agonista mu opioide, bloqueante de la recaptación de monoaminas, y morfina para el dolor fuerte relacionado con el cancer. *Ann Oncol* 1994; **4:** 336–41.
● 62. Dalal S, Melzack R. Potentiation of opioid analgesia by psychostimulant drugs: a review. *J Pain Symptom Manage* 1998; **16:** 245–53.
◆ 63. Bruera E, Chadwick S, Brenneis C, *et al.* Methylphenidate associated with narcotics for the treatment of cancer pain. *Cancer Treatment Reports* 1987; **71:** 67–70.
◆ 64. Wilderding MB, Loprinzi CL, Maillard JA, *et al.* A randomized crossover evaluation of methylphenidate in cancer patients receiving strong narcotics. *Support Care Cancer* 1995; **3:** 135–8.
65. Sawynok J, Yaksh TL. Caffeine as an analgesic adjuvant: a review of pharmacology and mechanisms of action. *Pharmacol Rev* 1993; **45:** 43–85.
66. Zacny JP, Lichtor JL, Flemming D, *et al.* A dose–response analysis of the subjective, psychomotor and physiological effects of intravenous morphine in healthy volunteers. *J Pharmacol Exp Ther* 1994; **268:** 1–9.
67. Zacny JP, Lichtor JL, Thapar P, *et al.* Comparing the subjective, psychomotor and physiological effects of intravenous butorphanol and morphine in healthy volunteers. *J Pharmacol Exp Ther* 1994; **270:** 579–89.
◆ 68. Bruera E, MacMillan K, Hanson J, MacDonald RN. The cognitive effects of the administration of narcotic analgesics in patients with cancer pain. *Pain* 1989; **39:** 13–16.
69. Lepzig RM, Goodman H, Gray G, *et al.* Reversible, narcotic-associated mental status impairment in patients with metastatic cancer. *Pharmacology* 1987; **35:** 47–54.
70. Sjogren P, Banning A. Pain, sedation and reaction time during long-term treatment of cancer patients with oral and epidural opioids. *Pain* 1989; **39:** 5–11.
71. Banning A, Sjogren P. Cerebral effects of long-term oral

opioids in cancer patients measured by continuous reaction time. *Clin J Pain* 1990; **6:** 91–5.

72. Banning A, Sjogren P, Kaiser F. Reaction time in cancer patients receiving peripherally acting analgesics alone or in combination with opioids. *Acta Anaesthesiol Scand* 1992; **36:** 480–2.

◆ 73. Vainio A, Ollila J, Matikainene E, *et al.* Driving ability in cancer patients receiving long-term morphine analgesia. *Lancet* 1995; **346:** 667–70.

◆ 74. Dertwinkel R, Zenz M, Strumpf M, *et al.* Drugs and driving. Abstracts of the IVth Congress of the EAPC, 6–9 December 1995, Barcelona (Spain). *Eur J Palliative Care* **15**.

75. Clemons M, Regnard C, Appleton T. Alertness, cognition and morphine in patients with advanced cancer. *Cancer Treat Rev* 1996; **22:** 451–68.

◆ 76. Bruera E, Miller MJ, MacMillan K, Kuehn N. Neuropsychological effects of methylphenidate in patients receiving a continuous infusion of narcotics for cancer pain. *Pain* 1992; **48:** 163–6.

77. Bruera E, Fainsinger R, MacEachern T, Hanson J. The use of methylphenidate in patients with incident cancer pain receiving regular opioids. A preliminary report. *Pain* 1992; **50:** 75–7.

78. American Psychiatric Association. *Diagnostic and Statistical Manual of Mental Disorders*, 4th edn. Washington, DC: American Psychiatric Association, 1994.

79. World Health Organization. *International Statistical Classification of Diseases and Related Health Problems*, 10th revision. Geneva: World Health Organization, 1992.

80. Caraceni A, Martini C, DeConno F, Ventafridda V. Organic brain syndromes and opioid administration for cancer pain. *J Pain Symptom Manage* 1994; **9:** 527–33.

◆ 81. Galer BS, Coyle N, Pasternak GW, Portenoy RK. Individual variability in the response to different opioids: report of five cases. *Pain* 1992; **49:** 87–91.

82. Paix A, Coleman A, Lees J, *et al.* Subcutaneous fentanyl and sufentanil infusion for substitution for morphine intolerance in cancer pain management. *Pain* 1995; **63:** 263–69.

◆ 83. Bruera E, Schoeller T, Montejo G. Organic hallucinosis in patients receiving high doses of opiates for cancer pain. *Pain* 1992; **48:** 397–99.

● 84. Caraceni A. Delirium in palliative medicine. *Eur J Palliative Care* 1995; **22:** 62–7.

● 85. Breitbart W, Chochinov HM, Passik S. Psychiatric aspects of palliative care. In: Doyle D, Hanks GWC, MacDonald N eds. *Oxford Textbook of Palliative Medicine*, 2nd edn. Oxford: Oxford University Press, 1998: 933–54.

86. Gagnon PR, Allard P, Masse B. Delirium in terminal cancer: a prospective study on incidence, prevalence and clinical course. Abstract, 12th International Congress on Care of the Terminally Ill, Montreal, 13–17 September 1998. *J Palliative Care* 1998; **143:** 106.

87. Poyhia R, Vainio A, Kalso E. A review of oxycodone's clinical pharmacokinetics and pharmacodynamics. *J Pain Symptom Manage* 1993; **8:** 63–7.

88. Heiskanen T, Kalso E. Controlled-release oxycodone and morphine in cancer related pain. *Pain* 1997; **73:** 37–45.

89. Bruera E, Belzile M, Pituskin E, *et al.* Randomized, double-blind, cross-over trial comparing safety and efficacy of oral controlled-release oxycodone with controlled-release morphine in patients with cancer pain. *J Clin Oncol* 1998; **16:** 3222–9.

90. Stiefel F, Fainsinger R, Bruera E. Acute confusional states in patients with advanced cancer. *J Pain Symptom Manage* 1992; **7:** 94–8.

91. Bruera E, Miller L, McCallion J, *et al.* Cognitive failure in patients with terminal cancer: a prospective study. *J Pain Symptom Manage* 1992; **7:** 192–5.

92. Lawlor P, Gagnon B, Mancini I, *et al.* Phenomenology of delirium and its subtypes in advanced cancer patients: a prospective study. Abstract, 12th International Congress on Care of the Terminally Ill, Montreal, 13–17 September, 1998. *J Palliative Care* 1998; **143:** 106.

93. Bruera E, Fainsinger R, Miller MJ, Juehn N. The assessment of pain intensity in patients with cognitive failure: a preliminary report. *J Pain Symptom Manage* 1992; **7:** 267–70.

◆ 94. Coyle N, Breitbart W, Weaber S, Portenoy R. Delirium as a contributing factor to "crescendo" pain: three case reports. *J Pain Symptom Manage* 1994; **9:** 44–7.

95. Folstein MF, Folstein SE, McHugh PR. "Mini Mental State": a practical method of grading the cognitive state of patients for the clinician. *J Psychiatr Res* 1975; **12:** 189–98.

● 96. Núñez Olarte JM. Control de la confusión en pacientes con cáncer en situación terminal. *Rev Soc Esp DOLOR* 1995; **2** (Suppl. II): 40–5.

97. Inouye SK, van Dyck CH, Alessi CA, *et al.* Clarifying confusion: the confusion assessment method. *Ann Intern Med* 1990; **113:** 941–8.

◆ 98. Breitbart W, Rosenfeld B, Roth A, *et al.* The Memorial Delirium Assessment Scale. *J Pain Symptom Manage* 1997; **13:** 128–37.

● 99. MacLeod AD. The management of delirium in hospice practice. *Eur J Palliative Care* 1997; **44:** 16–120.

◆100. Bruera E, Franco JJ, Maltoni M, *et al.* Changing pattern of delirium in patients with advanced cancer: association with cognitive monitoring, hydration and opiate rotation. *J Pain Symptom Manage* 1995; **10:** 287–91.

◆101. Maddocks I, Somogyi A, Abbott F, *et al.* Attenuation of morphine-induced delirium in palliative care by substitution with infusion of oxycodone. *J Pain Symptom Manage* 1996; **12:** 182–9.

◆102. de Stoutz N, Bruera E, Suarez-Almazor M. Opioid rotation for toxicity reduction in terminal cancer patients. *J Pain Symptom Manage* 1995; **10:** 378–84.

●103. Núñez JM. Síndromes neuropsicológicos: ansiedad, depresión y confusión. In: Gómez-Batiste X, Planas Domingo J, Roca Casas J, Viladiu Quemada P eds.

Cuidados Paliativos en Oncología. Barcelona: Editorial Jims, 1996: 229–36.

104. Passik SD, Cooper M. Complicated delirium in a cancer patient successfully treated with olanzapine. *J Pain Symptom Manage* 1999; **17:** 219–23.
105. Pereira J, Hanson J, Bruera E. The frequency and clinical course of cognitive impairment in patients with terminal cancer. *Cancer* 1997; **79:** 835–42.
106. Bruera E, Miller MJ, Kuehn N, *et al.* Estimate of survival of patients admitted to a palliative care unit: a prospective study. *J Pain Symptom Manage* 1992; **7:** 82–6.

●◆107. Núñez Olarte JM. Opioid-induced myoclonus. *Eur J Palliative Care* 1995; **24:** 146–50.

108. Hagen N, Swanson R. Strychnine-like multifocal myoclonus and seizures in extremely high-dose opioid administration: treatment strategies. *J Pain Symptom Manage* 1997; **14:** 51–8.
109. Núñez Olarte JM. Treatment of opioid-induced myoclonus. Abstract. 4th Congress of the European Association for Palliative Care, Barcelona, December 1995. *Eur J Palliative Care* 1995: 14–15.
110. Potter JM, Reid DB, Shaw RJ, *et al.* Myoclonus associated with treatment with high doses of morphine: the role of supplemental drugs. *Br Med J* 1989; **299:** 150–3.

◆111. Taboada R, Juez I, Conti M, Núñez Olarte JM. Papel de la hipomagnesemia en el mioclonus asociado a altas dosis de morfina. Abstract Book. 1st International Congress for Palliative Care, Madrid, February 1994: 78.

●112. Mercadante S. Pathophysiology and treatment of opioid-related myoclonus in cancer patients. *Pain* 1998; **74:** 5–9.

◆113. Kloke M, Bingel U, Seeber S. Complications of spinal opioid therapy: myoclonus, spastic muscle tone and spinal jerking. *Support Care Cancer* 1994; **2:** 249–52.

114. Kronenberg MF, Laimer I, Rifici C, *et al.* Epileptic seizure associated with intracerebroventricular and intrathecal morphine bolus. *Pain* 1998; **75:** 383–7.

◆115. Núñez Olarte JM. Opioid-induced myoclonus. Abstract Book. 6th Congress of the European Association for Palliative Care, Geneva, September 1999: 29.

116. Sjogren P, Jonsson T, Jensen NH, *et al.* Hyperalgesia and myoclonus in terminal cancer patients treated with continuous intravenous morphine. *Pain* 1993; **55:** 93–7.
117. Sjogren P, Jensen NH, Jensen TS. Disappearance of morphine-induced hyperalgesia after discontinuing or substituting morphine with other opioid agonists. *Pain* 1994; **59:** 313–16.

●◆118. Sykes N. The treatment of morphine-induced constipation. *Eur J Palliative Care* 1998; **51:** 12–15.

●119. Sykes NP. Constipation and diarrhoea. In: Doyle D, Hanks GWC, MacDonald N eds. *Oxford Textbook of Paliative Medicine,* 2nd edn. Oxford: Oxford University Press, 1998: 513–26.

120. Sykes NP. The relationship between opioid use and laxative use in terminally ill cancer patients. *Palliative Med* 1998; **12:** 375–82.

●121. Derby S, Portenoy RK. Assessment and management of opioid-induced constipation. In: Portenoy RK, Bruera E eds. *Topics in Palliative Care,* vol. 1. New York: Oxford University Press, 1997: 95–112.

◆122. Fallon MT, Hanks GW. Morphine, constipation and performance status in advanced cancer patients. *Palliative Med* 1999; **13:** 159–60.

123. Mancini I, Hanson J, Bruera E. Opioid type and other clinical predictors of laxative dose in advanced cancer patients: a retrospective study. *J Pain Symptom Manage* 1998; **15:** S16.

◆124. Megens AAHP, Artois K, Vermeire J, *et al.* Comparison of the analgesic and intestinal effects of fentanyl and morphine in rats. *J Pain Symptom Manage* 1998; **15:** 253–8.

◆125. Bruera E, Suárez-Almazor M, Velasco A, *et al.* The assessment of constipation in terminal cancer patients admitted to a palliative care unit: a retrospective review. *J Pain Symptom Manage* 1994; **98:** 515–19.

◆126. Sykes NP. Methods of assessment of bowel function in patients with advanced cancer. *Palliative Med* 1990; **4:** 287–92.

127. Donner B, Zenz M, Tryba M, Strumpf M. Direct conversion from oral morphine to transdermal fentanyl: a multicenter study in patients with cancer pain. *Pain* 1996; **64:** 527–34.
128. Donner B, Zenz M, Strumpf M, Raber M. Long-term treatment of cancer pain with transdermal fentanyl. *J Pain Symptom Manage* 1998; **15:** 168–75.
129. Zech DFJ, Grond SUA, Lynch J, *et al.* Transdermal fentanyl and initial dose-finding with patient-controlled analgesia in cancer pain. A pilot study with 20 terminally ill cancer patients. *Pain* 1992; **50:** 293–301.
130. Allan L, Hayes H, Jensen NH *et al.* Evidence for better analgesia with transdermal fentanyl in chronic pain treatment: comparison with sustained release morphine in a cross-over efficacy, safety and quality of life trial. Abstract Book. 17th Annual Scientific Meeting, American Pain Society, San Diego, November 1998: 132.
131. Davis A, Prentice W. Fentanyl, morphine and constipation [letter]. *J Pain Symptom Manage* 1998; **16:** 141–2.
132. Ahmedzai SH. Authors' response [letter]. *J Pain Symptom Manage* 1998; **16:** 142–4.
133. Daeninck PJ, Bruera E. Reduction in constipation and laxative requirements following opioid rotation to methadone: a report of four cases. *J Pain Symptom Manage* 1999; **18:** 303–9.
134. Bruera E, Brenneis C, Michand M, MacDonald N. Continuous subcutaneous infusion of metoclopramide for treatment of narcotic bowel syndrome. *Cancer Treat Rep* 1987; **71:** 1121–2.

◆135. Agra Y, Sacristan A, Gonzalez M, *et al.* Efficacy of senna versus lactulose in terminal cancer patients treated with opioids. *J Pain Symptom Manage* 1998; **15:** 1–7.

◆136. Ramesh PR, Kumar KS, Rajagopal MR, *et al.* Managing morphine-induced constipation: a controlled comparison of an ayurvedic formulation and senna. *J Pain Symptom Manage* 1998; **16:** 240–4.

◆137. Sykes NP. A volunteer model for the comparison of laxatives in opioid-related constipation. *J Pain Symptom Manage* 1996; **11:** 363–9.

138. Attar A, Lemann M, Ferguson A, *et al.* Comparison of a low dose polyethylene glycol electrolyte solution with lactulose for treatment of chronic constipation. *Gut* 1999; **44:** 226–30.

◆139. Culpepper-Morgan JA, Inturrisi CE, Portenoy RK, *et al.* Treatment of opioid-induced constipation with oral naloxone: a pilot study. *Clin Pharmacol Ther* 1992; **52:** 90–5.

◆140. Sykes NP. Oral naloxone in opioid-associated constipation. *Lancet* 1991; **337:** 1475.

◆141. Sykes NP. An investigation of the ability of oral naloxone to correct opioid-related constipation in patients with advanced cancer. *Palliative Med* 1996; **102:** 135–44.

◆142. Yuan CS, Foss FJ, O'Connor M, *et al.* Methylnaltrexone prevents morphine-induced delay in oral–cecal transit time without affecting analgesia: a double-blind randomized placebo-controlled trial. *Clin Pharmacol Ther* 1996; **59:** 469–75.

◆143. Yuan CS, Foss JF, Osinski J, *et al.* The safety and efficacy of oral methylnaltrexone in preventing morphine-induced delay in oral-cecal transit time. *Clin Pharmacol Ther* 1997; **61:** 467–75.

144. Hagen NA, Foley KM, Cerbone DJ, *et al.* Chronic nausea and morphine-6-glucuronide. *J Pain Symptom Manage* 1991; **6:** 125–8.

●145. Twycross R, Back I. Nausea and vomiting in advanced cancer. *Eur J Palliative Care* 1998; **52:** 39–45.

◆146. Campora E, Merlini L, Pace M, *et al.* The incidence of narcotic-induced emesis. *J Pain Symptom Manage* 1991; **6:** 428–30.

147. Aparasu R, McCoy RA, Weber C, *et al.* Opioid-induced emesis among hospitalized non-surgical patients: effect on pain and quality of life. *J Pain Symptom Manage* 1999; **18:** 280–8.

148. Ferris FD, Kerr IG, Sone M, Marcuzzi M. Transdermal scopolamine use in the control of narcotic-induced nausea. *J Pain Symptom Manage* 1991; **6:** 389–93.

149. Mercadante S, Sapio M, Serretta R. Ondansentron in nausea and vomiting induced by spinal morphine. *J Pain Symptom Manage* 1998; **16:** 259–62.

◆150. Mystakidou K, Befon S, Liossi C, Vlachos L. Comparison of tropisetron and chlorpromazine combinations in the control of nausea and vomiting in patients with advanced cancer. *J Pain Symptom Manage* 1998; **15:** 176–84.

◆151. Borgbjerg FM, Nielsen K, Franks J. Experimental pain stimulates respiration and attenuates morphine-induced respiratory depression: a controlled study in human volunteers. *Pain* 1996; **64:** 123–8.

◆152. Benedetti F, Amanzio M, Baldi S, *et al.* The specific effects of prior opioid exposure on placebo analgesia and placebo respiratory depression. *Pain* 1998; **75:** 313–19.

153. Quevedo F, Walsh D. Morphine-induced ventilatory failure after spinal cord compression. *J Pain Symptom Manage* 1999; **18:** 140–2.

154. Hanks GC, Twycross RG, Lloyd JM. Unexpected complication of successful nerve block (morphine-induced respiratory depression precipitated by removal of severe pain). *Anaesthesia* 1981; **36:** 37–9.

◆155. Bruera E, Schoeller T, Wenk R, *et al.* A prospective multi-center assessment of the Edmonton staging system for cancer pain. *J Pain Symptom Manage* 1995; **10:** 348–55.

◆156. Collin E, Poulain P, Gauvain-Piquard A, *et al.* Is disease progression the major factor in morphine "tolerance" in cancer pain treatment. *Pain* 1993; **55:** 319–26.

◆157. Porter J, Jick H. Addiction rare in patients treated with narcotics. *N Engl J Med* 1980; **302:** 123.

158. Kanner RM, Foley K. Patterns of narcotic drug use in a cancer pain clinic. *Ann NY Acad Science* 1981; **362:** 161–72.

◆159. Davies AN, Daniels C, Pugh R, Sharma K. A comparison of artificial saliva and pilocarpine in the management of xerostomia in patients with advanced cancer. *Palliative Med* 1998; **12:** 105–11.

160. Davies A, Gibbs L, Broadley K. An investigation into the relationship between xerostomia and hyposalivation in patients with advanced cancer. Abstract. 6th Congress of the European Association for Palliative Care, Geneva, September 1999: 21.

161. Waller A, Bercovitch M, Dori S, *et al.* Sialometry and its relationship to oral symptoms and quality of life parameters in terminally ill patients. Abstract. 6th Congress of the European Association for Palliative Care, Geneva, September 1999: 44.

162. Davies AN. A comparison of chewing gum and artificial saliva in the management of xerostomia in patients with advanced cancer. Abstract. 6th Congress of the European Association for Palliative Care, Geneva, September 1999: 20.

●163. Bamigbade TA, Langford RM. The clinical use of tramadol hydrochloride. *Pain Rev* 1998; **5:** 155–82.

◆164. Dunteman E, Karanikolas M, Filos KS. Transnasal butorphanol for the treatment of opioid-induced pruritus unresponsive to antihistamines. *J Pain Symptom Manage* 1996; **12:** 255–60.

◆165. Katcher J, Walsh D. Opioid-induced itching: morphine sulfate and hydromorphone hydrochloride. *J Pain Symptom Manage* 1999; **17:** 70–2.

166. Bruera E, Miller MJ. Non-cardiogenic pulmonary edema after narcotic treatment for cancer pain. *Pain* 1989; **39:** 297–300.

14

Nonopioid analgesic drugs

PETER RAVENSCROFT

Salicylates and salicylic acid are the first of the drugs to have become known as the nonsteroidal anti-inflammatory drugs (NSAIDs). They were first used and then recommended in the *Ebers papyrus* as dried leaves of myrtle to dispel rheumatic pain. One thousand years later Hippocrates wrote of the use of poplar juices to treat eye disease and willow bark to treat fever and the pain of childbirth. The first "clinical trial" of willow bark was reported by Edward Stone, a clergyman from Oxfordshire, in 1763 to the Royal Society. Salicylic acid was synthesized in 1860 in Germany and then Felix Hoffman synthesized aspirin in order to treat his father's rheumatism.

By the 1900s the main therapeutic actions of aspirin (and sodium salicylates themselves) were recognized as being antipyretic, anti-inflammatory, and analgesic.[1] Vane and colleagues did much of the pioneering work on establishing the role of the prostaglandins in the 1960s and 1970s and the role of NSAIDs in inhibiting them.[2,3] Cyclo-oxygenase was isolated in 1976 by Hemler *et al.*,[4] and more recently the COX-2 isoform was identified and the difference in its pharmacology demonstrated[5] (Table 14.1).

Over the intervening years a large number of drugs have been synthesized principally to try to overcome the adverse effects and improve efficacy. These drugs have become known as the nonsteroidal anti-inflammatory drugs (NSAIDs) to distinguish them from the other group of drugs used in inflammatory conditions, the glucocorticosteroids or steroids.[6] Members of the NSAID group of drugs are quite dissimilar chemically, but share similar effects and adverse effects to a greater or lesser degree.

MODE OF ACTION

Research has not shown a definite relationship between the extent of inhibition of prostaglandin *in vitro* and their effect on pain.[7]

NSAIDs have their main effect by inhibition of cyclo-oxygenase, with a secondary reduction in the synthesis of proinflammatory prostaglandins from arachidonic acid. This may occur in the periphery or in the central nervous system. NSAIDs have been shown to have a centrally mediated effect. They have a direct spinal action in blocking excessive sensitivity to pain induced by the activation of spinal glutamate and substance P receptors.[8]

These same mechanisms are also responsible for the adverse effects associated with NSAID use. The other

Table 14.1 *Classification of NSAIDs*

1 Nonselective inhibitors of COX-1 and COX-2 (NSI),
  1.1 Effect predominantly in the central nervous system, e.g. acetaminophen (paracetamol)
  1.2 Effective in the central nervous system and in the periphery, e.g. aspirin and other NSAIDs
2 Preferential inhibitors of COX-2 over COX-1 (PI), e.g. meloxicam, nimesulide
3 Specific inhibitors of COX-2 (the coxibs), e.g. celecoxib and rofecoxib

variables which have been implicated in causing toxicity are the presence of an enterohepatic circulation, as this means that the drug crosses the mucosa twice, leading to a higher gastrointestinal toxicity in laboratory animals,[9] and a long half-life, which has been associated also with a higher rate of gastrointestinal adverse effects as well as a greater potential to inhibit platelet aggregation.[10,11]

Recent evidence suggests that NSAIDs may differentially inhibit subforms of cyclo-oxygenase and therefore their anti-inflammatory and toxic effects may vary.[5,12,13] A classification of the NSAIDs is included in Table 14.1.

The NSAIDs may be classified into three groups based on current information. However, the discovery of two isoforms of cyclo-oxygenase, COX-1 and COX-2, gives hope of reduced toxicity. The isoforms have been reviewed by a number of authors.[2,14,15] COX-1 has been described as performing "housekeeping" duties by maintaining normal gastrointestinal blood flow and renal blood flow. COX-2 is induced by inflammatory stimuli and cytokines.[16–18] This rather simple concept will undoubtedly yield to further research as there are indications that this system is much more complex than first thought.

NSAIDs that are nonselective inhibitors bind to both COX-1 and COX-2 sites to inhibit the entry of arachidonic acid, thereby blocking prostaglandin synthesis. Most commonly used NSAIDs at the time of writing are of this type. The mechanism for selectivity seems to be dependent on the configuration of the binding site. The COX-2 site has a "pocket" in the hairpin structure of the COX-2 binding site (Fig. 14.1). This pocket appears to be the result of a smaller valine molecule being present in the amino acid structure of COX-2. COX-2-selective agents selectively bind at this pocket. In addition, the kinetics of the interactions between NSAIDs and the COX-1 and COX-2 receptors are different. The inhibition of COX-1 is instantaneous and reversible, but the inhibition of COX-2 is time dependent, with selectivity developing over 15–20 min, after which time the inhibition becomes essentially irreversible.[15]

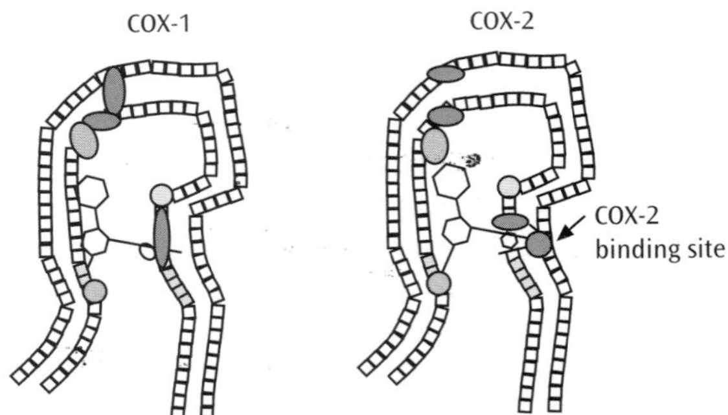

Figure 14.1 *A schematic representation of the COX-1 and COX-2 receptors. The COX-2 binding site has a "pocket" that allows for the specific ginding of COX-2 agents. See text for explanation. From Hawkey[15] with permission.*

Evidence is accumulating that the COX-2 inhibitors are clinically associated with less gastrointestinal bleeding. There seems to be a direct correlation between COX-2 selectivity and the risk of bleeding and perforation. However, it seems that in many tissues COX-1 and COX-2 coexist, so it is important to conduct clinical trials to demonstrate that selectivity does not adversely affect effectiveness or the prevalence of adverse effects.

NONSELECTIVE INHIBITORS OF COX, PRIMARILY ACTING IN THE CENTRAL NERVOUS SYSTEM

Acetaminophen (paracetamol)

Acetaminophen (paracetamol), a derivative of para-aminophenol, has analgesic and antipyretic actions on the central nervous system, where it inhibits prostaglandin synthetase in the hypothalamus.[6,19] Inhibition does not occur significantly at therapeutic doses in peripheral tissues so acetaminophen has minimal, if any, anti-inflammatory or antirheumatic actions.

Acetaminophen is rapidly absorbed so that its peak concentration is reached in about 30–90 min.[20] Therapeutic plasma concentrations range from 5 to 20 μg/ml, whereas toxic concentrations are in the range of 150 μg/ml and above. Its elimination half-life is 2–3 h and its protein binding is insignificant.[21] It crosses readily into the cerebrospinal fluid (CSF) and into the brain, where it has its major effect.

Metabolism of acetaminophen takes place in the liver, where it undergoes extensive first-pass metabolism and then is excreted by the kidneys. Metabolite production in overdose may lead to severe hepatic toxicity by the depletion of hepatic glutathione levels and subsequent hepatic necrosis. In adults, a dose of about 7.5–15 g, ingested and fully absorbed, is considered potentially toxic.[22,23] The smallest fatal dose recorded in adults is 18 g. The recognition and management of acetaminophen overdose is dealt with elsewhere; it should be regarded as a medical emergency and intravenous acetylcysteine or methionine should be considered without delay.[22]

Acetaminophen appears to exhibit a "ceiling effect," i.e. its dose–response curve levels out and does not continue to rise with increasing doses of the drug.[24] Tolerance or dependence with its use has not been reported.

Indications

The indications for acetaminophen are:

- analgesia for mild pain, particularly soft-tissue and musculoskeletal pain;
- relief of mild procedural pain;
- management of fever;
- management of more severe pain in association

with opioids, which may allow a reduction in opioid dosage;
- pain relief in patients hypersensitive to aspirin and the NSAIDs or in situations where aspirin and NSAIDs have caused adverse effects, e.g. bleeding or peptic ulceration;
- when mild analgesia is required but hyperuricemia and thrombocytopenia need to be avoided.

Acetaminophen is safe in pregnancy and lactation and undergoes no significant drug interactions.

Contraindications

Patients who have active liver disease, including alcoholic liver disease and glucose-6-phosphate dehydrogenase deficiency, should not be given the drug. In doses over 4 g/day some patients who have been starving or have had alcoholic liver disease have shown signs of a rise in hepatic enzymes.

In overdose (single doses of more than 100 mg/kg), acetaminophen can produce severe hepatotoxicity, hypoglycemia, and acute renal tubular necrosis. Clinical signs of the severity of the overdose may take some days to develop, so tests of hepatic and renal function and serum acetaminophen should be performed immediately followed by monitoring. Detoxification treatment should be commenced at the earliest opportunity. The management of acetaminophen toxicity is discussed in a number of references that are reviewed by Jackson *et al.*[22] and Rumack *et al.*[25]

Rarely, patients may experience urticarial or erythematous rashes, fever, or blood dyscrasias. Chronic use of acetaminophen alone does not seem to cause analgesic nephropathy.

Doses and treatment paradigms

In adults the recommended dose is 500–1,000 mg every 6 h to a maximum dose of 4 g/day. Doses of up to 1 g every 4 h have been recommended for chronic cancer pain.[26] This dosage may lead to reversible elevation of hepatic enzymes with long-term therapy.

In children 1 mg/kg orally or rectally every 4–6 h is recommended, with a maximum daily dose of 90 mg/kg and a single dose of 30 mg/kg at bedtime (Table 14.2).

Acetaminophen is available as tablets, capsules, syrup, or rectal suppositories. The doses are the same regardless of the route, but the suppository may be absorbed more slowly and less completely. Absorption of acetaminophen can be slow in about 25% of patients but can be enhanced by the addition of sorbitol, which is present in some preparations of the drug.[27]

Adverse effects and their management

Only about 5% of patients exhibit cross-allergy with aspirin or the NSAIDs, so acetaminophen can be used as a substitute for NSAIDs in this situation.[28] Sporadic cases of allergy to acetaminophen have been reported, and the symptoms usually occur shortly after ingestion of the drug.[29]

Table 14.2 *Recommended doses of acetaminophen with respect to age*

Age[a]	Single dose (mg)[b]
<4 months	40
4–11 months	80
12–23 months	120
2–3 years	160
4–5 years	240
6–8 years	320
9–10 years	400
11–12 years	480
>12 years (adult)	650–1,000

a. In children less than 2 years old acetaminophen should be used with the supervision of a doctor.
b. Doses may be repeated every 6 h.

Acetaminophen is not associated with the gastrointestinal, hemopoietic, or renal complications of aspirin or the NSAIDs.[30] However, care needs to be taken in patients taking anticoagulants as prolongation of the prothrombin time has been reported.[31]

There is little evidence that pre-existing chronic liver disease increases the risk of toxicity; prolongation of the half-life of acetaminophen may occur but has little clinical significance. No changes in liver function, compared with placebo, were seen in a 2-week trial with placebo.[32]

Pharmaceutical considerations

Preparations available include tablets, oral liquids, and suppositories.

Practical tips

Patients with chronic pain should take 4 g/day for a week before the drug is abandoned or another drug added.

Evidence for efficacy

Acetaminophen is recommended for cancer pain syndromes.[33]* The long-term use of acetaminophen in doses of 1.2–3.2 g/day has been shown to allow a reduction in the dosage of more potent analgesics or discontinuance of them altogether. Acetaminophen is considered equipotent in analgesic effect to aspirin.[34]** Although in the original studies 650-mg doses were administered, subsequent studies of the effect in dental pain have shown that 1,000-mg doses have greater efficacy.[35]**

The effectiveness of acetaminophen has been established principally in nonmalignant pain. Double-blind, randomized controlled trials have been conducted in patients with dental pain[36]** and pain following episiotomy.[37]** It is also valuable for headache alone [38]** or in combination with aspirin and codeine,[39]** but acetaminophen plus dextropropoxyphene was not found to be superior to acetaminophen alone in a review of 26 randomized controlled trials in patients with postsurgical pain, arthritis, and musculoskeletal pain.[40]**

In a randomized clinical trial in 50 athletes with football-related injuries, acetaminophen and codeine was found to be as effective as diflunisal.[41]** Single doses of ibuprofen (400 mg), acetaminophen (300 mg) plus codeine (30 mg), and placebo had similar effects in 120 postorthopedic patients with moderate to severe pain. Overall, the drugs were distinguishable from the placebo. Ibuprofen was more effective than acetaminophen and codeine.[42]**

The American College of Rheumatology recommends acetaminophen as a first-line drug in the management of osteoarthritis of the hip or knee.[43,44]** The evidence supporting this comes from a randomized, double-blind trial in patients with osteoarthritis, which demonstrated that acetaminophen 4 g/day was more effective than placebo and as effective as commonly used NSAIDs for pain relief and restoration of function.[45]**

In another randomized, double-blind, multicenter study, the efficacy of acetaminophen (2,600 mg/day) was compared with that of naproxen (750 mg/day). The analgesic efficacy of the two regimens was similar, but a considerable proportion of the patients in the study experienced suboptimal pain relief.[46]**

NONSELECTIVE INHIBITORS OF COX IN THE CENTRAL NERVOUS SYSTEM AND IN THE PERIPHERY

In this section the NSAIDs are dealt with as a general group as they share many properties. In Australia, the use of these drugs has fallen 25% in the last few years as a result of an educational campaign that has highlighted the adverse reactions to these drugs.[47]

Indications for NSAIDs

Indications for NSAIDs include:

- metastatic bone pain;
- mild to moderate pain due to inflammation and tissue injury, e.g. pain and pruritus associated with carcinoma en cuirass;
- inflammatory arthropathies;
- neoplastic fever;
- postoperative pain;
- headache;
- dysmenorrhea;
- acute gout;
- biliary and ureteric colic.

No single NSAID has been shown to be superior to any other.[48] The choice should be the NSAID that is the cheapest and safest that the patient will tolerate. Despite the fact that these drugs have the same apparent mode of action, some patients with arthropathies seem to respond to one of these drugs better that the others.[49] It may be worthwhile to change to another NSAID if the one that the patient is on does not seem to be effective. It is also important to give NSAIDs an adequate therapeutic trial of 2–4 weeks as their maximal effect may be delayed.[50] These factors may be important when considering the treatment of cancer pain.

NSAIDs are included on the World Health Organization (WHO) ladder for the management of pain in its publication *Cancer Pain Relief*.[33] In this book, the authors recommend that "NSAIDs, including ASA (acetylsalicylic acid), are particularly important in the treatment of pain caused by bone metastases." NSAIDs are generally considered effective for pain, especially for bone pain, although it has been recommended that when NSAIDs do not control the pain opioids should be added.[51,52]

Bone pain has been the major indication for the NSAIDs since it was found in experimental studies that prostaglandins are involved in the breakdown of bone associated with tumor deposits. Considerable work in animals shows that NSAIDs can inhibit the bone reabsorption associated with tumors. Subsequent work has not confirmed this hypothesis, and it seems that many factors are involved in metastatic bone destruction, some of which are not influenced by inhibition of prostaglandin synthesis. The general opinion is that NSAIDs do not slow the progression of bony metastases. However, NSAIDs can be very effective analgesics for bone pain, and a therapeutic decision taking into account risks and benefits is important for each patient.

Anecdotal opinions range from those that NSAIDs are no more useful than acetaminophen to those that these drugs have a major role in the management of bone pain, approaching the efficacy of opioids, and that NSAIDs have a place in all stages of malignancy.[53,54] Oncologists are on record as saying that NSAIDs do not have a place in the management of pain associated with bone metastases, nor is their pain-relieving effect predictable in patients with bone metastases.[55] Definite clinical evidence supporting their use has been relatively sparse, and their use has been based more on clinical impression or trials in nonmalignant pain, for example in arthritis.

Which NSAIDs are to be preferred? The "model list of essential drugs"[56] includes acetylsalicylic acid, acetaminophen, ibuprofen, and indomethacin. The evidence suggests that ibuprofen at doses of less than 1,600 mg/day or possibly less than 2,400 mg/day is a reasonable initial choice because of its low gastrointestinal side-effect profile.

Irreversible acetylation of platelets by aspirin significantly increases the risk of bleeding. Thirty percent of patients with a history of aspirin-related gastrointestinal bleeding have an exaggerated prolongation of skin bleeding time in response to aspirin, but the association of aspirin use and peptic ulcer has not been reported at doses less than 975 mg/day.[57,58] One study found that there were some differences in aspirin-related gastrointestinal complications compared with those experienced with nonaspirin NSAIDs, but others have not found this to be so.[59]

NSAIDs with high rates of gastrointestinal complications, such as piroxicam, ketoprofen, and tolmetin, should be avoided as first-line drugs. Other agents such as indomethacin (which causes confusion and drowsiness), meclofenate (which causes diarrhea), or phenylbutazone (which causes blood dyscrasias) should not be used.

A meta-analysis of 16 studies showed that the greatest risk of NSAID-associated gastrointestinal toxicity was in the first month of therapy.[60] Heartburn, pain, or dyspepsia may occur in up to 60% of patients taking NSAIDs, but there is no relationship between these symptoms and endoscopic findings.[61] Adverse effects of NSAIDs on the gastrointestinal tract occur in about 20–25% of patients taking these agents. Gastric ulcer occurs in about 10% of patients while duodenal ulcer occurs in about 15%.[61] About 10% of patients taking NSAIDs have complications such as hemorrhage, perforation, or obstruction.[18] There is also a 1% incidence of serious complications in the esophagus, intestine, and colon. These may take the form of ulcerations, strictures, colitis, or exacerbation of inflammatory bowel disease.[62] The prevalence of subclinical small bowel enteropathy is about 70% in patients receiving NSAIDs for 6 months or longer.[63–65]

Contraindications

These drugs should not be given to patients who have shown adverse reactions to them previously.

Hypersensitivity to NSAIDs may develop occasionally as an idiosyncratic reaction. This syndrome may develop in minutes after even small amounts of the drug are given. Vasomotor rhinitis, urticaria, angioedema, and bronchial asthma may extend to laryngeal edema, hypotension, loss of consciousness, and shock.

See the section on gastrointestinal adverse reactions below.

Doses and treatment protocols

See Table 14.3 for dosage guidelines.

Adverse effects and their management

The major problem with the NSAIDs is their adverse effects, which are summarized in Table 14.4. The adverse effects associated with the gastrointestinal tract, renal, and cardiovascular systems give most cause for concern.[66] The elderly are particularly affected, as the prevalence of adverse effects increases with age.[67]

Gastrointestinal adverse effects

Chronic administration of NSAIDs causes gastroduodenal mucosal erosions in approximately 35–60% of patients, gastric or duodenal ulceration in 10–25% of patients, and severe complications, such as gastrointestinal hemorrhage or perforation, in <1% of patients.[68] NSAIDs impair mucosal defense and delay the healing of peptic ulcers by interfering with the action of growth factors, decreasing epithelial cell proliferation in the ulcer margin, decreasing angiogenesis in the ulcer bed, and slowing maturation of the granulation tissue.[69]

The greatest risk for these complications is in the first month of therapy.[66] The risk is associated with age and with the drug itself. The likelihood of the drugs causing gastrointestinal adverse effects is given in Table 14.5. In summary, NSAIDs such as ibuprofen, diclofenac, and sulindac are associated with a relatively low risk, whereas the risk is intermediate for naproxen and high for ketoprofen.[60,66,70,71]

Patients over 65 years who require long-term NSAID therapy or those with a history of peptic ulcer disease should receive prophylactic therapy.[72]

Gastrointestinal complications and prophylaxis

A number of agents have been studied as prophylaxis. Sucralfate has been studied and found to be ineffective.[73,74] Two large multicenter trials were conducted to assess the effect of ranitidine (150 mg twice daily) in preventing peptic ulcer associated with NSAIDs. Ranitidine significantly reduced the incidence of duodenal ulcer but not gastric ulcer rates compared with placebo.[75,76] Famotidine, a H_2-receptor antagonist, prevents duodenal ulceration as well as gastric ulceration compared with placebo when given to patients taking NSAIDs.[77] Enteric coating or suppository formulations have little effect on the incidence of ulceration or bleeding but may reduce dyspepsia. Administration of NSAIDs with food may also reduce dyspepsia.

There is evidence that prophylactic use of antacids and H_2-receptor blockers is of limited value in patients receiving long-term treatment with NSAIDs. Misoprostol has been reviewed in detail.[78] It has been shown to prevent gastric and duodenal ulcers associated with NSAIDs.[79] However, there may be some problems with co-prescribing misoprostol. Misoprostol is expensive, is only partially effective (reduction by 40%), causes dose-dependent diarrhea, and may not relieve the ulcer symptoms.[66,80]

Gastric ulcers

Studies looking at the effectiveness of omeprazole, misoprostol, ranitidine, and placebo have shown that treatment failure rates for gastric ulcers are 7.8% for omeprazole (20 mg once daily), 10.5% for misoprostol (200 μg twice

Table 14.3 *Typical COX-1 NSAIDs and their pharmacokinetic data*

Drug	Time to peak (h)	Elimination half-life	Dose range (mg/day)	Dosing interval (h)	Maximum daily dose (mg)
Oral formulations					
Salicylates					
Aspirin	1–2	0.25[a]	300–600	4	3,600
Diflunisal	2–4	8–12	250–500	12	1,000
Acetic acids					
Indomethacin	1–2	6	50–100	6–12	200
Diclofenac	?	1	25–50	8–12	150
Sulindac (fulfide)	2–4	7	100–200	12	400
Ketorolac					
<65 years	1	4–6	10	4–6	40
>65 years	?	?	10	6–8	30
Proprionic acids					
Ibuprofen	0.5–1.5	2–2.5	200–400	6–8	1,600
Ketoprofen	0.5–2.0	1.5	100	12–24	200
Naproxen	1–2	15	250–500	12	1,000
Oxicams					
Piroxicam	2–4	53	10–20	24	20
Tenoxicam	1–2.6	72	10–20	24	20
Anthranilic acids					
Mefenamic acid	2–4	3–4	500	8	1,500
Para-aminophenols					
Acetaminophen	0.5–1.0	2	500–1,000	4–6	4,000
Parenteral formulations					
Acetic acids					
Ketorolac					
<65 years	1	4–6	10–30	4–6	90
>65 years	1		10–15	4–6	60

a. Metabolized to salicylate, which has a dose-dependent half-life.

daily), 16.3% for ranitidine (150 mg twice daily),[81–84] and 19.7% for placebo.[73] This suggests that omeprazole and misoprostol are the drugs of choice for preventing gastric complications associated with NSAIDs, though the adverse effects of misoprostol may preclude its use in some patients.

Duodenal ulcers

For the treatment of duodenal ulcers, omeprazole is superior to placebo and to misoprostol. The relapse rate of duodenal ulcers treated with omeprazole and misoprostol was reported to be 1.8% and 9.1% respectively in one study[83] and 0.5% and 3.3% for the same drugs in another study.[84]

The role of Helicobacter pylori *Helicobacter pylori* and NSAIDs are probably independent factors for the development of peptic ulcers. It remains controversial whether *H. pylori* is involved in the genesis of NSAID-associated peptic ulcers or if *H. pylori* protects in this situation through its stimulation of prostaglandin formation. Certainly, *H. pylori* seems to aggravate the symptoms of dyspepsia in these patients.[85] In spite of these uncertainties, it has been suggested that in patients with peptic ulcers who are taking NSAIDs, and in whom NSAIDs cannot be discontinued, eradication treatment for the *H. pylori* should be given and a proton pump inhibitor, such as omeprazole, should be added.[86–88]

With respect to the patient at risk of developing a peptic ulcer who is about to begin NSAIDs therapy, the evidence is not so clear. It would not be unreasonable to eradicate the *H. pylori* in this situation, particularly with respect to duodenal ulcers, which are exacerbated by NSAIDs.[77] However, this is subject to confirmation by further studies.

Adverse effects in the kidneys and urinary tract

NSAIDs may cause acute renal failure, an exacerbation of renal insufficiency, hyperkalemia, and interstitial nephritis. The mechanism appears to be inhibition

Table 14.4 *Adverse reactions and interactions of NSAIDS*

Gastrointestinal
Nausea, vomiting, dyspepsia, diarrhea, constipation
Gastric mucosal irritation, superficial erosions, peptic ulceration, esophagitis and strictures, increased fecal blood loss
Major gastrointestinal hemorrhage, penetrating ulcers
Small bowel erosions

Cardiovascular
Rise in blood pressure and fluid retention
Antagonism of β-adrenoreceptor blockers, angiotensin-converting enzyme (ACE) inhibitors and diuretics

Respiratory
Precipitation of asthma in patients with nasal polyps and skin rashes

Hepatic
Hepatotoxicity, hepatitis, fulminant hepatic failure

Renal
Glomerulopathy, interstitial nephritis, changes in renal blood flow leading to a fall in glomerular filtration rate, alterations in tubular function, reduction in diuretic-induced natriuresis, inhibition of renin release, edema

Central nervous system
Drowsiness, confusion, headaches, confusion, hallucinations, depersonalization reactions, depression, and tremor
Aseptic meningitis, tinnitus, vertigo, neuropathy, toxic amblyopia, transient transparent corneal deposits

Hematological
Anemia, bone marrow depression, Coombs-positive anemia, decreased platelet aggregation

Hypersensitivity
Asthma, asthma/urticaria syndrome, urticaria, rashes, photosensitivity, Stevens–Johnson syndrome

Other
Drug interactions, e.g. displacement of oral hypoglycemics and warfarin from protein binding sites and from sites of metabolism
Interference with the actions of β-blockers, ACE inhibitors

Pregnancy and lactation
In the third trimester of pregnancy there is a risk of closure of the fetal ductus arteriosus, tricuspid incompetence, and pulmonary hypertension and bleeding disorders, which make NSAIDs contraindicated in this part of pregnancy
There is very little information on studies in pregnancy and it is generally recommended that they not be given in pregnancy
NSAIDs are excreted in breast milk, and it is recommended that they are not given to lactating women

Children
Very little information is available on the use of NSAIDs in children. It is generally recommended that they are not given to children

Table 14.5 *Risk factors for developing NSAID-associated gastrointestinal toxicity (from McCarthy[61])*

Factor	Relative risk/ odds ratio
History of previous peptic ulcer	9.5
History of previous gastrointestinal bleed	6.7
History of prior use of H_2-receptor antagonist	3.9
Concomitant use of corticosteroids	4.4
Concomitant use of anticoagulants	12–16
High NSAID dose (> 120% of average daily dose)	7.7
Concomitant use of two or more NSAIDs	23.3
Regular use of NSAIDs + aspirin	3.6
Presence of an alcohol-related diagnosis	5.0
Irregularity of feeding	14.3

of renal prostaglandins. There is no risk among persons with normal renal function who have no other risk factors, such as dehydration. On the other hand, patients who continue administration of NSAIDs in the setting of acute hemodynamic effects caused by NSAIDs, which can be detected by rises in serum creatinine or blood urea nitrogen, risk permanent damage to the kidney. COX-2 inhibitors may provide a more favorable risk profile in this setting.[89] Ketorolac has been associated with deterioration when given at the time of surgery, and the risk increases with duration of treatment.[90,91] Cystitis may occur with tiaprofenic acid.

Cardiovascular adverse effects

These adverse effects are more commonly seen in the elderly. A meta-analysis found that NSAIDs were associated with an average rise in the mean blood pressure of 5 mmHg. NSAIDs antagonized the antihypertensive effects of β-adrenoreceptor blockers more than those of vasodilators and diuretics.[92] Antihypertensive drugs that act by affecting renal prostaglandins, such as β-adrenoreceptor blockers and angiotensin-converting enzyme inhibitors, will have their effects modified by NSAIDs. In addition, NSAIDs can also cause fluid retention, which may make cardiac failure worse.[93] There has been recent concern about the risk of cardiac failure in patients taking NSAIDs. The relative risk for cardiac failure in patients taking NSAIDs in the previous 7 days was 2.3 (95% confidence interval 1.2–4.4).[94]

Other adverse effects

Hepatotoxicity is reported as a side-effect of the NSAIDs; elevation of transaminases occurs but will generally be reversed when the drug is ceased. The range of hepatic injury may vary from cholestatic injury to severe hepatocellular injury and has been extensively reviewed by Boelsterli *et al.*[95] and Bjorkman.[62] The most common form of hepatotoxicity is an idiosyncratic reaction associated with an immunological response characterized by fever, rash, and eosinophilia. Examples of drugs which have caused this type of toxicity are ibuprofen, sulindac, and piroxicam. The other type of hepatotoxicity seems to be due to the accumulation of toxic metabolites, and drugs which have been associated with this type are diclofenac, indomethacin, and naproxen.

Asthma episodes may be precipitated by NSAIDs, particularly in those with nasal polyps and skin rashes.

Central nervous system adverse effects such as drowsiness and confusion are probably more frequent than realized by the clinician.

Pharmaceutical considerations

For pharmacokinetics see Table 14.3. For adverse reactions and drug interactions see Tables 14.4 and 14.5.

Practical tips

- It is prudent to begin with a relatively low dose and titrate the dose up at weekly intervals until there are adverse effects evident or to about 1.5–2 times the starting dose.
- The effect of NSAIDs is a "class effect," and the cheapest and most available should be satisfactory.
- The addition of acetaminophen to an NSAID may enhance its pain control and limit NSAID side-effects.
- Individual patients may respond to one NSAID rather than another.
- A prolonged plasma half-life of NSAIDs is associated with an increased risk of renal impairment, gastrointestinal complications, and bleeding.
- Specific inhibitors of COX-2 should be potentially safer drugs than COX-1 inhibitors.
- Drugs with an enterohepatic circulation, i.e. which are excreted in the bile, may be associated with a higher incidence of gastrointestinal adverse effects.
- There is generally a "ceiling effect" with these drugs. Going above this ceiling generally leads to adverse effects out of proportion with little improvement in effect.
- If pain is not well controlled with an NSAID, an opioid drug should be considered when treating cancer pain.
- In patients with impaired platelet function as a result of their disease, use acetaminophen or a nonacetylated salicylate or consider using one of the COX-2 inhibitors.
- NSAIDs may mask the usual signs of infection.

Evidence for efficacy

Variability in the response to NSAIDs seems to be a feature of the use of the drug in individual patients, although the cause of this variability has not been clarified. Individual patient response is one important variable. Other factors, such as plasma half-life, urinary excretion, protein binding, enantiomeric conversion, and pharmacodynamic variation, are also important. If these drugs are used in patients with arthropathy, the concentration in the synovial fluid is less variable than the plasma concentration. If the pain comes from other locations, for example bone pain, the plasma concentration may correlate better.[49]

One study on the symptomatic treatment of nociceptive pain in cancer reported statistically significant pain relief with naproxen 1,500 mg/day.[96**] In a review of 25 studies published up to 1992, Eisenberg *et al.*[97] noted that 13 studies were on single-dose effect, nine on multiple-dose effects, and three on both single and multiple dose effects.[97***] They included over 1,500 patients and 16 different NSAIDs. Because of methodological problems only single-dose studies underwent meta-analysis. A summary of the findings are included below.

- In single-dose studies NSAIDs showed greater efficacy than placebo.
- NSAIDs (650 mg aspirin) were approximately equivalent to 5–10 mg of intramuscular morphine.
- Aspirin was equivalent to indoprofen, ketoprofen, and naproxen in single-dose studies.
- Studies of recommended doses compared with supramaximal doses of ketoprofen, zomepirac (now withdrawn), and ketorolac confirmed a "ceiling analgesic effect" for these drugs.
- Adverse effects were more common with increasing dose without a "ceiling analgesic effect" and were more frequent with multiple doses.
- The addition of a weak opioid (pentazocine, codeine, oxycodone, or dextropropoxyphene) to the NSAID did not produce greater analgesia than NSAIDs alone but increased the prevalence of adverse effects.

In another randomized, nonplacebo-controlled trial over 3 days, no significant difference between high- and low-dose naproxen could be found, despite the fact that 83 of the 100 patients achieved significant pain relief from the loading dose of 550 mg of naproxen.[98**]

Studies of postoperative pain have shown the efficacy of NSAIDs, although the consensus is that they are not powerful enough alone to be used for severe pain.[99**,100**] The drugs that have been shown to be effective in this situation are indomethacin, intenoxicam, and ketorolac.[99**,101**,102**103**]

INDIVIDUAL NONSELECTIVE INHIBITORS OF COX-1 AND COX-2 EFFECTIVE IN THE CENTRAL NERVOUS SYSTEM AND IN THE PERIPHERY

Aspirin

Aspirin (acetylsalicylic acid, ASA) is produced from the naturally occurring salicylic acid. Aspirin's action is partially dependent on dose; in smaller doses aspirin has antiplatelet, analgesic, and antipyretic actions, but in larger doses (>3.6 g/day) the drug has anti-inflammatory effects.

Aspirin has a half-life of about 15 min, but it is metabolized to salicylate. Salicylate has dose-dependent kinetics with a half-life of about 2–3 h at lower doses and about 12 h at higher therapeutic concentrations. At toxic levels, the half-life may be up to 30 h. Factors enhancing excretion are alkaline urine and high urine flow rates. Considerable variation occurs in the blood levels after a fixed dose of aspirin because of variations in metabolism in the wall of the gastrointestinal tract, liver, and in the plasma itself, and the drug can be detected in the plasma for only about 30 min after a dose. Other variables such as pH in the gut, the formulation of the product, and gastric emptying time also play a role. The rectal route is relatively unreliable, but skin absorption is rapid.

Indications

Indications for aspirin are:

- mild to moderate pain, e.g. bone pain from metastases, musculoskeletal pain;
- fever (in patients over 12 years of age to avoid Reye's syndrome);
- migraine and tension headache;
- inhibition of platelet aggregation;
- mild to moderate pain, e.g. bone pain from metastases, musculoskeletal pain;
- dysmenorrhea;
- renal colic.

Contraindications

Contraindications to aspirin therapy are:

- active peptic ulcer disease;
- previous severe adverse reactions to aspirin;
- bleeding disorders, e.g. hemophilia.

In addition, aspirin should be avoided in the third trimester of pregnancy because of possible bleeding and aspirin should be withdrawn 7 days before surgery to prevent bleeding diathesis. Care should be taken when prescribing aspirin in patients with coexisting conditions such as asthma or vasomotor rhinitis (see below).

Doses and treatment protocols

The usual dose of aspirin is 500–1,000 mg every 4–6 h. Doses should not exceed 1,000 mg, and the total dose should not exceed 4 g/day. Going beyond this dose range is more likely to produce adverse effects without any increase in analgesia.

Aspirin inhibits both isoforms of COX, and the effects of aspirin depend on the rate of turnover of COX in different tissues. Platelets, in particular, are susceptible to the action of aspirin. The COX in platelets is inhibited by aspirin in the presystemic circulation and will not be regenerated during the life of the platelet.

Antiplatelet doses are much smaller than analgesic and anti-inflammatory doses. Irreversible acetylation of platelets by aspirin significantly increases the risk of bleeding. The risk of upper gastrointestinal bleeding significantly increases with doses >80 mg of aspirin per day.[57] The association of aspirin use and peptic ulcer has not been reported at doses less than 975 mg/day.[58] The antiplatelet effects of aspirin have been reviewed by Patrono.[104]

Adverse effects and their management

Toxicity is beyond the scope of this review. The adverse effects are listed below. Severe salicylic medical emergency and the management is reviewed elsewhere.[105]

Adverse effects of salicylates include:

- gastrointestinal: intolerance, peptic ulceration, and bleeding;
- hypersensitivity (see below);
- hepatotoxicity (see below);
- renal dysfunction;
- skin reactions including erythema multiforme;
- inhibition of uterine motility;
- salicylism, which may range from tinnitus to deafness and headache.

Adverse effects disappear when the drug is ceased. Serious intoxication can lead to disturbance to acid–base balance, convulsions, and death (10–30 g of salicylate or aspirin or 4 ml of methyl salicylate has caused death in children).

Two forms of hepatotoxicity are associated with salicylates.[106] The first is associated with elevated plasma transaminase concentrations, hepatocellular degeneration, and hepatic necrosis. Elevation in transaminases is common (up to 50% in some series), but clinically significant hepatotoxicity is rare. The hepatotoxicity is reversed when the drug is stopped. The second form is referred to as Reye's syndrome. This syndrome is fulminant hepatic failure following a viral infection in children associated with the administration of aspirin.

Aspirin hypersensitivity generally may occur within minutes of dosing, and most episodes have occurred within the hour. The mechanism is unknown. Patients suffering these episodes fall into two groups. Hypersensitivity reactions fall into groups: rhinitis, nasal polyps, and asthma; and urticaria, wheals, angiedema, hypotension, shock, and syncope.[107]

Evidence of efficacy

See NSAIDs.

Diclofenac

Diclofenac is a phenylacetic acid derivative structurally similar to both the phenylalkanoic acid and the anthranilic acid compounds.

Indications

As for the NSAIDs.

Contraindications

As for the NSAIDs.

Doses and treatment paradigms

The recommended dose for adults is 75–150 mg orally or rectally in two or three divided doses. The maximum dose is 200 mg daily in adults and 1–3 mg/kg in children (older than 1 year).

An enteric-coated formulation (25 and 50 mg) and a suppository of 100 mg are available.

Side-effects and their management

See NSAIDs.

Pharmaceutical considerations

Diclofenac is rapidly absorbed by the oral, rectal, and intramuscular routes and is highly protein bound. Antacids may delay absorption. First-pass effect accounts for about 50% of an oral dose. Diclofenac is eliminated following hepatic metabolism and is excreted in the urine and bile. Less than 1% is excreted unchanged in the bile.

Age and renal and hepatic diseases do not appear to have a great effect on the plasma concentrations, though metabolites may be increased with severe disease.[108] However, caution is indicated when giving this drug, as with other NSAIDs, to elderly patients. There seems to be minimal interaction with oral anticoagulants.[109]

Practical tips

- For cancer pain it is usually necessary to give diclofenac every 8 h to achieve optimal control of pain.
- Tablets should be taken whole with fluid or after food.
- Suppositories are useful for pain during the night.
- Dosage does not appear to be dependent on age or disease state.

Evidence for efficacy

In a study of patient-controlled analgesia, administration of diclofenac with oral methadone appeared to have an opioid-sparing effect.[110]** It is interesting to note that misoprostol may increase the therapeutic effect of diclofenac.[111]**

One hundred patients with advanced cancer were included in a randomized single-blind study to compare the analgesic efficacy and side-effects of oral ketorolac and diclofenac sodium in somatic and/or visceral pain. The study showed that both drugs were effective and tolerability was similar except that sleepiness was four times more frequent in the diclofenac-treated group.[112]**

Diflunisal

Diflunisal is a diflurophenyl derivative of salicylic acid but is not metabolized to salicylic acid.

Indications

As for NSAIDs. Diflunisal has a duration of analgesic activity of 12 h or more.

Contraindications

As for NSAIDs.

Doses and treatment protocols

The recommended dose is 250–500 mg twice daily as tablets. The maximum daily dose is 1,000 mg.

Side-effects and their management

As for NSAIDs. Life-threatening hypersensitivity has been reported.

Pharmaceutical considerations

Diflunisal is rapidly and completely absorbed. Food has no effect on bioavailability. Ninety percent is excreted in the urine, and almost none in the feces. Thus, impaired renal function leads to accumulation of the drug. It has dose-dependent kinetics, which means that, as the dose increases, the serum concentration rises disproportionately. This means rapid onset of toxicity if the dose exceeds the maximum recommended dose in some patients.

The coadministration of indomethacin and diflunisal has led to fatal bleeding.

Practical tips

- Take with adequate fluid or with or after food.
- The tablets should not be chewed or cut.
- Changing dose may take 2–3 days to have full effect.

- Diflunisal is relatively free from central nervous system adverse effects.
- Diflunisal has a uricosuric effect at therapeutic doses.
- Dose needs to be modified in renal failure.

Evidence for efficacy

See NSAIDs.

Diflunisal was evaluated and compared with dipyrone in moderate to severe cancer pain. In patients given 500 mg of diflunisal orally twice a day it was found to be superior to 500 mg of dipyrone three times a day. Adverse reactions were rare.[113**]

Flurbiprofen

Flurbiprofen is one of the most potent members of the phenylalkanoic acid series, and is effective orally.[114]

Indications

As for NSAIDs.

Flurbiprofen has been reported to be useful for the treatment of tissue inflammation pain and neoplastic fever.[26]

Contraindications

As for the NSAIDs.

Doses and treatment protocols

Dosage is 50–100 mg b.i.d. or t.i.d. Suppositories can be used.

Side-effects and their management

As for the NSAIDs.

Pharmaceutical considerations

Flurbiprofen is absorbed rapidly after oral intake. Its half-life is about 5.5 h. It is rapidly metabolized and 95% of a daily dose is excreted in the urine within 24 h.[114]

Ibuprofen

Ibuprofen is a proprionic acid derivative.

Indications

As for the NSAIDs.

Contraindications

As for the other NSAIDs. In studies of normal humans, ibuprofen had no effect on the binding of coumarin to albumin or on the coagulation factors; however, caution needs to be maintained if contemplating using these two drugs together.[115] Prothrombin production is not interfered with and platelet aggregation triggered by contact with bare collagen fibers is more potent with aspirin and naproxen than with ibuprofen.[116]

Doses and treatment protocols

The recommended dose is one 400-mg tablet four times daily. Doses up to 2,400 mg/day may be required. Suppositories are also available.

Side-effects and their management

See NSAIDs.

Pharmaceutical considerations

Ibuprofen is a proprionic acid derivative that has a short half-life of about 2 h and a duration of action of 4–6 h. Absorption is slightly delayed by food, but the drug is well tolerated on an empty stomach. It has two inactive metabolites and is eliminated completely by the kidney within 24 h.[117,118] Ibuprofen does not accumulate with regular dosing. Its onset of action is 20–30 min and duration of action 4–6 h.[26] The pharmacokinetics of ibuprofen are only minimally influenced by advanced age, the presence of alcoholic liver disease, or rheumatoid arthritis. The amount of ibuprofen in breast milk is negligible.

Drug interactions

There is some evidence that ibuprofen inhibits those liver enzymes responsible for N-demethylation, but there are no clinical studies to prove any significant interaction.[119] Ibuprofen can be combined with paracetamol without altering its pharmacokinetic profile.[120] There are some data to suggest that the combination of ibuprofen with aspirin may be associated with a reduction to less than half of the ibuprofen plasma serum concentrations.[120]

Practical tips

- Ibuprofen should be given a trial for 14–21 days before the trial is aborted.[21]
- There does not seem to be a problem with co-prescribing ibuprofen with diuretics or β-adrenoreceptor blockers.[121]
- Ibuprofen in lower therapeutic doses seems to be associated with the fewest gastrointestinal problems of the nonspecific NSAIDs.
- For low back pain, a dosing regimen of 1,200 mg in the morning, 800 mg at midday, and 400–600 mg in the early evening is recommended.[121]

Evidence for efficacy

See NSAIDs.

Ibuprofen has been shown to have analgesic action in single doses greater than 400 mg in dental extraction pain,[122] postpartum pain,[123] dysmenorrhea,[124] and soft-tissue injury.

Indomethacin

Indomethacin is a derivative of indole-acetic acid.

Indications

As for the NSAIDs. May be more effective than other NSAIDs for relieving the pain of ankylosing spondylitis.

Contraindications

See NSAIDs.

Doses and treatment protocols

For doses see Table 14.6.

Indomethacin is available as capsules (25 and 50 mg) or suppositories (100 mg) The recommended dose in adults is 50–200 mg daily in 2–4 divided doses.

Adverse effects and their management

See NSAIDs.

Pharmaceutical considerations

See NSAIDs.

Indomethacin is rapidly absorbed with a bioavailability approaching 100%. It is eliminated by metabolism and renal and biliary excretion. There is appreciable enterohepatic circulation. Its half-life is about 4.5 h and protein binding exceeds 90%.

Practical tips

- Headaches and vertigo are relatively more frequently seen with indomethacin than with other NSAIDs.
- Take with fluids or after food or with antacids.
- Fatal hepatotoxicity has been reported in children, and monitoring of hepatic function is necessary if children are to be given the drug.

Evidence for efficacy

See NSAIDs.

Ketoprofen

Ketoprofen is a derivative of proprionic acid.

Indications

See NSAIDs.

Contraindications

See NSAIDs.

Doses and treatment protocols

The recommended dosage is 100–200 mg, 2–4 times per day. Available formulations are 25- and 50-mg tablets, 100-mg sustained-release capsules (recommended dose 100–200 mg once daily), and 100-mg suppositories.

Side-effects and their management

See NSAIDs.

Pharmaceutical considerations

Absorption is 95% complete in 1–2 h and bioavailability following administration in suppository form is also good.[125] The half-life of ketoprofen is 1.5–2 h and protein binding is 60–90%. Metabolites are not biologically active.

With the sustained-release formulation, maximum serum concentrations occur about 6 h after the dose and absorption continues for up to 16 h.

Ketoprofen does not appear to alter the pharmacokinetics of other protein-bound drugs, e.g. anticoagulants.

Practical tips

- Give with food, fluids, or meals.

Ketorolac

Ketorolac is a heteroaryl acetic acid derivative. It is a potent analgesic but has limited anti-inflammatory activity.

Table 14.6 *Pharmacokinetics of the preferential inhibitors of COX-2 (after Hawkey[15])*

Drug	COX-2/ COX-1[a]	F^b	$t_{max}{}^c$ (h)	t^d (h)	Adult dose[e] (mg/day)	Comments
Meloxicam	3:77	~100	5–6	20	7.5–15	Hepatic or renal insufficiency does not alter pharmacokinetics
Numesulide	5:16	~100	1.2–3.2	1.8–4.7	100–200	Extensive metabolism and active metabolite

a. Approximate selectivity.
b. Bioavailability.
c. Time to maximum concentration.
d. Terminal half-life.
e. Approximate dose.

Indications

Ketorolac is generally recommended for short-term use, particularly for the pain of soft-tissue and bone metastases. Long-term use, such as would be required for cancer pain, increases the risk of adverse effects. However, individual patients with cancer have been maintained on ketorolac by infusion for up to 11 months.[126]

Contraindications

See NSAIDs.

Doses and treatment protocols

Intravenous administration should be over 15 s.

For continuous subcutaneous infusion, give 60 mg per 24 h; increase by 15 mg per 24 h if necessary.[26]

Side-effects and their management

See NSAIDs. For dosage guidelines, see Table 14.7.

The risk of bleeding is associated with the older age group, high doses, and treatment for more than 5 days.[127]

Pharmaceutical considerations

Ketorolac is marketed as the racemate but the *S*(−)-enantiomer is more active *in vitro*. Oral bioavailability is 80–100%. Peak plasma concentration after oral or parenteral administration occurs in 30–60 min. Food reduces the rate, but not the extent, of absorption. Ketorolac is plasma bound (> 99%) and has a terminal half-life of 5 h.[127] In the elderly, plasma clearance of the drug is reduced because of the age-dependent decline in renal function.

Interactions

Co-administration with lithium has resulted in lithium toxicity.[128]

Practical tips

- Ketorolac may reduce the amount of opioids required to control pain and reduce opioid side-effects.[129]

Evidence for efficacy

For the relief of dental pain a single oral dose of ketorolac has been found to be significantly more effective than aspirin or acetaminophen and at least as effective as ibuprofen and acetaminophen combined with either codeine or hydrocodone.[35]** When compared with meperidine (pethidine) (50 or 100 mg intramuscularly), ketorolac 10 mg was equally effective. Higher doses of ketorolac (30 or 90 mg) were significantly more efficacious than meperidine.[130]**

In a randomized, double-blind crossover trial comparing cancer pain treated with morphine (10 mg every 6 h) with a similar regimen of ketorolac in 51 patients, pain control was better with morphine. Adverse effects were higher with morphine, but prophylactic drugs for nausea and vomiting were not given with morphine.[131]**

In a meta-analysis reported by McCormack,[132]*** ketorolac (10–20 mg) provided better analgesia than diclofenac (50–100 mg), aspirin (600–650 mg), and diflunisal (250–1000 mg), but not ibuprofen (400 mg) or ketoprofen (25–100 mg).

Mefenamic acid

Mefenamic acid is an anthranilic acid derivative.

Indications

See NSAIDs. Mefenamic acid has been used extensively for the treatment of dysmenorrhea and menorrhagia.

Contraindications

See NSAIDs.

Doses and treatment protocols

The recommended dose for adults is 500 mg three times daily. The formulation is 250-mg capsules.

Side-effects and their management

May cause diarrhea and occasional intestinal ulceration.[133]

Pharmaceutical considerations

After oral administration peak plasma concentrations occur in 2 h. The drug is excreted as conjugates in amounts of about 50% in urine in 48 h.[134] Peak plasma concentration in 2–4 h and half-life about 2 h.

Table 14.7 *Dosage guidelines for ketorolac*

Age group	i.m. or i.v. administration	Oral administration
> 16, < 65 years	10 mg *stat*, 10–30 mg, 4–6 hourly, NTE 90 mg/day for 2 days or less	10 mg, 4–6 hourly, NTE 40 mg/day for 7 days or less
Age > 65[a]	As above, but NTE 60 mg/day for 2 days or less	As above, except NTE 40 mg/day for 7 days or less

NTE, not to exceed.

a. The dose should be reduced in patients weighing less than 50 kg and in patient with mild renal impairment (creatinine clearance less than 1.2–3 l/h). Avoid in patients with moderate or severe renal impairment.

Practical tips

- If a patient develops diarrhea on this drug, cease the drug without delay.
- Administer with fluids, with or following food.
- Patients with renal insufficiency are at risk of toxicity because the drug is excreted primarily by the kidneys.

Evidence for efficacy

See NSAIDs.

Nabumetone

Nabumetone is a prodrug; the active metabolite is 6-methoxy-2-naphthylacetic acid (6-MNA). It was initially proposed as a preferential COX-2 inhibitor, but studies have failed to confirm this.[135]

Indications

As for NSAIDs, principally for osteoarthritis and rheumatoid arthritis.

Contraindications

As for NSAIDs.

Doses and treatment protocols

The recommended dose is 1,000 mg once daily to a maximum daily dose of 2,000 mg. The drug is available in tablets of 500 and 750 mg.

Side-effects and their management

Virtually all clinical trials have confirmed the rarity of gastrointestinal adverse effects, which are not different to those associated with placebo treatment for doses of up to 2,000 mg/day.

Pharmaceutical considerations

The onset of action varies from 30 min to several hours. Maximum concentrations are seen 2.5–4 h after a dose. The nonacidic prodrug nabumetone is metabolized to 6-MNA, which does not undergo enterohepatic circulation and is predominantly excreted by the kidneys. Half-life is 22–30 h. It is a highly protein-bound drug.

Evidence for efficacy

A review of some 4,500 patients taking the drug for up to 2 years estimated the prevalence of gastrointestinal adverse effects to be 0.03%, about one-tenth of the rates with diclofenac, indomethacin, piroxicam, naproxen, and ibuprofen.[136**]

Naproxen

Naproxen is a proprionic acid derivative.

Indications

As for NSAIDs.

Naproxen has been recommended to control neoplastic fever.[137] Naproxen sodium is recommended for migraine headaches

Contraindications

As for NSAIDs.

Doses and treatment protocols

For pain syndromes the recommended dose is 250–500 mg b.i.d. to a maximum daily dose of 1,100 mg. Naproxen sodium is available in 250- and 500-mg capsules and 273- and 550-mg capsules.

Side-effects and their management

See NSAIDs.

Pharmaceutical considerations

Effective serum concentrations are achieved after 20–30 min and are maximum after 2 h. Absorption is slightly delayed with the rectal formulation. It is available in two forms – the free acid and the sodium salt. The sodium salt is absorbed more rapidly in gastric juices and therefore can be used for the treatment of acute pain syndromes, e.g. headaches.

The half-life of naproxen is 12–15 h, and is independent of dose, plasma concentration, continued administration, or age. Steady-state plasma concentrations are achieved within 2–3 days.[138] Mild to moderate renal impairment produces little change in pharmacokinetics.

Practical tips

Naproxen sodium contains 50 mg of sodium in each 550-mg capsule; this may mean that it should be avoided in patients with cardiac failure or edematous states.

The pharmacokinetics of naproxen are unaffected to any clinically significant extent by age or disease.

Naproxen and naproxen sodium both circulate as the naproxen ion so that these two drugs should not be given together.

Evidence for efficacy

The efficacy and safety of two dosages of naproxen sodium were compared in 100 patients with bone pain due to metastatic cancer in a multicenter, double-blind, randomized, parallel study. Pain was rated from 0 to 99. If the pain score was greater than 40 (moderate to severe pain), then a high-dose regimen of 550 mg every 8 h for

3 days ($n = 51$) was given; if the score was 40 or less, then patients were given the low-dose regimen. This consisted of 550 mg on day 1 then 275 mg every 8 h until day 3 ($n = 49$). Among patients who responded to naproxen, pain relief with the high-dose regimen was significantly greater than with the low-dose regimen; the prevalence of adverse effects, which were mainly mild gastrointestinal symptoms, was not significantly different in the two groups.[98]**

A single-blind, randomized study carried out simultaneously by five pain therapy and palliative care centers compared the analgesic power and side-effects of sodium naproxen and sodium diclofenac in a group of 100 advanced cancer patients who complained of somatic and/or visceral pain. The dose was 550 mg every 12 h for sodium naproxen and 100 mg every 12 h for diclofenac. The two drugs exhibited similar analgesic effect, with pain intensity and duration decreased by half in the first week of treatment; the morbidity rate was low.[54]**

Piroxicam

Indications

See NSAIDs.

Contraindications

See NSAIDs.

Doses and treatment protocols

The recommended dose in adults is 10–20 mg/day as a single dose.

Side-effects and their management

See NSAIDs. There is some controversy as to whether piroxicam is associated with higher rates of gastrointestinal toxicity than other NSAIDs. Meisel's[139] review of the published evidence suggests that the answer may be negative; other studies suggest an affirmative answer.[140]

Pharmaceutical considerations

Piroxicam is readily absorbed from the oral and rectal routes and absorption is not influenced by fasting or food.[141] Its half-life is 36–45 h, and therefore steady-state serum concentrations take 5–7 days to be achieved. Piroxicam is extensively metabolized, with less than 5% eliminated unchanged in the urine and feces.

Practical tips

- Overall gastrointestinal complications may be higher with this drug.
- Administer with food or fluids.
- If 1 day's dose missed after 7 days (steady state) there is little fall in plasma concentrations, in contrast to the situation with diclofenac, indomethacin, or flurbiprofen.[141,142]
- Piroxicam 20 mg daily is comparable to aspirin 3–6 g, indomethacin 75–150 mg, phenylbutazone 400 mg, naproxen 500 mg, ibuprofen 1,200–2,400 mg, and diclofenac 75 mg in rheumatoid arthritis.[141]

Evidence for efficacy

Sunshine *et al.*[143]*** reviewed two randomized, double-blind, single-dose studies looking at the efficacy and safety of piroxicam in moderate to severe postoperative pain. The first study concluded that both piroxicam 20 mg and codeine 60 mg were superior to placebo. In the second study, piroxicam 20 and 40 mg was compared with aspirin 648 mg and placebo. Both doses of piroxicam and the aspirin were superior to placebo for the first 12 h. The effects of piroxicam lasted longer than those of codeine, with a significantly longer time to remedication for piroxicam.

Comparative studies in Norway involving 2,640 patients on piroxicam and 2,694 on similar drugs, e.g. indomethacin, ibuprofen, naproxen, and diclofenac, as well as worldwide clinical trials and postmarketing surveillance studies show that the incidence of overall gastrointestinal adverse drug reactions is lower. The incidence of ulcers and/or bleeds appears to be about 1% for all NSAIDs, but the incidence of gastrointestinal adverse reactions increases with age.[139]**

TRANSDERMAL NSAIDS

Topical NSAIDs have not been taken seriously in the past, but they are modestly effective and their use may limit the toxicity of the oral preparations.[144] Comparisons of topical NSAIDs with acetaminophen, rest, elevation, or compresses do not appear to have been carried out.

From a quantitative review of 86 randomized controlled clinical trials (10,160 patients) of NSAIDs evaluating acute pain (strains, sprains, and sports injuries) and chronic conditions (arthritis and rheumatism), Moore *et al.*[145]** drew the following conclusions:

- Topical NSAIDs are effective in relieving both acute and chronic pain. The overall relative benefit for acute pain conditions was calculated at 1.7 and the number needed to treat to obtain one responder (NNT) was 3.9. For chronic conditions the relative benefit was 2.0 and the NNT was 3.1.
- Analysis by drug revealed that ketoprofen (relative benefit 2.6) was most effective, with the others in the following order: felbinac (3.0), ibuprofen (3.5), and piroxicam (4.2). Benzydamine and indomethacin were not different from placebo.
- For acute conditions, small trials (patient numbers

less than 40) exaggerated the effectiveness of topical NSAIDs by 33%.
- Adverse effects for the topical steroids were low and similar to placebo rates.

Five studies compared topical with oral NSAIDs. None showed a benefit for the oral over topical preparations

PREFERENTIAL INHIBITORS OF COX-2 OVER COX-1

Dosage considerations may determine the selectivity of these agents, but at the doses recommended they show preferential inhibition of COX-2. Some of the information in this section comes from the manufacturers as research is still in progress for a number of these drugs.

Meloxicam

Meloxicam is a NSAID of the oxicam class.

Indications

As for NSAIDs.

Contraindications

As for the NSAIDs. Adverse reactions to any drugs of the oxicam group is a contraindication.

Dose and treatment protocols

The recommended dose is 7.5–15 mg once daily. Suppositories of 15 mg may be given once daily.

Adverse effects and their management

Experience with meloxicam in large studies suggests that its gastrointestinal adverse reaction rate is low compared with diclofenac, naproxen, and piroxicam, but other studies have suggested that there may be little difference between meloxicam and piroxicam.[146–148] Overall, the adverse effects of meloxicam seem at the present time to be low, but a final assessment will need to be made when there has been much experience with the use of this drug.

Bevis *et al.*[149] published a study of 25 patients treated with meloxicam for 1 month. These patients had existing renal impairment that did not worsen with treatment.

Pharmaceutical considerations

Meloxicam has a half-life of 20 h, making it convenient for once-daily administration. Elimination is by four inactive metabolites that are excreted in the urine and feces. Neither hepatic nor renal insufficiency alters the pharmacokinetics. Dosage adjustment does not seem to be required in the elderly.[150]

Evidence for efficacy

Most of the evidence, so far, relates to arthritis and similar disorders. In a controlled, randomized, parallel-group, multicenter study, meloxicam (15 mg i.m. on day 1 and then 7 days of oral meloxicam at 15 mg/day) was compared with piroxicam (20 mg i.m. on day 1 then oral piroxicam, 20 mg/day for 7 days) in 160 patients with lumbago. The drugs were equally highly effective, but adverse gastrointestinal effects occurred in 1.2% of the meloxicam-treated patients compared with 7% of the piroxicam-treated patients.[151**]

In a double-blind study comparing the efficacy and toxicity of 15 mg of meloxicam and piroxicam, 20 mg, over 6 weeks in ambulant patients with osteoarthritis of the hip, there were no significant differences in pain or adverse events.[148] Goei The *et al.*[152**] studied the effect and tolerability of 15 mg meloxicam compared with 100 mg of slow-release diclofenac over 6 weeks in 258 patients with osteoarthritis of the knee. The differences between these two drugs did not reach significance and both drugs were regarded as effective and well tolerated.

Similarly, a double-blind study over 6 months in osteoarthritis patients comparing meloxicam 7.5 mg with slow-release diclofenac 100 mg revealed no significant difference in pain relief.[153**] In a double-blind, parallel group trial of meloxicam in 379 rheumatoid arthritis patients, 7.5 mg meloxicam once daily was compared with naproxen 750 mg once daily. There was no difference in most of the indicators of efficacy of the two drugs, but meloxicam was better tolerated. Significantly more patients in the naproxen group than in the meloxicam group withdrew because of gastrointestinal adverse effects.

One study showed an equivalence between the 7.5-mg dose and the 15-mg dose in rheumatoid arthritis, but other studies have favored the 15-mg dose over the 7.5-mg dose.[154**,155**,156**] Some longer studies have cast doubt on the efficacy of meloxicam (7.5 mg) compared with naproxen (750 mg/day), suggesting that more information is required to establish its place among the NSAIDs.[157**]

Nimesulide

Nimesulide is an NSAID of the sulfonanilide class.

Indications

As for NSAIDs.

In patients intolerant to NSAIDs, often because of urticaria, angioedema, asthma, and anaphylaxis, nimesulide is well tolerated.[158]

Nimesulide is also suitable for the treatment of fever

in children and adults. The drug has been studied in patients with nonbacterial acute inflammation of the ear, nose, and throat with some promising results, but further studies will be required to confirm these data.

Contraindications

As for NSAIDs.

Dose and treatment paradigms

The usual dose is 100 mg b.i.d. The drug is available as 100-mg tablets. Granules, suspension, and suppositories have been studied.

Side-effects and their management

In a large multicenter study of short-term treatment of osteoarthritis, the gastrointestinal adverse reaction rate was 8% in a group of nearly 23,000 patients treated for 1–3 weeks.[159]

Nimesulide has been reported as causing both hepatocellular and cholestatic liver damage and some of the patients had evidence of hypersensitivity with eosinophilia.[160]

Skin eruptions and bullous and erosive stomatitis have been reported.[161,162]

Pharmaceutical considerations

Nimesulide is rapidly and extensively absorbed, with maximum plasma concentration occurring between 1.2 and 2.75 h. Food has no effect on the rate or extent of bioavailability. Suppositories have a bioavailability about half that of the oral formulations. The half-life is 1.8–4.7 h. Steady-state plasma concentrations are achieved in 24–48 h. Minimal drug is excreted unchanged in urine and feces. Extensive metabolism occurs, with the 4-hydroxynimesulide being the major metabolite and slightly active.[163] Reviews of the pharmacokinetics and pharmacodynamic properties of nimesulide are available.[164]

No drug interactions reported with glibenclamide, cimetidine, antacids, theophylline, or digoxin have been reported. The magnitude and time course of the natriuretic, kaluretic, and diuretic effects of frusemide are attenuated by nimesulide, but dose-ranging studies have shown that up to 600 mg/day is tolerated in all respects.[165] Nimesulide does not usually affect the response to warfarin, but caution should be exercised and patients' coagulation status should be monitored.[166]

Practical tips

- Dose allowance for gender, children (> 7 years), and the elderly is not necessary.
- Dose adjustments are required in patients with hepatic failure.
- No adjustment is required in patients with renal failure provided the creatinine clearance is greater than 1.8 l/h.
- Nimesulide does not appear to interfere with clotting mechanisms, however caution is recommended and monitoring of the clotting mechanism is advisable.[167]

Evidence for efficacy

Nimesulide is as effective as acetaminophen in treating fever associated with upper or lower respiratory tract infections.[168]**

In a randomized study of 64 patients with cancer, who were given nimesulide (300 mg/day), oral diclofenac (150 mg/day), rectal nimesulide (400 mg/day), or rectal diclofenac (200 mg/day), no difference in analgesic effect was found.[169]** Similar results were obtained in cancer patients who were given either nimesulide (200 mg daily) or naproxen (500 mg twice daily).[112]**

Twenty patients intolerant to aspirin were given nimesulide in doses of 100 mg and showed no adverse reactions clinically or functionally. However, when the dose was increased to 400 mg three patients experienced mild bronchoconstriction that could be reversed by bronchodilators.[170]**

In a double-blind, placebo-controlled trial nimesulide was found to be effective for the treatment of dysmenorrhea.[171]** Nimesulide (200 mg t.i.d.) and diclofenac (100 mg t.i.d.) were found to be equally effective in relieving postoperative pain associated with hernioplasty or saphenectomy and hemorrhoidectomy.[172,173]** After oral surgery, nimesulide is as effective as other NSAIDs, such as ketoprofen and naproxen.[174]** Nimesulide has been shown to be effective in the management of acute sport injuries (compared with naproxen), after fractures in children, in osteoarthritis (compared with piroxicam and ketoprofen), and in superficial thrombophlebitis.[175–177]**

In a study of patients with bursitis and tendonitis, nimesulide (100 mg b.i.d.) showed similar effects to diclofenac (75 mg b.i.d.) but was better tolerated.[178]**

In a double-blind study comparing the gastrointestinal tolerability of nimesulide and diclofenac evaluated by endoscopy in osteoarthritic patients, Porto *et al.*[179]** found that there was no significant difference between the treatments. A similar finding was reported by Lecomte *et al.*[180]** in a study of tendonitis and bursitis over 14 days.

In a 3-month study of osteoarthritic patients, nimesulide (200 mg/day) was compared with etodalac (600 mg/day). There was no significant difference in efficacy and adverse events between the two compounds.[181]**

Etodolac

Etodolac is a nonacidic prodrug formulation with a short half-life that does not undergo enterohepatic circulation and is a preferential inhibitor of COX-2.[182]

Indications

As for NSAIDs.

Contraindications

As for NSAIDs.

Doses and treatment protocols

The recommended dose is 200 mg b.i.d. It is available as 200-mg tablets. A sustained-release preparation has been studied.[183]

Side-effects and their management

In healthy volunteers, gastrointestinal blood loss following administration of etodolac SR in doses of 600 mg and 1,200 mg/day was similar to that associated with placebo treatment.[184] A gastroscopic evaluation of 44 rheumatic patients treated with etodolac (200 mg b.i.d.) or naproxen (500 mg b.i.d.) for 4 weeks found that 15% of the etodolac-treated patients had gastric mucosal lesions compared with 46% of naproxen-treated patients. The two agents were equally efficacious.[185]

In a 4-week study in healthy volunteers, etodolac (400 mg/day) was compared with naproxen (500 mg b.i.d.) and placebo. The gastric injury seen in etodolac-treated volunteers was similar to that in placebo-treated subjects but was significantly greater in those receiving naproxen.[186]

Acute colitis and benign strictures of the colon have been reported.[187,188] A case of hypersensitivity vasculitis has been reported, and one of etodolac-associated agranulocytosis.[3,17]

Pharmaceutical considerations

Etodolac has a high oral bioavailability. Its half-life is about 7 h. It is almost completely metabolized, and little is excreted unchanged. It is marketed as the racemate, though the *S*-enantiomer is active. It is highly protein bound, but its pharmacokinetics are not affected by concomitantly administered drugs. Dosage modification is not needed for those with moderate renal impairment or stable hepatic disease or in the elderly.[183]

The sustained-release formulation has the similar pharmacokinetics as the conventional formulation, but a longer time to peak concentration and a lower peak. Food did not affect absorption of the sustained-release formulation.[189] The suppository formulation has also been shown to be bioequivalent with the tablets in one study.[190]

A comprehensive review of the pharmacokinetics has been reported by Brocks and Jamali.[191]

Interactions

Etodolac slightly alters methotrexate kinetics, but this was not considered significant.[192] It does not augment the pharmacological affect of warfarin.[193]

Practical tip

- Etodolac can be given to patients who are elderly, those with moderate renal impairment, and patients with stable hepatic disease, e.g. cirrhosis, without dosage modification.[189]

Evidence for efficacy

Many studies have shown that etodolac (400 mg b.i.d. and 200 mg b.i.d.), naproxen (500 mg b.i.d.), nabumetone (1500 mg/day), and indomethacin (50 mg t.i.d.) are equally effective and efficacious in osteoarthritis[194–196]** and rheumatoid arthritis (etodolac 300 mg b.i.d. was equivalent to sulindac, aspirin, ibuprofen, nimesulide, and piroxicam in standard doses).[181,197–199]**

Sustained-release (SR) etodolac at a dose of 600 mg once daily was compared with tenoxicam 20 mg once daily in patients with osteoarthritis of the knee. Treatment efficacy was found to be similar, but gastrointestinal toxicity was higher in the tenoxicam-treated group.[200]** Both etodolac and naproxen were found to be equally effective for symptoms of acute gout.[201]** In patients with osteoarthritis of the knee, etodolac was equivalent in efficacy to diclofenac SR, tenoxicam, and piroxicam.[202]** Etodolac SR and conventional etodolac are equieffective for rheumatoid arthritis and osteoarthritis and have similar safety profiles.[177,203]**

SPECIFIC INHIBITORS OF COX-2 – THE COXIBS

Celecoxib

Celecoxib's chemical name is benzenesulfonamide. At therapeutic doses, celecoxib inhibits COX-2 and not COX-1. There are limited publications available about this drug.

Indications

As for NSAIDs.

Contraindications

As for the NSAIDs. Celecoxib does not adversely affect platelet function after 10 days' therapy and does not cause gastrointestinal ulceration after 7 days' therapy.

Doses and treatment protocols

The recommended dose is 100–200 mg twice daily. Some studies have used up to 400 mg twice daily.

Side-effects and their management

In the early studies, the safety profile was similar to that of placebo. In patients with osteoarthritis of the knee, the most common adverse reactions are headache, diarrhea, abdominal discomfort, and dizziness, but the incidence of these is low.[204]

Pharmaceutical considerations

This drug is administered as a capsule. Absorption is delayed and the bioavailability increased by 40% when given with a high-fat meal. Maximum concentration after absorption occurs at about 1.7–2.1 h. Terminal half-life is 9–10.5 h in adults. The drug has linear kinetics to a dose of 900 mg. See Table 14.8 for the pharmacokinetic profile and Table 14.9 for drug interactions.

Evidence for efficacy

In phase II and III studies, celecoxib is as effective as naproxen for the treatment of osteoarthritis and rheumatoid arthritis and in relieving pain.[205]**

In a 4-week, double-blind, placebo-controlled study of patients with rheumatoid arthritis, patient global assessment, morning stiffness, and the number of painful and tender joints were improved compared with placebo treatment. The incidence of adverse effects was similar in the treated and control groups.[206]** Celecoxib has been shown to be more efficacious than placebo in reducing pain and joint swelling in patients with rheumatoid arthritis.[206]** Celecoxib has not been shown to be superior to the other NSAIDs in relieving postoperative pain.[207]**

Rofecoxib

Rofecoxib is a furone derivative.

indications

As for NSAIDs.

Contraindications

As for NSAIDs.

Doses and treatment protocols

The recommended starting dose is 12.5 mg once daily, and the maximum recommended daily dose is 50 mg. Tablets of 12.5 or 25 mg are available. Rofecoxib is also available as a suspension: each 5 ml contains either 12.5 or 25 mg of rofecoxib.

Table 14.8 *Pharmacokinetics of the coxibs (after Hawkey[15])*

Drug	COX-2/ COX-1[a]	t_{max}[b] (h)	Protein binding (%)	t^c (h)	Dose (mg/day)	Comments
Celecoxib	375	1.7–2.1	97	9–10.5	200–400	Usually given b.i.d. Linear kinetics to 900 mg
Rofecoxib	>800	2–3	85	17	12.5–50	Can be given once daily

a. Approximate selectivity.
b. Time to maximum concentration.
c. Terminal half-life.

Table 14.9 *Drug interactions of the coxibs (after Brooks and Day[212])*

Drug	Affects celecoxib	Affects rofecoxib	Effect of interaction	Clinical significance
Warfarin	+	+	↑ Prothrombin time	Yes
Methotrexate	–	+	↑ Methotrexate levels	Probably not
Lithium	+	+	↑ Lithium levels	Yes
ACE inhibitors	+	+	↓ Antihypertensive effects	Yes, potential for renal impairment
Inhibitors of CYP2C9[a]	+	–	↑ Celecoxib levels	Yes
Substrates of CYP2D6[b]	+	–	↑ Levels of substrate	Probably
Frusemide, thiazides	+	+	↓ Diuretic effect	Yes
Codeine, oxycodeine	+	–	Potential for reduced efficacy of substrates	Possibly
Antacids	+	?	↓ Celecoxib levels	Probably

a. Amiodarone, cimetidine, fluoxitine, fluconazole, metronidazole, fluvastatin.
b. β-Blockers, antidepressants (amitriptyline, desipramine, clomipramine, fluoxetine), and antipsychotics (haloperidol, thioridazine), perhexiline.

Side-effects and their management

After 4 weeks' treatment with 25 mg or 50 mg/day, fecal occult blood loss is similar to that associated with placebo treatment and significantly less than with ibuprofen 2,400 mg/day. These studies do not rule out some increase in the incidence of gastroduodenal ulcers compared with placebo treatment.

Pharmaceutical considerations

The bioavailability of rofecoxib is over 90%, and the median time to maximum concentrations is 2–3 h. The tablets and suspension are bioequivalent. Food has little effect on the bioavailability. It is approximately 90% bound to proteins. Rofecoxib is metabolized to inactive metabolites and over half the drug is excreted in the urine as metabolites. A small amount is excreted unchanged in the feces. Its half-life is approximately 17 h. Renal insufficiency does not influence the pharmacokinetics of rofecoxib, but no safety data for patients with renal insufficiency are available.

The pharmacokinetics are similar in men and women, and no racial differences of consequence have been found. Dosage does not have to be adjusted in the elderly. Initial studies indicated that probably no dosage adjustment is required in patients with mild stable hepatic insufficiency, but patients with more severe hepatic disease have not been studied. The use of rofecoxib in patients with advanced renal disease or renal insufficiency has not been studied. It is not known if the drug is excreted in human milk. See Table 14.8 for the pharmacokinetic profile and Table 14.9 for drug interactions.

Practical tip

- Rofecoxib is effective for pain relief and is not associated with the gastrointestinal adverse reactions of the nonselective NSAIDs. However, it does cause the other adverse reactions associated with prostaglandin inhibition.

Evidence for efficacy

Morrison *et al.*[208]** found that 50 mg of rofecoxib was the effective dose in the management of acute dental pain.

Rofecoxib 50 mg, celecoxib 200 mg, and ibuprofen 400 mg were compared with placebo for analgesic effect in patients with postoperative dental pain. Rofecoxib showed superior analgesic activity to celecoxib and was equal to ibuprofen (400 mg). Time to onset of analgesic effect (30 vs. 60 min), peak pain relief, and duration of effect (> 24 vs. 5.1 h) all favored rofecoxib. Safety profiles were similar.[209]**

For the pain of osteoarthritis, a randomized study of 809 patients carried out over 6 weeks showed that rofecoxib 12.5 mg and 25 mg were similar to ibuprofen 800 mg three times a day. All treatments were well tolerated.[210]**

Rofecoxib and celecoxib were compared for the relief of postoperative pain after spinal fusion surgery. Similar effects were found up to 4 h after surgery, but rofecoxib had an extended effect, lasting throughout the 24 h of the study.[211]**

SUMMARY

Acetaminophen is effective and relatively free from adverse reactions and should be the first drug tried for mild to moderate pain syndromes. It is also relatively cheap.

The nonselective NSAIDs are effective for pain relief, but because of their inhibition of the COX-1 isoform, they are associated with higher rates of gastrointestinal adverse reactions than the selective NSAIDs. These drugs are cheaper than the specific inhibitors.

The specific inhibitors of COX-2, the coxibs, seem to be associated with similar rates of gastrointestinal toxicity as placebo. They are certainly indicated for those people who have experienced previous toxicity with nonselective NSAIDs. Rofecoxib seems to have a better analgesic profile than celecoxib. Their expense may be one factor that limits their use in some countries.

REFERENCES

◆ 1. Vane J. Inhibition of prostaglandin synthesis as a mechanism of action for aspirin-like drugs. *Nature* 1971; **231:** 232–5.

● 2. Vane J, Botting R. Mechanism of action of nonsteroidal anti-inflammatory drugs. *Am J Med* 1998; **104(3A):** 1S–8S.

3. Ferreira S, Moncada S, Vane J. Indomethacin and aspirin abolish prostaglandin release from spleen. *Nature* 1971; **231:** 237–9.

4. Hemler M, Lands W, Smith W. Purification of the cyclooxygenase that forms prostaglandins; demonstration of the two forms of iron in the holoenzyme. *J Biol Chem* 1976; **251:** 5575–9.

5. Mitchell J, Akarasereenont P, Thiemermann C, *et al.* Selectivity of non-steroidal antiinflammatory drugs as inhibitors of constitutive and inducible cyclooxygenase. *Proc Natl Acad Sci USA* 1993; **90:** 11693–7.

6. Flower R, Vane J. Inhibition of prostaglandin synthetase in brain explains the anti-pyretic activity of paracetamol (4-acetamidophenol). *Nature* 1972; **240:** 410–11.

7. Abramson S. Therapy with and mechanisms of nonsteroidal anti-inflammatory drugs. *Curr Opin Rheumatol* 1991; **3:** 336–40.

8. Malmberg A, Yaksh T. Hyperalgesia mediated by spinal glutamate or substance P receptor blocked by spinal cyclooxygenase inhibition. *Science* 1992; **257:** 1276–8.

9. Reuter B, Davies N, Wallace J. Nonsteroidal anti-inflammatory drug enteropathy in rats: role of permeability, bacteria and enterohepatic circulation. *Gastroenterology* 1997; **112:** 109–17.

◆ 10. Henry D, Dobson A, Turner C. Variability in the risk of major gastrointestinal complications from nonaspirin nonsteroidal anti-inflammatory drugs. *Gastroenterology* 1993; **104:** 1078–88.

11. Schafer A. Effects of nonsteroidal antiinflammatory drugs on platelet function and systemic hemostasis. *J Clin Pharmacol* 1995; **35:** 209–19.

12. Meade E, Smith W, De Witt D. Expression of the murine prostaglandin (PGH) synthase-1 and PGH synthase-2 isoenzymes in cos-1 cells. *J Lipid Mediators* 1993; **6:** 119–29.

13. De Witt D, Meade E. Serum and glucocorticoid regulation of gene transcription of the prostaglandin H synthase-1 and prostaglandin H synthetase isoenzymes. *Arch Biochem Biophys* 1993; **306:** 94–102.

14. Byron C, Feldman M. Cyclooxygenase-1 and cyclooxygenase-2 selectivity of widely used nonsteroidal antiinflammatory drugs. *Am J Med* 1998; **104:** 413–21.

15. Hawkey C. Cox-2 inhibitors. *Lancet* 1999; **353:** 307–14.

16. Kargman S, Charleson S, Cartwright M. Characterization of prostaglandin G/H synthase 1 and 2 in rat, dog, monkey, and human gastrointestinal tracts. *Gastroenterology* 1996; **111:** 445–54.

17. Ristimaki A, Honkanen N, Jankala H, *et al*. Expression of cyclooxygenase-2 in human gastric carcinoma. *Cancer Res* 1997; **57:** 1276–80.

18. Cryer B, Feldman M. Effects of nonsteroidal antiinflammatory drugs on endogenous gastrointestinal prostaglandins and therapeutic strategies for prevention and treatment of nonsteroidal anti-inflammatory drug-induced damage. *Arch Int Med* 1992; **152:** 1145–55.

◆ 19. Piletta P, Porchet H, Dayer P. Central analgesic effect of acetaminophen but not of aspirin. *Clin Pharmacol Ther* 1991; **49:** 350–4.

20. Clements J, Heading R, Nimmo W, Prescott L. Kinetics of acetaminophen absorption and gastric emptying in man. *Clin Pharmacol Ther* 1978; **24:** 420–31.

● 21. Forrest J, Clements J, Prescott L. Clinical pharmacokinetics of paracetamol. *Clin Pharmacokinet* 1982; **7:** 93–107.

22. Jackson C, MacDonald N, Cornett J. Acetaminophen: a practical overview. *Can Med Assoc J* 1984; **131:** 25–33.

23. Prescott L. Effects of non-narcotic analgesics on the liver. *Drugs* 1986; **32** (Suppl. 4): 129–47.

24. Skelbred P, Album B, Lokken P. Acetylsalicylic acid vs paracetamol: effects on postoperative course. *Eur J Clin Pharmacol* 1977; **12:** 257–64.

25. Rumack B, Peterson R, Koch G, Amara I. Acetaminophen overdose; 662 cases with evaluation of oral acetylcysteine treatment. *Arch Intern Med* 1981; **141:** 380–5.

26. Twycross R. *Pain Relief in Advanced Cancer*. Edinburgh: Churchill Livingstone, 1994.

27. Gwilt J. The absorption characteristics of paracetamol tablets in man. *J Pharmacy Pharmacol* 1963; **15:** 445–53.

● 28. Settipane G. Adverse reactions to aspirin and related drugs. *Arch Int Med* 1981; **141:** 328–32.

29. Stricker B, Mayboom R, Lingquist M. Acute hypersensitivity reactions to paracetamol. *Br Med J* 1985; **291:** 938–9.

30. Vickers F. Mucosal effects of aspirin and acetaminophen: report of a controlled gastroscopic study. *Gastrointest Endosc* 1967; **14:** 94–9.

◆ 31. Boeijinga J, Boestra E, Ris P, *et al*. Interaction between paracetamol and coumarin anticoagulants. *Lancet* 1982; **i:** 506.

● 32. Benson G. Hepatotoxicity following the therapeutic use of antipyretic analgesics. *Am J Med* 1983; **75:** 85–93.

33. WHO. *Cancer Pain Relief*. Geneva: World Health Organization, 1996.

34. Mehlisch D. Review of the comparative analgesic efficacy of salicylates, acetaminophen and pyrazolones. *Am J Med* 1983; **75(5A):** 47–52.

35. Forbes J, Butterworth G, Burchfield W. Evaluation of ketorolac, aspirin and an acetaminophen-codeine combination in postoperative oral surgery pain. *Pharmacotherapy* 1990; **10(6):** 77S–93S.

36. Korberly B, Schreiber G, Kikuts A, *et al*. Evaluation of acetaminophen and aspirin in the relief of preoperative dental pain. *J Am Dent Assoc* 1980; **100:** 39–42.

37. Hopkinson III J, Bartlett Jr F, Stefens A, *et al*. Acetaminophen versus propoxyphene hydrochloride for relief of pain in episiotomy patients. *J Clin Pharmacol* 1973; **13:** 251–63.

38. Matts S. Headache. *Br J Clin Pract* 1972; **26:** 361–2.

39. Lipton R, Stewart W, Ryan Jr R, *et al*. Efficacy and safety of acetaminophen, aspirin and caffeine in alleviating migraine headache pain: three double-blind, randomised, placebo-controlled trials. *Arch Neurol* 1998; **55:** 210–17.

40. Li Wan Po A, Zhang W. Systematic overview of co-proxamol to assess analgesic effects of addition of dextropropoxyphene to paracetamol. *Br Med J* 1980; **315:** 1565–71.

41. Indelicato P. Comparison of diflunisal and acetaminophen with codeine in the treatment of mild to moderate pain due to strains and sprains. *Clin Ther* 1986; **8:** 269–24.

42. Heidrich G, Slavic-Svircev V, Kaiko R. Efficacy and quality of ibuprofen and acetaminophen plus codeine analgesia. *Pain* 1985; **22:** 385–97.

● 43. Hockberg M, Altman R, Brandt K, *et al*. Guidelines of the medical management of osteoarthritis. Part II: osteoarthritis of the knee. *Arthritis Rheum* 1995; **38:** 1541–6.

● 44. Hockberg M, Altman R, Brandt K, *et al*. Guidelines of the medical management of osteoarthritis. Part I: osteoarthritis of the hip. *Arthritis Rheum* 1995; **38:** 1535–40.

45. Bradley J, Brandt K, Katz B, *et al*. Treatment of knee osteoarthritis: relationship of clinical features of joint inflammation to the response to a nonsteroidal antiinflammatory drug or pure analgesic. *J Rheumatol* 1992; **19:** 1550–4.

46. Williams H, Ward J, Egger J, *et al.* Comparison of naproxen and acetaminophen in a two-year study of treatment of osteoarthritis of the knee. *Arthritis Rheum* 1993; **36:** 1196–206.

47. McManus P, Primrose J, Henry D, *et al.* Pattern of non-steroidal anti-inflammatory drug use in Australia 1990–1994. A report from the Drug Utilization Sub-Committee of the Pharmaceutical Benefits Committee. *Med J Aust* 1996; **164:** 589–92.

● 48. Jacox A, Carr D, Payne R. New clinical guidelines of the management of pain in patients with cancer. *N Engl J Med* 1994; **330:** 651–5.

◆ 49. Brooks P, Day R. Nonsteroidal anti-inflammatory drugs – differences and similarities. *N Engl J Med* 1991; **324:** 1716–25.

50. Beaver W. *Advances in Pain Research and Therapy*. New York, NY: Raven Press, 1990.

● 51. Inturissi C. Management of cancer pain. *Cancer Res* 1989; **63:** 2308–20.

52. Ashburn M, Lipman A. The management of pain in the cancer patient. *Anesth Analg* 1993; **76:** 402–16.

● 53. Payne R. Pharmacological management of bone pain in the cancer patient. *Clin J Pain* 1989; **5** (Suppl. 2): S43–S50.

54. Ventafridda V, Fochi C, DeConno D, Sganzerla E. Use of non-steroidal anti-inflammatory drugs in the treatment of pain in cancer. *Br J Clin Pharmacol* 1980; **10:** 343S–346S.

55. Coombs R, Munro N, Gazet J-C, *et al. Cancer Chemother Pharmacol* 1979; **3:** 41–4.

56. World Health Organization. The *Use of Essential Drugs*. Sixth report of the WHO Expert Committee. Geneva: World Health Organization, 1995.

◆ 57. Lanas A, Arroyo M, Esteva F, *et al.* Aspirin related gastrointestinal bleeders have an exaggerated bleeding time response to aspirin use. *Gut* 1996; **39:** 654–60.

58. Levy M, Miller D, Kaufman D, *et al.* Major upper gastrointestinal tract bleeding: relation to the use of aspirin and other nonnarcotic analgesics. *Arch Intern Med* 1988; **148:** 281–5.

● 59. Henry D, Lim L-Y, Garcia Rodriguez L. Variability in risk of gastrointestinal complications with individual non-steroidal anti-inflammatory drugs: results of a collaborative meta-analysis. *Br Med J* 1996; **312:** 1563–6.

● 60. Gabriel S, Jaakkimainen L, Bombadier C. Risk for serious gastrointestinal complications related to use of non-steroidal anti-inflammatory drugs: a metaanalysis. *Ann Intern Med* 1991; **115:** 787–96.

61. McCarthy D. Nonsteroidal antiinflammatory drug-induced ulcers: management by traditional therapies. *Gastroenterology* 1989; **96** (Suppl.): 662–74.

● 62. Bjorkman D. Nonsteroidal anti-inflammatory drug-associated toxicity of the liver, lower gastrointestinal tract, and esophagus. *Am J Med* 1998; **105(5A):** 17S–21S.

63. Banjee A. Enteropathy induced by non-steroidal antiinflammatory drugs. *Br Med J* 1989; **298:** 1539–40.

64. Kikendall J, Friedman A, Oyewole M. Pill-induced esophageal injury: case reports and review of the medical literature. *Dig Dis Sci* 1983; **28:** 174–82.

65. Langman M, Morgan L, Worrall A. Use of anti-inflammatory drugs by patients admitted with small or large bowel perforations and haemorrhage. *Br Med J* 1985; **290:** 347–9.

66. Griffin M, Piper J, Daugherty J. Non-steroidal anti-inflammatory drug use and increased risk for peptic ulcer disease in elderly persons. *Ann Intern Med* 1991; **114:** 257–63.

67. Johnson A, Day R. The problems and pitfalls of NSAID therapy in the elderly. Part IV. *Drugs Aging* 1991; **1:** 130–43.

● 68. Hawkey C. Non-steroidal anti-inflammatory drugs and peptic ulcers. *Br Med J* 1990; **300:** 278–84.

69. Schmassmann A. Mechanisms of ulcer healing and effects of nonsteroidal anti-inflammatory drugs. *Am J Med* 1998; **104(3A):** 43S–51S.

70. Bateman D. NSAIDs: time to re-evaluate gut toxicity. *Lancet* 1994; **343:** 1051–2.

71. Piper J, Ray W, Daugherty J, Griffin M. Corticosteroid use and peptic ulcer disease: role of non-steroidal anti-inflammatory drugs. *Ann Intern Med* 1991; **114:** 735–40.

● 72. Ad Hoc Committee, American College of Rheumatology. Guidelines for monitoring drug therapy in rheumatoid arthritis. *Arthritis Rheum* 1996; **39:** 723–1.

73. Lanza F. Prophylaxis against nonsteroidal anti-inflammatory drug-associated ulcers and erosions: a commentary on the new data. *Am J Med* 1998; **104(3A):** 75S–78S.

74. Agrawal N, Roth S, Graham D. Misoprostol compared with sucralfate in the prevention of nonsteroidal anti-inflammatory drug-induced gastric ulcer. *Ann Intern Med* 1991; **115:** 195–200.

75. Ehsanullah R, Page M, Tildesley G, Wood J. Prevention of gastroduodenal damage induced by non-steroidal anti-inflammatory drugs: controlled trial of ranitidine. *Br Med J* 1988; **297:** 1017–21.

76. Robinson M, Griffin J, Bowers J, *et al.* Effect of ranitidine on gastroduodenal mucosal damage induced by nonsteroidal antiinflammatory drugs. *Dig Dis Sci* 1989; **34:** 424–8.

77. Taha A, Russel R. *Helicobacter pylori* and non-steroidal anti-inflammatory drugs: uncomfortable partners in peptic ulcer disease. *Gut* 1993; **34:** 580–3.

78. Scheiman J, Isenberg J. Agents used in the prevention and treatment of nonsteroidal anti-inflammatory drug-associated symptoms and ulcers. *Am J Med* 1998; **105(5A):** 32S–38S.

79. Silverstein F, Graham D, Senior J, *et al.* Misoprostol

reduces serious gastrointestinal complications in patients with rheumatoid arthritis receiving non-steroidal anti-inflammatory drugs: a randomized, double-blind, placebo-controlled trial. *Ann Intern Med* 1995; **105(5A):** 241–9.

◆ 80. Raskin J, White R, Jackson E, *et al.* Misoprostol dosage in the prevention of nonsteroidal anti-inflammatory drug-induced gastric and duodenal ulcers: a comparison of three regimens. *Ann Intern Med 1995*; **123:** 344–50.

◆ 81. Ekstrom P, Carling L, Wetterhus S, *et al.* Prevention of peptic ulcer and dyspeptic symptoms with omeprazole in patients receiving continuous non-steroidal anti-inflammatory drug therapy: a Nordic multicentre study. *Scand J Gastroenterol* 1996; **31:** 753–8.

82. Cullen D, Bardhan K, Eisner M, *et al.* Primary gastroduodenal prophylaxis with omeprazole for non-steroidal anti-inflammatory users. *Aliment Pharmacol Ther* 1998; **12:** 135–140.

83. Hawkey C, Karrasch L, Szczepanski L, *et al.* Omeprazole compared with misoprostol for ulcers associated with nonsteroidal antiinflammatory drugs, omeprazole versus misoprostol for NSAID-induced ulcer management (OMNIUM) study group. *N Engl J Med* 1998; **338:** 727–34.

● 84. Yeomans N, Tulassay Z, Juhasz L, *et al.* A Comparison of omeprazole with ranitidine for ulcers associated with nonsteroidal antiinflammatory drugs. Acid Suppression Trial: Ranitidine versus Omeprazole for NSAID-Associated Ulcer Treatment (ASTRONAUGHT) Study Group. *N Engl J Med* 1998; **338:** 719–26.

85. Goggin P, Collins D, Jazrawi R, *et al.* Prevalence of *Helicobacter pylori* infection and its effects on symptoms and nonsteroidal antiinflammatory drug-induced gastrointestinal damage in patients with rheumatoid arthritis. *Gut* 1993; **34:** 1677–1680.

86. Bianchi Porro G, Parente F, Imbesi V. Role of “Helicobacter pylori” in ulcer healing and recurrence of gastric and duodenal ulcers in longterm NSAID users: response to omeprazole dual therapy. *Gut* 1996; **39:** 22–6.

87. Chan F, Sung J, Chung S. Randomised trial of eradication of “helicobacter pylori” before non-steroidal anti-inflammatory drug therapy to prevent peptic ulcers. *Lancet* 1997; **350:** 975–9.

● 88. NIH Consensus Development Panel. *Helicobacter pylori* in peptic ulcer disease. *JAMA* 1994; **272:** 65–9.

● 89. Murray M, Brater D. Effects of NSAIDs on the kidney. *Progr Drug Res* 1997; **49:** 155–71.

90. Power I, Cumming A, Pugh G. Effect of diclofenac on renal function and prostacylin generation after surgery. *Br J Anaesth* 1992; **69:** 451–6.

91. Feldman H, Kinman J, Berlin J, *et al.* Parenteral ketorolac: the risk for acute renal failure. *Ann Intern Med* 1997; **126:** 193–9.

92. Johnson A, Nguyen T, Day R. Do nonsteroidal anti-inflammatory drugs affect blood pressure? A meta-analysis. *Ann Intern Med* 1994; **121:** 289–300.

93. Friedman P, Brown Jr E, Gunther S. Coronary vasoconstrictor effect of indomethacin in patients with coronary artery disease. *N Engl J Med* 1981; **305:** 1171–5.

94. Brooks P. Recent advances: rheumatology. *Br Med J* 1998; **316:** 1810–12.

● 95. Boelsterli U, Zimmeerman H, Kretz-Rommel A. Idiosyncratic liver toxicity of nonsteroidal antiinflammatory drugs: molecular mechanisms and pathology. *Crit Rev Toxicol* 1995; **25:** 207–35.

96. Dellemijin P, Verbiest H, van Vliet J, *et al.* Medical therapy of malignant nerve pain. A double-blind explanatory trial with naproxen and slow-release morphine. *Eur J Cancer* 1994; **30:** 1244–250.

● 97. Eisenberg E, Berkey C, Carr D, *et al.* Efficacy and safety of nonsteroidal antiinflammatory drugs for cancer pain: a meta-analysis. *J Clin Oncol* 1994; **12:** 2756–65.

98. Levick S, Jacobs C, Loukas D, *et al.* Naproxen sodium in treatment of bone pain due to metastatic cancer. *Pain* 1988; **35:** 253–8.

99. Power I, Noble D, Douglas E, Spence A. Comparison of intramuscular ketorolac trometerol and morphine sulphate for pain relief after cholecystectomy. *Br J Anaesth* 1990; **65:** 448–55.

100. Cepeda S, Vargas L, Ortegon G, *et al.* Comparative analgesic efficacy of patient-controlled analgesia with ketorolac versus morphine after elective intra-abdominal operations. *Anesth Analg* 1995; **80:** 1150–3.

101. Turner G, Gorringe J. Indomethacin as adjunct analgesia following open cholecystectomy. *Anaesth Intensive Care* 1994; **22:** 25–9.

102. Brown C, Mazzulla J, Mok M, *et al.* Comparison of repeat doses of intramuscular ketorolac trimethamine and morphine sulphate for analgesia after major surgery. *Pharmacotherapy* 1990; **10:** 455–505.

103. Elkahim M, Nafie M. Intravenous tenoxicam for analgesia during caesarian section. *Br J Anaesth* 1995; **74:** 643–6.

104. Patrono C. Aspirin as an antiplatelet drug. *N Engl J Med* 1994; **330:** 1287–14.

105. Insel P. *Antipyretic and Antiinflammatory Agents and Drugs Employed in the Treatment of Gout*. New York, NY: McGraw-Hill, 1995.

●106. Brass E. Hepatic toxicity of antirheumatic drugs. *Cleveland Clin J Med* 1993; **60:** 466–72.

107. Clissold S. Aspirin and related derivatives of salicylic acid. *Drugs* 1986**; 32** (Suppl. 4): 8–26.

●108. Todd P, Sorkin E. Diclofenac Sodium. A reappraisal of its pharmacodynamic and pharmacokinetc. properties, and therapeutic efficacy. *Drugs* 1988; **35:** 244–85.

◆109. Davies N, Anderson K. Clinical pharmacokinetics of diclofenac. Therapeutic insights and pitfalls. *Clin Pharmacokinet* 1997; **33:** 184–213.

110. Mercadante S, Sapio M, Caligara M, *et al.* Opioid-sparing effect of diclofenac in cancer pain. *J Pain Symptom Manage* 1997; **14:** 15–20.

●111. Sheild M. Misoprostil: new frontiers; benefits beyond

the gastrointestinal tract. *Scand J Rheumatol* 1992; **92:** 31–52.

112. Toscani F, Gallucci M, Scaricabarozzi I. Numesulide in the treatment of advanced cancer pain. Double-blind comparison with naproxen. *Drugs* 1993; **46:** 156–8.

113. Yalcin S, Gullu I, Tekuzman G, *et al.* A Comparison of two nonsteroidal antiinflammatory drugs (diflunisal versus dipyrone) in the treatment of moderate to severe cancer pain: a randomized crossover study. *Am J Clin Oncol* 1998; **21:** 185–8.

●114. Kantor T. Physiology and treatment of pain and inflammation. *Am J Med* 1986; **80:** 3–9.

115. Penner J, Albrecht P. Lack of interaction between ibuprofen and warfarin. *Curr Ther Res* 1975; **18:** 862–71.

116. McIntyre B, Philp R. Effect of three non-steroidal anti-inflammatory agents on platelet function and prostaglandin synthesis in vitro. *Thromb Res* 1978; **12:** 67–77.

117. Mills R, Adams S, Cliffe E, *et al.* The metabolism of ibuprofen. *Xenobiotica* 1973; **3:** 589–98.

118. Adams S, Bough R, Cliff E, *et al.* Absorption, distribution and toxicity of ibuprofen. *Toxicol Appl Pharmacol* 1969; **15:** 10–330.

119. Reinicke C, Klinger W. Influence of ibuprofen on drug metabolizing enzymes in rat liver in vivo and in vitro. *Biochem Pharmacol* 1975; **24:** 145–7.

120. Albert K, Gernaat C. Pharmacokinetics of ibuprofen. *Am J Med* 1984; **70:** 40–6.

121. Busson M. Update of Ibuprofen. *J Int Med Res* 1986; **14:** 53–62.

122. Cooper S, Needle S, Kruger G. Comparative analgesic potency of aspirin and ibuprofen. *J Oral Surg* 1977; **35:** 898–903.

123. Bloomfield S, Barden T, Mitchell J. Comparative efficacy of ibuprofen and aspirin in episiotomy pain. *Clin Pharmacol Ther* 1974; **16:** 565–70.

124. Pulkinnen M, Csapo A. The effect of ibuprofen on the intrauterine pressure and menstrual pain of dysmenorrheic patients. *Prostaglandins* 1978; **15:** 1055–62.

125. Kantor T. Ketoprofen: a review of its pharmacologic and clinical properties. *Pharmacotherapy* 1986; **6:** 93–103.

126. Middleton R, Lyle J, Berger D. Ketorolac continuous infusion: a case report and review of the literature. *J Pain Symptom Management* 1996; **12:** 190–4.

127. Gillis J, Brogden R. Ketorolac: a reappraisal of its pharmacodynamic and pharmacokinetic properties and therapeutic use in pain management. *Drugs* 1997; **53:** 139–88.

128. Langlois R, Paguette D. Increased serum lithium levels due to ketorolac therapy. *Can Med Assoc J* 1994; **150:** 1455–6.

129. Myers K, Trotman I. Use of ketorolac by continuous subcutaneous infusion for the control of cancer-related pain. *Postgrad Med J* 1994; **70:** 359–62.

130. Fricke Jr J, Angelocci D, Fox K, *et al.* Comparison of the efficacy and safety of ketorolac and meperidine in the relief of dental pain. *J Clin Pharmacol* 1992; **32:** 376–84.

131. Jameel A, Stein R, Rawson N. Comparative study of intramuscular ketorolac tromethamine and morphine in patient experiencing cancer pain (clinical study). *Int J Oncol* 1995; **6:** 1307–11.

132. McCormack K. Non-steroidal anti-inflammatory drugs and spinal nociceptive processing. *Pain* 1994; **59:** 9–43.

133. Beaver W. The pharmacologic basis for the choice of an analgesic. II. Mild analgesics. *Pharmacol Physicians* 1970; **4:** 1–7.

134. Parkhouse J. Simple analgesics. *Drugs* 1975; **10:** 366–93.

◆135. Riendeau D, Percival M, Boyce S, *et al.* Biochemical and pharmacological profile of a tetrasubstituted furanone as a highly selective COX-2 inhibitor. *Br J Pharmacol* 1997; **121:** 105–17.

136. Lipani J, Poland M. Clinical update of the relative safety of nabumetone in long-term clinical trials. *Immunopharmacology* 1995; **3:** 351–61.

●137. Todd P, Clissold S. Naproxen. A reappraisal of its pharmacology, and therapeutic use in rheumatic diseases and pain states. *Drugs* 1990; **40:** 91–137.

138. Dahl H. Naproxyn (Naprosyn). Pharmacokinetics: therapeutical relevance and tolerance profile. *Cephalalgia* 1986; **6** (Suppl. 4): 69–75.

139. Meisel A. Clinical benefits and comparative safety of piroxicam. *Am J Med* 1986; **81:** 15–21.

140. Henry D, Page J, Whyte I, *et al.* Consumption of non-steroidal anti-inflammatory drugs and the development of functional renal impairment in elderly subjects: results of a case–control study. *Br J Clin Pharmacol* 1997; **44:** 85–90.

●141. Brogden R, Heel R, Speight T, Avery G. Piroxicam: a review of its pharmacological properties and therapeutic efficacy. *Drugs* 1981; **22:** 165–87.

142. Calin A. Therapeutic focus: piroxicam. *Br J Clin Pract* 1988; **42:** 161–4.

143. Sunshine A, Roure C, Colon A, *et al.* Analgesic efficacy of piroxicam in the treatment of postoperative pain. *Am J Med* 1988; **84(5A):** 16–22.

●144. Henry D. Review: topical nonsteroidal anti-inflammatory drugs are effective and safe for pain. *ACP J Club* 1998; **129:** 10.

●145. Moore R, Tramer M, Carroll D, *et al.* Quantitative systematic review of topically applied non-steroidal anti-inflammatory drugs. *Br Med J* 1998; **316:** 333–8.

146. Fenn G, Morant S. Safety of meloxicam: a global analysis of clinical trials. *Br J Rheumatol* 1997; **36:** 817–19.

●147. Furst D. Meloxicam: selective COX-2 inhibition in clinical practice. *Semin Arth Rheum* 1997; **26:** 21–7.

148. Linden B, Distel M, Bluhmki M. A double-blind study to compare the efficacy and safety of meloxicam 15 mg with piroxicam 20 mg in patients with osteoarthritis of the hip. *Br J Rheumatol* 1996; **35:** 35–8.

149. Bevis P, Bird H, Lapham G. An open study to assess the

safety and tolerability of meloxicam 15 mg in subjects with rheumatic disease and mild renal impairment. *Br J Rheumatol* 1996; **35:** 56–60.

◆150. Davies N, Skjodt N. Clinical pharmacokinetics of meloxicam: a cyclo-oxygenase-2 preferential nonsteroidal anti-inflammatory drug. *Clin Pharmacokinet* 1999; **36:** 115–26.

151. Bosch H, Sigmund R. Efficacy and tolerability of intramuscular and oral meloxicam in patients with acute lumbago: a comparison with intramuscular and oral prixociam. *Curr Med Res Opin* 1997; **14:** 29–38.

152. Goei The H, Lund B, Distel M, Bluhmki E. A double-blind, randomized trial to compare meloxicam 15 mg with diclofenac 100 mg in the treatment of osteoarthritis of the knee. *Osteoarthritis Cartilage* 1997; **5:** 283–8.

153. Hosie J, Distel M, Bluhmki E. Meloxicam in osteoarthritis: a 6-month, double-blind comparison with diclofenac sodium. *Br J Rheumatol* 1996; **35:** 39–43.

154. Reginster J, Distel M, Bluhmki E. A double-blind, three-week study to compare the efficacy and safety of meloxicam 7.5 mg and meloxicam 15 mg in patients with rheumatoid arthritis. *Br J Rheumatol* 1996; **35:** 17–21.

155. Lund B, Distel M, Bluhmki E. A double-blind, randomized, placebo-controlled study of efficacy and tolerance of meloxicam treatment in patients with osteoarthritis of the knee. *Scand J Rheumatol* 1998; **27:** 32–37.

156. Lemmel E, Bolten W, *et al.* Efficacy and safety of meloxicam in patients with rheumatoid arthritis. *J Rheumatol* 1997; **24:** 282–90.

157. Wojtulewski J, Schattenkirchner M, Barcelo P, *et al.* A six-month double-blind trial to compare the efficacy and safety of meloxicam 7.5 mg daily and naproxen 750 mg daily in patients with rheumatoid arthritis. *Br J Rheumatol* 1996; **35:** 22–8.

158. Senna G, Passalacqua G, Andri G, *et al.* Nimulsulide in the treatment of patients intolerant of aspirin and other NSAIDs. *Drug Safety* 1996; **14:** 94–103.

159. Pochobradsky M, Mele G, Beretta A, Montagnani G. Post-marketing survey of nimesulide in the short-term treatment of osteoarthritis. *Clin Res* 1991; **17:** 197–204.

160. Van Steenbergen W, Peeters P, De Bondt J, *et al.* Nimesulide-induced acute hepatitis: evidence from six cases. *J Hepatol* 1998; **29:** 135–41.

●161. Anonymous. Cutaneous reactions to analgesic–antipyretics and nonsteroidal anti-inflammatory drugs. *Dermatology* 1993; **186:** 164–9.

162. Valsecchi R, Reseghetti A, Cainelli T. Bullous and erosive stomatitis induced by nimesulide. *Dermatology* 1992; **185:** 74–5.

163. Bernareggi A. Clinical pharmacokinetics of nimesulide. *Clin Pharmacokinet* 1998; **35:** 247–74.

164. Davis R, Brogden R. Nimesulide. An update of its pharmacodynamic and pharmacokinetic properties, and therapeutic efficacy. *Drugs* 1994; **48:** 431–454.

165. Steinhauslin F, Nunafo A, Buclin T, *et al.* Renal effects of nimesulide in furosemide-treated subjects. *Drugs* 1993; **46:** 257–62.

166. Perucca E. Drug interaction with nimesulide. *Drugs* 1993; **46:** 79–82.

167. Marbet G, Yasikoff Strub M, Macceocchi A, Tsakiris D. The effect of nimesulide versus placebo on hemostasis in healthy volunteers. *Eur J Clin Pharmacol* 1998; **54:** 383–7.

168. Cunietti E, Monti M, Vigano A, *et al.* A comparison of numesulide vs paracetamol in the treatment of pyrexia in the elderly. *Drugs* 1993; **46:** 124–6.

169. Corli O, Cozzolino A, Scaricabarozzi I. Nimesulide and diclofenac in the control of cancer-related pain. Comparison between oral and rectal administration. *Drugs* 1993; **46:** 152–5.

170. Bianco S, Robuschi M, Petrigni G, *et al.* Efficacy and tolerability in asthmatic patient intolerant to aspirin. *Drugs* 1993; **46:** 115–20.

171. Pulkkinen M. Nimesulide in dysmenorrhoea. *Drugs* 1993; **46:** 129–33.

172. Zuckermann M, Panconesi R, Scaricabarozzi I, *et al.* Clinical efficacy and tolerability of nimesulide compared with naproxen in the treatment of posthaemorrhoidectomy pain and inflammation. *Drugs* 1993; **46:** 177–9.

173. Ramella G, Costagli V, Vetere M, *et al.* Comparison of numesulide and diclofenac in the prevention and treatment of painful inflammatory postoperative complications of general surgery. *Drugs* 1993; **46:** 159–61.

174. Pierleoni P, Tonelli P, Scaricabarozzi I. A double-blind comparison of numesulide and ketoprofen in dental surgery. *Drugs* 1993; **46:** 168–70.

175. Facchini R, Selva G, Peretti G. Tolerability of nimesulide and ketoprofen in paediatric patients with traumatic or surgical fractures. *Drugs* 1993; **46:** 238–41.

176. Agus G, de Angelis R, Mondani P, Moia R. Double-blind comparison of numesulide and diclofenac in the treatment of superficial thrombophlebitis with telethermographic assessment. *Drugs* 1996; **46:** 200–3.

177. Dreiser R, Riebenfeld D. A double-blind study of the efficacy of nimesulide in the treatment of ankle sprain in comparison with placebo. *Drugs* 1993; **46:** 183–6.

178. Wober W, Rahlfs V, Bchl N, *et al.* Comparative efficacy and safety of the non-steroidal anti-inflammatory drugs numesulide and diclofenac in patients with acute subdeltoid bursitis and bicipital tendinitis. *Int J Clin Pract* 1998; **52:** 169–75.

179. Porto A, Almeida H, Cunha M, Macciocchi A. Double-blind study evaluating by endoscopy the tolerability of nimesulide and diclofenac on the gastric mucosa in osteoarthritic patients. *Eur J Rheumatol Inflamm* 1994; **14:** 33–8.

180. Lecomte J, Buyse H, Taymans J, Monti T. Treatment of tendinitis and bursitis: a comparison of numesulide and natroxen sodium in a double-blind parallel trial. *Eur J Rheumatol Inflamm* 1994; **14:** 29–32.

181. Lucker P, Pawlowski C, Friedrick I, *et al.* Double-blind,

randomised, multi-centre clinical study evaluating the efficacy and tolerability of nimesulide in comparison with etodalac in patients suffering from osteoarthritis of the knee. *Eur J Rheumatol Immun* 1994; **14:** 29–38.

●182. Rothstein R. Safety profiles of leading nonsteroidal anti-inflammatory drugs. *Am J Med* 1998; **105(5A):** 39S–43S.

●183. Benet L. Pharmacokinetics of sustained-release etodolac. *Rheumatol Int* 1993; **13(2):** S3–S5.

184. Leese P. Comparison of the effects of etodolac SR and naproxen on gastro-intestinal blood loss. *Curr Med Res Opin* 1992; **13:** 13–20.

185. Bianchi Porro G, Caruso I, Petrillo M, *et al.* A double-blind gastroscopic evaluation of the effects of etodolac and naproxen on the gastrointestinal mucosa of rheumatic patients. *J Intern Med* 1991; **229:** 5–8.

186. Laine L, Sloane R, Ferretti M, Cominelli F. A randomised double-blind comparison of placebo, etodolac and naproxen on gastrointestinal injury and prostaglandin production. *Gastrointest Endosc* 1995; **42:** 428–33.

187. Wilcox G, Porensky R. Acute colitis associated with etodolac. *J Clin Gastroenterol* 1997; **25:** 367–8.

188. Eis M, Watkins B, Philip A, Willing R. Nonsteroidal-induced benign strictures of the colon: a case report and review of the literature. *Am J Gastroenterol* 1998; **93:** 120–1.

◆189. Benet L. Pharmacokinetic profile of etodolac in special populations. *Eur J Rheumatol Inflamm* 1994; **14:** 15–18.

190. Molina-Martinez I, Herrero R, Gutierrez J, *et al.* Bioavailability and bioequivalence of two formulations of etocolac (tablets and suppositories). *J Pharm Sci* 1993; **82:** 211–13.

191. Brocks D, Jamali F. Etodolac clinical pharmacokinetics. *Clin Pharmacokinet* 1994; **26:** 259–74.

192. Anaya J, Fabre D, Bressolle F, *et al.* Effect of etodolac on methotrexate pharmacokinetics in patients with rheumatoid arthritis. *J Rheumatol* 1994; **21:** 203–8.

193. Ermer J, Hicks D, Wheeler S, *et al.* Concomitant etodolac affects neither the unbound clearance nor the pharmacologic effect of warfarin. *Clin Pharmacol Ther* 1994; **55:** 305–16.

●194. Schnitzer T, Constantine G. Etodolac (Lodine) in the treatment of osteoarthritis: recent studies. *J Rheumatol* 1997; **47:** 23–31.

195. Dore R, Ballard I, Constantine G, Mcdonald P. Efficacy and safety of etodolac and naparoxen in patients with osteoarthritis of the knee: a double-blind, placebo-controlled study. *Clin Ther* 1995; **17:** 656–66.

196. Karbowski A. Double-blind, parallel comparison of etodolac and indomethacin in patients with osteoarthritis of the knee. *Curr Med Res Opin* 1991; **12:** 309–17.

197. Lightfoot R. Comparison of the efficacy and safety of etodolac and piroxicam in patients with rheumatoid arthritis. Etodolac Study 326 Rheumatoid Arthritis Investigators Group. *J Rheumatol* 1997; **47:** 10–16.

198. Neustadt D. Double blind evaluation of the long-term effects of etodolac versus ibuprofen in patients with rheumatoid arthritis. *J Rheumatol* 1997; **47:** 17–22.

199. Spencer-Green G. Low dose etodolac in rheumatoid arthritis: a review of early studies. *J Rheumatol* 1997; **47:** 3–9.

200. Perpignano G, Bogliolo A, Puccetti L. Double-blind comparison of the efficacy and safety of etodolac SR 600 u.i.d. and of tenoxicam 20 mg u.i.d. in elderly patient with osteoarthritis of the hip and of the knee. *Int J Clin Pharmacol Res* 1994; **14:** 203–16.

201. Maccagno A, Di Giorgio E, A R. Effectiveness of etodloac (Lodine) compared with naproxen in patients with acute gout. *Curr Med Res Opin* 1991; **12:** 423–9.

◆202. Porzio F. Meta-analysis of three double-blind comparative trials with sustained-release etodolac in the treatment of osteoarthritis of the knee. *Rheumatol Int* 1993; **13:** S19–S24.

203. Khan F, Williams P. Double-blind comparison of etodolac SR and dicolfenac SR in the treatment of patients with degenerative joint disease of the knee. *Curr Med Res Opin* 1992; **13:** 1–12.

204. Simon L, Lanza F, Lipsky P, *et al.* Preliminary study of the safety and efficacy of SC-58635, a novel cyclooxygenase 2 inhibitor: efficacy and safety in two placebo-controlled trials in osteoarthritis and rheumatoid arthritis, and studies of gastrointestinal and platelet effects. *Arthritis Rheum* 1998; **41:** 1591–1602.

205. Cameron A. Selective COX-2 inhibitors gather speed. *Inpharma* 1998; **1122:** 9–10.

206. Lipsky P, Isakson P. Outcome of specific COX-2 inhibition in rheumatoid arthritis. *J Rheumatol* 1997; **24:** 9–14.

207. Ault A. First COX-2 inhibitor clears initial FDA hurdle. *Lancet* 1998; **352:** 1912.

●208. Morrison B, Fricke Jr J, Brown J, *et al.* The optimal analgesic dose of rofecoxib: overview of six randomized controlled trials. *J Am Dent Assoc* 2000; **131:** 1729–37.

209. Malmstrom K, Daniels S, Kotey P, *et al.* Comparison of rofecoxib and celecoxib, two cyclooxygenase-2 inhibitors, in postoperative dental pain: a randomized, placebo- and active-comparator-controlled clinical trial. *Clin Ther* 1999; **21:** 1653–63.

210. Day R, Morrison B, Luza A, Castaneda O, *et al.* A randomized trial of the efficacy and tolerability of the COX-2 inhibitor rofecoxib vs ibuprofen in patients with osteoarthritis. Rofecoxib/Ibuprofen Comparator Study Group. *Arch Intern Med* 2000; **160**: 1781–7.

211. Reuben S, Connelly N. Postoperative analgesic effects of celecoxib and rofecoxib after spinal fusion surgery. *Anesth Analg* 2000; **91:** 1221–5.

212. Brooks P, Day R. COX-2 inhibitors. *Med J Aust* 2000; **173:** 433–6.

15

Adjunct therapies, e.g. antidepressants

JOHN CAVENAGH AND RICHARD BURSTAL

Several terms are applied to those pharmacological agents that "help" the opioid and nonopioid analgesics to be more effective in relieving pain, e.g. adjuvants, co-analgesics, concomitants, and "adjunct therapy," the title of this chapter. We have defined adjunct therapy as follows:

> Those pharmacological agents which have a primary role other than the relief of pain and are used to supplement analgesic agents (opioids, NSAIDs, etc.) to make pain-relieving strategies more effective for patients.

Discussions about adjunct drugs have been important features of many reviews on the management of cancer pain[1–7] over the last decade. Some of these agents may have intrinsic analgesic properties in their own right. They may also reduce opioid side-effects by enabling lower doses of analgesics to be used to achieve acceptable pain control for patients. They may control symptoms that have exacerbated the perception of pain, thus reducing analgesic requirements. Adjunct drugs occupy an important place in the World Health Organization's analgesic ladder,[8] being an important option for each of the three steps.

Generally speaking, anesthetists, palliative care physicians, rheumatologists, oncologists, etc. might include many agents in this category, e.g. antidepressants, antibiotics, anxiolytics, muscle relaxants, corticosteroids, anticonvulsants, antiarrhythmics, bisphosphonates, and perhaps even laxatives. In everyday practice, clinicians are well aware that seriously ill patients can have multiple symptoms apart from pain. These are not separate entities that can be eliminated one by one in our quest for good pain and symptom control, but are all inter-related.

The International Association for the Study of Pain[9] (IASP) defines pain as a "sensory and emotional experience ....," and the same could apply to many of the nonpain symptoms affecting patients with cancer. Desbiens *et al.*[10] demonstrated that patients with nausea and dyspnea experience more pain than patients free of these symptoms. If this is the case with dyspnea and nausea, then it is possible that other symptoms also influence the perception of pain and need to be effectively controlled if pain management is to be optimal. The logical position to adopt might therefore be to include all nonanalgesic drugs as adjunct drugs, but this would obviously be stretching the point. The definition of adjunct therapy needs to be restricted from this potentially large list, and in this chapter we will discuss the following groups, realizing that there may be readers who could have argued correctly for the inclusion of many other agents.

1. α_2-adrenergic agonists (clonidine);
2. oral or parenteral local anesthetics [lidocaine (lignocaine), mexiletine, flecainide];
3. anticonvulsants (carbamazepine, phenytoin, sodium valproate, clonazepam, gabapentin, lamotrigine);
4. antidepressants (tricyclic antidepressants, selective serotonin reuptake inhibitors, monoamine oxidase inhibitors);
5. corticosteroids (dexamethasone, prednisolone);
6. drugs causing muscle relaxation (diazepam, baclofen, dantrolene, quinine, glyceryl trinitrate, hyoscine, oxybutynin);
7. *N*-methyl-D-aspartate (NMDA) receptor blockers (ketamine, dextromethorphan);
8. miscellaneous (drugs affecting calcium metabolism – calcitonin; bisphosphonates – pamidronate, clodronate; calcium channel blockers – nifedipine, nimodipine; capsaicin).

Several of these agents may be required for the effective control of pain in some patients. In the case of patients with neuropathic pain, for example, we may find ourselves prescribing multiple combinations of these agents because several different pain mechanisms may be identified at the same time in an individual patient.

Unless careful monitoring is undertaken by the prescriber, the patient may be condemned to swimming in a pharmacological soup, albeit with the best of intentions! The issue of drug interactions and increasingly complex side-effects must therefore always be considered in all therapeutic endeavors. An excellent review of drug interactions in this circumstance has been published[11] and is recommended reading.

A recent study by Grond *et al.*[12] surveyed 593 cancer patients treated by a pain service that adhered to the World Health Organization (WHO) guidelines for relief of cancer pain.[8] These patients were clinically assessed and placed into three groups according to their underlying pain types (nociceptive, neuropathic, or mixed). Treatments included nonopioid or opioid analgesics, antidepressants, anticonvulsants, and corticosteroids. In addition, some patients in each group received antineoplastic therapy, nerve blocks, psychotherapy, physiotherapy, and transcutaneous electrical nerve stimulation. Antidepressants were used in 8% of the patients with nociceptive pain, 25% of the patients with neuropathic pain, and 19% of the patients with mixed pain. According to Grond *et al.*, there was a better than 50% reduction in mean pain severity scores in all three groups, suggesting that, if the WHO guidelines are followed, substantial pain relief can be achieved in patients with cancer pain irrespective of the type of pain. This study clearly emphasizes the role of adjunct analgesic therapy in pain relief. A sound working knowledge of the adjunct analgesics is essential for effective pain management in cancer patients.

This chapter will discuss each of the groups listed using the following headings.

- indications;
- contraindications;
- doses and treatment paradigms;
- side-effects and management;
- pharmaceutical considerations;
- practical tips;
- efficacy.

ADJUNCT THERAPIES OF SPECIFIC DRUG GROUPS

α_2-Adrenergic agonists

There are two classes in this group:

- partial agonists, e.g. clonidine hydrochloride;
- full agonists, e.g. medetomidine.

Although medetomidine has been used to produce anesthesia in both human[13] and veterinary medicine,[14] most research has focused on the partial agonist clonidine. This drug was initially marketed as an antihypertensive agent. It is a centrally acting partial α_2-adrenergic agonist, producing its antihypertensive effects by stimulation of the sympathetic cardioaccelerator and constrictor mechanisms. This results in a decrease in sympathetic outflow.[15,16] Its analgesic action was first described in 1984, when it was inserted into the epidural space.[17] Clonidine's analgesic action is thought to be the result of stimulation of α_2-receptors in the dorsal horn of the spinal cord[18,19] and brainstem,[20] which attenuates the ongoing transmission of nociceptive impulses.[21] In addition, because clonidine reduces sympathetic activity, it has the potential to help control sympathetically maintained pain. The mechanisms of its action, however, are complex and not clear. Bryas-Smith *et al.*,[22] in a randomized controlled trial using transdermal clonidine in patients with diabetic neuropathy, found that some patients exhibited a better response than other, similar patients. The mechanisms of analgesia here did not involve reduction in sympathetic activity. Eisenach *et al.*[23] drew attention to the role of epidural clonidine in patients with neuropathic pain. In the case of neuropathic pain, the mechanism of action of clonidine is probably increased spinal release of acetylcholine.[24] Gentili *et al.*[25] showed, by the use of intra-articular injection of clonidine, that this drug has analgesic effects unrelated to systemic uptake. In a double-blind randomized controlled trial, Glynn and O'Sullivan[26] found that clonidine had an additive effect on the analgesia produced by lidocaine. Kayser *et al.*[27] demonstrated a differential effect in the pain-relieving ability of clonidine depending on the pain stimulus. Clonidine produced a dissociative effect with mechanical stimuli and a heightened pain sensation with hot and cold stimuli. Middleton *et al.*[28] showed that clonidine had the ability to relieve muscle spasms of spinal origin when a standard muscle relaxant, i.e. baclofen, was ineffective. Khan *et al.*[28a] have recently published a review article on the α-receptor agonists, which is recommended reading.

Indications

Clonidine's main use is in the management of neuropathic pain in combination with opioids and local anesthetic drugs, usually via spinal administration.[29,30] The oral route has been used effectively in patients with proctalgia fugax.[31] There is evidence that orally administered clonidine can be effective as maintenance treatment after pain has initially been controlled with epidural clonidine.[32,33] Clonidine has been administered in combination with baclofen to reduce muscle spasms after spinal cord injury.[28] It has also been used to manage the withdrawal symptoms of alcohol and opioid dependency.[34,35] Clonidine has been administered together with bupivicaine to prolong caudal analgesia associated with pediatric surgery.[36]

Contraindications

Contraindications to clonidine are a known hypersensitivity to the drug and situations in which reduction of sympathomimetic output could be critical, e.g. bradyarrhythmias[37] resulting from conduction disturbances of the heart.

Doses and treatment paradigms

The involvement of a pain specialist or an anesthetist is strongly recommended when the use of clonidine is being considered. This is because this drug is mainly administered via spinal catheters. The epidural dose is similar to the oral dose because the drug is well absorbed orally with bioavailability close to 100%.[38] Doses of 2 μg/kg/day have been used[39] in combination with opioids and local anesthetic agents. Similar doses given intramuscularly have been shown to be effective for the management of postoperative pain.[40] Epidural administration is usually achieved by infusion using portable pumps. Recent opinion suggests that intrathecal catheters are more appropriate than epidural catheters and are associated with fewer complications.[41] Intrathecal doses are similar to epidural doses.

Side-effects and management

Drowsiness, dry mouth, bradycardia, constipation, headache, fatigue, and weakness result from the reduction in sympathetic tone. Hypotension following the use of clonidine usually does not require any treatment. In the initial stabilization period, an i.v. cannula with a crystalloid infusion in progress would be wise. The use of drugs predisposing to hypotension, e.g. tricyclic antidepressants, is contraindicated. Depression may be exacerbated by clonidine, and a rise in blood sugar may be noted initially. In patients with cardiac disease, peripheral vascular disease, or renal impairment the use of clonidine is potentially contraindicated, and significant dose reduction may be required.[16]

Pharmaceutical considerations

Clonidine is rapidly absorbed orally and has a half-life of 12–20 h (18–48 h if there is poor renal function). Sixty to seventy percent is excreted by the kidney. Tablets of 100 and 150 μg (scored) are usually administered twice daily.

Ampoules (150 μg/ml) are used as part of epidural or intrathecal infusion techniques. A more concentrated solution for spinal technique is available in some centers.

Practical tips

Seek advice from a pain specialist or anesthetist experienced in pain management about the use of this agent. Consider its use for neuropathic pain poorly responsive to other regimens. Clonidine in combination with baclofen has been reported to be useful as a muscle relaxant in patients in whom spinal cord damage has occurred as a complication of cancer.

Efficacy

Eisenach *et al.*[23] have clearly shown that the most effective use of clonidine is in patients with neuropathic pain, with success being expected in more than 50% of these patients compared with placebo.

Key points

- Clonidine has a clear indication for use in the treatment of neuropathic pain.
- Infusion into a spinal catheter is the preferred method of administration of clonidine.
- Withdraw the drug gradually at least over 7 days to prevent rebound hypertension.

Antiarrhythmic drugs

Antiarrhythmic drugs are usually classified into four classes as follows:[38]

1. Class 1 – sodium channel blockade. This class includes class 1B drugs, e.g. lidocaine and mexiletine, and class 1C drugs, e.g. flecainide.
2. Class 2 – β-adrenergic blockade. This class includes propranolol.
3. Class 3 – prolongation of repolarization. This class includes amiodarone and sotalol.
4. Class 4 – calcium channel blockade. This class includes verapamil, nifidepine, and diltiazem.

The class 1 drugs lidocaine, mexiletine, and flecainide will be discussed in this section.

Local anesthetic drugs reversibly interrupt nerve transmission by blockade of sodium channels in the cellular membrane.[42] Mexiletine and flecainide are orally active sodium channel blockers.

Lidocaine infusions have been investigated as both therapeutic and diagnostic strategies in the management of chronic pain.[43–48] Lidocaine infusion tests are sometimes performed in specialized pain management centers to aid in determining which adjunct drugs may be more effective in particular patients. Because of the very narrow therapeutic window, the "lidocaine test" has to be regarded as a specialized procedure. This test may have a role in determining optimal therapy. Ferrante *et al.*[45] describe the effect of i.v. lidocaine as a precipitous "break in pain" over a narrow dosage and concentration range. Lidocaine has been used with effect in complex regional pain syndromes[47] delivered as a subcutaneous infusion. Woolf and Weisenfeld-Hallin[49] showed that systemic administration of drugs (lidocaine) that increase the inactivation of sodium channels could produce a selective central block of certain types of stimuli in the spinal cord. Boas *et al.*[50] evaluated the effect of i.v. lidocaine in a small number of patients with pain of varying etiologies. Their results suggested that better analgesia was produced in those patients with deafferentation pain than in those with pain of peripheral origin. Tanelion and MacIver[51] showed that analgesia resulting from lidocaine was the result of the suppression of tonic neural discharge in injured peripheral Aδ- and C-fiber nociceptors and also showed that neuropathic pain could be relieved by drugs blocking sodium channels, such as lidocaine, carbamazepine, and mexiletine.[52] However, Elleman *et al.*[53] found no difference between infusion of saline and infusion of 5 mg/kg lidocaine in the relief of neuropathic pain among cancer patients. Although favorable outcomes with i.v. lidocaine infusions have been reported in some painful states, e.g. central pain, migraine, arthritis, the use of i.v. lidocaine infusions in the management of neuropathic pain in cancer is not common.

Of greater interest in cancer pain is the use of the oral antiarrhythmics – flecainide and mexiletine. These oral agents, like lidocaine infusions, are in a similarly uncertain position with many clinicians, showing no consistent results in the management of neuropathic pain. They are mostly used when there has been tumor infiltration of a major nerve plexus, e.g. lumbosacral plexopathy. Mexiletine is structurally similar to lidocaine and is a class 1B antiarrhythmic. Flecainide is a class 1C antiarrhythmic and slows conduction more powerfully than mexiletine.[38] These agents have major toxic effects and must be used cautiously. They are usually administered in small doses to begin with, dosage being increased steadily over 1–2 weeks to gauge response. The use of flecainide in the management of neuropathic pain in 21 patients has been described.[54] Almost half the patients achieved a good result, with higher dosing being more effective. The authors have experience of several patients who have responded remarkably well to flecainide, but also of many who have not.

Flecainide has suffered from its association with the cardiac arrhythmia suppression trial,[55] in which evidence was obtained that flecainide is proarrhythmogenic. Mexiletine has not been implicated in arrhythmia, and therefore may be a more appropriate first choice. Flecainide has a place in the treatment of many difficult neuropathic pain problems in patients with advanced cancer, but experienced opinion[56] suggests that mexiletine should be used as first choice, unless evidence is produced verifying the safety of flecainide in cancer pain management.

Indications

Lidocaine (lignocaine) may be indicated in the management of neuropathic pain that has responded poorly to opioids and other adjunct therapy, e.g. antidepressants, anticonvulsants. It is important to seek specialist advice. The use of lidocaine infusion as a diagnostic test in the assessment of refractory cancer pain may be justified in a specialized pain management unit under close supervision.[56a]

Contraindications[37]

Contraindications to the use of lidocaine include compromised cardiac contractility and conduction disturbances. Caution should be exercised in patients with renal and hepatic function as the drug metabolism and/or excretion may be delayed. Concurrent use of other drugs, e.g. tricyclic antidepressants, may increase the possibility of arrhythmias.

Doses and treatment paradigms[57]

Lidocaine (lignocaine) infusion is a specialist procedure and advice must be obtained from a pain specialist or palliative care specialist if this treatment is being considered. Commence mexiletine using a low dose of 50 mg three times daily and increase the dose by 50 mg three times daily every 4 days to a maximum dose of 10 mg/kg.

Commence flecainide 50 mg b.i.d. and increase every 3 days to a maximum dose of 200 mg b.i.d. The usual dose is 150 mg b.i.d.

Side-effects and management

Mexiletine

Side-effects are related to blood levels and therefore monitoring is advised. A large number of adverse reactions[37] have been mentioned in the literature, including the gastrointestinal side-effects of nausea, gastric discomfort, vomiting, unpleasant taste, hiccups, and esophageal ulcer if a capsule becomes lodged in the esophagus. Chong *et al.*[58] found that the gastrointestinal side-effects of mexiletine were much worse than those associated with flecainide. Central nervous system side-effects include drowsiness, dizziness, inarticulate speech, ataxia, tremor, and confusional states. Cardiovascular side-effects include hypotension, and arrhythmogenicity. Severe skin reactions have been reported with mexiletine.[59]

Flecainide

There is some evidence[58] that flecainide is better tolerated than mexiletine as far as the gastrointestinal tract is concerned. Other side-effects include dizziness, visual disturbances, signs of heart failure (decrease in contractility), nausea, vomiting, peripheral neuropathy, pneumonitis, and delirium. Paranoid psychosis has been reported.[60]

Pharmaceutical considerations

Mexiletine has a half-life of approximately 10 h and is 70% protein bound. Therapeutic monitoring is suggested (0.8–2 mg/l). Flecainide has a half-life of 19 h in cardiac patients, which is likely to be the case for patients with advanced cancer as well. It is 52% protein bound. Therapeutic monitoring is also advisable with flecainide, and the dose should be kept below 0.8 mg/l.[57] In some countries, flecainide is difficult to prescribe, and in Australia it must be commenced in a hospital. Intractable pain is not an approved indication. However, the potential effectiveness of flecainide in the management of difficult pain problems warrants a trial of this agent on occasions. Mexiletine is much more accessible to community practitioners.

Practical tips

Stop tricyclic antidepressants at least 48 h prior to commencing mexiletine. Flecainide solution administered per rectum has been shown to be better absorbed than oral tablets.[61] Therapeutic monitoring is very important.

Because these agents are used less frequently than opioid analgesics and other adjunct drugs it is wise to refresh your knowledge by reading major drug information texts prior to prescribing and carefully excluding important drug interactions.

It is advisable to perform an ECG prior to commencing these drugs to check for a prolonged QT interval.

Efficacy

The response to this class of drugs is not easily predictable but they should be given a trial in those patients with pain that is poorly responsive to opioids and other adjunct drugs.

Key points

- Use as a third choice after opioids and other adjunct therapies.
- The main indication is in those patients with neuropathic pain.
- Therapeutic monitoring is indicated to avoid side-effects from these agents.
- Review the patient's response very regularly in the initial stages of use.

Evidence for particular drugs

*Flecainide, mexiletine.

Anticonvulsants

Until recently, the anticonvulsants most used in pain management were phenytoin, carbamazepine, sodium valproate, and clonazepam;[62] however, in recent years some of the newer anticonvulsants have also found some application, e.g. gabapentin[63–68] and lamotrigine.[69–72] Anticonvulsants have been used extensively in the management of refractory cancer pain over the years, although clear evidence for their effectiveness is sparse. In contrast, there is good evidence for their effectiveness in nonmalignant pain. McQuay *et al.*[62] examined the effectiveness of anticonvulsants in the management of pain using a systematic review. These authors examined the evidence from 1966 through to 1994. They reported that anticonvulsant drugs were effective for the treatment of trigeminal neuralgia and diabetic neuropathy and for migraine prophylaxis. Anticonvulsant drugs have been used in many painful conditions in which there is a descriptive element of a sharp, shooting, or lancinating sensation. Many painful states cause patients to use these descriptors, e.g. diabetic neuropathy, trigeminal neuralgia, glossopharyngeal neuralgia, postherpetic neuralgia, multiple sclerosis, phantom limb pain, and many cancer pains, often involving the malignant infiltration of a nerve plexus or nerve root compression. Our own experience suggests that the clinical effectiveness of the anticonvulsants is unpredictable in cancer patients. The main drugs used in cancer pain management have been sodium valproate, carbamazepine, and clonazepam, with gabapentin use now being increasingly popular with pain and palliative care specialists.

The mechanism of action of anticonvulsants is complex, and their effectiveness in controlling convulsions is not necessarily associated with their effectiveness as analgesics. Berde[73] reviewed anticonvulsants and their use in pain management, and provided a useful summary of their mechanisms of action. Drugs developed before 1980 appear to act on sodium channels, γ-aminobutyric acid (GABA) type A receptors, or calcium channels.[74] Macdonald and Kelly[74] suggest that benzodiazepines and barbiturates enhance $GABA_A$ receptor-mediated inhibition and that phenytoin, carbamazepine, and possibly sodium valproate decrease high-frequency repetitive firing of action potentials by enhancing sodium channel inactivation.[75] Gabapentin binds to a high-affinity site on neuronal membranes in a restricted regional distribution of the central nervous system.[76] Binding to this site may result in the active transport of gabapentin into neurons, but this is uncertain. Rose and Kam[76a] have recently reviewed the pharmacology of gabapentin and suggest that its action may be on voltage-dependent calcium ion channels at the postsynaptic dorsal horn. Lamotrigine blocks neuronal sodium channels in a use-dependent manner, and it inhibits excessive release of glutamate.[77] Excessive glutamate has been implicated in the development of central sensitization. Lamotrigine was found to be effective in relieving nonmalignant pain[78] in a double-blind crossover study of 14 patients with trigeminal neuralgia. Vigabatrin[74] irreversibly inhibits GABA transaminase, the enzyme that degrades GABA, thereby producing greater available pools of presynaptic GABA for release in central synapses. Increased activity of GABA at postsynaptic receptors may underline the clinical efficacy of vigabatrin.

Indications

McQuay *et al.*,[62] in a systematic review, found that anticonvulsants were effective in relieving any neuropathic pain provided there was a descriptor suggesting lancinating, shooting, sharp, or stabbing pain.

Contraindications

Obviously, these drugs are contraindicated where there is a known hypersensitivity. Care must also be taken when used with the selective serotonin reuptake inhibitors and the tricyclic antidepressants.[11]

Doses and treatment paradigms

The following information is adapted from Brodie and Dichter,[79] Dichter and Brodie,[80] and Berkovic.[75] There is a suggestion that analgesic doses are lower than those required for the management of epilepsy,[81] but this has not been verified. The doses mentioned here reflect similar doses used in the control of epilepsy. Emphasis is placed on starting at low doses and increasing gradually while observing for clinical effect. The most commonly used agents in cancer include:

- Carbamazepine (half-life 8–24 h) is commenced at 5 mg/kg/day, and this is gradually increased to 15 mg/kg/day. This approximates to 200–600 mg daily for cancer patients with neuropathic pain.
- Sodium valproate (half-life 7–17 h) is commenced at 10 mg/kg/day and is gradually increased to 25 mg/kg/day. This approximates to 200–500 mg twice daily and occasionally to 500 mg three times daily.
- Clonazepam (half-life 30–40 h) is commenced at 0.025 mg/kg/day and increased to 0.05–0.1 mg/kg/day very slowly, e.g. at weekly intervals, because of its long half-life.
- Gabapentin (half-life 6 h) is commenced at 7.5 mg/kg/day and increased to 40 mg/kg/day. The dose can be increased more rapidly because of the short half-life.
- Lamotrigine is commenced at 1 mg/kg/day and increased to 15 mg/kg/day. Dose increases should not be more frequent than once weekly. The half-life is 25 h, but this may decrease with enzyme-inducing drugs, e.g. phenobarbital, phenytoin, and carbamazepine, to 12–14 h. If used with enzyme inhibitors, e.g. sodium valproate, the half-life may increase to 50–60 h. Doses of lamotrigine up to 200 mg daily were not effective in relieving neuropathic pain in a controlled trial.[82]

Side-effects and management

Anticonvulsant drugs have many potential side-effects.

The side-effects of carbamazepine are dose related and include diplopia, dizziness, headache, nausea, drowsiness, neutropenia, and hyponatremia. Idiosyncratic reactions include exfoliative dermatitis, Stevens–Johnson syndrome, systemic lupus erythematosus, thrombocytopenia, and agranulocytosis.[79]

The side-effects of sodium valproate include tremor, weight gain, dyspepsia, nausea, vomiting, alopecia, and peripheral edema. Idiosyncratic reactions include hepatotoxic effects, thrombocytopenia, and pancreatitis.[79] Sodium valproate inhibits the metabolism of tricyclic antidepressant drugs.[83]

The side-effects of clonazepam include excessive sedation, fatigue, and dizziness. The idiosyncratic reactions include rash and thrombocytopenia.[79]

The side-effects of gabapentin include somnolence, fatigue, ataxia, dizziness, and nausea. It can rarely cause thrombocytopenia and neutropenia.[80] It has been reported that the incidence of side-effects is much lower with gabapentin than with other anticonvulsants.[84] However, there has been a recent report of probable gabapentin-induced polyneuropathy.[85]

The side-effects of lamotrigine include rash, dizziness, diplopia, ataxia, tremor, headache, nausea, and vomiting. The Stevens–Johnson syndrome is a rare idiosyncratic reaction.[80]

These side-effects all involve the gastrointestinal, central nervous, and hematological systems. Treatment involves stopping the drug, but prevention is more important, and side-effects can be minimized by commencing at low doses and gradually increasing the dose while carefully monitoring the patient. Obviously, the Stevens–Johnson syndrome requires urgent specialized assessment and management.

There are some important drug interactions if two anticonvulsants are used simultaneously because some may induce while others may inhibit hepatic enzymes. In our opinion combinations of anticonvulsants should not be used for pain management. Anticonvulsants can interact with the selective serotonin reuptake inhibitors (antidepressants). Paroxetine may be the least likely to cause problems.[86] There are interactions with many other drugs, e.g. corticosteroids, warfarin, felodipine, cyclosporine, and doxycycline.[75] Therapeutic levels of a particular anticonvulsant may be affected, causing decreased effectiveness. This again emphasizes the importance of therapeutic monitoring to give a particular drug the best chance of being effective.

Vigabatrin is another relatively new anticonvulsant used in children and patients with refractory epilepsy. It has been reported to cause psychiatric symptoms and visual field defects.[87]

Pharmaceutical considerations[16,37]

Carbamazepine is slowly and irregularly absorbed from the gut and is metabolized in the liver, producing an active metabolite. The metabolites are renally excreted. It is 75% protein bound. It is a liver enzyme inducer, and its half-life shortens with use, as well as if other enzyme inducers are also being taken simultaneously. The therapeutic range is in the vicinity of 16–50 μmol/l.

Sodium valproate is rapidly and completely absorbed from the gut but its absorption is influenced by food intake. Unlike carbamazepine, it is not an enzyme inducer, but other medications can influence its rate of metabolism. It is excreted in the urine as metabolites. It is 95% protein bound. The therapeutic range is in the vicinity of 280–700 μmol/l.

Clonazepam is rapidly absorbed from the gut and can be given sublingually, which is of advantage in patients who cannot swallow. It is metabolized and the metabolites are renally excreted. It is 86% protein bound and has a half-life of about 20–40 h.

Gabapentin is not metabolized in humans. Its absorption is not influenced by food. It is renally excreted. It is less than 3% protein bound. Its half-life is 5–7 h. Rose and Kam[76a] state that gabapentin is conspicuous among anticonvulsant drugs for its lack of clinically relevant drug interactions, its lack of hepatic metabolism and ability to induce or inhibit hepatic microsomal enzymes, and its low protein binding.

Lamotrigine is rapidly absorbed from the gut and is extensively metabolized in the liver; the metabolites are also renally excreted. It is 55% protein bound. Its half-life is 29 h, but this is greatly prolonged by enzyme inducers such as some of the other anticonvulsants.

Vigabatrin is rapidly absorbed from the gut and its absorption is not influenced by food. It has a half-life of 5–8 h. It is not bound to plasma proteins and is not extensively metabolized. It is not an enzyme inducer. Drug interactions are unlikely with this drug.

In most countries anticonvulsants are not approved for the management of neuropathic pain. Until recently, the one exception was carbamazepine, which had a recognized place in the management of trigeminal neuralgia. A recently published randomized, double-blind, placebo-controlled study by Rice *et al.*[87a] has now provided the evidence that gabapentin is also effective in the management of postherpetic neuralgia.

Practical tips

It is important to commence at a low dose and titrate gradually upward depending on the half-life of the drug. It is advisable to perform therapeutic monitoring if this is available.

Efficacy

Sequential trials may be required in individual patients. In palliative care patients with advanced illness we usually start with carbamazepine, valproate, or clonazepam. We have rarely used phenytoin for neuropathic pain. Experience with the newer agents is largely confined to specialized units.

Key points

- The effectiveness of these drugs can only be assessed by clinical trial in a particular patient.
- Commence treatment using low doses and increase gradually.
- It is advisable to trial one drug thoroughly before stopping it and starting a trial of another drug as there are unpredictable interactions between anticonvulsants.
- Doses used are often similar to those required for the treatment of epilepsy.
- Therapeutic drug monitoring is recommended to optimize dosage and limit side-effects.

Evidence for particular drugs

***Carbamazepine.
**Gabapentin.
*Valproate, clonazepam, vigabatrin, lamotrigine.

Antidepressants

Antidepressant medications can be divided into the following groups:[88]

- tricyclic antidepressants (TCAs) (amitriptyline, clomipramine, desipramine, dothiepin, doxepin, imipramine, nortriptyline);
- tetracycline derivatives (mianserin);
- monoamine oxidase inhibitors (MAOIs) (phenelzine, tranylcypromine);
- reversible monoamine oxidase inhibitors (RMAOIs) (moclobemide);
- selective serotonin reuptake inhibitors (SSRIs) (citalopram, fluoxetine, fluvoxamine, paroxetine, sertraline);
- selective serotonin and norepinephrine (noradrenaline) reuptake inhibitors (SSNRI) (nefazodone, venlafaxine).

The use of antidepressants in chronic pain states has been discussed in the literature from the early 1980s.[89–100] Antidepressant medications have been used increasingly in patients with neuropathic pain states resulting from both malignant and nonmalignant conditions. In a meta-analysis of 39 controlled studies examining antidepressants in chronic nonmalignant pain, Onghena and Van Houdenhove[101] stated that the average chronic pain patient who received antidepressant treatment had less pain than the 74% of the chronic pain patients who received a placebo.

Antidepressants have for many years been known to exert analgesic effects, but their mechanism of action is still debated. Several mechanisms have been postulated, e.g. antidepressant activity *per se*,[96] or some sort of potentiation of the effects of opioids.[102] However, Watson *et al.*[103] suggested that the state of an individual's neurotransmitter systems, as well as the particular agent used, are important factors. Both the serotoninergic as well as the noradrenergic properties of the TCAs seem to be important. Watson *et al.* showed that amitriptyline (a mixed noradrenergic and serotoninergic reuptake inhibitor) was more effective than maprotiline (a specific noradrenergic reuptake inhibitor) in relieving the pain of postherpetic neuralgia.

Analgesic effects of many antidepressant drugs have

been demonstrated in patients with either chronic non-malignant or cancer pain syndromes. Such drugs include tricyclic antidepressants (amitriptyline, imipramine, doxepin, clomipramine, desipramine, and nortriptyline) and some of the SSRIs (paroxetine and citalopram). Comparisons of the pain-relieving effects of individual tricyclic antidepressants have not shown any significant differences in effectiveness. Imipramine,[104] desipramine,[105] nortriptyline,[106,107] doxepin,[108] and clomipramine[109,110] have all been shown to have analgesic effectiveness. Amitriptyline[103,105,111–118] seems to be the agent that has been examined most thoroughly.

McQuay *et al.*[119] performed a systematic review of all controlled trials that investigated the effectiveness of antidepressants in neuropathic pain. The review supported the view that antidepressants are effective in relieving neuropathic pain. McQuay *et al.* suggested that if 100 patients with neuropathic pain were given antidepressants, 30 would obtain more than 50% pain relief, 30 would have minor adverse reactions, and four would have to stop treatment because of major adverse effects compared with a placebo. Much of the research work has concentrated on the management of nonmalignant painful conditions, e.g. diabetic neuropathy, trigeminal neuralgia, chronic low back pain, and postherpetic neuralgia. However, a few studies have suggested that these agents are also effective for the treatment of neuropathic pains experienced by cancer patients.[12,94,95,120–123] Both burning and shooting pain syndromes respond to TCAs.[124] The newer SSRIs citalopram and paroxetine have been shown to be effective in patients with diabetic neuropathy.[125,126] In chronic pain their use may be more attractive because they do not show the many side-effects seen with tricyclic antidepressants (sedation or anticholinergic or hypotensive effects).

Indications

Indications for antidepressants are neuropathic pain states, e.g. lumbar, sacral, and brachial plexopathies.

Contraindications

Contraindications to the use of tricyclic antidepressants are:

- heart block;
- glaucoma;
- urinary hesitancy.

In the case of SSRIs, the main contraindications occur with coadministration of other drugs:

- The QT interval may be affected when astemizole (antihistamine), terfenadine (antihistamine), or cisapride (prokinetic agent) is coadministered.
- The plasma level of coadministered carbamazepine and phenytoin (anticonvulsants) may rise, resulting in the need to adjust their dose downwards.
- SSRIs may cause a rise in the plasma concentration of tricyclic antidepressants, which may result in the serotonin syndrome.
- The coadministration of MAOIs and SSRIs is contraindicated because reversible inhibition of monoamine oxidase leads to an increase in serotonin, which is additive to the action of the SSRI.
- Coadministration of an SSSRI and lithium may lead to neurotoxicity of lithium or the serotonin syndrome.
- MAOI use with meperidine (pethidine) and TCAs is contraindicated.
- SSRI use with tramodol, buspirone, and bromocriptine is contraindicated.
- Coadministration of flecainide may result in a rise in the plasma levels of this agent.
- Plasma levels of propanolol and metoprolol can be increased if SSRIs are also prescribed.
- SSRIs may increase the effect of warfarin.

Doses and treatment paradigms

The doses used in the past have often been considerably lower than those required for treating depression. Zitman *et al.*[127] showed that there was only a small analgesic effect at low doses, but that it helped patients. It has been shown that analgesic effects relate to serum levels of the drug and that doses of TCAs up to 150 mg daily may be required to secure effective analgesia in patients able to tolerate these doses.[105,124] The authors have seen effective responses in patients with advanced malignancy with much lower doses, e.g. amitriptyline 10–30 mg *nocte*. It has been suggested by Breitbart *et al.*[128] that this may be explained by impaired metabolism. Breitbart *et al.* also suggest that there is a biphasic effect in the onset of action of TCAs as analgesics. The early effect usually occurs within a few days and is thought to be the result of inhibition of synaptic reuptake of norepinephrine. A later effect may occur at 2–4 weeks, and this is possibly the result of receptor effects by the TCAs.

Side-effects and their management

Many side-effects,[57] including sedation, delirium, postural hypotension, hyponatremia, and various muscarinic effects (blurred vision, constipation, bladder relaxation, etc.), are caused by the TCAs. Sedation is probably the main concern for many patients. However, side-effects are dose related, and analgesic effects may be achieved at doses considerably less than those required for the treatment of depression, as mentioned previously. To prevent side-effects the clinician should start with low doses and titrate upwards at weekly intervals to try to achieve pain relief. This can be continued until unacceptable side-effects occur. This technique has the advantage of not "frightening off" patients from the potential benefits of the drug, as several weeks or more of titration may be required to achieve an effective dose. Side-effects may be limited by careful selection of the tricyclic antidepressant.[88] Orthostatic hypotension is least likely with clomipramine, desipramine, and nortriptyline. These agents may be preferable if continuing mobility in debilitated patients is desirable. Anticholinergic side-effects are less troublesome with desipramine and nortriptyline, and sedative effects are least likely with desipramine, imipramine, and nortriptyline.

The SSRIs are free of the anticholinergic, antimuscarinic, and hypotensive effects of the tricyclic antidepressants but may cause movement disorders, nausea, and vomiting. In the authors' experience, movement disorders (akathisia) may occur with the coadministration of SSRIs and major tranquilizers such as haloperidol, pericyazine, or thioridazine and some antiemetics, e.g. metoclopramide. Although these effects tend to subside over time, they can be sufficiently unpleasant for some patients to want to cease the medication. The potential drug interactions of the SSRIs are many and are detailed by Virani *et al.*[11] One of the major concerns is the serotonin syndrome, which is seen in some patients who have received combined serotoninergic drugs.[129] Sporer[129] describes this syndrome as being characterized by many symptoms such as confusion, fever, shivering, diaphoresis, ataxia, hyper-reflexia, myoclonus, or diarrhea, while others[130] describe four classic signs of fever, rigidity, autonomic instability, and altered consciousness. Sporer[129] states that the syndrome is caused by excessive serotonin (5-hydroxytryptamine) availability in the nervous system, particularly at the 5-HT_{1A} receptor, and there may also be some interaction with dopamine and 5-HT_2 receptors. It is vital to avoid combinations of the following drugs:

- MAOIs and SSRIs;
- MAOIs and TCAs;
- MAOIs and tryptophan; and
- MAOIs and pethidine and tramadol.
- SSRIs or TCAs and tramadol.

The most likely clinical situation in cancer pain management is to find a tricyclic antidepressant that reduces the reuptake of serotonin, e.g. clomipramine, and a SSRI being used simultaneously. This situation may arise when multiple clinicians are involved in a particular patient's management, e.g. oncologists, pain specialists, palliative medicine specialists, and general practitioners. Constant evaluation of a patient's therapeutic drug list should be a routine aspect of all cancer pain management by all involved.

Pharmaceutical considerations[16]

Amitriptyline is rapidly absorbed from the gut and is extensively metabolized by the liver to form its active metabolite nortriptyline and other metabolites. Its absorption may be delayed because of delayed gastric emptying as a consequence of the antimuscarinic effects of the drug. The half-life is between 13 and 36 h. The plasma level varies widely between individuals and is not related to the therapeutic effect. How the tricyclic antidepressants are metabolized may depend on genetic factors. Amitriptyline is a reasonable first-choice tricyclic antidepressant, but the clinician may need to change to another tricyclic with a lower side-effect profile, e.g. clomipramine or desipramine.

Citalopram is rapidly absorbed from the gut and the absorption is not influenced by food. It is less than 80%. bound to plasma proteins It is metabolized to other SSRIs, but these are less potent than the parent compound. The half-life is 36 h. Impaired liver function will increase the half-life significantly.

Paroxetine is readily absorbed from the gut and is approximately 95% protein bound. It is extensively metabolized by the liver, and these metabolites have almost no activity compared with the parent substance. Impaired renal and hepatic function results in higher plasma levels. The half-life is about 24 h. There is no correlation between plasma levels and clinical effect.

Of the SSRIs, paroxetine and citalopram are reasonable first choices.

Practical tips

For the tricyclic antidepressants, it is advisable to give the initial dose once daily at night commencing at a low dose, e.g. 10 mg. The timing of the dose can be varied depending on the degree of drowsiness in the morning.

The same principle of initial low dose applies to the SSRIs, with frequent clinical monitoring advisable in the initial stages. A careful check must be made of all possible drug interactions for a particular patient prior to commencing a trial of one of these drugs.

Psychiatric consultation to better understand how best to manage possible depression may be of great benefit in drug selection.

Efficacy

These agents have proven efficacy in nonmalignant conditions involving neuropathic pain syndromes.[119,131] Few studies have been undertaken in the management of cancer pain syndromes, but their effectiveness in the management of noncancer neuropathic pain has also been successfully extrapolated to the treatment of patients with cancer pain.

Key points

- Exclude any possible drug interactions with the SSRIs before use.
- Commence at low dosage and increase gradually to achieve effect or until unacceptable side-effects necessitate a cessation of the trial.

Evidence for particular drugs

***Tricyclic antidepressants.
**Selective serotonin reuptake inhibitors.

Corticosteroids

Corticosteroids have been used extensively in patients with cancer-related pain.[12,132,133] These drugs are used for the management of pain resulting from headache due to raised intracranial pressure as a result of cerebral metastases,[134] expanding pelvic malignancies, spinal cord compression, peripheral nerve compression, bone metastases, as well as, for example, pain resulting from liver capsule distension. They also have multiple uses in other symptom control[135–138] and contribute to the control of nausea and vomiting related to chemotherapy.[139] Twycross[140] has reviewed the use of corticosteroids in cancer patients and reminds us of the importance of using these agents carefully. When considering their use it is important to state clearly at the outset exactly what it is hoped to achieve and over what period of time. There may be a sense of complacency among clinicians in the use of corticosteroids in patients with advanced cancer, and once these agents are commenced they tend to be continued, often without clear justification.[141] Patients may benefit from an improved sense of well-being and mild euphoria, and relatives often feel all is well on seeing the "healthy" facial appearance in their relative. It is important that these effects are placed in perspective and that it is carefully explained to both patients and relatives that the apparent improvement is not the result of cancer remission.

Indications

Indications for corticosteroids include:

- increased intracranial pressure as a result of edema surrounding cerebral metastases;
- nerve compression (particularly involving the lumbosacral plexus);
- spinal cord compression, as an initial therapy until radiation therapy treatments take effect;
- bone pain;
- organ capsular distension.

Contraindications

Contraindications to the administration of corticosteroids include sepsis and previous exposure causing severe mood disturbances.

Doses and treatment paradigms

Dexamethasone is traditionally used for suspected spinal cord compression and is usually given in a large initial dose followed by a substantial maintenance dosage until radiation therapy and/or surgical treatments have been undertaken. In the authors' experience the initial dose is 24 mg given by i.v. injection, followed by 16–24 mg daily by mouth. In North America, higher doses have been described, e.g. a 100-mg i.v. bolus followed by 24 mg orally four times daily for 3 days, then tapered over 10 days.[142] These doses are used for those patients presenting with already impaired function of the cord or a low spinal lesion, e.g. cauda equina syndrome, in an effort to preserve as much neurological function as possible. These doses are stated to be more effective – 81% compared with 63% if smaller doses are used.[142] The difficulty is deciding whether the risks of side-effects of these very high doses are acceptable to both patients and carers, as these doses can be associated with substantial morbidity.[143] The decision to use steroids is based on the risk–benefit ratio and the appropriateness for the individual patient.

A trial of steroids may be appropriate for many types of refractory cancer pains, and a common starting dose is prednisolone 25 mg twice daily or dexamethasone 4mg twice daily for 3 days. Subsequently, the dose should be reduced to the minimal effective dose, and possibly ceased completely if other pain-relieving strategies have subsequently become successful.

Side-effects and management

In patients with advanced disease, the risk of accelerated proximal myopathy can be a major problem necessitating extensive home nursing support and perhaps even prolonged hospitalization. Bowyer *et al.*[144] described evidence of myopathy in 48% of patients with asthma taking 40 mg or more of prednisolone per day, but importantly noted that this effect was practically nonexistent in patients taking 30 mg or less per day. The occurrence of myopathy may be related to the use of fluorinated corticosteroids, e.g. dexamethasone as opposed to prednisolone. Dekhuijzen *et al.*[145] have demonstrated a clear difference between the effects of triamcinalone (a fluorinated corticosteroid) and prednisolone on the fiber diameter of muscle tissue in the rat diaphragm. It is disappointing that, as yet, this effect has not, to our knowledge, been demonstrated in cancer patients. If this is ever shown to be the case then prednisolone should be the drug of choice rather than dexamethasone except when mineralocorticoid effects are considered harmful to the patient's comfort. Evidence of myopathy should be assessed in all ambulatory cancer patients requiring corticosteroids, and the lowest effective dose should be used.

Neuropsychiatric side-effects, e.g. depression and delirium, are associated with corticosteroid therapy.[146,147] Wolkowitz[148] administered prednisone, 80 mg/day for 5 days, in a double-blind manner to healthy volunteers. Seventy-five percent developed mild behavioral side-effects. In addition, he demonstrated deterioration in cognitive performance in these volunteers. This is yet another reason for using the minimal effective dose. Corticosteroids can result in the impairment of glucose metabolism. This may unmask diabetes mellitus in predisposed individuals and make diabetes more difficult to control.[149]

Corticosteroids, even inhaled corticosteroids, are often associated with the appearance of distressing oral, esophageal, and vaginal candidiasis.[150] This effect is probably the result of suppression of monocyte activity. Heidenreich *et al.*[151] demonstrated that corticosteroids suppress the formation of tumor necrosis factor-α, which is required for full monocyte activation. Effective management of candidiasis should include reduction of the corticosteroid dose if possible, as well as topical and possibly systemic antifungal drugs in severe cases.

Pharmaceutical considerations[16,38,57]

Prednisolone and prednisone are both rapidly absorbed from the gut. Prednisone is converted in the liver to prednisolone, the active component. The half-life is 3.5h and the duration of action is 12–36h. This contrasts with dexamethasone, which has a half-life of 4.5h and a duration of action of 36–72h. Both prednisolone and dexamethasone can be given as a single daily dose. Dexamethasone seems to be the drug most used because of the absence of mineralocorticoid effects. However, the development of peripheral edema can have other causes, e.g. low serum albumin levels. Assuming that the evidence concerning fluorinated steroids and myopathy also applies to humans, then the use of prednisolone rather than dexamethasone may be advisable.

Practical tips

Try to state clearly the reason for using a corticosteroid and plan a review date. Aim to reduce the dosage to the minimal effective dose.

Efficacy

Corticosteroids usually produce improvements in pain control as well as an elevation in mood, tending to create a sense of optimism in all involved. While this is a useful effect in most circumstances, the clinician has an important responsibility to ensure that the minimum effective dose is used and that dosage is reviewed frequently.

Key points

- Use a trial of steroids for a specific period and reduce to the minimum effective dose as quickly as possible.
- Understand clearly the aims of treatment.
- Monitor side-effects.
- Consider using the nonfluorinated corticosteroids to lessen the possibility of myopathy.

Evidence for particular drugs

*Dexamethasone, prednisolone.

Muscle relaxants

Cancer patients with muscle spasm may experience considerable distress. This may occur when surrounding muscles attempt to protect a part of the skeletal structure weakened as a result of metastatic bone disease, e.g. vertebral body, femur, humerus. There may or may not be pain attributable to the bone pathology itself, but frequently the major pain results from intense muscle spasm. Waldman[152] reviewed the use of these drugs in 1994 and listed the following drugs in this group:

- Drugs reducing skeletal muscle tone
  - diazepam
  - baclofen
  - dantrolene
  - quinine
- Smooth muscle relaxants
  - glyceryl trinitrate
  - hyoscine butylbromide
  - oxybutynin.

Other agents mentioned in the literature include orphenadrine, a drug usually known for its use as an antiparkinsonian agent, which has been used as the citrate salt in various preparations as a muscle relaxant, and cyclobenzaprine, an agent similar in structure to the tricyclic antidepressants.[38] The evidence for these agents is weak and they will not be discussed further.

Diazepam is a benzodiazepine that has multiple medical applications (anticonvulsant, muscle relaxant, psychotropic). Over the years it has been used to help reduce muscle tone.

Diazepam acts by helping the neurotransmitter GABA bind to its receptor, which results in neuronal inhibition.[153] Baclofen is a $GABA_B$ receptor agonist that also results in neuronal inhibition.[154] Both these agents result in the suppression of spinal cord activity, which results in skeletal muscle relaxation. These agents are effective for those patients with spinal cord damage in whom disinhibition has resulted in increased neuronal activity. Baclofen is used intrathecally for this purpose as well as orally.[155–157] Baclofen has also found a use in the treatment of intractable hiccup along with other muscle relaxants, e.g. midazolam. Dantrolene works very differently to diazepam and baclofen, by uncoupling muscle contraction. This is achieved by interfering with calcium release from sarcoplasmic reticulum.[158] Dantrolene has been used in the life-threatening conditions of malignant hyperthermia[159] and neuroleptic malignant syndrome[160] as well as in the treatment of muscle spasms and opioid-related myoclonus in cancer patients.[161] Quinine has been used in the management of nocturnal muscle cramps for many years, and a recent review suggested that, although quinine reduces the frequency of nocturnal cramps, it does not reduce their severity.[162] There is a risk of severe adverse effects from quinine following inadvertent administration of excessive doses.[162–168] Quinine acts by increasing the refractory period of muscle, causing a diminished response to a tetanic stimulation, and the excitability of the motor end plate is also diminished. Nitroglycerin has been used effectively in the management of anal sphincter spasm resulting from thrombosed external hemorrhoids and/or anal fissure.[169] This is not an uncommon complaint, particularly in patients with advanced cancer requiring opioid analgesics, who often have constipation requiring rectal laxatives, and even disimpaction. Hyoscine butylbromide has been used to treat painful colic resulting from malignant bowel obstruction in patients with advanced cancer. It is also used in diagnostic radiological investigations.[170,171] Its use in the medical management of malignant bowel obstruction seems quite appropriate as it also reduces gastrointestinal secretions.[172] Oxybutynin is used in the management of bladder spasm associated with urinary catheters.[173]

Indications

The indications for use of this diffuse group of drugs are outlined in the previous section.

Contraindications

Contraindications to individual muscle relaxants are as follows:

- Diazepam: known allergy, myasthenia gravis, sleep apnea, severe hepatic impairment, and respiratory depression.
- Baclofen: known allergy, peptic ulcer, severe psychiatric disorders, epilepsy.
- Dantrolene: known allergy, active hepatic disease.
- Quinine: known allergy, glucose-6-phosphate dehydrogenase deficiency, myasthenia gravis, tinnitus, optic neuritis.
- Nitroglycerin: known allergy, marked anemia; silidenafil use is contraindicated.
- Oxybutynin: closed-angle glaucoma, gastrointestinal obstruction, paralytic ileus, colitis, myasthenia gravis, obstructive uropathy.

Doses and treatment paradigms

Diazepam

This drug (half-life 30–56 h) has a metabolically active metabolite with an even longer half-life of 3–4 days. The active metabolite accumulates in the body over time. Commence at 2 mg b.i.d. orally and increase slowly. Larger doses seem to be well tolerated in cancer patients.

Baclofen

Baclofen (half-life 3.5 h) is usually commenced at 5 mg t.i.d. orally and increased every 3 days to a maximum dose of 15 mg ti.d. It should be withdrawn slowly as abrupt cessation can result in agitation, delirium, and even convulsions.[174] The dose should be reduced slowly over 2 weeks. Intrathecal administration should be considered when oral doses exceed 100 mg.

Dantrolene

The starting dose of dantrolene (half-life 9 h) is 25 mg orally daily, and this can be gradually increased every 5–6 days to a maximum dose of 100 mg q.i.d. It has an specialized use in malignant hyperthermia, when it is administered by anesthetists and intensive care specialists at a dose of 1 mg/kg. A total dose of 10 mg/kg may eventually be required.

Quinine

The usual use of this drug (half-life 14 h) is to treat night cramps, when 300 mg *nocte* is administered. The use of quinine is questionable, but there are some patients who have convincing stories to relate about its effectiveness.

Nitroglycerin

Nitroglycerin (half-life 2.5 min) can be applied around the anus to act as a nitric oxide donor to mediate the anorectal inhibitory reflex. Pain relief is reported to last 4–6 h.[169] The amount of ointment applied is probably less than that required for the treatment of angina, in which case 1 cm of 2% nitroglycerin ointment applied topically is recommended.

Hyoscine hydrobromide

Hyoscine hydrobromide (half-life 2.5 h) is usually administered as an injection of 20 mg subcutaneously or as a continuous infusion in higher doses.

Oxybutynin

The usual dosage of oxybutynin (half-life < 2 h) is 2.5 mg b.i.d. orally, increasing to 5 mg t.i.d. It can also be used as an intravesical solution in a dose of 0.1 mg/kg twice daily for bladder spasm.

Side-effects and management

Diazepam

Excessive drowsiness necessitates a reduction in dose. Infrequent side-effects include headache, vertigo, dizziness, delirium, paradoxical excitation and hostility, and very rarely blood disorders, e.g. leukopenia. The essential strategy is to cease the drug. A competitive antagonist, flumazenil, can reverse the effects of diazepam in the event of benzodiazepine intoxication. However, this drug has only a short effect.

Baclofen

This drug commonly causes gastrointestinal upsets and may cause delirium and muscle weakness. Rarely, it causes ataxia, depression, deterioration in liver function, and a paradoxical spasticity. The effective use of this agent necessitates low doses initially with gradual increases and clinical monitoring to observe for side-effects.

Dantrolene

Side-effects usually occur shortly after starting treatment and are normally short-lived. They include drowsiness, malaise, muscle weakness, and troublesome diarrhea, but central nervous system side-effects are generally fewer than with baclofen. Urinary retention, dyspnea, and headache may be the result of excessive dose. Commence at low doses and increase gradually. Rarely, this drug can cause severe liver toxicity,[175] usually in subjects older than 30.

Quinine

Evidence of diminished visual acuity (optic neuritis), tinnitus, or anemia necessitates the immediate cessation of the drug. Evidence of hemolysis requires specialist hematological advice and management.

Glyceryl trinitrate

The main side-effect here is headache as a result of vascular dilation.

Hyoscine butylbromide

The advantage of this drug is it does not cross the blood–brain barrier, and therefore central nervous system side-effects are limited compared with its relative hyoscine hydrobromide.

Oxybutynin

Like hyoscine, this drug is also an anticholinergic, but it causes more central effects. The usual anticholinergic side-effects of dry mouth, blurred vision, confusion, and urinary difficulties are all dose related and can be minimized if the drug is used carefully.

Pharmaceutical considerations

These have been largely covered in the preceding sections.

Practical tips

An important principle is to commence at a low dose and titrate the dose slowly according to response and the presence of side-effects.

Efficacy

These agents are usually helpful but it is often difficult to assess their efficacy, particularly in patients with advanced cancer.

Key points

- Careful history-taking is essential for detecting symptoms resulting from muscle spasms.
- Commence all muscle relaxants at a low dose.
- Withdraw baclofen and benzodiazepines *slowly* over 2 weeks to avoid side-effects.
- Monitor liver function for patients on dantrolene.

Evidence for particular drugs

*All muscle relaxants.

N-methyl-D-aspartate (NMDA) receptor blockers

Lipton and Rosenberg[176] suggest that the excitatory amino acids glutamate and aspartate are important in the development of plasticity in the central nervous system. They explain that there are two main types of receptors that may be stimulated by these excitatory amino acids – ionotropic receptors (associated with membrane ion channels) and metabotropic receptors (associated with G-proteins, which result in second-messenger activity within the cell). The NMDA receptor is one of the ionotropic receptors, and overstimulation of this receptor (normally blocked by a plug of magnesium) has been implicated in the state of central sensitization. The NMDA receptor is also involved in memory,[177,178] motor activity,[179] visual development,[180–182] and epilepsy,[183,184] thus explaining the diverse range of side-effects of NMDA receptor blockers. A recent review[185] of neuropathic pain mechanisms emphasizes the role of the NMDA receptor. Central sensitization can be attenuated by the use of NMDA antagonists, which abolish pain hypersensitivity in patients with neuropathic pain. The NMDA receptor has been intensively studied over the last 15 years because of its role in central sensitization.[184,186–191] Research has suggested that blockade of this receptor is an effective strategy in the prevention of central sensitization, also known as "windup."[192] The administration of an NMDA antagonist may reverse opioid tolerance.[193] The noncompetitive NMDA antagonists ketamine[194–204] and dextromethorphan[205–211] have attracted much interest resulting in clinical application. Ketamine has been administered intravenously and subcutaneously as well as orally.[194,212–217] More recently, it has become apparent that some opioids, e.g. the D-isomer of methadone, have the ability to block NMDA receptors, as do other drugs, e.g. nonsteroidal anti-inflammatory drugs.[218–221] Ketamine is used to relieve cancer pain,[203,204] particularly in patients receiving palliative care. The administration of dextromethorphan has also been attempted but with less consistent results.[205,211]

Indications

NMDA blockers are indicated in patients with neuropathic pain.

Contraindications

The only contraindication is a known hypersensitivity to the drug.

Doses and treatment paradigms

Ketamine (half-life 3 h) is metabolized by the liver. It is generally commenced at a low dose and the dose slowly increased because of the frequency of adverse effects experienced by some patients. Ketamine has been administered by subcutaneous, oral, and intravenous routes. The subcutaneous route is most commonly used in palliative care settings; however, this may evolve with time. Recommended adult starting doses are

- 0.1 mg/kg/h subcutaneously;
- 30 mg i.v. in 500 ml of normal saline over 3 h;
- 10 mg orally up to q.i.d.

These doses are similar to those suggested by Portenoy,[222] who proposed 0.1–0.15 mg/kg/h for palliative care patients. Quite high subcutaneous doses (>2,000 mg daily) have been used.[223] Oral administration has been described with doses of up to 200 mg four times daily.[203] Prolonged oral use has also been reported in doses of 100–240 mg daily.[194] The drug has also been administered by the epidural route.[224]

Dextromethorphan is administered orally at an initial dose of 45–60 mg daily, increasing to a maximum dose of 1,000 mg daily if side-effects are acceptable.[222]

Side-effects and management

Side-effects are dose related,[225] and at low doses are much less of a problem than were experienced with ketamine anesthesia in the past. However, in our experience patients may complain of vivid dreams, which can be severe enough to warrant dose reduction. Twycross *et al.*[57] report that the incidence of adverse effects in patients receiving a continuous subcutaneous infusion of ketamine is 40%. Usually, ketamine is administered with midazolam in an effort to limit these side-effects following on from the experiences in pediatric anesthesia and painful pediatric procedures.[226–228] The doses of midazolam are in the range of 5–10 mg/24 h as a continuous subcutaneous infusion. Haloperidol is an alternative to midazolam.

Pharmaceutical considerations

This drug is available only as a solution for injection, but the same solution can be given orally.[212] When administered orally, it is more extensively metabolized by the liver than after i.v. administration, and this results in greater amounts of the active metabolite norketamine. This is less potent than the parent substance (30%).[229,230]

The solution can be quite irritant to the tissues when administered by continuous subcutaneous infusion, and maximal dilution with saline is advisable.

Ketamine is compatible with morphine and midazolam when mixed in the same syringe for use in an infusion pump.[57] Its oral availability is 20–30%. It has a half-life of 2–3 h and is only 12% protein bound.[38]

Practical tips

Use in a continuous subcutaneous infusion. Dilute the solution with saline as much as possible. Commence at a low dose and increase gradually. Bolus injection may produce unacceptable side-effects. A different approach, using a "burst" ketamine technique, has recently been described by Jackson *et al.*[230a]

Efficacy

The effects are often unpredictable, probably because there may be a mixed nociceptive–neuropathic pain component.

Key points

- Ketamine, an NMDA receptor antagonist, has an established role in the management of neuropathic pain.
- The drug is usually administered by continuous subcutaneous infusion and less often by mouth.
- The coadministration of midazolam in a continuous subcutaneous infusion is useful to prevent adverse effects of vivid dreams, etc.

Evidence for particular drugs

**Ketamine.
*Dextromethorphan.

MISCELLANEOUS DRUGS

This group includes a number of drugs which have had limited application. In certain circumstances they may be particularly useful. The following list is not exhaustive.

- drugs associated with calcium metabolism –calcitonin and bisphosphonates (pamidronate, clodronate);
- calcium channel blockers – nifedipine, nimodipine;
- capsaicin.

Drugs associated with calcium metabolism – calcitonin and bisphosphonates (pamidronate, clodronate)

Calcitonin is an endogenous polypeptide hormone released by the parafollicular C-cells of the thyroid, parathyroid, and thymus glands (Ref. 38, p. 1507). Along with parathyroid hormone, which is released by the parathyroid gland, calcitonin is involved with the regulation of plasma calcium.[16] Calcitonin theoretically lowers serum calcium by reducing calcium absorption from the gut, increasing renal clearance, and inhibiting osteoclast activity. However, in humans the amount of calcitonin released does not appear to be sufficient to lower serum calcium,[231] and its precise role in calcium metabolism is not clear. If calcitonin is administered in larger amounts to patients with Paget's disease or osteoporosis, bone resorption is curtailed.

Whether calcitonin has a specific role in the prevention of pain transmission is uncertain. Guidobono and co-workers[232–234] investigated the action of calcitonin within the central nervous system, demonstrating the existence of many binding sites. It was also suggested that catecholamines might be associated with its action.[232] There have been a number of reports that calcitonin has a role in the management of patients with generalized cancer pain,[235] pain due to osteolytic lesions from breast cancer,[236] phantom limb pain,[237,238] reflex sympathetic dystrophy and causalgia (now known as complex regional pain syndrome),[239] and pain associated with hypercalcemia of malignancy.[240] Apart from its effect on bone, the mechanism of action of calcitonin as an analgesic is still not clear. In the management of bone pain it has largely been replaced by the bisphosphonates. Lowering raised serum calcium levels often seems to re-establish effective pain management in cancer patients.[241]

The bisphosphonates have now become the major pharmacological weapon used in the management of hypercalcemia of malignancy and in the management of bone pain *per se*. They act as potent inhibitors of osteoclastic bone resorption. The bisphosphonates differ from each other according to the side-chains attached to the basic molecular structure of phosphorus–carbon–phosphorus,[242] with very powerful third-generation drugs now becoming available. Recent reviews[243,244] indicate that the bisphosphonates represent a major therapeutic advance in the management of the skeletal morbidity caused by metastatic breast cancer or multiple myeloma and are the standard treatment for tumor-associated hypercalcemia. These drugs slow down the progression of disease, have analgesic effects, and they improve the quality of life for patients. There is evidence that the intravenous formulation, pamidronate, is more effective than oral clodronate.[245,246] High doses of pamidronate seem to be very effective in relieving painful bone metastases.[247] There is a suggestion that the bisphosphonates have a direct antineoplastic effect by inducing neoplastic cell apoptosis.[248] There has been a clear demonstration of the effectiveness of these agents in metastatic bone disease of breast cancer[249,250] and multiple myeloma.[251] There is also evidence for the use of bisphosphonates in prostate cancer,[252] and the results of definitive trials are awaited. In a report of three cases, pamidronate was reported to be effective in relieving resistant bone pain associated with hypertrophic pulmonary osteoarthropathy.[253]

Indications

Indications for these drugs include:

- multiple myeloma;
- metastatic bone disease in breast cancer;
- possibly prostate cancer;
- tumor-induced hypercalcemia.

Contraindications

Known hypersensitivity is the only contraindication.

Doses and treatment paradigms

Pamidronate

The usual dosage is 90 mg by slow i.v. infusion in saline (over 4 h) for the average adult with a frequency of once every 4 weeks.[37] Pamidronate should *never* be given as a bolus.

Clodronate

The usual dose is 300 mg by slow i.v. infusion diluted with saline (over 4 h). It can also be given orally in a dose of 2,400–3,200 mg daily to treat hypercalcemia and then reduced to 1,600 mg daily as a maintenance dose to maintain serum calcium at normal levels.

Side-effects and management

Pyrexia for 48 h associated with flu-like symptoms, transient bone pain, nausea, and headache are the main side-effects. Hypocalcemia may occur, as evidenced by hypotension, tetany, and paresthesias, and can be readily treated with the infusion of calcium gluconate.

Pharmaceutical considerations[37]

The half-life of pamidronate in the plasma is about 0.8 h. Approximately 50% of the infused material remains in the skeleton for years. After infusion, about 20–55% of the dose is recovered in the urine within 72 h. There is no hepatic or renal transformation. The oral preparation of clodronate should be taken on an empty stomach in the morning and never with milk, and an interval of 2 h should be allowed both before and after dosing. The oral absorption of clodronate is low (2%) and the half-life is in two phases. The distribution phase takes about 2 h and is followed by a very long second phase because of its intense binding to bone; the rate of this absorption phase is proportional to bone turnover.

Practical tips

There has been extensive experience in the use of bisphosphonates by hematologists and oncologists, and discussion with them is recommended for any patients under joint management.

Efficacy

Bisphosphonates have an established role in the management of bone pain associated with multiple myeloma and breast cancer and possibly also prostate cancer.

Key points

- Calcitonin has been largely replaced by the bisphosphonates in the management of bone pain associated with breast cancer and multiple myeloma and possibly prostate cancer.
- Intravenous infusion of pamidronate is more effective than oral bisphosphonates.
- Pamidronate is usually well tolerated in a dose of 90 mg infused in 500–1,000 ml of saline over 4 h.
- Mild pyrexia and flu-like symptoms are seen in up to 10% of patients.

Evidence for particular drugs

***Pamidronate, clodronate.

Calcium channel blockers – nifedipine, nimodipine

Calcium channel blockers block the inward current of calcium into cells and are used in the treatment of angina, arrhythmias (particularly paroxysmal supraventricular atrial tachycardia), hypertension, and, less commonly, migraine, Raynaud's phenomenon, and hemorrhagic cerebral vasospasm.[254] Birdsey *et al.* list four classes:

- dihydropyridines (nifedipine, nimodipine);
- benzothiapines (diltiazem);
- phenylalkylamines (verapamil)
- T-type calcium channel blockers (mibefradil).

Since the mid-1980s there has been interest in the role of calcium channel blockers in the control of pain.[255,256] It has been suggested[257–259] that nimodipine, a dihydropyridine calcium channel blocker, suppresses electrically induced seizures in the rabbit and that calcium influx into neurons is related to seizure activity. It was also suggested that centrally acting calcium channel blockers might have an application as anticonvulsants. Contreras *et al.*[260] argued that these drugs may enhance the effect of morphine and reduce morphine tolerance. Miranda *et al.*[261] suggested that a drug with a calcium blocking effect therefore probably has an analgesic effect. Although Roca *et al.*[262] showed that nimodipine fails to enhance the analgesic effects of morphine in the early phases of morphine treatment, Santillan *et al.*[263] showed that the use of nimodipine in patients chronically treated with morphine attenuates the development of morphine tolerance. This effect supports the accepted belief that increased calcium uptake is involved in the development of opioid tolerance. Nifedipine has also been used successfully in patients with pain related to muscle spasm, e.g. proctalgia fugax,[264] tenesmus,[265] intractable hiccups with concurrent administration of fludrocortisone to limit hypotension,[266] esophageal spasm,[267] and in patients with pain possibly resulting from vascular mechanisms, e.g. multiple leiomyomas[268] and melorheostosis, a painful sclerotic dysplasia of bone.[256]

Indications

Nimodipine has a specific indication in subarachnoid hemorrhage to limit cerebral damage by dilating cerebral blood vessels, but it may also have a role in pain management to limit tolerance and prevent opioid dose escalation.

Nifedipine has a role in pain management in the treatment of painful muscle spasms, e.g. tenesmus and esophageal spasm, and is an alternative to glyceryl trinitrate.

Contraindications

Obviously, these drugs are not to be used in patients with cardiogenic instability, and their use in patients with advanced cancer needs to be carefully considered.

Doses and treatment paradigms

Nimodipine has been used to limit opioid tolerance in a dose of 30 mg four times daily for 4 weeks.[263] Nifedipine has been used to relieve muscle spasm in doses of 10 mg *stat* followed by 10–20 mg three times daily with or after food, with a maximum dose of 60–80 mg daily.[57]

Side-effects and management

Fludrocortisone has been used to counter the side-effects of high-dose nifidepine for intractable hiccups.[266] The main side-effects[254] include bradycardia, headache, flushing, edema, and raised liver enzymes; rash, nausea, and vomiting are other side-effects. Management consists initially in circulatory support, followed by the reduction of dosage or even cessation of the drug.

Pharmaceutical considerations[16]

Nifedipine has a half-life of 2–5 h and nimodipine 1–2 h. Both are rapidly absorbed from the gut and undergo extensive first-pass metabolism in the liver, resulting in an oral bioavailability of 45–75% for nifedipine and 13% for nimodipine. Peak blood concentrations for nifedipine are achieved between 1 and 2 h. Both are 95–97% protein bound. Nimodipine readily crosses the blood–brain barrier.

Practical tips[16]

Beware of the extensive drug interactions with calcium channel blockers, e.g. digoxin, cimetidine, and sodium valproate, which raise plasma levels, and hepatic enzyme inducers, e.g. carbamazepine and phenytoin, which lower plasma levels. Alpha-blockers and beta-blockers may increase the risk of hypotension and heart failure. Concurrent use with i.v. dantrolene may cause atrial fibrillation.

Efficacy

Nimodipine has a limited application in opioid tolerance, but nifedipine is worth considering in the management of muscle spasm pain.

Key points

- Multiple drug interactions may occur.
- Calcium channel blockers are useful in muscle spasm painful states (nifedipine).
- These drugs have a possible use in limiting the development of opioid tolerance.

Evidence for particular drugs

**Nifedipine.
*Nimodipine.

Capsaicin

Capsaicin is the main component of red pepper and is administered as a topical cream for various painful states, e.g. diabetic neuropathy[269–271] and postherpetic neuralgia.[272] A meta-analysis[273] has demonstrated its effectiveness in diabetic neuropathy and osteoarthritis. It has also been suggested as an option for the management of neurogenic bladder by diminishing bladder sensitivity to various stimuli causing blockade at the afferent level rather than using anticholinergics to block the efferent pathways to the bladder.[274–276] Capsaicin has been studied extensively over the last 15 years both as an analgesic and as a research tool in the investigation of the mechanisms of painful states.[275–289] It acts by antagonizing the effects of one or more neuropeptides involved in peripheral sensitization, e.g. by affecting the synthesis, storage, transport, and release of substance P. In the recent past, the receptor for capsaicin, known as the vanilloid receptor (VR1), has been identified and is thought to be involved in the activation and sensitization of nociceptors.[290] Capsaicin application causes the release of substance P, which results in its main adverse effect, a burning sensation at the site of application. However, continued use causes depletion of substance P and the burning sensation becomes less and less of a problem as the treatment continues. As substance P is depleted there is a reduction in pain transmission and analgesia increases. Research is hampered by the difficulty of conducting blind trials due to the burning sensation of this compound following application. Shuster[291] has claimed that the pain produced after application of capsaicin cream is identical to that experienced by patients with a diagnosis of causalgia.

Indications

The use of capsaicin in cancer-related pain is limited to coexisting conditions such as those mentioned above, most notably diabetic neuropathy and postherpetic neuralgia.

Contraindications

Hypersensitivity to capsaicin is the only contraindication.

Doses and treatment paradigms

Capsaicin is available as 0.025% and 0.075% cream. For specific conditions it is applied at least three times daily.

Side-effects and management

Burning sensation in the skin after application is the main problem and this can be lessened by an initial application of a topical local anesthetic cream for the initial applications, e.g. EMLA cream. EMLA (eutectic mixture of local anesthetics) is a 1:1 oil–water misture of lidocaine (lignocaine) and prilocaine.

Pharmaceutical considerations

Capsaicin is available as a topical agent only.

Practical tips

Prior application of EMLA cream or amethocaine gel may be appropriate to encourage patient compliance for the first few applications.

Efficacy

Capsaicin is effective in the treatment of diabetic neuropathy and postherpetic neuralgia

Key points

- Patients need to be well informed about the side-effect of a burning sensation after application.

Evidence for particular drugs

***Capsaicin.

REFERENCES

● 1. Schug SA, Dunlop R, Zech D. Pharmacological management of cancer pain. *Drugs* 1992; **43 (1):** 44–53.

● 2. De Conno F, Ripamonti C, Sbanotto A, *et al.* The pharmacological management of cancer pain. Part 1: The role of non opioid and adjuvant drugs. *Ann Oncol* 1993; **4 (3):** 187–93.

● 3. Portenoy RK. Pharmacologic management of cancer pain. *Semin Oncol* 1995; **22** (2 Suppl. 3): 112–20.

● 4. Cherny NI, Portenoy RK. The management of cancer pain. *CA: Cancer J Clinicians* 1994; **44:** 263–303.

● 5. Cherny NI, Portenoy RK. Cancer pain management. Current strategy. *Cancer* 1993; **72** (11 Suppl.): 3393–415.

● 6. Portenoy RK. Cancer pain management. *Semin Oncol* 1993; **20** (2 Suppl. 1): 19–35.

● 7. Portenoy RK. Pain management in the older cancer patient. *Oncology* 1992; **6** (2 Suppl.): 86–98.

8. World Health Organization. *Cancer Pain Relief and Palliative Care*. Technical Report Series No. 804. Geneva: World Health Organization, 1986, 1990.

9. IASP S-CoT. Classification of chronic pain. *Pain* 1986; Suppl. 3: 216–21.

10. Desbiens A, Mueller-Rizner N, Connors A, Wenger N. The relationship of nausea and dyspnoea to pain in seriously ill patients. *Pain* 1997; **71:** 149–56.

● 11. Virani A, Mailis A, Shapiro LE, Shear NH. Drug interactions in human neuropathic pain pharmacotherapy. *Pain* 1997; **73:** 3–13.

● 12. Grond S, Radbruch L, Meuser T, *et al*. Assessment and treatment of neuropathic cancer pain following WHO guidelines. *Pain* 1999; **79:** 15–20.

13. Aho MS, Erkola OA, Scheinin H, *et al*. Effect of intravenously administered dexmedetomidine on pain after laparoscopic tubal ligation. *Anesth Analges* 1991; **73:** 112–18.

● 14. Tranquilli WJ, Benson GJ. Advantages and guidelines for using alpha-2 agonists as anesthetic adjuvants. *Vet Clin N Am – Small Animal Practice* 1992; **22:** 289–93.

15. Ferguson R, Vlasses P. Hypertensive emergencies. *JAMA* 1986; **255:** 1607–13.

16. Reynolds J, Parfitt K, Parsons A, Sweetman S eds. *Martindale: The Extra Pharmacopoeia,* 13th edn. London: Pharmaceutical Press, 1993.

17. Tamsen A, Gordh T. Epidural clonidine produces analgesia. *Lancet* 1984; **2:** 231–2.

18. Puke MJ, Wiesenfeld-Hallin Z. The differential effects of morphine and the alpha 2-adrenoceptor agonists clonidine and dexmedetomidine on the prevention and treatment of experimental neuropathic pain. *Anesth Analg* 1993; **77:** 104–9.

● 19. Yaksh TL. Pharmacology of spinal adrenergic systems which modulate spinal nociceptive processing. *Pharmacol Biochem Behav* 1985; **22:** 845–58.

20. Sagen J, Proudfit H. Evidence for pain modulation by pre- and postsynaptic noradrenergic receptors in the medulla oblongata. *Brain Res* 1985; **331:** 285–93.

21. Yaksh TL, Reddy SV. Studies in the primate on the analgesic effects associated with intrathecal actions of opiates, alpha-adrenergic agonists and baclofen. *Anesthesiology* 1981; **54:** 451–67.

22. Byas-Smith MG, Max MB, Muir J, Kingman A. Transdermal clonidine compared to placebo in painful diabetic neuropathy using a two-stage "enriched enrollment" design. *Pain* 1995; **60:** 267–74.

23. Eisenach JC, DuPen S, Dubois M, *et al*. Epidural clonidine analgesia for intractable cancer pain. The Epidural Clonidine Study Group. *Pain* 1995; **61:** 391–9.

24. Pan H, Chen S, Eisenach J. Intrathecal clonidine alleviates allodynia in neuropathic rats: interaction with spinal muscarinic and nicotinic receptors. *Anesthesiology* 1999; **90:** 509–14.

25. Gentili M, Juhel A, Bonnet F. Peripheral analgesic effect of intra-articular clonidine. *Pain* 1996; **64:** 593–6.

◆ 26. Glynn C, O'Sullivan K. A double-blind randomised comparison of the effects of epidural clonidine, lignocaine and the combination of clonidine and lignocaine in patients with chronic pain. *Pain* 1996; **64:** 337–43.

27. Kayser V, Desmeules J, Guilbaud G. Systemic clonidine differentially modulates the abnormal reactions to mechanical and thermal stimuli in rats with peripheral mononeuropathy. *Pain* 1995; **60:** 275–85.

28. Middleton J, Siddall P, Walker S, *et al*. Intrathecal clonidine and baclofen in the management of spasticity and neuropathic pain following spinal cord injury: a case study. *Arch Phys Med Rehabil* 1996; **77:** 824–6.

28a. Khan Z, Ferguson, C, Jones R. Alpha-2 and imidazoline receptor agonists. Their pharmacology and therapeutic role. *Anaesthesia* 1999; **54:** 14–65.

◆ 29. Tumber PS, Fitzgibbon DR. The control of severe cancer pain by continuous intrathecal infusion and patient controlled intrathecal analgesia with morphine, bupivacaine and clonidine. *Pain* 1998; **78:** 217–20.

30. Mercadante S, Serretta R, Sapio M, *et al*. When all else fails: stepwise multiple solutions for a complex cancer pain syndrome. *Support Care Cancer* 1999; **7:** 47–50.

31. Swain R. Oral clonidine for proctalgia fugax. *Gut* 1987; **28:** 1039–40.

32. Glynn C, Dawson D, Sanders R. A double-blind comparison between epidural morphine and epidural clonidine in patients with chronic non-cancer pain. *Pain* 1988; **34:** 123–8.

33. Petros AJ, Wright RM. Epidural and oral clonidine in domiciliary control of deafferentation pain [letter]. *Lancet* 1987; **1:** 1034.

34. Gold MS, Redmond DE, Jr, Kleber HD. Clonidine in opiate withdrawal [letter]. *Lancet* 1978; **1:** 929–30.

35. Gold MS, Redmond DE, Jr, Kleber HD. Clonidine blocks acute opiate-withdrawal symptoms. *Lancet* 1978; **2:** 599–602.

36. Russell S, Doyle E. Recent advances: paediatric anaesthesia. *Br Med J* 1997; **314:** 201–3.

37. Caswell A ed. *MIMS Annual*, 23rd edn, Australian Edition. Sydney: MIMS Annual, 1999.

38. Goodman LS, Gillman AG, Nies A, Taylor P eds. *Goodman and Gillman's The Pharmacological Basis of Therapeutics*, 8th edn. New York, NY: Pergamon Press, 1990.

39. Bonnet F, Boico O, Rostaing S, *et al*. Postoperative analgesia with extradural clonidine. *Br J Anaesth* 1989; **63:** 465–9.

40. Bonnet F, Boico O, Rostaing S, *et al*. Clonidine-induced analgesia in postoperative patients: epidural versus intramuscular administration. *Anesthesiology* 1990; **72:** 423–7.

● 41. Mercadante S. Neuraxial techniques for cancer pain: an ◆ opinion about unresolved therapeutic dilemmas. *Regional Anesth Pain Med* 1999; **24:** 74–83.

42. Arthurson J, Gould M. Anaesthetics. In: Misan G, Bochner F eds. *Australian Medicines Handbook*. Adelaide: Australian Medicines Handbook; 1998: 2.1–2.5.

43. Bach FW, Jensen TS, Kastrup J, *et al*. The effect of intravenous lidocaine on nociceptive processing in diabetic neuropathy *Pain* 1990; **40:** 29–34.

44. Baranowski AP, De Courcey J, Bonello E. A trial of intravenous lidocaine on the pain and allodynia of postherpetic neuralgia. *J Pain Symptom Manage* 1999; **17:** 429–33.

45. Ferrante FM, Paggioli J, Cherukuri S, Arthur GR. The analgesic response to intravenous lidocaine in the treatment of neuropathic pain. *Anesth Analges* 1996; **82:** 91–7.

46. Kastrup J, Bach FW, Petersen P, *et al*. Lidocaine treatment of painful diabetic neuropathy and endogenous opioid peptides in plasma. *Clin J Pain* 1989; **5:** 239–44.

47. Linchitz RM, Raheb JC. Subcutaneous infusion of lidocaine provides effective pain relief for CRPS patients. *Clin J Pain* 1999; **15:** 67–72.

48. Wallace MS, Dyck JB, Rossi SS, Yaksh TL. Computer-controlled lidocaine infusion for the evaluation of neuropathic pain after peripheral nerve injury. *Pain* 1996; **66:** 69–77.

49. Woolf C, Wiesenfeld-Hallin Z. The systemic administration of local anaesthetics produces a selective depression of C-afferent fibre evoked activity in the spinal cord. *Pain* 1985; **23:** 361–74.

50. Boas R, Covino B, Shahnarian A. Analgesic responses to i.v. lignocaine. *Br J Anaesth* 1982; **54:** 501–505.

51. Tanelian DL, MacIver MB. Analgesic concentrations of lidocaine suppress tonic A-delta and C fiber discharges produced by acute injury. *Anesthesiology* 1991; **74:** 934–6.

52. Tanelian DL, Brose WG. Neuropathic pain can be relieved by drugs that are use-dependent sodium channel blockers: lidocaine, carbamazepine, and mexiletine. *Anesthesiology* 1991; **74:** 949–51.

53. Ellemann K, Sjogren P, Banning A, *et al*. Trial of intravenous lidocaine on painful neuropathy in cancer patients. *Clin J Pain* 1989; **5:** 291–4.

54. Anonymous. Flecainide in cancer nerve pain [letter; comment]. *Lancet* 1991; **337:** 1347.

55. Anonymous. Preliminary report: effect of encainide and flecainide on mortality in a randomized trial of arrhythmia suppression after myocardial infarction. The Cardiac Arrhythmia Suppression Trial (CAST) Investigators. *N Engl J Med* 1989; **321:** 406–12.

● 56. Portenoy RK. Adjuvant analgesic agents. *Hematol–Oncol Clin N Am* 1996; **10:** 103–19.

56a. Mao J, Chen L. Systemic lidocaine for neuropathic pain relief. *Pain* 2000; **87** (July): 7–17.

● 57. Twycross R, Wilcock A, Thorp S. *PCF1 Palliative Care Formulary*. Oxford: Radcliffe Medical Press, 1998.

58. Chong SF, Bretscher ME, Mailliard JA, *et al*. Pilot study evaluating local anesthetics administered systemically for treatment of pain in patients with advanced cancer. *J Pain Symptom Manage* 1997; **13:** 112–17.

59. Higa K, Hirata K, Dan K. Mexiletine-induced severe skin eruption, fever, eosinophilia, atypical lymphocytosis, and liver dysfunction. *Pain* 1997; **73:** 97–9.

60. Bennett MI. Paranoid psychosis due to flecainide toxicity in malignant neuropathic pain. *Pain* 1997; **70:** 93–4.

61. Lie AHL, Proost JH, Kingma JH, Meijer DK. Absorption kinetics of oral and rectal flecainide in healthy subjects. *Eur J Clin Pharmacol* 1990; **38:** 595–8.

● 62. McQuay H, Carroll D, Jadad A, *et al*. Anticonvulsant ◆ drugs for management of pain: a systematic review. *Br Med J* 1995; **311:** 1047–1052.

63. Attal N, Brasseur L, Parker F, *et al*. Effects of gabapentin on the different components of peripheral and central neuropathic pain syndromes: a pilot study. *Eur Neurol* 1998; **40:** 191–200.

64. Rowbotham M, Harden N, Stacey B, *et al*. Gabapentin for the treatment of postherpetic neuralgia: a randomized controlled trial *JAMA* 1998; **280:** 1837–42.

65. Backonja M, Beydoun A, Edwards KR, *et al*. Gabapentin for the symptomatic treatment of painful neuropathy in patients with diabetes mellitus: a randomized controlled trial. *JAMA* 1998; **280:** 1831–6.

66. Merren MD. Gabapentin for treatment of pain and tremor: a large case series. *Southern Med J* 1998; **91:** 739–44.

67. Wetzel CH, Connelly JF. Use of gabapentin in pain management. *Ann Pharmacother* 1997; **31:** 1082–3.

68. Rosner H, Rubin L, Kestenbaum A. Gabapentin adjunctive therapy in neuropathic pain states. *Clin J Pain* 1996; **12:** 56–8.

69. Nakamura-Craig M, Follenfant RL. Effect of lamotrigine in the acute and chronic hyperalgesia induced by PGE2 and in the chronic hyperalgesia in rats with streptozotocin-induced diabetes. *Pain* 1995; **63:** 33–7.

70. Hunter JC, Gogas KR, Hedley LR, *et al*. The effect of novel anti-epileptic drugs in rat experimental models of acute and chronic pain. *Eur J Pharmacol* 1997; **324:** 153–60.

71. Harbison J, Dennehy F, Keating D. Lamotrigine for pain with hyperalgesia. *Irish Med J* 1997; **90:** 56.

72. Canavero S, Bonicalzi V. Lamotrigine control of central pain. *Pain* 1996; **68:** 179–81.

73. Berde C. New and old anticonvulsants for management of pain. *IASP Newsletter* 1997 (Jan–Feb): 3–5.

● 74. Macdonald RL, Kelly KM. Antiepileptic drug mechanisms of action. *Epilepsia* 1995; **36** (Suppl. 2): S2–12.

75. Berkovic S, Eadie M, Fung V, *et al*. Neurological drugs – antiepileptics. In: Misan G, Bochner F eds. *Australian Medicines Handbook*. Adelaide: Australian Medicines Handbook; 1998: 16.2–16.18.

● 76. Macdonald RL, Kelly KM. Mechanisms of action of currently prescribed and newly developed antiepileptic drugs. *Epilepsia* 1994; **35** (Suppl. 4): S41–50.

●76a. Rose M, Kam C. Gabapentin: pharmacology and its use ◆ in pain management. *Anaesthesia* 2002; **57:** 451–62.

● 77. Nurmikko TJ, Nash TP, Wiles JR. Recent advances: ◆ control of chronic pain. *Br Med J* 1998; **317:** 1438–41.

78. Zakrzewska JM, Chaudhry Z, Nurmikko TJ, *et al.* Lamotrigine (lamictal) in refractory trigeminal neuralgia: results from a double-blind placebo controlled crossover trial. *Pain* 1997; **73:** 223–30.

79. Brodie M, Dichter M. Drug therapy: antiepileptic drugs. *N Engl J Med* 1996; **334:**168–75.

80. Dichter M, Brodie M. Drug therapy: new antiepileptic drugs. *N Engl J Med* 1996; **334:** 1583–90.

81. Snare A, Tett S, Kaye K, Lickiss N. Retrospective analysis of neuropathic pain control in patients with advanced cancer. *J Pharmacy Technol* 1993; **9** (May/June): 114–17.

82. McCleane G. 200mg of Lamotrigine has no analgesic effect in neuropathic pain: a randomized, double blind, placebo controlled trial. *Pain* 1999; **83:** 105–7.

83. Fu C, Katzman M, Goldbloom D. Valproate/nortriptyline interaction [letter]. *J Clin Psychopharmacol* 1994; **14:** 205–6.

● 84. Andrews CO, Fischer JH. Gabapentin: a new agent for the management of epilepsy. *Ann Pharmacother* 1994; **28:** 1188–96.

85. Gould H. Gabapentin induced polyneuropathy. *Pain* 1998; **74:** 341–3.

86. Andersen BB, Mikkelsen M, Vesterager A, *et al.* No influence of the antidepressant paroxetine on carbamazepine, valproate and phenytoin. *Epilepsy Res* 1991; **10:** 201–4.

87. Eke T, Talbot J, Lawden M. Severe persistent visual field constriction associated with vigabatrin. *Br Med J* 1997; **314:** 180.

87a. Rice A, Maton S, Group PNAS. Gabapentin in postherpetic neuralgia: a randomised, double blind, placebo controlled study. *Pain* 2001; **94:** 215–24.

88. Bassett D, Braddon J, Hill R, *et al.* Psychotropics. In: Misan G, Bochner F eds. *Australian Medicines Handbook*. Adelaide: Australian Medicines Handbook; 1998: 18.1–18.36.

89. Walsh T. Antidepressants in chronic pain. *Clin Neuropharmacol* 1983; **6:** 271–95.

90. France R, Houpt J, Ellinwood E. Therapeutic effects of antidepressants in chronic pain. *Gen Hosp Psychiatry* 1984; **6:** 55–63.

91. Clifford D. Treatment of pain with antidepressants. *Am Family Phys* 1985; **31:** 181–5.

● 92. Feinmann C. Pain relief by antidepressants: possible modes of action. *Pain* 1985; **23:** 1–8.

● 93. Stimmel GL, Escobar JI. Antidepressants in chronic pain: a review of efficacy. *Pharmacotherapy* 1986; **6:** 262–7.

94. Magni G, Arsie D, De Leo D. Antidepressants in the treatment of cancer pain. A survey in Italy. *Pain* 1987; **29:** 347–53.

95. Ventafridda V, Bonezzi C, Caraceni A, *et al.* Antidepressants for cancer pain and other painful syndromes with deafferentation component: comparison of amitriptyline and trazodone. *Ital J Neurol Sci* 1987; **8:** 579–87.

● 96. France RD. The future for antidepressants: treatment of pain. *Psychopathology* 1987; **20** (Suppl. 1): 99–113.

● 97. Getto CJ, Sorkness CA, Howell T. Issues in drug management. Part I. Antidepressants and chronic nonmalignant pain: a review. *J Pain Symptom Manage* 1987; **2:** 9–18.

98. Ventafridda V, Ripamonti C, De Conno F, *et al.* Antidepressants increase bioavailability of morphine in cancer patients [letter]. *Lancet* 1987; **1:** 1204.

99. Harris M, Feinmann C. Tricyclic antidepressants and the treatment of facial pain. *TMJ Update* 1988; **6:** 65–8.

●100. Krishnan KR, France RD. Antidepressants in chronic pain syndromes. *Am Family Phys* 1989; **39:** 233–7.

101. Onghena P, Van Houdenhove B. Antidepressant-induced analgesia in chronic non-malignant pain: a meta-analysis of 39 placebo-controlled studies. *Pain* 1992; **49:** 205–19.

102. Ventafridda V, Bianchi M, Ripamonti C, *et al.* Studies on the effects of antidepressant drugs on the antinociceptive action of morphine and on plasma morphine in rat and man. *Pain* 1990; **43:** 155–62.

103. Watson CP, Chipman M, Reed K, *et al.* Amitriptyline versus maprotiline in postherpetic neuralgia: a randomized, double-blind, crossover trial. *Pain* 1992; **48:** 29–36.

104. Young RJ, Clarke BF. Pain relief in diabetic neuropathy: the effectiveness of imipramine and related drugs. *Diabetic Med* 1985; **2:** 363–6.

105. Max MB, Lynch SA, Muir J, *et al.* Effects of desipramine, amitriptyline, and fluoxetine on pain in diabetic neuropathy. *N Engl J Med* 1992; **326:** 1250–6.

106. Gomez-Perez FJ, Rull JA, Dies H, *et al.* Nortriptyline and fluphenazine in the symptomatic treatment of diabetic neuropathy. A double-blind cross-over study. *Pain* 1985; **23:** 395–400.

107. Gomez-Perez FJ, Choza R, Rios JM, *et al.* Nortriptyline-fluphenazine vs. carbamazepine in the symptomatic treatment of diabetic neuropathy. *Archiv Med Res* 1996; **27:** 525–9.

●108. Godfrey RG. A guide to the understanding and use of tricyclic antidepressants in the overall management of fibromyalgia and other chronic pain syndromes. *Archiv Intern Med* 1996; **156:** 1047–52.

●109. Philipp M, Fickinger M. Psychotropic drugs in the management of chronic pain syndromes. *Pharmacopsychiatry* 1993; **26:** 221–34.

110. Kurokawa K, Tanino R. Effectiveness of clomipramine for obsessive-compulsive symptoms and chronic pain in two patients with schizophrenia [letter]. *J Clin Psychopharmacol* 1997; **17:** 329–30.

111. Zitman F, Linssen A, Edelbroek P, Van Kempen G. Clinical effectiveness of antidepressants and antipsychotics in chronic benign pain. *Clin Neuropharmacol* 1992; **15** (Suppl. 1 Pt A): 377A–78A.

112. Vrethem M, Boivie J, Arnqvist H, *et al.* A comparison of amitriptyline and maprotiline in the treatment of painful polyneuropathy in diabetics and nondiabetics. *Clin J Pain* 1997; **13:** 313–23.

113. Ventafridda V, Caraceni A, Saita L, *et al.* Trazodone for deafferentation pain. Comparison with amitriptyline. *Psychopharmacology* 1988; **95** (Suppl.): S44–9.

114. Sandford PR, Lindblom LB, Haddox JD. Amitriptyline and carbamazepine in the treatment of dysesthetic pain in spinal cord injury. *Archiv Phys Med Rehabil* 1992; **73:** 300–1.

115. McQuay HJ, Carroll D, Glynn CJ. Dose–response for analgesic effect of amitriptyline in chronic pain. *Anaesthesia* 1993; **48:** 281–5.

116. McQuay HJ, Carroll D, Glynn CJ. Low dose amitriptyline in the treatment of chronic pain. *Anaesthesia* 1992; **47:** 646–52.

●117. Bryson HM, Wilde MI. Amitriptyline. A review of its pharmacological properties and therapeutic use in chronic pain states. *Drugs Aging* 1996; **8:** 459–76.

118. Brenne E, van der Hagen K, Maehlum E, Husebo S. Treatment chronic pain with amitriptyline. A double-blind dosage study with determination of serum levels [in Norwegian]. *Tidsskrift for Den Norske Laegeforening* 1997; **117:** 3491–4.

●◆119. McQuay HJ, Tramer M, Nye BA, *et al.* A systematic review of antidepressants in neuropathic pain. *Pain* 1996; **68:** 217–27.

●120. Magni G. The use of antidepressants in the treatment of chronic pain. A review of the current evidence. *Drugs* 1991; **42:** 730–48.

121. Panerai AE, Bianchi M, Sacerdote P, *et al.* Antidepressants in cancer pain. *J Palliative Care* 1991; **7:** 42–4.

●122. Cameron LB. Neuropsychotropic drugs as adjuncts in the treatment of cancer pain. *Oncology* 1992; **6:** 65–72; discussion **72:** 77–80.

●123. McKay WR. Pain management for urological malignancies. *Urol Int* 1991; **46:** 252–8.

124. Max MB, Culnane M, Schafer SC, *et al.* Amitriptyline relieves diabetic neuropathy pain in patients with normal or depressed mood. *Neurology* 1987; **37:** 589–96.

125. Sindrup SH, Bjerre U, Dejgaard A, *et al.* The selective serotonin reuptake inhibitor citalopram relieves the symptoms of diabetic neuropathy. *Clin Pharmacol Ther* 1992; **52:** 547–52.

126. Sindrup SH, Gram LF, Brosen K, *et al* The selective serotonin reuptake inhibitor paroxetine is effective in the treatment of diabetic neuropathy symptoms. *Pain* 1990; **42:** 135–44.

127. Zitman FG, Linssen AC, Edelbroek PM, Stijnen T. Low dose amitriptyline in chronic pain: the gain is modest. *Pain* 1990; **42:** 35–42.

128. Breitbart W, Rosenfeld B, Passik S, *et al.* A comparison of pain report and adequacy of analgesic therapy in ambulatory AIDS patients with and without a history of substance abuse. *Pain* 1997; **72:** 235–43.

●◆129. Sporer K. The serotonin syndrome. Implicated drugs, pathophysiology and management. *Drug Safety* 1995; **13:** 94–104.

130. Bristow M, Kohen D. How “malignant” is the neuroleptic malignant syndrome? *Br Med J* 1993; **307:** 1223–4.

●131. McQuay HM, RA. Antidepressants and chronic pain: effective analgesia in neuropathic pain and other syndromes [Editorial]. *Br Med J* 1997; **314:** 763–4.

132. Twycross R. Corticosteroids in advanced cancer [editorial; comment]. *Br Med J* 1992; **305:** 969–70.

●133. Ettinger AB, Portenoy RK. The use of corticosteroids in the treatment of symptoms associated with cancer. *J Pain Symptom Manage* 1988; **3:** 99–103.

●134. Oneschuk D, Bruera E. Palliative management of brain metastases. *Support Care Cancer* 1998; **6:** 365–72.

●135. Herrstedt J, Aapro MS, Smyth JF, Del Favero A. Corticosteroids, dopamine antagonists and other drugs. *Support Care Cancer* 1998; **6:** 204–14.

●136. Bruera E. Current pharmacological management of anorexia in cancer patients. *Oncology* 1992; **6:** 125–30; discussion 132, 137.

●137. Bruera E. Is the pharmacological treatment of cancer cachexia possible? *Support Care Cancer* 1993; **1:** 298–304.

●138. Vigano A, Watanabe S, Bruera E. Anorexia and cachexia in advanced cancer patients. *Cancer Surveys* 1994; **21:** 99–115.

●139. Aapro MS. Corticosteroids as antiemetics. *Recent Results Cancer Res* 1988; **108:** 102–11.

●140. Twycross R. The risks and benefits of corticosteroids in advanced cancer. *Drug Safety* 1994; **11:** 163–78.

141. Needham PR, Daley AG, Lennard RF. Steroids in advanced cancer: survey of current practice. *Br Med J* 1992; **305:** 999.

142. Sorensen S, Helweg-Larsen S, Mouridsen H, Hansen HH. Effect of high-dose dexamethasone in carcinomatous metastatic spinal cord compression treated with radiotherapy: a randomized trial. *Eur J Cancer* 1994; **30A:** 22–7.

143. Heimdal K, Hirschberg H, Slettebo H, *et al.* High incidence of serious side-effects of high-dose dexamethasone treatment in patients with epidural spinal cord compression. *J Neuro-oncol* 1992; **12:** 141–4.

144. Bowyer SL, LaMothe MP, Hollister JR. Steroid myopathy: incidence and detection in a population with asthma. *J Allergy Clin Immunol* 1985; **76** (2 Pt 1): 234–42.

◆145. Dekhuijzen P, Richard, Gayan-Ramirez G, *et al.* Triamcinolone and prednisolone affect contractile properties and histopathology of rat diaphragm differently. *J Clin Invest* 1993; **92:** 1534–42.

146. Patten S, Williams J, Love E. Self-reported depressive symptoms following treatment with corticosteroids

and sedative-hypnotics. *Int J Psychiatry Med* 1996; **26:** 15–24.

●147. Brown E, Suppes T. Mood symptoms during corticosteroid therapy: a review. *Harvard Rev Psychiatry* 1998; **5:** 239–46.

●148. Wolkowitz OM. Prospective controlled studies of the behavioral and biological effects of exogenous corticosteroids. *Psychoneuroendocrinology* 1994; **19:** 233–55.

●149. Chan JC, Cockram CS, Critchley JA. Drug-induced disorders of glucose metabolism. Mechanisms and management. *Drug Safety* 1996; **15:** 135–57.

150. Hanania NA, Chapman KR, Kesten SMD. Adverse effects of inhaled corticosteroids. *Am J Med* 1995; **98:** 196–208.

◆151. Heidenreich S, Kubis T, Schmidt M, Fegeler W. Glucocorticoid-induced alterations of monocyte defense mechanisms against Candida albicans. *Cell Immunol* 1994; **157:** 320–7.

●152. Waldman HJ. Centrally acting skeletal muscle relaxants and associated drugs. *J Pain Symptom Manage* 1994; **9:** 434–41.

●153. Snyder S. Drug and neurotransmitter receptors. New perspectives with clinical relevance. *JAMA* 1989; **261:** 3126–9.

154. Schwarz M, Klockgether T, Wullner U, *et al.* Delta-aminovaleric acid antagonizes the pharmacological actions of baclofen in the central nervous system. *Exp Brain Res* 1988; **70:** 618–26.

155. Latash ML, Penn RD, Corcos DM, Gottlieb GL. Short-term effects of intrathecal baclofen in spasticity. *Exp Neurol* 1989; **103:** 165–72.

156. Latash ML, Penn RD, Corcos DM, Gottlieb GL. Effects of intrathecal baclofen on voluntary motor control in spastic paresis. *J Neurosurg* 1990; **72:** 388–92.

157. Lazorthes Y, Sallerin-Caute B, Verdie JC, *et al.* Chronic intrathecal baclofen administration for control of severe spasticity. *J Neurosurg* 1990; **72:** 393–402.

●158. Ward A, Chaffman MO, Sorkin EM. Dantrolene. A review of its pharmacodynamic and pharmacokinetic properties and therapeutic use in malignant hyperthermia, the neuroleptic malignant syndrome and an update of its use in muscle spasticity. *Drugs* 1986; **32:** 130–68.

●159. Tomarken JL, Britt BA. Malignant hyperthermia. *Ann Emergency Med* 1987; **16:** 1253–65.

●160. Shalev A, Hermesh H, Munitz H. Mortality from neuroleptic malignant syndrome. *J Clin Psychiatry* 1989; **50:** 18–25.

161. Mercadante S. Dantrolene treatment of opioid-induced myoclonus. *Anesth Analges* 1995; **81:** 1307–8.

●162. Brasic JR. Should people with nocturnal leg cramps drink tonic water and bitter lemon? *Psychol Rep* 1999; **84:** 355–67.

163. Feeney GF, Lee GA, O'Connor PA. Quinine-induced blindness during attempted heroin withdrawal. *Med J Aust* 1999; **170:** 449.

164. Farver DK, Lavin MN. Quinine-induced hepatotoxicity. *Ann Pharmacother* 1999; **33:** 32–4.

●165. Glynne P, Salama A, Chaudhry A, *et al.* Quinine-induced immune thrombocytopenic purpura followed by hemolytic uremic syndrome. *Am J Kidney Dis* 1999; **33:** 133–7.

166. Schattner A. Quinine hypersensitivity simulating sepsis. *Am J Med* 1998; **104:** 488–90.

167. Mackie MA, Davidson J, Clarke J. Quinine – acute self-poisoning and ocular toxicity. *Scottish Med J* 1997; **42:** 8–9.

●168. McDonald SP, Shanahan EM, Thomas AC, *et al.* Quinine-induced hemolytic uremic syndrome. *Clin Nephrol* 1997; **47:** 397–400.

169. Gorfine S. Treatment of benign anal disease with topical nitroglycerin. *Dis Colon Rectum* 1995; **38:** 453–7.

170. McLoughlin RF, Mathieson JR, Chipperfield PM, *et al.* Effect of hyoscine butylbromide on gastroesophageal reflux in barium studies of the upper gastrointestinal tract. *Can Assoc Radiol J* 1994; **45:** 452–4.

171. Kozak RI, Bennett JD, Brown TC, Lee TY. Reduction of bowel motion artifact during digital subtraction angiography: a comparison of hyoscine butylbromide and glucagon. *Can Assoc Radiol J* 1994; **45:** 209–11.

172. De Conno F, Caraceni A, Zecca E, *et al.* Continuous subcutaneous infusion of hyoscine butylbromide reduces secretions in patients with gastrointestinal obstruction. *J Pain Symptom Manage* 1991; **6:** 484–6.

●173. Wein AJ. Pharmacologic options for the overactive bladder. *Urology* 1998; **51** (2A Suppl.): 43–7.

174. Barker I, Grant IS. Convulsions after abrupt withdrawal of baclofen [letter]. *Lancet* 1982; **2:** 556–7.

175. Utili R, Boitnott J, Zimmerman H. Dantrolene-associated hepatic injury. Incidence and character. *Gastroenterology* 1977; **72** (4 Pt 1): 610–16.

●◆176. Lipton S, Rosenberg P. Excitatory amino acids as a final common pathway for neurologic disorders. *N Engl J Med* 1994; **330:** 613–22.

●177. Muller WE, Scheuer K, Stoll S. Glutamatergic treatment strategies for age-related memory disorders. *Life Sci* 1994; **55:** 2147–53.

●178. Izquierdo I. Role of NMDA receptors in memory. *Trends Pharmacol Sci* 1991; **12:** 128–9.

●179. Carter AJ. Antagonists of the NMDA receptor-channel complex and motor coordination. *Life Sci* 1995; **57:** 917–29.

●180. Kirkwood A, Bear MF. Elementary forms of synaptic plasticity in the visual cortex. *Biol Res* 1995; **28:** 73–80.

●181. Hofer M, Constantine-Paton M. Regulation of N-methyl-D-aspartate (NMDA) receptor function during the rearrangement of developing neuronal connections. *Prog Brain Res* 1994; **102:** 277–85.

●182. Fox K, Daw NW. Do NMDA receptors have a critical function in visual cortical plasticity? *Trends Neurosci* 1993; **16:** 116–22.

●183. Rogawski MA. The NMDA receptor, NMDA antagonists and epilepsy therapy. A status report. *Drugs* 1992; **44:** 279–92.

●184. Meldrum BS. Excitatory amino acid receptors and disease. *Curr Opin Neurol Neurosurg* 1992; **5:** 508–13.

●185. ◆ Woolf C, Mannion R. Neuropathic pain: aetiology, symptoms, mechanisms, and management. *Lancet* 1999; **353:** 1959–1964.

186. Davies SN, Lodge D. Evidence for involvement of N-methylaspartate receptors in "wind-up" of class 2 neurones in the dorsal horn of the rat. *Brain Res* 1987; **424:** 402–6.

187. Dickenson AH, Sullivan AF. Evidence for a role of the NMDA receptor in the frequency dependent potentiation of deep rat dorsal horn nociceptive neurones following C fibre stimulation. *Neuropharmacology* 1987; **26:** 1235–8.

188. Lodge D, Davies SN, Jones MG, *et al.* A comparison between the in vivo and in vitro activity of five potent and competitive NMDA antagonists. *Br J Pharmacol* 1988; **95:** 957–65.

189. Haley JE, Sullivan AF, Dickenson AH. Evidence for spinal N-methyl-D-aspartate receptor involvement in prolonged chemical nociception in the rat. *Brain Res* 1990; **518:** 218–26.

190. Woolf CJ, Thompson SW. The induction and maintenance of central sensitization is dependent on N-methyl-D-aspartic acid receptor activation; implications for the treatment of post-injury pain hypersensitivity states. *Pain* 1991; **44:** 293–9.

191. Mao J, Price DD, Hayes RL, Lu J, Mayer DJ. Differential roles of NMDA and non-NMDA receptor activation in induction and maintenance of thermal hyperalgesia in rats with painful peripheral mononeuropathy. *Brain Res* 1992; **598:** 271–8.

●192. Dickenson AH. A cure for wind up: NMDA receptor antagonists as potential analgesics. *Trends Pharmacol Sci* 1990; **11:** 307–9.

●193. Wiesenfeld-Hallin Z. Combined opioid–NMDA antagonist therapies. What advantages do they offer for the control of pain syndromes? *Drugs* 1998; **55:** 1–4.

194. Enarson MC, Hays H, Woodroffe MA. Clinical experience with oral ketamine. *J Pain Symptom Manage* 1999; **17:** 384–6.

195. Rabben T, Skjelbred P, Oye I. Prolonged analgesic effect of ketamine, an N-methyl-D-aspartate receptor inhibitor, in patients with chronic pain. *J Pharmacol Exp Ther* 1999; **289:** 1060–6.

196. Takahashi H, Miyazaki M, Nanbu T, *et al.* The NMDA-receptor antagonist ketamine abolishes neuropathic pain after epidural administration in a clinical case. *Pain* 1998; **75:** 391–4.

197. Stubhaug A, Breivik H. Long-term treatment of chronic neuropathic pain with the NMDA (N-methyl-D-aspartate) receptor antagonist ketamine [editorial; comment]. *Acta Anaesthesiol Scand* 1997; **41:** 329–31.

198. Wood T, Sloan R. Successful use of ketamine for central pain [letter]. *Palliative Med* 1997; **11:** 57.

199. Rostaing-Rigattieri S, Cesaro P, N'Guyen J-P, *et al.* Preliminary report on the effect of ketamine in patients with central pain. *Pain Res Manage* 1997; **2:** 95–100.

200. Felsby S, Nielsen J, Arendt-Nielsen L, Jensen TS. NMDA receptor blockade in chronic neuropathic pain: a comparison of ketamine and magnesium chloride. *Pain* 1996; **64:** 283–91.

201. Eide PK, Stubhaug A, Breivik H, Oye I. Reply to S.T. Meller: Ketamine: relief from chronic pain through actions at the NMDA receptor [letter; comment]. *Pain* 1997; **72:** 289–91.

202. Mathisen LC, Skjelbred P, Skoglund LA, Oye I. Effect of ketamine, an NMDA receptor inhibitor, in acute and chronic orofacial pain. *Pain* 1995; **61:** 215–20.

●203. ◆ Mercadante S. Ketamine in cancer pain: an update. *Palliative Med* 1996; **10:** 225–30.

204. Mercadante S, Lodi F, Sapio M, *et al.* Long-term ketamine subcutaneous continuous infusion in neuropathic cancer pain. *J Pain Symptom Manage* 1995; **10:** 564–8.

205. Nelson KA, Park KM, Robinovitz E, *et al.* High-dose oral dextromethorphan versus placebo in painful diabetic neuropathy and postherpetic neuralgia. *Neurology* 1997; **48:** 1212–18.

206. Kauppila T, Xu XJ, Yu W, Wiesenfeld-Hallin Z. Dextromethorphan potentiates the effect of morphine in rats with peripheral neuropathy. *Neuroreport* 1998; **9:** 1071–4.

●207. Elliott K, Kest B, Man A, *et al.* N-methyl-D-aspartate (NMDA) receptors, mu and kappa opioid tolerance, and perspectives on new analgesic drug development. *Neuropsychopharmacology* 1995; **13:** 347–56.

208. Church J, Jones MG, Davies SN, Lodge D. Antitussive agents as N-methylaspartate antagonists: further studies. *Can J Physiol Pharmacol* 1989; **67:** 561–7.

209. Advokat C, Rhein FQ. Potentiation of morphine-induced antinociception in acute spinal rats by the NMDA antagonist dextrorphan. *Brain Res* 1995; **699:** 157–60.

210. Klepstad P, Borchgrevink PC. Four years' treatment with ketamine and a trial of dextromethorphan in a patient with severe post-herpetic neuralgia. *Acta Anaesthesiol Scand* 1997; **41:** 422–6.

211. Mercadante S, Casuccio A, Genovese G. Ineffectiveness of dextromethorphan in cancer pain. *J Pain Symptom Manage* 1998; **16:** 317–22.

212. Broadley KE, Kurowska A, Tookman A. Ketamine injection used orally. *Palliative Med* 1996; **10:** 247–50.

213. Mao J, Price DD, Hayes RL, Lu J, *et al.* Intrathecal treatment with dextrorphan or ketamine potently reduces pain-related behaviors in a rat model of peripheral mononeuropathy. *Brain Res* 1993; **605:** 164–8.

214. Max MB, Byas-Smith MG, Gracely RH, Bennett GJ. Intravenous infusion of the NMDA antagonist, ketamine, in chronic posttraumatic pain with allodynia: a double-blind comparison to alfentanil and placebo. *Clin Neuropharmacol* 1995; **18:** 360–8.

215. Nikolajsen L, Hansen PO, Jensen TS. Oral ketamine

therapy in the treatment of postamputation stump pain. *Acta Anaesthesiol Scand* 1997; **41:** 427–9.

216. Park KM, Max MB, Robinovitz E, *et al.* Effects of intravenous ketamine, alfentanil, or placebo on pain, pinprick hyperalgesia, and allodynia produced by intradermal capsaicin in human subjects. *Pain* 1995; **63:** 163–72.

217. Sethna NF, Liu M, Gracely R, *et al.* Analgesic and cognitive effects of intravenous ketamine–alfentanil combinations versus either drug alone after intradermal capsaicin in normal subjects. *Anesth Analges* 1998; **86:** 1250–6.

218. Davis AM, Inturrisi CE. d-Methadone blocks morphine tolerance and N-methyl-D-aspartate-induced hyperalgesia. *J Pharmacol Exp Ther* 1999; **289:** 1048–53.

●219. Ebert B, Thorkildsen C, Andersen S, *et al.* Opioid analgesics as noncompetitive N-methyl-D-aspartate (NMDA) antagonists. *Biochemical Pharmacol* 1998; **56:** 553–9.

220. Gorman AL, Elliott KJ, Inturrisi CE. The d- and l-isomers of methadone bind to the non-competitive site on the N-methyl-D-aspartate (NMDA) receptor in rat forebrain and spinal cord. *Neurosci Lett* 1997; **223:** 5–8.

221. Oxenham D, Farrer K. Methadone: opioid, N-methyl-D-aspartate antagonist or both? [letter]. *Palliative Med* 1998; **12:** 302.

●222. ◆ Portenoy R. Adjuvant analgesics in pain management. In: Doyle D, Hanks G, MacDonald N eds. *Oxford Textbook of Palliative Medicine.* Oxford: Oxford University Press; 1998: 361–90.

223. Clark JL, Kalan GE. Effective treatment of severe cancer pain of the head using low-dose ketamine in an opioid-tolerant patient. *J Pain Symptom Manage* 1995; **10:** 310–4.

224. Lin TC, Wong CS, Chen FC, *et al.* Long-term epidural ketamine, morphine and bupivacaine attenuate reflex sympathetic dystrophy neuralgia. *Can J Anaesth* 1998; **45:** 175–7.

225. Ghoneim M, Hinrichs J, Mewaldt S, Petersen R. Ketamine: behavioral effects of subanesthetic doses. *J Clin Psychopharmacol* 1985; **5:** 70–7.

226. Roelofse JA, Louw LR, Roelofse PG. A double blind randomized comparison of oral trimeprazine–methadone and ketamine-midazolam for sedation of pediatric dental patients for oral surgical procedures. *Anesth Prog* 1998; **45:** 3–11.

227. Slonim AD, Ognibene FP. Sedation for pediatric procedures, using ketamine and midazolam, in a primarily adult intensive care unit: a retrospective evaluation. *Crit Care Med* 1998; **26:** 1900–4.

●228. Bissonnette B, Swan H, Ravussin P, Un V. Neurolept-anesthesia: current status. *Can J Anaesth* 1999; **46:** 154–68.

229. Clements JA, Nimmo WS, Grant IS. Bioavailability, pharmacokinetics, and analgesic activity of ketamine in humans. *J Pharmaceut Sci* 1982; **71:** 539–42.

230. Clements JA, Nimmo WS. Pharmacokinetics and analgesic effect of ketamine in man. *Br J Anaesth* 1981; **53:** 27–30.

230a. Jackson K, Ashby M, Martin P, *et al.* "Burst" ketamine for refractory cancer pain: an open-label audit of 39 patients. *J Pain Symptom Manage* 2001; **22:** 834–42.

231. Mankin J. Instructional Course Lectures, The American Academy of Orthopedic Surgeons. Metabolic bone disease. *J Bone Joint Surg* 1994; **76A**: 760–88.

232. Guidobono F, Netti C, Sibilia V, *et al.* Role of catecholamines in calcitonin-induced analgesia. *Pharmacology* 1985; **31:** 342–8.

233. Guidobono F, Netti C, Pecile A, *et al.* Calcitonin binding site distribution in the cat central nervous system: a wider insight of the peptide involvement in brain functions. *Neuropeptides* 1987; **10:** 265–73.

234. Guidobono F, Netti C, Pagani F, *et al.* Evidence for different classes of calcitonin binding sites in rat CNS: an autoradiographic study with carbo-calcitonin. *Neurosci Lett* 1987; **79:** 91–6.

235. Hindley AC, Hill EB, Leyland MJ, Wiles AE. A double-blind controlled trial of salmon calcitonin in pain due to malignancy. *Cancer Chemother Pharmacol* 1982; **9:** 71–4.

236. Roth A, Kolaric K. Analgetic activity of calcitonin in patients with painful osteolytic metastases of breast cancer. Results of a controlled randomized study. *Oncology* 1986; **43:** 283–7.

237. Kessel C, Worz R. Immediate response of phantom limb pain to calcitonin. *Pain* 1987; **30:** 79–87.

238. Jaeger H, Maier C. Calcitonin in phantom limb pain: a double-blind study. *Pain* 1992; **48:** 21–7.

239. Gobelet C, Waldburger M, Meier JL. The effect of adding calcitonin to physical treatment on reflex sympathetic dystrophy. *Pain* 1992; **48:** 171–5.

240. Ralston SH, Gallacher SJ, Patel U, *et al.* Cancer-associated hypercalcemia: morbidity and mortality. Clinical experience in 126 treated patients. *Ann Intern Med* 1990; **112:** 499–504.

●241. Heath D. The treatment of hypercalcaemia of malignancy. *Clin Endocrinol* 1991; **34:** 155–7.

●242. ◆ Fleisch H. Bisphosphonates. Pharmacology and use in the treatment of tumour-induced hyper calcaemic and metastatic bone disease. *Drugs* 1991; **42:** 919–44.

●243. Body JJ, Bartl R, Burckhardt P, *et al.* Current use of bisphosphonates in oncology. International Bone and Cancer Study Group. *J Clin Oncol* 1998; **16:** 3890–9.

●244. ◆ Fulfaro F, Casuccio A, Ticozzi C, Ripamonti C. The role of bisphosphonates in the treatment of painful metastatic bone disease: a review of phase III trials. *Pain* 1998; **78:** 157–69.

245. Brincker H, Westin J, Abildgaard N, *et al.* Failure of oral pamidronate to reduce skeletal morbidity in multiple myeloma: a double-blind placebo-controlled trial. Danish–Swedish co-operative study group. *Br J Haematol* 1998; **101:** 280–6.

246. Coleman RE, Houston S, Purohit OP, *et al.* A randomised phase II study of oral pamidronate for the treatment of

bone metastases from breast cancer. *Eur J Cancer* 1998; **34:** 820–4.

247. Cascinu S, Graziano F, Alessandroni P, *et al.* Different doses of pamidronate in patients with painful osteolytic bone metastases. *Support Care Cancer* 1998; **6:** 139–43.

●248. Musto P. The role of bisphosphonates for the treatment of bone disease in multiple myeloma. *Leukemia Lymphoma* 1998; **31:** 453–62.

●249. Lipton A. Bisphosphonates and breast carcinoma. *Cancer* 1997; **80** (8 Suppl.): 1668–73.

250. Hultborn R, Gundersen S, Ryden S, *et al.* Efficacy of pamidronate in breast cancer with bone metastases: a randomized double-blind placebo controlled multicenter study. *Acta Oncol* 1996; **35** (Suppl. 5): 73–4.

●251. Berenson JR. Bisphosphonates in multiple myeloma. *Cancer* 1997; **80** (8 Suppl.): 1661–7.

●252. Adami S. Bisphosphonates in prostate carcinoma. *Cancer* 1997; **80** (8 Suppl.): 1674–9.

253. Speden D, Nicklason F, Francis H, Ward J. The use of pamidronate in hypertrophic pulmonary osteoarthropathy (HPOA). *Aust New Zealand J Med* 1997; **27:** 307–10.

254. Birdsey G, Campbell T, Halstead P, *et al.* Cardiovascular drugs. In: Misan G, Bochner F eds. *Australian Medicines Handbook*. Adelaide: Australian Medicines Handbook, 1998: 6.1–6.85.

255. Prough DS, McLeskey CH, Poehling GG, *et al.* Efficacy of oral nifedipine in the treatment of reflex sympathetic dystrophy. *Anesthesiology* 1985; **62:** 796–9.

256. Semble EL, Poehling GG, Prough DS, *et al.* Successful symptomatic treatment of melorheostosis with nifedipine. *Clin Exp Rheumatol* 1986; **4:** 277–80.

257. Meyer F, Tally P, Anderson R, *et al.* Inhibition of electrically induced seizures by a dihydropyridine calcium channel blocker. *Brain Res* 1986; **384:** 180–3.

258. Meyer F, Anderson R, Sundt T, *et al.* Suppression of pentylenetetrazole seizures by oral administration of a dihydropyridine Ca^{2+} antagonist. *Epilepsia* 1987; **28:** 409–14.

259. Ots ME, Yaksh TL, Anderson RE, Sundt TM, Jr. Effect of dihydropyridines and diphenylalkylamines on pentylenetetrazol-induced seizures and cerebral blood flow in cats. *J Neurosurg* 1987; **67:** 406–13.

260. Contreras E, Tamayo L, Amigo M. Calcium channel antagonists increase morphine-induced analgesia and antagonize morphine tolerance. *Eur J Pharmacol* 1988; **148:** 463–6.

261. Miranda HF, Bustamante D, Kramer V, *et al.* Antinociceptive effects of Ca^{2+} channel blockers. *Eur J Pharmacol* 1992; **217:** 137–41.

262. Roca G, Aguilar JL, Gomar C, *et al.* Nimodipine fails to enhance the analgesic effect of slow release morphine in the early phases of cancer pain treatment. *Pain* 1996; **68:** 239–43.

263. Santillan R, Hurle MA, Armijo JA, *et al.* Nimodipine-enhanced opiate analgesia in cancer patients requiring morphine dose escalation: a double-blind, placebo-controlled study. *Pain* 1998; **76:** 17–26.

264. Celik AF, Katsinelos P, Read NW, *et al.* Hereditary proctalgia fugax and constipation: report of a second family. *Gut* 1995; **36:** 581–4.

265. McLoughlin R, McQuillan R. Using nifedipine to treat tenesmus [letter]. *Palliative Med* 1997; **11:** 419–20.

266. Brigham B, Bolin T. High dose nifedipine and fludrocortisone for intractable hiccups [letter]. *Med J Aust* 1992; **157:** 70.

267. Cargill G, Theodore C, Paolaggi JA. Nifedipine for relief of esophageal chest pain [letter]. *N Engl J Med* 1982; **307:** 187–8.

268. George S, Pulimood S, Jacob M, Chandi SM. Pain in multiple leiomyomas alleviated by nifedipine. *Pain* 1997; **73:** 101–2.

●269. Wright JM. Review of the symptomatic treatment of diabetic neuropathy. *Pharmacotherapy* 1994; **14:** 689–97.

270. Anonymous. Treatment of painful diabetic neuropathy with topical capsaicin. A multicenter, double-blind, vehicle-controlled study. The Capsaicin Study Group. *Archiv Intern Med* 1991; **151:** 2225–9.

271. Tandan R, Lewis GA, Krusinski PB, *et al.* Topical capsaicin in painful diabetic neuropathy. Controlled study with long-term follow-up. *Diabetes Care* 1992; **15:** 8–14.

272. Watson CP, Tyler KL, Bickers DR, *et al.* A randomized vehicle-controlled trial of topical capsaicin in the treatment of postherpetic neuralgia. *Clin Ther* 1993; **15:** 510–26.

273. Zhang W, Li Wan Po A. The effectiveness of topically applied capsaicin. A meta-analysis. *Eur J Clin Pharmacol* 1994; **46:** 517–22.

274. Durant PA, Yaksh TL. Micturition in the unanesthetized rat: effects of intrathecal capsaicin, N-vanillylnonanamide, 6-hydroxydopamine and 5,6-dihydroxytryptamine. *Brain Res* 1988; **451:** 301–8.

275. Dasgupta P, Chandiramani V, Parkinson MC, *et al.* Treating the human bladder with capsaicin: is it safe? *Eur Urol* 1998; **33:** 28–31.

●276. Maggi CA. Therapeutic potential of capsaicin-like molecules: studies in animals and humans. *Life Sci* 1992; **51:** 1777–81.

●277. Watson CP. Topical capsaicin as an adjuvant analgesic. *J Pain Symptom Manage* 1994; **9:** 425–33.

●278. Winter J, Bevan S, Campbell EA. Capsaicin and pain mechanisms. *Br J Anaesth* 1995; **75:** 157–68.

●279. Surh YJ, Lee SS. Capsaicin, a double-edged sword: toxicity, metabolism, and chemopreventive potential. *Life Sci* 1995; **56:** 1845–55.

●280. Rumsfield JA, West DP. Topical capsaicin in dermatologic and peripheral pain disorders. *Drug Intell clin Pharmacy* 1991; **25:** 381–7.

●281. Dickenson AH. Capsaicin: gaps in our knowledge start to be filled. *Trends Neurosci* 1991; **14:** 265–6.

●282. Dray A. Mechanism of action of capsaicin-like molecules on sensory neurons. *Life Sci* 1992; **51:** 1759–65.

●283. Fitzgerald M. Capsaicin and sensory neurones – a review. *Pain* 1983; **15:** 109–30.

●284. Fusco BM, Giacovazzo M. Peppers and pain.
◆ The promise of capsaicin. *Drugs* 1997; **53:** 909–14.

●285. Karlsten R, Gordh T. How do drugs relieve neurogenic pain? *Drugs Aging* 1997; **11:** 398–412.

●286. Lipman AG. Analgesic drugs for neuropathic and sympathetically maintained pain. *Clin Geriatric Med* 1996; **12:** 501–15.

●287. Lynn B. Capsaicin: actions on nociceptive C-fibres and therapeutic potential. *Pain* 1990; **41:** 61–9.

●288. Monsereenusorn Y, Kongsamut S, Pezalla PD. Capsaicin – a literature survey. *Crit Rev Toxicol* 1982; **10:** 321–39.

289. Perkins M, Dray A. Novel pharmacological strategies for analgesia. *Ann Rheum Dis* 1996; **55:** 715–22.

●290. Nakamura A, Shiomi H. Recent advances in neuropharmacology of cutaneous nociceptors. *Jap J Pharmacol* 1999; **79:** 427–31.

291. Shuster S. Capsaicin and the cause of causalgia. *Lancet* 1995; **345:** 160–1.

16

Nerve blocks – chemical and physical neurolytic agents

JOHN E WILLIAMS

Numerous different chemical substances and physical techniques have been applied to elements of the central and peripheral nervous systems in efforts to disrupt pain transmission in a durable yet safe fashion.

Destructive chemical substances include alcohol, phenol, glycerol, and hypertonic saline. Physical methods range from heating the nerve with lasers and electricity to cooling the nerves with topical sprays or locally induced ice balls (Table 16.1).

Neurolytic procedures with chemical and physical agents have been successfully applied to treat pain since the early part of the twentieth century. Table 16.2 outlines some of the major early historical developments in the use of neurolytic agents. Over the last two decades, dramatic improvements in the pharmacologic management of pain, such as the development of long-acting opioid preparations and alternative strong opioids, an improved understanding of the role of adjuvant analgesics, and better access to analgesics and acceptance of their role, as well as improvements in anticancer therapies, argue for a more circumscribed role for neurolytic agents in contemporary practice.

Additionally, developments in our understanding of the interactions between nociceptive input and the plasticity of the nervous system suggest that pain is not dependent on hard-wired line-labeled linkages but is capable of change and modification at all levels throughout the nervous system. This new understanding implies that neurolytic interruption of discrete pathways is unlikely to provide complete pain relief for prolonged intervals. Nevertheless, the varied and complex patterns of pain present in patients with progressive cancer, and the compelling mandate for achieving pain relief in such settings, ensure an essential, although limited, role for neurolysis when pain is intractable.

Although the recent emphasis on the importance of evidence-based medicine has outstripped the availability of controlled trials that accurately depict the relative effect of alternative interventions, potentially useful therapies cannot ethically be withheld while awaiting such data.

The aim of this chapter is to describe the different chemical and physical agents and to outline their role in modern pain management.

Table 16.1 *Chemical and physical agents used in current clinical practice*

Chemical agents	Physical agents
50–100% alcohol – intrathecal, sympathetic (especially celiac), peripheral (especially intercostal)	*Cryoneurolysis* – facet joint, selected peripheral nerves, (especially intercostal)
5–15% phenol – intrathecal, epidural, selected peripheral nerves (especially intercostal)	*Radiofrequency lesioning* – facet joint, selected peripheral nerves, percutaneous cordotomy
Glycerol – trigeminal ganglion	*Laser*

Table 16.2 *History of chemical neurolysis*

1903 – Schloesser	Use of alcohol for trigeminal neuralgia
1919 – Kappis	Percutaneous celiac plexus block
1926 – Swetlow	Neurolytic sympathetic block with alcohol to relieve angina
1929 – De Beule	Alcohol celiac plexus block
1931 – Dogliotti	Absolute alcohol used intrathecally
1947 – Mandl	Phenol for lumbar sympathetic block

Another difficulty relates to ensuring accurate placement of the chemicals or physical agents at the target area. In the case of alcohol and phenol, image intensification is used to ensure accurate localization of the needle tip before injection. Physical lesioning using instruments such as the cryoprobe or radiofrequency generator requires accurate localization of the probe tip and should take account of measurement of temperature and duration of application.

PATHOPHYSIOLOGY OF NEUROLYSIS

Chemical and physical agents have a final common pathway in their action on the nerve cells. They are employed with the aim of producing nerve injury sufficient to result in degeneration of the nerve fiber distal to the lesion along with its myelin sheath. This process is called Wallerian degeneration.[1] This temporarily interferes with nerve cell transmission and thus results in nociceptive block. This type of degeneration does not completely disrupt the nerve cell; persistence of the basal lamina of the Schwann cells potentially allows for axonal regrowth with reconnection to the proximal end of the nerve fiber.

If, however, the nerve is surgically cut, there is complete disruption of the neuron and basal lamina. This is more likely to result in disorganized regrowth without reconnection of the cut nerve endings, possibly resulting in production of painful neuromata and dysesthetic pain.[2] This difference (Table 16.3) justifies reliance on the use of neurolytic agents over surgical interruption of peripheral nerve fibers for the treatment of chronic pain.

Selective neurolysis

It was postulated that neurolytic chemicals and physical methods of nerve interruption would produce a differential effect on small nociceptive fibers without interfering with sensory, motor, or autonomic function. Unfortunately, a reliable differential effect has not been shown for any of these methods. Neural tissue appears to be affected nonselectively, with consequent risk of injury to motor and sensory nerves and surrounding tissue. With most modalities, however, there is a concentration effect such that lower concentrations tend to produce a more reversible, less profound degeneration than higher concentrations (Table 16.4).

CHEMICAL NEUROLYTIC AGENTS

Alcohol, phenol, and glycerol are the only neurolytic agents employed in current clinical practice. Their optimal use depends on producing sufficient damage to result in Wallerian degeneration but not excessive nerve cell disorganization, resulting in adverse effects.

Alcohol

Alcohol is the classic neurolytic agent, though today phenol is more commonly used for peripheral neurolysis as it is potentially less toxic. Alcohol is used in concentrations from 3% to 100%. It damages sensory, motor, and autonomic nerves in a nonselective way and is injurious to surrounding soft tissue. It is readily soluble in body fluids, and is hypobaric with respect to cerebrospinal fluid (CSF) and thus will rise, diffusing rapidly from the injection site.[3] Careful positioning of the patient is required to allow the alcohol to act predominantly on the posterior, sensory nerve roots for the treatment of pain (patient in supine position) or anterior motor nerve roots for treatment of spasticity (patient in prone position).

Alcohol works by extracting fatty substances from the myelin sheath and precipitating proteins.[4] This results in degeneration of the nerve fiber and myelin sheath distal to the lesion (Wallerian degeneration). Providing the nerve cell is not completely destroyed (i.e. the basal lamina of the Schwann cell is preserved), regeneration usually begins within 3–4 months. If the entire nerve cell is completely disrupted, regeneration does not occur and effects are prolonged. Despite this, there is a risk of the development of dysesthetic pain as a result of central nervous system (CNS) plasticity or neuroma formation.

Damage to the nerve cells is proportional to the concentration and volume of alcohol used, as well as the

Table 16.3 *Chemical or physical neurolysis versus surgical sectioning of nerve cell*

	Neurolysis with chemical or physical agent	Surgical cutting of nerve
Pathological process	Wallerian degeneration Preservation of basal lamina Axonal regrowth	Complete nerve cell disruption
Possible clinical effect	Temporary (1–3 months) block of nociception Dysesthetic pain	Painful neuromata

Table 16.4 *Pathophysiological effects of physical and chemical neurolysis*

Agent	Effect on nerve conduction
Minimal heat applied to peripheral nerve	Enhanced nerve conduction
Local anesthetic drug applied to peripheral nerve 2% lidocaine (lignocaine) 0.5% bupivacaine	Totally reversible reduction in nerve conduction
5–7.5% phenol 50% alcohol 50% glycerol	Reduction in nerve conduction – usually reversible after weeks or months
10–15% phenol 100% alcohol Radiofrequency lesions <44°C Cryoprobe causing ice ball	Depression of nerve conduction – may be reversible
Radiofrequency lesion temperature >44°C Cryoprobe causing intraneural ice crystals	Potentially irreversible nerve block – permanent lesion
Surgical nerve sectioning Any physical neurolytic measure taken to extreme limits of time and/or temperature	Permanent neural lesion, non-Wallerian nerve degeneration, neuroma formation

rate of instillation, but there is no evidence for selective destruction of nociceptive, motor or sensory fibers (Table 16.5).

Phenol

Phenol is commonly used in concentrations of 5–15% for neurolysis. Five percent phenol is roughly equivalent to 40% alcohol in neurolytic potency. When dissolved in glycerine, it is hyperbaric compared with CSF and therefore patients need to be positioned contrary to that described above for alcohol. It is also less water soluble than alcohol and therefore may spread less liberally from the injection site.[5]

For neuraxial use phenol is formulated in glycerine, which acts as a base from which theoretically the glycerine slowly is released, potentially resulting in higher local concentrations. Used peripherally or near the sympathetic axis, phenol is typically compounded with water or saline.

Originally believed to preferentially destroy sensory neurons, destruction is now thought to be nonspecific, although when lower concentrations of phenol are used (e.g. <3%) destruction is mild, temporary, and similar to the type of block achieved with a local anesthetic agent. Believed to produce less neuritis, phenol is more widely used than alcohol (Table 16.6) because the duration and intensity of block are thought to be less than with alcohol and, therefore, there is a wider margin of safety and complications are more frequently reversible. An exception is that traditionally alcohol is used for neurolytic celiac plexus blockade; this may be because alcohol has theoretically less affinity for vascular structures that are present in the vicinity of the celiac plexus. Phenol may cause ulceration of soft tissues if injected subcutaneously.

Glycerol

Glycerol is used only for peripheral nerve blockade. It is used in the treatment of trigeminal neuralgia, when it is injected onto branches of the trigeminal nerve. It may produce less sensory deficit than alcohol, though repeat blocks may be required after a few months.

Ammonium compounds

Ammonium chloride and ammonium hydroxide have been used in 6% solutions to produce neurolytic block

Table 16.5 *Effect of different alcohol concentrations on nerve cell destruction*

Alcohol concentration	Effect
3%	Mild local anesthetic effect, usually self-limited
33%	Sensory nerve damage, little effect on motor neurons
50%	Motor damage, concentration used for celiac plexus blocks
100%	Persistent motor paralysis; risk of damage to skin and surrounding tissues

Table 16.6 *Neurolytic chemicals in current clinical use*

	Alcohol	Phenol	Glycerol
Concentration	50–100%	4–15%	50–100%
Diluent	Nil	Glycerine Saline Water	Nil
Baricity in cerebrospinal fluid (CSF)	Hypobaric	Hyperbaric	Not used in CSF
Pain on injection	Yes ++	No, local anesthetic effect	Yes +
Onset	Immediate	15–20 min slow release from glycerine	15–20 min
Position for nociceptive block	Painful side up	Painful side down	–
Complications	Neuritis (common)	Neuritis (uncommon) Toxicity is volume dependent	
Use	Celiac plexus block (50% conc.) Intrathecal Peripheral	Intrathecal Peripheral	Trigeminal neuralgia, facial pain

for pain control. Initially it was thought that a selective, sensory block was achieved, but results are unreliable and unpredictable, and microscopically it was shown that the neurolysis affected all types of nerve fiber.

Hypertonic and hypotonic solutions

Intrathecal injections of these solutions have been used to treat pain. They cause a localized osmotic swelling of the nerve bundle, which reduces nerve conduction. Prolonged exposure may produce more permanent impairment of neurological function, systemic toxicity, and death

CLINICAL APPLICATIONS OF CHEMICAL NEUROLYSIS

Use of neurolytic chemicals in clinical practice is a balance between yielding potentially beneficial effects and the risk of adverse effects. This balance is dependent on clinical factors such as:

- patient life expectancy;
- the degree to which reasonable systemic analgesic treatments have been unsuccessful;
- pre-existing levels of autonomic or motor impairment.

There may be a role for the use of these blocks as adjuncts to systemic treatments, such as the use of intercostal blocks for thoracic pain and glycerol blocks in the treatment of facial pain.

Neurolytic celiac plexus block

Celiac plexus block using local anesthetic was first used in 1914 as an adjunct to surgical anesthesia. The neurolytic block using alcohol was first used in 1919 to treat the pain of upper abdominal malignancy (Table 16.1). Since then there have been numerous case reports attesting to its efficacy in the treatment of cancer-related pancreatic pain.[6]

Any pain originating from visceral structures innervated by the celiac plexus can be alleviated by blockade of the plexus (Table 16.7). This includes malignant disease of the pancreas, liver, gallbladder, and alimentary tract from the distal esophagus to the transverse colon, including the adrenal glands, although efficacy is poor with ascites and carcinomatosis.

This block may also relieve pain from other upper abdominal malignancies and has been used to treat pain from pancreatitis, but efficacy and durability are reported as being much lower.[7,8]

There may be additional beneficial effects apart from pain relief, including decreased constipation, decreased nausea, increased appetite, and less sedation as a result of a reduced systemic opioid requirement.

Indications

This block is indicated for patients with visceral pain due to malignancy in one of the sites listed above. Many abdominal malignancies present with mixed visceral and somatic pains as a result of retroperitoneal extension or metastatic spread. The celiac block may unmask pains of somatic origin. This may result in a reduction in systemic opioid requirement, but it is preferable to determine the

Table 16.7 *Sites of abdominal pain for which neurolytic celiac plexus block may be indicated*

Pancreatic carcinoma
Retroperitoneal metastasis
Colon or stomach carcinoma
Capsular distension of liver or spleen

etiologies of the pain prior to blockade. This can be done with a diagnostic, temporary block using local anesthetic, when feasible.

Procedure

Traditionally, the posterior route is taken, using two 7-inch needles to approach the celiac plexus posterolateral to the vertebral bodies under radiographic image intensification. More recently, the anterior approach under computed tomographic (CT) or ultrasound guidance has been described.[9,10]

Complications

Complications have been divided into major and minor. Major complications include paralysis and autonomic dysfunction due to damage to a feeder artery of the spinal cord. The incidence of this may be as high as 1 in 700.[11] Minor complications include hypotension and diarrhea, and are usually transient.

Efficacy

Case reports on neurolytic celiac plexus block (NCPB) give an efficacy of 57–95%.[6,12–14] However, most are retrospective in nature and have been criticized for poor methodology[15] (Table 16.8).

Data from randomized controlled trials comparing the efficacy of the NCPB with oral morphine showed equal visual analog scores in the two groups but significantly fewer opioid-induced side-effects such as sedation and constipation in patients treated with NCPB.[16]** A meta-analysis of NCPB reported long-lasting benefit (< 3months) in 70–90% of patients.[17]***

There is some controversy over the timing of the block, with some authors advocating early use of the block and others use only if systemic opioids are ineffective or are associated with toxicity (Table 16.9).

A full assessment of the potential risks versus benefit of the block needs to be discussed with each patient. Duration of block has been variously reported. It is possible that regeneration of new pain pathways or development of deafferentation syndromes may result in pain returning after 6–12 months.[18,19]

Intrathecal neurolysis

Clinical considerations

The use of intrathecal neurolysis has declined over the past two decades. This may be because of the increased use of reversible techniques such as neuraxial and opioid delivery systems and because of fears over the side-effects of neurolysis, in particular motor, autonomic, and sensory effects. However, in carefully selected patients this type of block appears to play an important role, particularly when other treatments have not been successful.

Table 16.8 *Evidence for the efficacy of the neurolytic celiac plexus block*

Mercadante[16]	Randomized controlled trial (n = 20) No difference in pain scores between celiac block group and oral morphine group, but fewer side-effects with NCPB
Sharfmann and Walsh[15]	Review article Efficacy 87% in 418 patients in 15 published series Case series studies criticized for methodology
Eisenberg[17]***	Meta-analysis; efficacy in 70–90% of patients
Mean of nine case series (n = 333)[6]	Pain relief – good 78% Pain relief – fair 16% Pain relief – poor 6%

Table 16.9 *Controversies in neurolytic celiac block*

Timing	The block has been performed relatively early in the course of malignant disease; others reserve its use for pain unrelieved by systemic opioids
Efficacy	Case series report high efficacy (60–95%)
	A comparative trial has shown that the efficacy is similar to that of oral opioids
Balance of risk versus benefit	There is a significant risks of paraplegia in a small proportion of patients
Duration of blockade	Block has been reported to last 6–12 months, which is often adequate Longer-term follow-up is lacking

Permanent neurolytic procedures should only be considered after more conservative treatments have proven ineffective or been found to result in unacceptable side-effects (Table 16.10).

Technique

The effectiveness of this procedure depends on bathing the posterior, sensory, nerve root with neurolytic solution. Either alcohol or phenol can be used. If alcohol is used the patient is placed on his or her side with the painful side uppermost to allow the hypobaric solution to spread onto the posterior nerve roots. The reverse position, painful side down, is used for phenol, and is often too demanding of patients.

Outcomes

No controlled data exist comparing the effectiveness of this treatment with other analgesic interventions. Case reports indicate a success rate of between 50% and 75%. Success is improved by careful patient selection and meticulous technique and is inversely proportional to the number of dermatomes that need to be blocked. Some patients with a partially effective block may require supplemental oral analgesics.

Complications

Complications following neurolysis include motor paralysis, sensory disturbance, autonomic disturbance, and minor problems such as pain on injection (Table 16.11). No controlled data exist regarding the use of intrathecal neurolysis, so it is difficult to estimate the exact incidence of these complications. However, the incidence of complications is likely to be reduced by accurate needle placement using image intensification where appropriate. The higher concentrations of alcohol, 50% and above, are more likely to cause motor paralysis. Dysesthetic pains such as neuralgias are infrequent after injection. After intrathecal neurolysis an area of numbness may replace the painful area. Some patients will find this distressing.

Alcohol is irritant and painful on injection. After injection it is important to flush the alcohol through the needle with saline to prevent fistula formation.

Table 16.10 *Indications for intrathecal neurolysis (modified from Patt[20])*

Systemic pharmacotherapy and antineoplastic treatments have not been effective or have resulted in excessive side-effects
Severe pain, likely to persist, well localized The pain should be somatic or visceral in origin. Neuropathic pain is less likely to respond favorably. However many cancer-related pains are of mixed etiology
Patient has limited life expectancy, less than 12 months In practice, this usually means patients with cancer-related pain. In patients with a longer life expectancy, side-effects such as deafferentation pain and motor impairment would potentially have a far greater implication. Additionally, the duration of effect of neurolysis is reported as being from 3 to 6 months, thus repeated blocks would be needed for patients with a longer life expectancy

Epidural neurolytic blockade

Phenol has been injected via the epidural route to achieve a neurolytic sensory block. Theoretical advantages include a lower incidence of autonomic impairment and potentially a less dramatic, more easily titratable, effect.

Single bolus injections of phenol (2 ml of 7%) have been used, with some reports of pain relief for as long as 9 months.

Racz *et al.*[21] have developed an epidural catheter that is resistant to the corrosive effects of the neurolytic solution, thus allowing repeated epidural dosing. They reported good pain relief in over 50% of patients persisting for 3–6 months. Repeated dosing was possible if the block receded. Unlike intrathecal administration there is greater latency to effect, and topographic spread is more variable.

Neurolytic sympathetic blocks

The sympathetic chain can be blocked with a neurolytic substance at any point along its course.

In the treatment of complex regional pain syndromes and other painful neuropathic syndromes of the upper limb the sympathetic nerve supply to the upper limb can be blocked by injection of phenol or alcohol into the stellate ganglion. This is a risky procedure, however, with the potential to produce a prolonged Horner syndrome and damage to the brachial plexus and recurrent laryngeal nerve, and is conducted with dilute (3–5%) phenol.

Neurolytic blockade of the sympathetic supply to the chest, abdomen, and pelvis has also been described. All of these techniques are associated with infrequent complications and may be suitable for patients with intractable pain and limited life expectancy because sympathetic denervation should not interfere with sensory or motor function.

Neurolytic block of peripheral nerves

The use of peripheral nerve neurolysis in cancer pain patients with intractable pain and limited life expectancy has been described.[6] However, these neurolytic blocks may result in neuralgia as the nerves regenerate after neurolysis or in a deafferentation pain syndrome. An exception to this is that neurolytic blockade of the branches of the trigeminal nerve does not usually produce neuralgia during regeneration.

Table 16.11 *Complications of intrathecal neurolysis*

Dysesthetic pain	Painful neuralgias, burning pain, and dysesthetic pain can last for weeks or months, but are rare May be related to damage to somatic nerves
Motor paresis	More common with higher volumes
Anesthesia or hypoesthesia	Areas of numbness can occur, which can be distressing
Sphincter disturbance	Bowel and bladder disturbance can occur after intrathecal neurolysis in the sacral area Accurate placement of solution is important
Irritation of surrounding tissue	Alcohol is injurious to surrounding tissue; accurate needle placement and injection important
Alcohol toxicity	Alcohol is rapidly absorbed systemically, however it is unlikely to cause a major problem with the small doses that are used clinically
Pain on injection	Transient

Other neurolytic nerve blocks include paravertebral injections, block of individual branches of the lumbar plexus, ilioinguinal and iliohypogastric blocks, and block of the intercostal nerves.

PHYSICAL NEUROLYTIC AGENTS

Nerves can be cooled or heated in an attempt to interrupt pain transmission. Modern methods of application of these physical techniques include the cryprobe (cooling) and lasers and radiofrequency lesioning (heating).

Hypothermia

The application of cold to peripheral nerves results in a reversible block of nerve conduction. This phenomenon has been used to treat pain for many years. Hippocrates described the use of ice and snow packs to relieve pain, and painful limbs were frozen prior to amputation during the Napoleonic wars. Ethyl chloride spray has been used to produce local anesthesia since 1890. Today cooling is achieved with the use of a cryoprobe.

Cryoanalgesia

In 1976, Lloyd *et al.*[22] described the use of a probe to apply extreme cold locally to nerves to achieve pain relief by a long-term reversible nerve block called cryoanalgesia. This technique uses the rapid expansion of nitrous oxide or carbon dioxide to produce a temperature of –20°C at the probe tip, which is applied to the nerve. This produces an ice ball, which interferes with nerve cell conduction, and if the probe is placed on the nerve for long enough the interior of the cell turns into ice crystals, causing a more permanent Wallerian degeneration of the nerve cell. The analgesic effect may last for weeks or months. Providing the basal lamina of the neuron has not been damaged, axonal regeneration of the nerve takes place within 3 months and normal neural function returns. It is possible that the analgesic effect will be more prolonged, and this may be because there has been a more permanent disruption of the nerve cell interior.

One of the disadvantages of the cryoprobe is the size of the probe tip itself, usually more than 3 mm; this can make accurate placement on a nerve difficult (Table 16.12).

Cryoneurolysis of the intercostal nerves during surgery is the best-known application of cryotherapy for the treatment of acute post-thoracotomy pain.[23] A number of reports have described effective pain management in this situation, especially when combined with other analgesic treatments.[24,25] However, the occurrence of chronic dysesthetic pain has led a number of surgeons to abandon its routine use.

Cryolesions have been described for a number of facial nerves, including supraorbital, infraorbital, mandibular, and mental nerves, and in the treatment of groin pain via the iliohypogastric and ilioinguinal nerves.

Hyperthermia

Heating of peripheral nerves initially causes nerve conduction enhancement; if the heat application is continued a reversible depression is produced (the neuron can regrow following Wallerian degeneration) followed by an irreversible depression if the entire nerve is disrupted. Induction heating is a process whereby heated pellets can be inserted into brain tissue and then destroy surrounding tissue. This method has been used in neurosurgery to destroy brain tissue. Because of its relatively nonspecific effects, it is not a technique that has been used for pain control.

Lasers

Lasers can be used to heat and cut nerve tissue in the brain and spinal cord. The laser disrupts the interior of the nerve cell, which subsequently undergoes Wallerian degeneration. The perineurium may not be damaged, and regeneration of the nerve cell can take place. Direct visualization of the nerve is required for effective laser treatment. Dorsal root entry zone (DREZ) lesions have been made using a laser. Potential problems include difficulties in quantifying the extent and rapidity of nerve cell destruction and thus variable clinical defects may be produced.[26]

Radiofrequency lesioning

This is the use of electricity to generate heat, which can then create a lesion in the nervous system. The radiofrequency probe provides a discrete controllable heat source, which creates a neural lesion when placed directly into the brain or onto peripheral nerves. The size of the lesion is dependent on the temperature of the probe and duration of application. There is some suggestion that the smaller Aδ- and C-fibers may be preferentially affected by the lesioning. One of the advantages of radiofrequency lesioning is a precise and measurable application of heat, thus avoiding unwanted and uncontrolled side-effects such as sticking, charring, and formation of explosive gas (Table 16.13).

The radiofrequency probe can be applied to the brain (temperatures up to 42°C), or directly onto peripheral nerves (up to 60–70°C).

Clinical application of radiofrequency lesioning

The best-known indication for radiofrequency lesioning is lumbar pain emanating from the lumbar facet joints. There are also an increasing number of publications concerning the application of these procedures in thoracic and cervical pain syndromes.[27]

Facet joint pain

The aim of radiofrequency lesioning is to destroy the nerve supply to the facet joints at multiple vertebral levels. The radiofrequency probe is placed on the nerve to the facet joints; lesions are generated after about 1 min at 80°C. The reported efficacy is about 50–60%. One randomized, controlled study has shown a benefit.[28**]

Lumbar diskogenic pain

Radiofrequency lesions have been used to treat lumbar disk pain. Either the gray ramus communicans or the nerves within the disk itself are the targets for radiofrequency lesioning.

Trigeminal neuralgia

Radiofrequency lesions have been used to treat facial pain by targeting the trigeminal (Gasserian) ganglion.

Sympathetic chain

Percutaneous radiofrequency lesioning of the thoracic or lumbar sympathetic chain has been used to treat pain due to sympathetically maintained pain syndromes. Under

Table 16.12 *Advantages and disadvantages of cryoneurolysis*

Advantages	Disadvantages
Potential role in acute and chronic pain	Reports of neuritis and dysesthetic pain
Reversible nerve destruction; duration of analgesia 1–5 months	Lack of comparative studies on efficacy (case reports only)
Relatively easy to use	Large probe tip may make accurate application difficult
Precise placement of probe is necessary, usually under direct vision	

Table 16.13 *Advantages and disadvantages of radiofrequency lesioning*

Advantages	Disadvantages
More consistent production of lesions than some other physical methods such as lasers	Potential damage to surrounding tissue, including sensory or motor nerves
Possible to specifically target peripheral nerves, such as trigeminal nerve	Paucity of controlled data describing efficacy
Quantifiable and measurable effects	Paucity of recent descriptions of efficacy
Potentially can selectively destroy pain fibers rather than Aβ-fibers	Requires purchase of expensive equipment and training in its use
Small tip allows discreet placement, and avoids uncertainties of the spread of injected solutions	Pain after lesioning
	Lesion is produced within seconds; accurate placement is required

image intensification, the sympathetic chain is visualized and the radiofrequency lesion generator applied directly to it.

SUMMARY

A variety of different chemical (phenol and alcohol) and physical (heat and cold) neurolytic agents have been used to destroy nerves and reduce afferent nociceptive impulse transmission in the treatment of chronic pain. However, these nerves can regenerate, and the pain can return or a new pain can develop due to deafferentation. Thus, careful consideration of the risk–benefit ratio of the procedure and appropriate patient selection is important. The use of chemical intrathecal neurolysis has diminished over the past 10–20 years with the advent of improved analgesic drugs and the use of reversible infusional pumps and techniques. However, there may still be a role for this technique in intractable pain, especially in cancer pain patients with limited prognosis and functional ability. The neurolytic celiac plexus block is comprehensively described in numerous research studies and may have an important role in the management of intractable upper abdominal pain due to malignancy. However, as with all these techniques, good-quality controlled evidence is lacking. Physical techniques such as cryotherapy and radiofrequency lesioning are well recognized as treatments for chronic pain problems, but again evidence for efficacy is lacking.

REFERENCES

1. Waller A. Experiments on the section of the glossopharyngeal and hypoglossal nerves of the frog and observations of the alterations produced thereby in the structure of their primitive fibres. *Phil Trans R Soc* 1850; **40:** 423.
2. Sunderland S. The anatomical basis of nerve repair. In: Jewett DL, McCaroll Jr HR eds. *Nerve Repair and Regeneration.* St Louis, MO: Mosby, 1980: 14.
3. Swerdlow M. Current views on intrathecal neurolysis. *Anesthesia* 1978; **33:** 733–40.
4. ◆ Rumbsy MG, Finean JB. The action of organic solvents on the myelin sheath of peripheral nerve tissue. *J Neurochem* 1966; **13:** 1509.
5. Politis MJ , Schaumburg HH, Spencer PS. Neurotoxicity of selected chemicals. In: Spencer PS, Schaumburg eds. *Experimental and Chemical Neurotoxicity.* Baltimore, MD: William & Wilkins, 1980: 613.
6. ● Bonica JJ, Buckley FP, Moricca G, Murphy TM. Neurolytic blockade and hypophysectomy. In: Bonica JJ, Loeser JD, Chapman CR, Fordyce WE eds. *The Management of Pain.* Philadelphia, PA: Lea & Febiger, 1990: 1980–2040.
7. Bell SN, Cole R, Roberts-Thompson IC. Celiac plexus block for control of pain in chronic pancreatitis. *Br Med J* 1980; **281:** 1604.
8. ● Waldmann SD. Celiac plexus block. In: RS Weiner ed. *Innovations in Pain Management.* Orlando, FL: PMD Press, 1990: 10–15.
9. Matamala AM, Lopez FV, Martinez LI. The percutaneous anterior approach to the celiac plexus using CT guidance. *Pain* 1988; **34:** 285–8.
10. Leiberman RP, Nance PN, Cuka DJ. Anterior approach to the celiac plexus during interventional biliary procedures. *Radiology* 1988; **167:** 562.
11. Davies DD. Incidence of major complications of neurolytic celiac plexus block. *J R Soc Med* 1993; **86:** 269.
12. Brown DL, Bulley CK, Quiel EL. Neurolytic celiac plexus block for pancreatic cancer pain. *Anesth Analg* 1987; **66:** 869–73.
13. Orwitz S, Sundararao K. Celiac plexus block: an overview. *Mount Sinai J Med* 1983; **50:** 486–90.
14. Bridenbaugh LD, Moore DC, Campbell DO. Management of upper abdominal cancer pain. *JAMA* 1964; **190:** 877–80.
15. Sharfman WH, Walsh TD. Has the analgesic efficacy of neurolytic celiac plexus block been demonstrated in pancreatic cancer pain? *Pain* 1990; **41:** 267–71.
16. ◆ Mercadante S. Celiac plexus block versus analgesics in pancreatic cancer pain. *Pain* 1993; **52:** 187–92.
17. ● Eisenberg E, Carr DB, Chalmers TC. Neurolytic celiac plexus block for treatment of cancer pain. A meta-analysis. *Anesth Analg* 1995; **80:** 290–7.
18. Gorbitz C, Laevens ME. Alcohol block of the celiac plexus for control of upper abdominal pain caused by cancer and pancreatitis. *J Neurosurg* 1971; **34:** 575–9.
19. Hegedus V. Relief of pancreatic pain by radiography-guided block. *Am J Roentgenol* 1979; **133:** 1101–3.
20. ● Patt RB. The current status of anesthetic approaches to cancer pain management. In: Payne R, Patt RB, Stratton Hill C eds. *Assessment and Treatment of Cancer Pain.* Seattle, WA: IASP Press, 1998: 195–213.
21. Racz GB, Heavner J, Haynsworth P. Repeat epidural phenol injections in chronic pain and spasticity. In: Lipton S ed. *Persistent Pain: Modern Methods of Treatment.* New York, NY: Grune & Stratton, 1985.
22. Lloyd JW, Barnard JDW, Glynn CJ. Cryoanalgesia: a new approach to pain relief. *Lancet* 1976; **2:** 982–4.
23. Glynn CJ, Lloyd JW, Barnard JD. Cryoanalgesia in the management of pain after thoracotomy. *Thorax* 1980; **35:** 325–327.
24. Saberski LR. Cryoneurolysis in clinical practice. In: Waldman SD, Winnie AP eds. *Interventional Pain Management.* Philadelphia, PA: WB Saunders, 1996.
25. Evans PJD. Cryoanalgesia. *Anaesthesia* 1981; **36:** 1003–13.
26. Kline MT. Radiofrequency techniques in clinical practice. In: Waldman SD, Winnie AP eds. *Interventional Pain Management.* Philadelphia, PA: WB Saunders, 1996.

27. Van Suijlekom JA, Weber WEJ, van Kleef M. Treatment of spinal pain by means of radiofrequency procedures – Part 2; thoracic and cervical area. *Pain Rev* 1999; **6:** 175–91.

28. Gallagher J, Vadi PLP, Wedley JR, *et al.* Radiofrequency facet joint denervation in the treatment of low back pain: a prospective controlled double-blind study to assess its efficacy. *Pain Clin* 1994; **7:** 193–8.

17

Stimulation-induced analgesia in cancer pain management

CATHY STANNARD

Sensory stimulation has been used in the management of pain since ancient times. The application of a painful stimulus to abolish pain dates back to the fourth century BC in ancient Greece and Rome,[1] and electrical stimulation similarly has been used by ancient peoples, with records suggesting that this was practiced as early as 2,500 BC, when the electric fish was used to treat pain.[2]

The use of stimulation techniques in modern pain medicine dates from the publication of the gate theory of Melzack and Wall in the 1960s,[3] which was verified clinically when it was demonstrated that prolonged percutaneous stimulation of peripheral nerves modified responses of healthy volunteers to noxious stimuli.[4] The use of transcutaneous nerve stimulation (TENS), stimulation of peripheral nerves (PNS), spinal cord stimulation (SCS), and deep brain stimulation (DBS) is now established in modern pain practice.

Pain in patients with cancer is common, occurring in 20–50% of patients with newly diagnosed malignancies, 30% during cancer treatment, and in 75–90% of patients with advanced disease.[5] Pharmacological therapy remains the mainstay of cancer pain therapy. Clinicians who care for patients with malignancy are experienced in dealing with the symptom of pain, and patients referred to pain clinics represent some of those with the most refractory pain problems.[6] Although there is an extensive world literature on the use of stimulation techniques, little of it stands up to rigorous scientific scrutiny. However, for patients intolerant or resistant to pharmacotherapy, pragmatism must prevail; if a therapy is safe and inexpensive a trial of treatment is worthwhile. More caution should be exercised when treatments are invasive and costly and where morbidity is potentially serious. It is in the use of these advanced techniques that robust evidence is urgently needed. Detailed history-taking, examination, and appropriate investigations should precede institution of any form of pain therapy, whatever the cause of the pain, but this is especially so in the case of patients with malignancy as the dynamic nature of the condition may mean that symptoms and signs can change rapidly. Any change in responsiveness to a therapy should prompt re-evaluation of the underlying condition.

TENS AND CANCER PAIN*

Mechanism of action

A detailed understanding of mechanisms involved in nociceptive processing have led to scientifically validated theories of how TENS provides analgesia. A number of different mechanisms contribute to the effect, particularly with the use of different modes of stimulation (see below).

Large myelinated (Aβ) afferent fibers that subserve the (innocuous) sensations of light touch and vibration enter the spinal cord in the dorsal root and ascend without synapse in the ipsilateral dorsal column. At the level at which they enter the cord they give rise to collateral branches to the dorsal horn which terminate in several laminae, particularly III–V and deeper.[7] They also synapse directly with terminals of unmyelinated C-fibers in lamina II. The use of TENS (segmentally) stimulates Aβ-fibers and via these collaterals modifies the onward transmission of nociceptive information, predominantly via a presynaptic mechanism involving the release of γ-aminobutyric acid (GABA),[8] although postsynaptic mechanisms have also been postulated.[9] In addition to this segmental effect involving local inhibitory circuits, activation of descending inhibitory mechanisms may contribute to the analgesic effect, although this is more likely with the use of high-intensity stimulation.[10] The role of endogenous opioid peptides in TENS analgesia has been investigated and, although naloxone was shown to reverse TENS analgesia in one study,[11] other studies have shown that naloxone does not reverse the effect of high-frequency TENS.[12,13] This may be related to the differing effects of the drug at mu, kappa, and delta receptors.[14] In addition, TENS has a modulating effect on the autonomic system, which in turn modifies the experience of pain and is probably responsible for the beneficial effects of the technique in pain of cardiac origin.[15]

Indications

TENS has been used successfully to treat many sorts of pain. It is well known that patients with cancer may have a number of types of pain, with mixed pictures of nociceptive and neurogenic symptoms. These may be related to the underlying disease or to its treatment. In addition, these patients may have coincidental pain unrelated to their malignancy. In practice, it may be difficult to differentiate the different components of patients' pain experiences, for example the pain of bony metastases is thought to be predominantly nociceptive and that of infiltration of a nerve by tumor neurogenic, but more commonly a mixed picture prevails. It is not possible to predict which types of pain will respond to TENS therapy,[16] so a trial of TENS is reasonable in most cases. Many patients may be refractory to analgesic pharmacotherapy or may suffer from troublesome side-effects of medication. In many cases, TENS will provide a useful adjunct or alternative to pain-relieving drugs.[17]

Another group in whom this therapy may be useful are those with postsurgical pain syndromes, the commonest of which is post-thoracotomy pain. Persisting pain following thoracotomy for malignancy is most commonly due to recurrence or progression of malignancy but is occasionally benign.[18] A comparison of TENS and sham TENS in a small group of such patients demonstrated a reduction in opioid consumption in the TENS group.[19] Similarly, pain following mastectomy, neck dissection, or amputation of a limb may be usefully treated with TENS.

Important contraindications to the use of TENS

TENS should not be used to stimulate over a pregnant uterus, as there are no data relating to its safety in pregnancy except for its use as analgesia during labor. The presence of a cardiac pacemaker is a contraindication to the use of TENS, particularly demand pacemakers. Although use with fixed rate pacemakers may be safe, the therapy should always be discussed with the patient's cardiologist. Stimulation should not be applied to the anterior neck as this may stimulate the carotid sinus or laryngeal nerve supply.

Practical issues

The practical application of TENS therapy is common for many types of pain and is discussed elsewhere in this text but important aspects are summarized here.

The most important aspect of this treatment is that the patient is both willing and practically able to use the device. For patients who are enthusiastic about the therapy it has the added advantage of giving them control over their symptoms.[20] In debilitated patients with advanced cancer disease, TENS may be useful; however, additional practical support is likely to be necessary.

Equipment

A large number of TENS machines are commercially available. They comprise a stimulator connected via leads to electrodes which are applied to the patient's skin. The basic requirements of the stimulator are:

1. combined on/off amplitude control 0–50 mA;
2. frequency control 0–100 Hz.

Useful additional features include:

3. ability to change mode, e.g. from continuous to pulsed;
4. pulse width control 0.1–0.5 ms.

Electrodes are usually made of carbon rubber and are applied to the skin with conductive jelly and adhesive tape. Self-adhesive conductive polymer pads are also available.

Positioning electrodes

Optimal electrode positioning varies between patients, so patients should be allowed to try the machine for long enough to experiment with different sites. Electrodes should not be applied to irritated skin or hairy areas. Usually optimal stimulation is achieved by stimulating over the painful area or over nerves innervating the painful area. Limb electrodes are usually placed longitudinally and truncal electrodes in the axis of the dermatome. They are placed in pairs usually about 2 cm apart. If a large area is to be stimulated, more than one pair of electrodes may be used with either a dual channel stimulator or a double adaptor lead.

Modes of stimulation

Common modes of stimulation are summarized in Table 17.1.

Trial of TENS

Trial of TENS should be at least 1 h, but preferably much longer. Ideally, patients should be allowed to take equipment home as pain relief may increase over several weeks. TENS analgesia will occur within 30 min in around 75% of patients and will disappear within 30 min of cessation of stimulation in over half of patients.[22] Patients should try stimulation for various periods, e.g. 1 h thrice daily or continuously, and should try different stimulus parameters and modes of stimulation. The sensation produced should be comfortable. Some patients may continue to have pain relief after the machine has been switched off.[23] Patients should be followed up regularly, and should particularly be reassessed if symptoms worsen or change.

Problems with the use of TENS

TENS is generally a safe therapy compared with analgesic medication and interventional treatments but a number of problems may occur.

Skin irritation

This is probably the commonest complaint of those using TENS and may occur in up to one-third of users.[22,24] It may be the result of allergy to the jelly, electrode, or tape or of drying out of the electrode jelly.[24,25] These problems may be minimized by attention to skin hygiene, careful cleaning of the electrodes, and frequent changing of the electrode site.

Tolerance

The efficacy of TENS treatment tends to fall with time. This phenomenon is termed tolerance. The extent to which tolerance occurs varies considerably in published case series, ranging from series in which only 12.5% of patients achieved prolonged analgesia to series in which over half of patients appear to have useful analgesia after 1 year.[22,26,27] The neurophysiological basis of tolerance is not well worked out, although it seems not to be a placebo phenomenon. It may be related to diminished neurotransmitter release or downregulation of receptors for endogenous opioids or central nervous system (CNS) monoamines. Regular patterns of stimulation may encourage habituation of the nervous system.[14] Multielectrode devices to which pulses are randomly distributed have been developed in an attempt to overcome tolerance.[17,28] It may be more practical to withdraw TENS therapy for a period and then reinstitute it. When managing patients with malignancy it cannot be overemphasized that a change in the intensity or character of the pain during any type of previously successful analgesic therapy should prompt clinical re-evaluation of the patient.

Evidence for the efficacy of TENS

TENS is described as a useful tool in the management of cancer pain in large numbers of textbooks and review articles. There is a huge world literature on the use of TENS to manage many different types of pain, and most suggest that it is an effective form of pain relief. Despite this, most of the data do not stand up to rigorous scientific scrutiny. The only systematic reviews of the therapy conclude that the therapy has not undergone sufficiently rigorous clinical evaluation[29] and that, although the therapy may well be useful, it cannot be proven.[30] There are a number of particular difficulties in producing good-quality TENS research. Studies vary widely in relation to the use of suitable control therapy, a problem which may be related to difficulties with blinding.[31] Control groups are often given "sham" TENS in which batteries are removed from the machine or when subthreshold stimu-

Table 17.1 *Common modes of TENS stimulation*[21]

Mode	Stimulation characteristics
Conventional TENS	High frequency (40–50 Hz) (most patients prefer 40–70 Hz) Low intensity (10–30 mA) (patients should adjust amplitude to the maximum comfortable level – the sensation should be nonpainful)
Burst (pulsed) TENS	Trains of high frequency (bursts of 100 Hz at 1–2 Hz) Low intensity (10–30 mA)
Acupuncture-like TENS	Bursts of 100 Hz at 1–2 Hz High intensity (20–50 mA) May be useful for those not responding to conventional TENS More uncomfortable for patient Partly reversed by naloxone, so probably different mode of action from conventional TENS

lation is delivered. As the eliciting of paresthesia is so fundamental in instituting a trial of TENS, it is unsurprising that both investigators and patients are aware if adequate stimulation is not being achieved. The use of low-frequency submaximal stimulation has recently been suggested as an active TENS placebo.[32] In addition, the huge range of TENS equipment available, the large numbers of different modes of stimulation and electrode placement, and differing duration of therapy and length of follow-up make it very difficult to compare trials. However, the overall impression from most studies is that TENS provides superior analgesia to placebo.

There is very little literature specifically concerning the use of TENS in the management of cancer pain, and inferences must be drawn from the general literature. It would appear that overall TENS use for this indication is low, with one report suggesting that it is used in 3% of cases.[33] Several case series have been published on the use of TENS for a number of indications, but generally the numbers of patients with pain associated with neoplasia in these series is few.[22,34–37] The largest of these series studied 84 patients with cancer, although in addition to those patients in whom it was used for management of tumor pain it was used as an adjunct to general anesthesia and for the management of postoperative pain.[37] The apparent success of the therapy in these series is variously reported as being between 11%[36] and 99%,[37] with the largest series reporting that useful analgesia was achieved in around one-quarter of patients with advanced tumors and that opioid consumption was reduced.[38] One case series has examined its use in orofacial cancer, in which it was useful in 60% of patients.[39] One of the few controlled trials involving patients with cancer investigated the use of TENS for postoperative pain relief in patients following thoracotomy for malignant disease.[19] The conclusion of this paper was that TENS was superior to sham TENS for this indication, but the outcome measure was requirements for postoperative opioid therapy, which is a secondary outcome measure and therefore less satisfactory than measurement of pain intensity or pain relief.[40] A more recent study of post-thoracotomy pain suggests that TENS is ineffective.[41]

Long,[42] in a review of TENS therapy over a 15-year period, concluded that the pain of cancer is not reliably relieved with this treatment. More generally, a systematic review of the use of TENS for chronic pain concludes that the treatment may be of use but that the evidence to date is insufficient.[40]

PERIPHERAL NERVE STIMULATION AND CANCER PAIN*

The use of subcutaneously implanted electrodes in order to stimulate peripheral nerves directly was first described for clinical use in 1968.[43] Electrodes are applied to or placed around peripheral nerves in a surgical procedure.[44] The most usual indication for this therapy has been for patients with nerve injury.[45,46] Only one case series included patients with cancer.[47]

SPINAL CORD STIMULATION AND CANCER PAIN*

Spinal cord stimulation (SCS) was introduced for the control of pain in 1967.[48] Relief of chronic pain was achieved by means of radiofrequency stimulation of plate electrodes placed directly over the dorsal columns in a surgical procedure. The intention was to inhibit C-fiber activity by stimulation of Aβ-fibers in the dorsal column of the spinal cord. However, subsequent experience suggested that ventral stimulation of the cord was also effective in producing pain relief in cancer patients.[49] It is therefore unclear precisely how spinal cord stimulation provides analgesia. Other pathways, such as corticospinal and sympathetic pathways, are probably stimulated. Stimulation may cause segmental suppression of nociceptive transmission or may electrically interfere with ascending and descending polysynaptic pathways. Central neurohumoral mechanisms may be activated by electrical stimulation.[50,51] In addition, there is evidence for a visceral pathway in the dorsal columns of the cord,[52] and the dorsal columns may play an important role in the transmission of nociceptive visceral input to the thalamus and beyond.

Practical issues

The original systems for SCS involved laminotomy for electrode placement and implantation of a radiofrequency-coupled receiver, which was driven by an external power source. Fully implantable battery-powered pulse generators are now available. In addition, epidural electrodes may be placed percutaneously in the awake patient in order to produce stimulation in the region of reported pain. The electrodes may be unipolar, bipolar, or multipolar. It is recommended that the patient undergoes a trial stimulation period with an external pulse generator; only if this provides significant pain relief should an implantable pulse generator be inserted. Some patients find the induced paresthesia more painful than the condition that is being treated. The trial period has predictive value for the final success of a fully implanted system.[53,54] The principal complications of SCS are infection, which is usually reported as occurring in 1% of patients in whom optimal surgical conditions are used,[55] and technical failures such as electrode migration or breakage.

Efficacy

There are few data available relating to the use of SCS in cancer pain. In the UK in the past decade, no stimulators have been implanted for this indication (Medtronic Ltd, Watford, UK, personal communication). No randomized controlled trials are available. A number of case series have been described, but the numbers of patients with cancer in these series is small.[56–58] In one series it was concluded that the technique is not useful for the management of cancer pain,[59] and in another smaller series that the results for cancer pain were equivocal.[60]

DEEP BRAIN STIMULATION AND CANCER PAIN*

Stimulation of the brain for pain control was first used in the 1960s and in expert hands is now an accepted technique for the management of some chronic painful conditions refractory to conventional therapy. The most usual sites for stimulation are:

- In the caudal medial thalamic area around the third ventricle (periventricular gray, PVG) and at the junction of the third ventricle and aqueduct of Sylvius (periaqueductal gray, PAG) Early studies suggested that this was the optimal site of stimulation for the relief of cancer pain.[44] The analgesic effect was thought to be related to elevation of endogenous opioids,[61] but more recent literature is conflicting.[62]
- In the somatosensory areas of the ventrobasal thalamus, particularly the ventroposterior lateral (VPL) and ventroposterior medial (VPM) nuclei. The mechanism for analgesia is thought to be similar to that for spinal cord stimulation.

One paper described electrical stimulation of the pituitary in three patients with cancer pain.[63]

Target localization is achieved with magnetic resonance imaging, and electrodes may be implanted stereotactically via a burr hole under local anesthesia. When the target is reached, electrodes are externalized to allow a period of trial stimulation which, if successful, may lead to insertion of an implanted stimulator. The precise complication rates from these techniques is unknown but overall is probably in the region of 20%,[21] although one series of 17 patients with pain due to intractable malignancy identified no complications.[64] Side-effects may be related to electrode insertion such as hemorrhage, infection, or seizures or may be related to hardware problems.[62] Although not all side-effects are permanent, the potential for serious morbidity or mortality should reserve this highly invasive and expensive therapy for a tiny minority of patients who have otherwise intractable pain.

Efficacy

There have been no randomized controlled trials of brain stimulation in cancer pain. One review of world literature studied 916 patients receiving stimulation for a variety of indications and found that over half of patients gained satisfactory pain relief.[62] Young and Brechner[64] studied 17 patients with malignancy followed up for 1–21 months and found that four required narcotic analgesia on leaving hospital. All of these patients had been tolerant to large doses of opioids at the time of surgery. Six patients were still alive at the time of writing. Of those successfully treated, 14 eventually needed opioid medication in the last few weeks of their lives. In another case series of patients receiving stimulation for a range of pain conditions, a small number of whom had cancer, the analgesic efficacy in the cancer patients was found to be short-lived,[65] a finding reiterated in a longer term review by the same group.[66] A larger series of 141 patients, of whom six had cancer, indicates more encouraging results.[67] There is not sufficient information in the literature specifically addressing the use of this therapy in the cancer population to draw any conclusions as to its utility.

A PRAGMATIC APPROACH TO THE USE OF STIMULATION TECHNIQUES IN CANCER PAIN

The pharmacological management of cancer pain remains a problem in large numbers of patients, although this probably represents a small *proportion* of patients with malignant disease. The use of many effective analgesics is limited by side-effects, and adjunctive therapy is frequently necessary. Although the goal should be to base practice on robust scientific evidence, particularly when interventions may be costly or associated with significant morbidity, there may be a role for simple, safe, cheap, and easily applied treatments when the evidence is equivocal. A number of safeguards should be employed. Patients should have been appropriately investigated and diagnosed and the progress of the malignancy should be under regular review. Close liaison should be maintained between the pain therapist and the cancer care team. In most cases, stimulation techniques will provide an adjunct to other pain-relieving therapies, either enhancing the effect of medication or by allowing dose reduction of drugs with troublesome side-effects. Of the therapies described, clinical experience would suggest that TENS and acupuncture are worth offering to patients whose pain is not controlled. For these treatments the likely benefits outweigh the minimal risk. It would seem sensible to exercise more caution with more costly and invasive stimulation techniques. These should be reserved for the most refractory patients and should be carried out in centers with considerable experience of the therapies. Although there is some literature to inform a balanced and rational decision on the management of these difficult cases there is an urgent need for good-quality multicenter research to ensure that patients are not subjected to treatments which may be ineffective or may harm them.

REFERENCES

1. Melzack R. Folk Medicine and the sensory modulation of pain. In: Wall PD, Melzack R eds. *Textbook of Pain*, 3rd edn. Edinburgh: Churchill Livingstone, 1994: 1209–17.
2. Thompson JW, Filshie J. Transcutaneous electrical nerve stimulation (TENS) and acupuncture. In: Doyle D, Hanks GWC, Macdonald M eds. *Oxford Textbook of Palliative Medicine*. Oxford: Oxford University Press, 1993: 229–44.
3. ◆ Melzack R, Wall PD. Pain mechanisms: a new theory. *Science* 1965; **150:** 971–9.
4. ◆ Wall PD, Sweet WH. Temporary abolition of pain in man. *Science* 1967; **155:** 108–9.
5. Grossman SA, Staats P. Current management of pain in patients with cancer. *Oncology* 1994; **8(3):** 93–107.
6. ● Filshie J, Redman D. Acupuncture and malignant pain problems. *Eur J Surg Oncol* 1985; **11:** 389–94.
7. Stannard CF. Anatomy and physiology of pain. In: Stannard CF, Booth S eds. *Pocketbook of Pain*. Edinburgh: Churchill Livingstone, 1998: 4–11.
8. Garrison DW, Foreman RD. Decreased activity of spontaneous and noxiously evoked dorsal horn cells during transcutaneous electrical nerve stimulation (TENS). *Pain* 1994; **58:** 309–15.
9. Woolf CJ, King AE. The physiology and morphology of multireceptive neurons with C-afferent inputs in the deep dorsal horn of the rat lumbar spinal cord. *J Neurophysiol* 1987; **58:** 460–79.
10. ● Filshie J. The non-drug treatment of neuralgic and neuropathic pain of malignancy. *Cancer Surveys* 1988; **7(1):** 161–93.
11. Sjolund B, Eriksson M. The influence of naloxone on analgesia produced by peripheral conditioning stimulation. *Brain Res* 1979; **173:** 295–301.
12. Woolf CJ, Mitchell D, Myers RA, Barrett JD. Failure of naloxone to reverse peripheral transcutaneous electroanalgesia in patients suffering from acute trauma. *South Afr Med J* 1978; **53:** 179–80.
13. Abrams SE, Reynolds AC, Cusick JF. Failure of Naloxone to reverse analgesia from transcutaneous electrical stimulation in patients with chronic pain *Anesth Analg* 1981; **60:** 81–4.
14. Woolf CJ, Thompson JW. Stimulation induced analgesia: transcutaneous electrical nerve stimulation (TENS) and vibration In: Wall PD, Melzack R eds. *Textbook of Pain*, 3rd edn. Edinburgh: Churchill Livingstone, 1994: 1191–208.
15. Mannheimer C, Carlsson CA, Vedin A, Wilhelmssen C. Transcutaneous electrical nerve stimulation (TENS) in angina pectoris. *Pain* 1986; **26:** 291–300.
16. ◆ Johnson MI, Ashton CH, Thompson JW. An in-depth study of long term users of transcutaneous electrical nerve stimulators (TENS). Implication for clinical use of TENS. *Pain* 1981; **44:** 221–9.
17. ◆ Librach SL, Rapson LM. The use of transcutaneous electrical nerve stimulation (TENS) for the relief of pain in palliative care. *Palliative Med* 1988; **2:** 15–20.
18. D'Amours RH, Riegler FX, Little AG. Pathogenesis and management of persistent postthoracotomy pain. *Chest Surg Clin N Am* 1998; **8:** 703–22.
19. Rooney S, Jain S, Goldiner P. Effect of transcutaneous nerve stimulation on postoperative pain after thoracotomy. *Anesth Analg* 1983; **62:** 1010–12.
20. ● Portenoy RK. Optimal pain control in elderly cancer patients. *Geriatrics* 1987; **42(5):** 33–44.
21. Stannard CF. Neurostimulation. In: Stannard CF, Booth S eds. *Pocketbook of Pain*. Edinburgh: Churchill Livingstone, 1998: 112–20.
22. Johnson MI, Ashton CH, Thompson JW, *et al.* The clinical use of TENS. *J Orthop Med* 1992; **14:** 3–12.
23. Andersson SA, Hahsson G, Holmgren E. Evaluation of pain suppressing effect of different frequencies of peripheral electrical stimulation in chronic pain conditions. *Acta Orthop Scand* 1976; **47:** 149–57.
24. Mason JL, Mackay NAM. Pain sensations associated with electrocutaneous stimulation. *IEEE Trans Biomed Eng* 1976; **23:** 405–9.
25. Yamamoto T, *et al.* Formative mechanisms of current concentration and breakdown phenomena dependent on direct current flow through skin by a dry electrode. *IEEE Trans Biomed Eng* 1986; **33:** 396–404.
26. ◆ Loeser JD, Black RG, Christman RM. Relief of pain by transcutaneous stimulation. *J Neurosurg* 1975; **42:** 308–14.
27. Eriksson MBE, Sjolund BH, Sundberg G. Pain relief from conditioning stimulation in patients with chronic facial pain. *J Neurosurg* 1984; **61:** 149–55.
28. Pomeranz B, Niznick G. Codetron: a new electrotherapy device overcomes the habituation problems of conventional TENS devices. *Am J Electromed* 1987; **1:** 22–6.
29. ◆ Reeve J, Menon D, Corabian P. Transcutaneous electrical nerve stimulation (TENS); a technology assessment. *Int J Technol Assess Hlth Care* 1996; **12:** 299–324.
30. ◆ McQuay HJ, Moore A. Transcutaneous electrical nerve stimulation (TENS) in chronic pain. In: McQuay HJ, Moore A eds. *An Evidence-based Resource for Pain Relief*. Oxford: Oxford University Press, 1998; 207–12.
31. ◆ Deyo RA, Walsh NE, Schoenfeld LS, Ramanurthy S. Can trials of physical treatments be blinded? The example of transcutaneous electrical stimulation for chronic pain. *Am J Phys Med Rehabil* 1990; **69:** 6–10.
32. Chakour M, Gibson SJ, Neufeld M, *et al.* Development of an active placebo for studies of TENS treatment. In: Devor M, *et al.* eds. *Proceedings of the 9th World Congress on Pain, Progress in Pain Research and Management*, 2000: 987–92.
33. ◆ Zech DF, Grand S, Lynch J, *et al.* Validation of World

Health Organization Guidelines for cancer pain relief: a 10-year prospective study. *Pain* 1995; **63(1):** 65–76.

34. Bates JAV, Nathan PW. Transcutaneous electrical nerve stimulation for chronic pain. *Anaesthesia* 1980; **35:** 817–22.
35. Campbell JN, Long DM. Peripheral nerve stimulation in the treatment of intractable pain. *J Neurosurg* 1976; **45:** 692–9.
36. Ventafridda V. Transcutaneous nerve stimulation in cancer pain. In: Bonica JJ, Ventafridda V eds. *Advances in Pain Research and Therapy*. New York, NY: Raven Press, 1979: 509–15.
37. Dil'din AS, Tikhonova GP, Kozlov SV. Transcutaneous electrostimulation method leading to a permeation system of electroanalgesia in oncological practice. *VOPROSY onkologii* 1985; **31(8):** 33–6.
38. Avellanosa AM, West CR. Experience with transcutaneous nerve stimulation for relief of intractable pain in cancer patients. *J Med* 1982; **13:** 203–13.
39. Chiarini L, *et al.* Management of facial pain resulting from cancer in oral and maxillofacial surgery. *Minerva Stomatol* 1997; **46(1–2):** 27–38.
40. ◆ McQuay HJ, *et al.* Transcutaneous nerve stimulation. In: McQuay HJ, Moore RA, Eccleston C, *et al.* eds. Systematic review of outpatient services for chronic pain control. *Hlth Technol Assess* 1997; **1(6):** 43–50.
41. Benedetti F, Amanzio M, Casadio C, *et al.* Control of postoperative pain by transcutaneous electrical nerve stimulation after thoracic operations. *Ann Thorac Surg* 1997; **63:** 773–6.
42. Long DM. Fifteen years of transcutaneous electrical stimulation for pain control. *Stereotact Funct Neurosurg* 1991; **56(1):** 2–19.
43. ◆ Sweet WH, Wepsic JG. Treatment of chronic pain by stimulation of fiber of primary afferent neuron. *Trans Am Neurol Assoc* 1968; **93:** 103–5.
44. Loeser J. Neurosurgical approaches in palliative care. In: Doyle D, Hanks GWC, Macdonald M eds. *Oxford Textbook of Palliative Medicine.* Oxford: Oxford University Press, 1993: 221–9.
45. Law JD, Swett J, Kirsch WM. Retrospective analysis of 22 patients with chronic pain treated by peripheral nerve stimulation. *J Neurosurg* 1980; **52:** 482–5.
46. Nashold BS. Peripheral nerve stimulation for pain. *J Neurosurg* 1980; **53:** 132–3.
47. Campbell JN, Long DM. Peripheral nerve stimulation in the treatment of intractable pain. *J Neurosurg* 1976; **45:** 692–9.
48. ◆ Shealy CN, Mortimer JT, Reswick J. Electrical inhibition of pain by stimulation of the dorsal column: preliminary clinical reports. *Anesth Analg* 1967; **46:** 489–91.
49. Larsen SJ, Sances A, Cusick JF. A comparison between anterior and posterior spinal implant systems. *Surg Neurol* 1975; **4:** 180–6.
50. Duggan AW, Foong FW. Bicuculline and spinal inhibition produced by dorsal column stimulation in the cat. *Pain* 1985; **22(3):** 249–59.
51. Cui JG, O'Connor WT, Ungerstedt U, *et al.* Spinal cord stimulation attenuates augmented dorsal horn release of excitatory amino acids in mononeuropathy via a GABAergic mechanism. *Pain* 1997; **73:** 87–95.
52. Willis WD, Al-Chaer ED, Quast MJ, Westlund KN. A visceral pain pathway in the dorsal column of the spinal cord. *Proc Natl Acad Sci USA* 1999; **96:** 7675–9.
53. Burton C. Dorsal column stimulation: optimization of application. *Surg Neurol* 1975; **4:** 171–6.
54. North RS, Fischell TA, Long DM. Chronic dorsal column stimulation via percutaneously inserted epidural electrodes. *Appl Neurophysiol* 1977; **40:** 181–91.
55. Krainick J, Thoden U. Spinal cord stimulation. In: Wall PD, Melzack R eds. *Textbook of Pain,* 3rd edn. Edinburgh: Churchill Livingstone, 1994: 1219–23.
56. Shimoji K, Hokari T, Kano T. Management of intractable pain with percutaneous epidural spinal cord stimulation: differences in pain-relieving effects among diseases and sites of pain. *Anesth Analg* 1993; **77(1):** 110–16.
57. Lazorthes Y, Siegfried J, Verdic JC, Casaux J. Chronic spinal cord stimulation in the treatment of neurogenic pain. Cooperative and retrospective study on 20 years follow-up. *Neurochirurgie* 1995; **41(2):** 73–6.
58. North RB, Fischell TA, Long DM. Chronic stimulation via percutaneously inserted epidural electrodes. *Neurosurgery* 1977; **1:** 215–18.
59. Meglio M, Cioni B, Rossi GF. Spinal cord stimulation in management of chronic pain. A 9-year experience. *J Neurosurg* 1989; **70:** 519–24.
60. Krainick JU, Thoden U. Experience with dorsal column stimulation (DCS) in the operative treatment of chronic intractable pain. *J Neurosurg Sci* 1974; **18(3):** 187–9.
61. Hosobuchi Y, Adams JE, Bloom FE. Stimulation of human periaqueductal grey for pain relief increases immunoreactive β-endorphin in ventricular fluid. *Science* 1979; **203:**279–281.
62. Young RF, Rinaldi PC. Brain stimulation for relief of chronic pain In: Wall PD, Melzack R eds. *Textbook of Pain*, 3rd edn. Edinburgh: Churchill Livingstone 1994: 1225–33.
63. Yanagida H, Suwa K, Troouwborst A, *et al.* Electrical stimulation of the pituitary: its use in the treatment of cancer pain. *Pain Clin* 1988; **2/4:** 225–8.
64. Young RF, Brechner T. Electrical stimulation of the brain for relief of intractable pain due to cancer. *Cancer* 1986; **57(6):** 266–72.
65. Kumar K, Wyant GM, Nath R. Deep brain stimulation for alleviating chronic intractable pain. *Can J Surg* 1985; **28(1):** 20–2.
66. Kumar K, Wyant GM, Nath R. Deep brain stimulation for control of pain in humans, present and future: a ten year follow-up. *Neurosurgery* 1990; **26:** 774–81.
67. ● Levy RM, Lamb S, Adams JE. Treatment of chronic pain by deep brain stimulation: long term follow-up and review of the literature. *Neurosurgery* 1987; **21:** 885–93.

18

Radiotherapy in cancer pain management

PETER J HOSKIN

Radiotherapy has far-ranging application in the management of cancer pain. A feature of radiotherapy is that it is, with the exception of wide-field radiation and isotope therapy, a locoregional treatment. This means that as a result of the delivery of ionizing radiation in the form of beams of photons or electrons a selected anatomical region will be treated. It should therefore be considered in any situation in which a localized tumor mass is resulting in pain, for example bone metastasis or soft-tissue infiltration, or in the case of neuropathic pain arising from tumor encroaching upon sensory nerves.

The mechanism of the analgesic action of radiotherapy remains uncertain. Pain relief can often be achieved by low doses of radiation, exemplified by the treatment of bone metastasis, for which a nontumor effect on humoral mediators of pain has been proposed. It is, however, important to realize that after radiation doses of only 2 Gy 50–80% of the cell population in common cancers will fail to survive in experimental cultures. Where there is soft-tissue infiltration or neuropathic pain, tumor shrinkage reducing local pressure and thereby the physical pain stimulus may be important, but again a direct effect upon the release of chemical pain mediators and nerve conduction cannot be excluded. However, the degree of shrinkage required for symptomatic as distinct from radiographic response may be very small, and thus the concept of radiosensitivity as applied to the curative situation should not be used to deny patients local radiotherapy for cancer pain.

SPECIFIC INDICATIONS FOR RADIOTHERAPY IN CANCER PAIN MANAGEMENT

Bone pain is by far the commonest indication for radiotherapy in cancer pain management, accounting for up to 20% of all radiotherapy treatment given in some departments. This is discussed in detail in Chapter Ca21. The other two main indications for radiotherapy in cancer pain management are soft-tissue pain and nerve pain. The main indications for radiotherapy in soft-tissue pain are given in Table 18.1. By far the most common indications are local chest pain from carcinoma of the bronchus, reflecting its high incidence, and headache from cerebral metastasis.

The main indications for radiotherapy in nerve pain are given in Table 18.2.

Often it is not possible to distinguish readily the three categories of pain described above. For example, bone metastases in the spine are often associated with both local pain in the bone invaded and neuropathic pain from nerve root irritation; soft-tissue infiltration into the presacral space or pelvic side wall will result in both local pelvic pain and neuropathic pain radiating from the lumbosacral plexus.

Soft-tissue pain

Chest pain

Malignant chest pain may result from carcinoma of the bronchus, occurring in 40–70% of cases,[1**,2**,3] or where there is pleural infiltration from either a primary mesothelioma or blood-borne metastasis. In general, pleural infiltration is far more troublesome with regard to pain than a central chest tumor.

In the treatment of carcinoma of the bronchus there is published evidence from randomized trials using specific symptom score cards to show that radiotherapy is effective in controlling chest pain in over 70% of patients.[1**,2**] This can be achieved with simple prag-

Table 18.1 *Indications for radiotherapy in soft-tissue pain*

Site of pain	Cause of pain	Published response rate	Level of evidence
Chest pain	Primary bronchial carcinoma	70–80%[1,2]	**
	Mesothelioma	68%[14]	*
Headache	Primary glioma	Not stated[5]	
	Cerebral metastases	70–80%[6–8]	**
Liver pain	Primary hepatocellular cancer	Not available	
	Liver metastases	55–74%[9,10]	**
Splenic pain	Leukemia/lymphoma	91%[11]	*
Loin pain	Renal cancer	Not available	
Back pain	Para-aortic nodes	Not available	
Pelvic pain	Uterine cancer	83%[12]	*
	Ovarian cancer	44%[13]	*

Table 18.2 *Indications for radiotherapy in nerve pain*

Site of pain	Cause of pain	Published response rate	Level of evidence
Pelvic pain	Presacral mass, e.g. cancer of the rectum	70%[14]	*
	Lumbosacral plexus infiltration	100%[15]	*
Shoulder/ upper limb	Apical lung cancer (Pancoast's)	30–79%[16,17]	*
	Axillary nodes, e.g. breast cancer	77%[18]	*

matic courses of treatment, the randomized trials demonstrating that a dose of 17 Gy in two fractions is as good as 30 Gy in 10 fractions,[1]** and indeed in poor performance status patients equivalent pain control can be achieved with a single dose of 10 Gy.[2]**

There is less evidence to support the use of radiotherapy in pleural disease, although it is a relatively common practice when faced with symptomatic mesothelioma or metastatic deposits. One small series of 19 patients with pain from mesothelioma reported pain relief in 13 (68%) at 1 month, but longer term pain control was poor, with only four patients having sustained relief at 3 months.[4] An additional advantage for radiotherapy in this setting is the prevention of tumor growth through drain sites in the chest wall, although again evidence in support of this is largely anecdotal.

Headache

Headache may arise from an expanding mass within the skull, and in the context of malignant disease this may be either a primary or secondary tumor. In the population at large, primary brain tumors are rare, and the majority of intracranial neoplasms will be cerebral metastases. Radiotherapy may well have a role in the treatment of a primary brain tumor, but randomized controlled trials have focused principally upon survival rather than symptom control. Performance status and quality of life is undoubtedly improved with local radiotherapy for high-grade gliomas in selected patients who are aged under 65, present with fits alone, and have no major neurological deficits.[5]* Among older patients and those with more advanced disease at presentation, hypofractionated radiotherapy delivering 30 Gy in six fractions improved functional status as measured by the Barthel index in 38% of patients, with a further 39% remaining stable; specific data relating to pain were not reported.[19]

In contrast, prospective randomized data[6]**,[7]**,[8]** strongly support the use of radiotherapy in the management of headache due to cerebral metastasis. The two largest series performed by the Radiotherapy Therapy Oncology Group (RTOG) in the United States[6]** some years ago reported control of headache in 70–80% of patients, and across its series of studies including over 2,000 patients it was shown that this could be achieved with relatively low doses of radiation down to 20 Gy in five daily fractions over 1 week, with no difference when compared with longer treatments over 4 weeks. More recently, the UK Royal College of Radiologists' randomized trial[8]** compared 12 Gy in two fractions with 30 Gy in 10 fractions and again found equivalent responses and control of headache in over 90% of patients. This has therefore become the standard treatment in the UK for brain metastasis, and elsewhere 1- to 2-week courses of radiotherapy are generally given with good effect for control of headache.

Liver pain

Rapid expansion of the liver with progressive hepatic metastasis results in right-sided abdominal pain due to stretching of the liver capsule. In patients with tumors that are sensitive to chemotherapy or hormone therapy, this is usually the most appropriate treatment alongside systemic steroids. In many cases, however, progressive, painful liver metastases will reflect advanced disease either insensitive to systemic anticancer therapy or having relapsed after earlier exposure. Two randomized trials[9**,10**] have evaluated the role of hepatic irradiation in these circumstances and demonstrated control of liver pain in over 50% from relatively low doses of radiation delivering 20–30 Gy over 2–3 weeks to the liver. One of the major difficulties and reservations with regard to hepatic irradiation relates to the associated toxicity, and nausea, vomiting, and general malaise are recognized problems. The published data,[9**,10**] however, suggest that the benefits in terms of liver shrinkage and improved well-being as a result of improved liver function outweigh these toxicities, which can be minimized by avoiding irradiation to the whole liver if possible and using appropriate antiemetic cover.

Splenic pain

Pain from the spleen may arise because of progressive enlargement, typically due to hematological malignancies such as chronic granulocytic leukemia or non-Hodgkin's lymphoma. In many circumstances, the treatment of choice will be surgical removal or chemotherapy, but in advanced cases or when the patient is unfit for surgery splenic irradiation is entirely appropriate. Very low doses of irradiation will cause significant splenic shrinkage and considerable pain relief. A greater effect with doses above 5 Gy has been reported, and typical schedules will deliver doses of around 10 Gy in up to 10 daily treatments over 2 weeks. Reduction in splenic size was reported in 60%, and pain relief occurred in 91% and was maintained for up to 6 months.[11*]

Loin pain

Both primary renal cancer and retroperitoneal sarcoma can present severe loin and back pain. This will reflect infiltration of the retroperitoneal tissues, and generally such tumors are locally advanced and inoperable. In these circumstances, local radiotherapy may be of value, although the dose to be delivered will be limited by the surrounding tissues, which are relatively sensitive to radiation, in particular the small bowel, stomach, liver, and normal kidney. Nonetheless, useful pain control may be achieved, although published data to support this are scanty.

Para-aortic lymphadenopathy

Enlargement of the para-aortic lymph nodes causes a characteristic persistent backache. When due to chemotherapy-sensitive tumors such as lymphoma or germ cell tumors, then chemotherapy may well be the best approach, but in chemoresistant tumors local radiotherapy delivering doses of 20–30 Gy in 2–3 weeks is the traditional treatment. Anecdotally, good pain control can be achieved, although there are few published data to support this impression.

Pelvic pain

Advanced or recurrent tumors within the pelvis frequently present with local pain, which may be of a visceral nature or neuropathic (see below). Visceral pain is typically related to gynecological primary tumors, in particular of the cervix and ovary. Results from palliative radiotherapy to recurrent ovarian cancer delivering a median dose of 35 Gy report pain relief in 83% of 47 treatments,[13] and in advanced uterine cancer pain relief was seen in 44% after single-dose treatment with 10 Gy.[12]

Nerve pain

Bone metastasis may be a cause of nerve root compression and associated neuropathic pain. The management of this is generally no different to that of localized metastatic bone pain, as discussed previously.

Pelvic pain

Pelvic pain may be associated with pain in the sciatic nerve distribution radiating into the buttocks and down the leg because of infiltration of the lumbosacral plexus. A common situation in which this is encountered is presacral recurrence of colorectal tumor. In patients who have not received chemotherapy this should be considered, typically using 5-fluorouracil (5-FU)-based schedules, but if there are local symptoms pelvic radiotherapy may be of value. One series evaluated the response of pelvic pain, reporting success in 80% of patients who received either a single dose of 10 Gy or 35 Gy in 15 fractions, with no difference between the two radiation dose schedules.[14] One study of 13 patients with neuropathic pain from lumbosacral plexus involvement with tumor reported pain relief in all patients after doses of either 17 Gy in two fractions or 20 Gy in five fractions.[15]

Upper limb pain

Upper limb pain may arise because of local tumor growing in the apex of the lung, axilla, or lower neck. The typical situation is that of the Pancoast tumor, which is an apical primary tumor of the lung. Another common situation is metastatic lymph nodes, which may be axillary from carcinoma of the breast, low deep cervical lymph nodes from carcinoma of the bronchus, or left-sided supraclavicular nodes arising from intra-abdominal malignancy. A wide range of doses have been reported, ranging from single doses of 10 Gy to 58 Gy in 31 fractions.[18] "Significant" pain relief has been reported in up to 77% of patients with metastatic breast cancer, with similar response rates for Pancoast's tumor. However, one retrospective series of treatment to apical lung cancer suggests that no more than 30% of patients receiving radiotherapy will achieve durable pain control.[17] A dose–response effect has been reported with Pancoast's tumor,[16] although other studies report no improvement with increasing dose.[17]

PITUITARY ABLATION

This is rarely performed today but has been reported as a useful technique in the management of intractable pain. Local radiotherapy has been used as a means of achieving this. Similarly, thalamic ablation using stereotactic irradiation has been described,[20] and the proponents of this approach have reported response rates in patients with intractable pain of up to 90%.

SPECIAL COMMENTS

Radiotherapy will rarely be used as a sole agent in the management of cancer pain. Within the indications mentioned above, it will be used alongside analgesics and co-analgesics, as detailed in the relevant chapters. The relative merits of each approach remain uncertain. Clearly, there is a strong indication for local radiotherapy when simple drug schedules fail to control pain adequately. The need for radiotherapy in patients in whom regular analgesia can control pain is less certain unless there is undue toxicity associated with the drug regimen, in which case local radiotherapy may provide a means of reducing or even abolishing the need for regular systemic medication. Associated symptoms may also be an important consideration in seeking radiotherapy as an effective palliation. For example, in patients with chest pain and associated hemoptysis from nonsmall-cell lung cancer radiotherapy is indicated for both symptoms, and similarly the presence of motor weakness with headache due to brain metastases presents a situation in which local radiotherapy may have a dual indication, even if the headache can be controlled with steroids and analgesics.

Radiotherapy is, therefore, but one of several possible treatments for cancer pain, with specific indications as discussed above. The application of the basic principles of careful patient assessment, pain identification, and diagnosis of underlying pathological mechanisms will allow individualized treatment for each patient, incorporating radiotherapy where appropriate.

REFERENCES

◆ 1. Medical Research Council Lung Cancer Working Party. Prepared on behalf of the working party and all its collaborators by: Bleehen NM, Girling DJ, Machin D, Stephens RJ. Inoperable non-small-cell lung cancer (NSCLC): a Medical Research Council randomised trial of palliative radiotherapy with two fractions or ten fractions. *Br J Cancer* 1991; **63:** 265–70.

◆ 2. Medical Research Council Lung Cancer Working Party. Prepared on behalf of the working party and all its collaborators by Bleehen NM, Girling DJ, Machin D, Stephens RJ. A Medical Research Council (MRC) randomised trial of palliative radiotherapy with two fractions or a single fraction in patients with inoperable non-small-cell lung cancer (NSCLC) and poor performance status. *Br J Cancer* 1992; **65:** 934–41.

● 3. Collins TM, Ash DV, Close HJ, Thorogood J. An evaluation of the palliative role of radiotherapy in inoperable carcinoma of the bronchus. *Clin Radiol* 1988; **39:** 284–6.

4. Bissett D, Macbeth FR, Cram I. The role of palliative radiotherapy in malignant mesothelioma. *Clin Oncol* 1991; **3:** 315–17.

◆ 5. Bleehen NM, Stenning SP on behalf of the Medical Research Council Brain Tumour Working Party. A Medical Research Council trial of two radiotherapy doses in the treatment of grades 3 and 4 astrocytoma. *Br J Cancer* 1991; **64:** 769–74.

◆ 6. Borgelt B, Gelber R, Kramer S, *et al.* The palliation of brain metastases: final results of the first two studies by the Radiation Therapy Oncology Group. *Int J Radiat Oncol Biol Phys* 1980; **6:** 1–9.

7. Harwood AR, Simpson JW. Radiation therapy of cerebral metastases: a randomized prospective clinical trial. *Int J Radiat Oncol Biol Phys* 1977; **2:** 1091–4.

◆ 8. Priestman TJ, Dunn J, Brada M, *et al.* Final results of the Royal College of Radiologists' trial comparing two different radiotherapy schedules in the treatment of cerebral metastases. *Clin Oncol* 1996; **8:** 308–15.

9. Borgelt B, Gelber R, Brady LW, *et al.* The palliation of hepatic metastases: results of the Radiation Therapy Oncology Group pilot study. *Int J Radiat Oncol Biol Phys* 1981; **7:** 587–91.

10. Leibel SA, Pajak TF, Massullo V, *et al.* A comparison of Misonidazole sensitized radiation therapy to radiation therapy alone for the palliation of hepatic metastases: results of a Radiation Therapy Oncology Group randomized prospective trial. *Int J Radiat Oncol Biol Phys* 1987; **13:** 1057–64.

11. Paulino AC, Reddy SP. Splenic irradiation in the palliation of patients with lymphoproliferative and myeloproliferative disorders. *Am J Hospice Palliative Care* 1996; **13:** 32–5.

12. Halle JS, Rosenman JG, Varia MA, *et al.* 1000cGy single dose palliation for advanced carcinoma of the cervix or endometrium. *Int J Radiat Oncol Biol Phys* 1986; **12:** 1947–50.

13. Corn BW, Lanciano RM, Boente M, *et al.* Recurrent ovarian cancer. Effective radiotherapeutic palliation after chemotherapy failure. *Cancer* 1994; **74:** 2979–83.

14. Allum WH, Mack P, Priestman TJ, Fielding JWL. Radio-

therapy for pain relief in locally recurrent colorectal cancer. *Ann Roy Coll Surg Engl* 1987; **69:** 220–1.

15. Russi EG, Pergolizzi S, Gaeta M, *et al.* Palliative-radiotherapy in lumbosacral carcinomatous neuropathy. *Radiother Oncol* 1993; **26:** 172–3.
16. Morris RW, Abadir R. Pancoast tumour: the value of high dose radiation therapy. *Radiology* 1979; **132:** 717–19.
17. Watson PN, Evans RJ. Intractable pain with lung cancer *Pain* 1987; **29:** 163–73.
18. Ampil FL. Radiotherapy for carcinomatous brachial plexus plexopathy. *Cancer* 1985; **56:** 2185–8.
19. Thomas R, James N, Guerro D, *et al.* Hypofractionated radiotherapy as a palliative treatment in poor prognosis patients with high grade glioma. *Radiother Oncol* 1994; **33:** 113–16.
20. Leksell L, Meyerson BA, Forster DMC. Radiosurgical thalamotomy for intractable pain. *Confinia Neurol* 1972; **34:** 264.

19

Neurosurgical modalities in the management of cancer-related pain

EHUD ARBIT AND SUSAN PANNULLO

The majority of cancer patients experience pain during the course of their disease, especially in the advanced stages.[1***,2***,3***] In most patients, pain is directly related to the tumor but may also be the result of cancer therapy or an unrelated etiology. Unrelieved pain impairs physical and psychological functioning of patients and compromises quality of life. Antineoplastic therapy, pain management, and symptom palliation (both physical and psychological) are interrelated aspects of the global care of cancer patients that are best addressed simultaneously.

Contemporary pain management is based on a medication titration protocol and is effective in relieving 75–90% of cancer pain.[4***,5***] In a significant number of cancer patients, pain is refractory to pharmacotherapy and some form of intervention is indicated. Neurolysis, rhiziolysis, or gangliolysis performed with neurolytic agents, cryoablation, or radiofrequency ablation is the most common form of intervention. In a small minority of patients, ablative or modulatory neurosurgical procedures are indicated. There is a growing consensus that intrathecal opiate therapy, which has the advantage of reversibility and a more favorable risk–benefit ratio, may be warranted before irreversible neuroablative modalities are considered.

Based on anatomical and physiological data, many sites in the central nervous system (CNS) have been lesioned to produce analgesia. Except for cordotomy, a procedure that withstood the test of time, the role of other destructive procedures in the CNS is less well defined. However, small surveys of patients who have undergone cingulotomy, hypothalamotomy, thalamotomy of varied types, mesencephalotomy, pontine spinothalamic tractotomy, or trigeminal tractotomy suggest that these procedures can be safe and effective in patients with refractory pain.

This chapter addresses when to consider surgical intervention for cancer-related pain and how to select the most appropriate procedure for a specific pain situation. A detailed description of technical aspects is beyond the confines of this chapter, and readers are referred to appropriate texts on technical issues. The neurosurgical approaches and ablative procedures emphasized here reflect a personal bias of the authors and were chosen based on literature review, personal communications, and personal experience.

THE PHENOMENOLOGY OF CANCER PAIN

Pain, with its broad implications, is a dynamic and multifactorial phenomenon. Because the degree of nociceptive activation correlates with extent of tissue damage, pain intensity mirrors the degree of tissue injury. Furthermore, repeated activation by nociceptive stimuli of nuclei and tracts in the CNS may lead to structural and functional alterations in the system. Chronic pain in humans may be attributable to pathological changes in the CNS that result from repeated noxious stimuli. Neuropathic pain, as an example, refers to persistent pain which presumably results from pathological functioning of the nervous system, which then assumes the role of an autonomous spontaneous central generator of pain. The dynamics of pain in the cancer patient are not limited to changes in the CNS however. The cancer process itself may affect multiple sites, and pain may result from diverse etiologies as the disease evolves. Among patients with advanced cancer, 50% have more than one pain syndrome and 34% four or more.[6***]

Factors contributing to the diversity of pain syndromes include the site of the primary cancer, its biological behavior, its proclivity for specific sites (e.g. bone), its proximity to neural structures, and the generation by the tumor of pain-producing substances. Clearly, subjective variables such as personality, mood, and psychosocial comorbidity can profoundly influence the phenomenology and impact of pain in the cancer patient.

CLINICAL ASSESSMENT

The foundation of the decision-making process is thorough assessment and information gathering. Before meeting with the patient, information concerning the patient's cancer, grade, extent of concurrent disease, prior response to therapy and potential for further therapy and response, including from experimental therapies, should be obtained from the treating oncologist. A medication history should include the past and present use of analgesics and adjunctive drugs. The patient or family should be asked for a detailed history, including information about the onset, duration, severity, quality, location, temporal profile, and course of the pain as well as clarification of provoking and palliative factors. During this initial process it is important to obtain an impression of related emotional, behavioral, and social disturbances that might be affecting the patient. A general medical and neurological examination, along with appropriate laboratory tests and radiographic evaluation of the patient, is important to identify specific pain syndromes, determine the extent of disease, and clarify the specific etiology and type of pain. The search for an underlying etiology can be time-consuming and may cause unnecessary discomfort to the patient. It must therefore be placed in the context of the patient's illness and is justified only when the etiology is uncertain and the findings could lead to a change in therapy.

From the neurosurgical standpoint, consideration of topographic characteristics, pathophysiologic profile, and the functional status of the patient have important implications. Most patients have little difficulty in providing an accurate description of the topography of pain. Pain may be focal, multifocal, or generalized. This distinction is clinically relevant and may indicate or contraindicate specific interventions.

Cancer pain can be classified based on inferred pathophysiology, which broadly distinguishes nociceptive pain from neuropathic pain. Although this distinction is an oversimplification of a complex pathophysiology, it nevertheless has been found to be useful to clinicians as each requires a different approach.

The vast majority of pain in the cancer patient population is nociceptive. Nociceptive pain implies chronic pain commensurate with tissue damage associated with an identifiable somatic or visceral lesion. Its persistence is presumed to be related to the ongoing activation of primary afferent neurons responsive to noxious stimuli. Pain resulting from activation of nociceptors in skin or deep tissue is also termed somatic pain. Somatic pain is typically characterized as localized and constant and is described as aching, stabbing, throbbing, or pressure-like. Visceral pain occurs when visceral nociceptors are activated by stretch or distension of intrathoracic or intra-abdominal viscera. Visceral pain is typically poorly localized and experienced as gnawing or crampy, when due to the obstruction of a hollow viscus and aching, sharp, or throbbing when due to the involvement of organ capsules or mesentery. Visceral pain is often associated with nausea, vomiting, and diaphoresis, and may be referred to cutaneous sites distant from the nociceptive lesion.

In general, nociceptive pain is more responsive to opioids[7] and is more amenable to ablative procedures. Visceral pain is conducted afferently by visceronociceptive fibers, which ascend in the spinal cord bilaterally in crossed and uncrossed tracts. Because of this anatomical pattern, interruption of visceronociceptive pathways must be carried out either at the peripheral ganglionic level or bilaterally at more rostral segments in the spinal cord.

Neuropathic pain is a consequence of damage to the peripheral and/or CNS and is believed to be sustained by aberrant somatosensory processing in these system. Such damage is often caused by tumor infiltration or compression of peripheral nerves, nerve roots, or a nerve plexus, and not infrequently results from radiotherapeutic or chemotherapeutic interventions (Table 19.1). Neuropathic pain is described as a sensation similar to pins and needles, numbness, dysesthesia, or electric shock. Paroxysmal pain may be related to spontaneous and ectopic impulse conduction at axonal sites of damaged peripheral nerves. Ongoing nociception is not a requisite for the occurrence of neuropathic pain, as it is for nociceptive pain; neuropathic pain occurs presumably as the result

Table 19.1 *Neuropathic pain syndromes in malignancy*

Tumor-related neuropathic pain
Mononeuropathy
Polyneuropathy
Radiculopathy
Plexopathy (cervical, brachial, lumbosacral, sacral)
Spinal cord pathology
Treatment-related neuropathic pain
Radiation induced (radiation fibrosis, radiation myelopathy)
Chemotherapy induced (polyneuropathies)
Surgery induced (postmastectomy and post-thoracotomy syndromes)

of a central pain generator or mechanism, and thus the removal of the nociceptive lesion may not produce relief. Neuropathic pain is regarded as being less opioid responsive than somatic pain and may require specific adjuvant analgesics. From the surgical perspective, some neuropathic pain syndromes, including evoked pains such as allodynia, hyperpathia, and hyperesthesia, as well as spontaneous pains with neuralgic elements, may respond well to ablations by cordotomy, dorsal root entry zone (DREZ) lesions, or ablation in the brainstem or thalamus. The spontaneous, steady burning (causalgic) or dysesthetic type of pain is, to large extent, impervious to ablations.[8] This type of pain is more amenable to modalities based on chronic stimulation of peripheral nerves, the dorsal columns, or the medial lemniscal system.

Most cancer-related pain is predominantly nociceptive, at least initially, but many patients develop an underlying component of deafferentation pain as the cancer evolves. As the tumor mass increases and compresses or encases neural structures, irreversible neural damage and denervation may ensue, resulting in a dysesthetic, causalgic pain superimposed on the primary, original nociceptive pain. This component of deafferentation pain is often overlooked, leading to suboptimal results achieved by procedures aimed at nociceptive pain. By the same token, a component of deafferentation should not dissuade the surgeon from an ablative procedure. Only when the pain is predominantly of the deafferentation type should treatment procedures be focused on deafferentation-related problems as such.

The patient population under consideration may be placed in one of two groups: (1) patients with refractory cancer, possibly with widespread systemic disease that is likely to be fatal within weeks or a few months, and (2) individuals with potential protracted longevity, whose focal or systemic cancer may be eradicable or controllable for months to years by antineoplastic therapy.

The majority of patients for whom surgical interventions are sought belong to the first group. They are terminally ill with a short prospective survival time. Frequently, they are partially or completely functionally impaired because of neurological deficits, long bone fractures, spinal metastases, or other causes. These patients are unique in that the benefit of pain relief may well outweigh the risks and consequences of further loss of neurological function. Faced with one of these patients, the neurosurgeon has a choice between an ablative or an augmentative procedure. The decision depends on the likelihood of efficacy of augmentative procedures. As an example, patients who require very high doses of opiates and do not obtain significant relief are less likely to respond to intraspinal or intracerebroventricular opioids, although a trial may still be warranted. In patients with severe, acute movement or position-provoked pain, such as encountered with bony metastases, intraspinal opioids often fail to eliminate the pain as effectively as ablative procedures. An important advantage of ablative procedures in this clinical setting is that they are "once only" events and, unlike augmentative procedures, do not require ongoing attendance and service. This fact becomes an advantage inasmuch as the patient may be discharged home or to a hospice, where expertise in the management of infusion pumps or ports may be unavailable or inadequate.

The second group of patients, those with prospective long-term survival, may be further divided into highly functional or functionally impaired individuals. In the highly functional patient with a long prospective survival, ablative procedures are deferred for as long as nonablative, reversible augmentative procedures can be judiciously applied. In patients with a long prospective survival and functional impairment, the choice between destructive and nondestructive procedures, based on the rationales described above, is more challenging.[9]

TIMING AND COMMUNICATION

There is a general consensus among clinicians that interventional modalities should be applied only after medical noninterventional management has failed. The definition of "failure" remains both an ambiguous and controversial concept. Simply stated, failure is the point when treatment does not provide adequate pain relief and analgesia cannot be attained without side-effects (sedation, intractable nausea and vomiting) that profoundly interfere with the patient's quality of life. Most neurosurgical procedures for cancer-related pain are presently done stereotactically under local anesthesia, and therefore can be performed even on extremely ill patients. However, a prerequisite for performance of this type of minimally invasive procedure is a cooperative patient. Unnecessary delays in acknowledging the inadequacy of medical treatment (e.g. the encephalopathic patient) may adversely affect the results of neurosurgical interventions and will exclude some therapeutic options. The pain specialist needs to recognize early tell-tale signs of treatment inadequacy and the interventionalist needs to be prepared to institute a clear and comprehensive treatment plan. This timely and smooth transition of care – "anticipatory care" – serves the patient best.

Ongoing communication with the patient and family is considered among the most important and challenging aspects of cancer patient care. Ablative procedures carry a toll, replacing pain with loss of some perception, and present risks of which patients and families need to be fully apprised. Failure to discuss these risks judiciously may lead to disappointment and resentment. Similarly, ambiguities concerning the disease, its likely progression, the cause of pain, and the realistic treatment objectives, including the palliation of pain and the patient's expectations, are an invitation for misapprehension and mistrust.

SURGICAL APPROACHES

Surgical procedures for pain are divided into two broad categories: ablative and augmentative (Table 19.2). Ablative procedures are those in which an anatomical site subserving pain is denervated by physical means such as by surgery, neurolytics, radiofrequency, cryoablation. or radiation (Gamma knife). In augmentative procedures pain perception is modulated by instillation of drugs either into the epidural space or intrathecally to interact with nociceptors or by deep brain stimulation (DBS) of the thalamus or periaqueductal gray to produce analgesia via the endogenous opioid system and/or activation of a descending inhibitory system. Experience with DBS for refractory cancer pain is limited. The expertise, expensive equipment required, the need for ongoing care and the availability of less invasive methods have relegated DBS to a rarely considered option for the patient with intractable cancer pain.

Perhaps the greatest advance in the last decade in the management of cancer-related pain has been the introduction and evolution of spinal and ventricular opioid therapy and related technology (Table 19.3). The concept of direct instillation of opioids into the cerebrospinal fluid (CSF) was the logical consequence of the discovery of opioid receptors in the spinal cord and brain. There are many advantages to intraspinal or intraventricular opioids which are highly relevant for pain of malignant origin. Opioids are best suited for nociceptive and visceral pain, the types most prevalent in cancer patients. Although neuropathic pain is less sensitive to opioid drugs, a considerable reduction in pain is attainable with direct drug instillation into the CSF. Opioid therapy produces a reversible analgesia and is most suitable for pain in multiple sites and for diffuse, bilateral, or midline pain. The techniques involved in drug infusion procedures are relatively as compared with ablative modalities, and drug doses and drug choice can be readily modified as the disease and the pain evolve.[10–13] Furthermore, accurate and simple screening measures with temporary percutaneous catheters are reliable in predicting the likelihood of treatment efficacy and tolerability. The choice between spinal intrathecal and intracerebroventricular opioids depends on the topography of pain. Most authors concur that the spinal route is indicated for pain in the lower part of the body, pelvicoperineal region, and spine. Intracerebroventricular opioids are reserved for pain in the head and neck region, the thoracic region, upper extremities, brachial plexopathy, and pain that has not responded to spinal opioids. The doses of opioid necessary for instillation directly into the CSF are minuscule compared with systemic doses. For conversion from systemic to spinal route of administration the equianalgesic dose is usually considered to be 10% for epidural administration, 1% for intrathecal administration, and 0.1% for intracerebroventricular administration of the 24- h intravenous morphine dose.[14***,15***]

Contraindications to the insertion of spinal or cerebroventricular delivery systems include bleeding diathesis, septicemia, and lack of a support system to provide for ongoing care and daily injections if such are required. Risks of infection are increased in neutropenic patients, diabetic subjects, and patients with immune compromise of other etiologies; these patients require extra precautions. The presence of spinal involvement with tumor does not preclude the use of spinal opioids. Placement of the catheter cephalad to the tumor and the potential CSF obstruction site is necessary to ascertain adequate drug distribution. Ongoing radiotherapy or chemotherapy is not considered a contraindication for placement of drug infusion systems.

Potential side-effects of CSF opioids are relatively rare in cancer patients who have been exposed chronically to systemic opioids. The most frequent side-effects include respiratory depression, gastrointestinal hypomotility, urinary retention, nausea, vomiting, pruritus, sedation, and peripheral edema. Respiratory depression can be reversed without reversing analgesia with an infusion of naloxone. Very high doses of spinal opioids can produce convulsions, generalized rigidity, and myoclonic jerks as well as hyperalgesia. Failure of the device from migration, kinking, breakage, or disconnection can occur. Epidural catheters are prone to malfunction due to fibrosis in the epidural space. Minor infections of the subcutaneous tissue or catheter track are more common with external devices and can usually be managed without removing the catheter. Major infections involving the epidural space or causing meningitis are less frequent and require, at a minimum, temporary removal of the system.

Similar to treatment with systemic opioids, patients may require dose escalation during long-term intra-

Table 19.2 *Procedures for relief of cancer-related pain*

Modulatory
Opiate infusion: intraspinal, intraventricular
Periaqueductal/periventricular gray (PVG/PAG) stimulation
Hypothalamic stimulation
Ablative
Neurectomy
Ganglionectomy
Sympathectomy
Rhizotomy
Dorsal root entry zone procedures
Cordotomy
Myelotomy
Trigeminal nucleotractotomy
Medullary tractotomy
Pontine tractotomy
Mesencephalic tractotomy
Various thalamic procedures
Cingulotomy
Hypothalamotomy
Hypophysectomy

Table 19.3 *Delivery systems for spinal and intracerebroventricular drugs*

System	Comments
Spinal	
Percutaneous catheter	Placed in the epidural or subarachnoid space Least durable system and associated with highest incidence of infections Use generally limited to short-term treatment, drug trials, or screening
Tunneled catheter	For most of its length the catheter is internal, although the proximal end may be externalized or connected to an implantable port Durable system used for lengthy treatment Drugs can be administered by bolus injections or continuously via an external infusion pump
Implantable pump	Most durable and associated with the least risk of infection, costly and to be considered for long-term subarachnoid therapy Programmable pumps allow the rate of infusion to be adjusted System requires drug replenishing For long-term therapy most likely cost-effective
Intracerebroventricular	
Ports (e.g. Ommaya)	Allows for repeated percutaneous injections Long-term therapy (months) associated with high rate of infection
Tunneled catheters	Proximal end of system externalized in the neck or chest area More resilient to infections but requires utmost care
Implantable pump	Most durable and effective for long-term treatment Except for drug replenishment devoid of need for ongoing care or servicing

spinal therapy. The dose escalation usually occurs in the setting of increased pain due to disease progression. Long-term administration of opioids and dose escalation has been known to cause a sudden onset of dysesthetic pain–hyperalgesic syndrome that is not relieved with naloxone.[16] To decrease the incidence of hyperalgesic syndrome it is advisable to increase opioid dose in modest increments.

Alternatives to opioids or drugs that can be coadministered with opioids are under evaluation and include: clonidine, γ-aminobutyric acid, neostigmine, NMDA (*N*-methyl-D-aspartate) antagonists (dextromethorphan, dextrophan, and MK-801), somatostatin, and SNX 111.

ABLATIVE PROCEDURES FOR SPECIFIC PAIN

Neurosurgical options for cancer pain syndromes are outlined in Table 19.4.

Unilateral lower extremity and torso pain

For patients suffering from unilateral pain below the C5 dermatome – the highest level at which analgesia consistently persists – anterolateral cordotomy (ACC) is probably the most effective modality. The goal in ACC is the interruption of the neospinothalamic tract (STT), a discrete tract within the spinal cord that conducts mainly acute pain and temperature sensation. Afferent fibers originate in the DREZ and ascend one or more segments before decussating in the anterior white commissure to ascend in the contralateral anterolateral quadrant of the cord. Fibers in the STT are somatotopically arranged, with decussating axons settling on the medial edge of

Table 19.4 *Neurosurgical options for cancer pain syndromes*

Unilateral pain in lower extremity/torso
Spinal opiates infusion
Anterolateral cordotomy
Bilateral pain, axial, pelvic–perineal
Intrathecal opiate infusion
Bilateral cordotomy; C1–2 and low cervical
Myelotomy (limited or stereotactic)
Unilateral chest pain and arm pain – lower nerve roots
Intrathecal opiate infusion
Anterolateral cordotomy (contraindicated in some patients!)
Unilateral pain above C5 including pain in shoulder, head, and neck
Intrathecal opiate infusion
Mesencephalic tractotomy
Unilateral head and orofacial pain
Intrathecal opiate infusion
Stereotactic nucleotractotomy (including pain from cranial nerves V, VII, IX, and X)
Percutaneous freehand trigeminal tractotomy

the tract at each spinal cord level. Consequently, as the tracts ascend, the most lateral and posterior fibers represent the lower part of the body and the most medial the upper extremity and neck. The location of the STT and its somatotopic arrangement enable the creation of a selective lesion tailored specifically for the patient's pain location, sparing other sensory and motor functions.[17,18]

Anterolateral cordotomy is most frequently performed percutaneously at the C1–C2 interspace using radiofrequency lesioning.[19] The approach has been perfected by adding impedance recording, positive contrast imaging (minimyelogram), and, more recently, the performance of the procedure under computed tomography (CT) guidance.[20–22] The procedure is contraindicated if the only effective lung is ipsilateral to the side of the proposed cordotomy. The strictly ipsilateral reticulospinal tract responsible for autonomic respiration lies adjacent to the STT, and its loss will result in inadequate unconscious respiration in patients dependent on the ipsilateral lung alone. Using the same rationale, bilateral high cervical cordotomies in patients with normal lungs must be performed at two separate sittings (10 days apart) or the second procedure is created at a lower spinal segment, usually after laminectomy.[23]

Tasker,[24] based on his vast personal experience with ACC, reports long-term pain-free survival in 72% of patients. Seventy-two percent had significant pain relief after bilateral cordotomy. Complications included temporary paresis in 16.8%, permanent paresis (2%), bladder dysfunction (2%), dysesthesia (3%), temporary respiratory suppression (0.5%), and persistent respiratory suppression in 0.5%. Mortality was 0.3%. About 41% of patients developed contralateral pain and 2.6% recurrent ipsilateral pain from a receding or inadequate level of analgesia.

Bilateral, midline, and pelvic–perineal pain

Bilateral cordotomies are effective procedures for bilateral pain, including pain of pelvic–perineal origin and axial pain from spinal involvement by tumor.[25] Some authors believe that midline pain, because it is often accompanied by deafferentation elements, is more resistant to cordotomy and therefore expected results are inferior to those attainable with unilateral cordotomy.

An alternative procedure for bilateral and midline pain and visceral pain from cancer of the rectum, uterus, or bladder is commissural myelotomy. Originally pain relief was believed to result from interruption of decussating spinothalamic fibers, but it is now thought to occur through interruption of specialized spinothalamic neurons with complex bilateral receptive fields.[26]

Commissural myelotomy can be achieved through laminectomy with multilevel denervation for all segments intended plus two segments cephalad. Limited myelotomy is similar to commissural myelotomy but only one segment is denervated.[27] In the case of pelvic perineal pain, the exposure is through a T9 laminectomy whereby the T12 segment of the spinal cord is exposed. The results of limited myelotomy and commissural myelotomy are similar, with roughly 70% of patients experiencing significant pain relief, but the former is associated with a lower morbidity; the most common complications consist of loss of proprioception and ataxia.

A third variation of commissurotomy is the percutaneous stereotactic method, as described first by Hitchcock[28,29] and later Schvarcz.[30] The method involves application of a stereotactic frame. With the head fully flexed, the spinal cord is outlined with contrast medium and approached through the atlanto-occipital interspace. The lesion is created by radiofrequency with physiologic monitoring similar to anterolateral cordotomy. Seventy to eighty percent of patients attain a satisfactory result with stereotactic cervical myelotomy. Complications include gait disturbance and loss of proprioception, but generally these side-effects are transient.

A fourth variation is the punctate midline myelotomy.[31] In this procedure the anatomical target is a recently described major visceral pain pathway located in the midline of the posterior column. The cell bodies of this pathway lie in the spinal gray matter dorsal to the central canal near the base of the dorsal horn, where they are directly or indirectly in receipt of segmental primary afferents. The axons ascend ipsilaterally to terminate in the nucleus gracilis, and from there arcuate fibers transmit nociceptive input to the visceronociceptive neurons in the ventroposterolateral nucleus of the thalamus (VPL).

Pain above C5 including chest and upper extremity

For unilateral pain that involves the head, neck, and upper extremity, midbrain tractotomy is a highly effective approach. The anatomical target is the rostral extension of the spinothalamic tract. At midbrain level the spinothalamic tract from the body and the bulbothalamic or quintothalamic tracts originating from the nucleus caudalis of the trigeminal nucleus subserving the head and face are adjacent and form a compact target. The target can be readily extrapolated from thin-section axial magnetic resonance images. The target is 5–10 mm lateral to the midline and in line or slightly anterior to the aqueduct. The final site for lesioning is chosen by electrophysiologic stimulation. Stimulation of the STT produces paresthesiae in the contralateral face and body. The accuracy of magnetic resonance imaging (MRI) localization and the precision afforded by stereotaxis combined with the controlled discrete lesion produced by radiofrequency lesioning provide for excellent pain control with minimal morbidity. Lasting pain relief after mesencephalic tractotomy is attained in 85% of patients. The most common complications of the procedure are dysesthesiae (15%), ocular movement disorders (20%), most of which are transient, and a mortality of 1.8%.[32–34]

Alternatives for head, neck and arm pain include intracerebral opioid analgesia and trigeminal tractotomy. Stereotactic nucleotractotomy is effective for the treatment of nociceptive or deafferentation cancer pain of the orofacial and head region, including areas subserved by the fifth, seventh, ninth, and tenth cranial nerves.[35–38] It is more difficult to relieve head and neck and arm pain with opioid infusion than it is to relieve body pain with intraspinal opioids. This may be because of a more prominent element of deafferentation in head and neck pain syndromes and the fact that opioids are less effective for deafferentation pain than for nociceptive pain. For these reasons mesencephalic tractotomy or trigeminal nucleotractotomy should be considered appropriate for patients with malignant head and neck or arm pain who are not responding to pharmacological management.

CT- guided ablations

A recent innovative approach to performing ablative lesions in the spinal cord and medulla has been introduced by Kanpolat and Cosman.[39] In essence, in addition to impedance monitoring and physiological verification of the target, this method allows CT visualization of the target. For anterolateral cordotomy, for example, the shape, diameter, and the equator of the spinal cord can be clearly visualized and are important variables for correct target electrode positioning. Furthermore, direct visualization allows the surgeon to see the site and the depth of penetration of the electrode and can disclose problems emanating from displacement of the cord in advance of the electrode. A special radiofrequency electrode system has been designed to minimize imaging artifacts created by steel hubs and thick electrodes.[39] The technique using CT guidance has been used to create lesions in the anterolateral spinal cord and trigeminal tract and to perform extralemniscal myelotomy.[40–42] The authors have adopted the Kanpolat technique, varied by using C-arm fluoroscopy and CT in concert. The authors believe that C-arm fluoroscopy facilitates and saves time during placement and establishes the general trajectory of the electrode in the initial stage of the procedure. CT guidance is then used upon entry of the subarachnoid space for fine trajectory and placement adjustments. CT guidance facilitates performing ablative procedures on the spinal cord and medulla but, more importantly, adds the critical dimension of visualization to impedance and physiological monitoring of the electrode position in its intended target.

Rhizotomies of the trigeminal and glossopharyngeal nerves have been significantly facilitated by using CT guidance. The advantages of CT-guided procedures include direct and clear delineation and visualization of the neural foramina, especially when bony destruction at the base of skull secondary to cancer is present. Furthermore, patients maintain a neutral head position during the procedure as CT gantry changes can be made for optimal anatomical visualization.[43,44]

OTHER ABLATIVE MODALITIES

For multiple reasons, neurectomies and rhizotomies have generally been supplanted by nondestructive interventions for refractory pain, such as spinal drug infusion. Pain is rarely confined to the distribution of a few nerves or roots, involved nerves are often mixed, and denervation may compromise motor or sphincter function. Furthermore, neuropathic pain is believed to be predominantly sustained by central mechanisms. Exceptions to this generalization include the use of neurolytic blocks for somatic pain (e.g. neurolysis of the Gasserian ganglion), visceral blocks of the celiac plexus and superior hypogastric plexus, and sympathectomy when pain is believed to be sympathetically maintained.[45–48] Dorsal rhizotomies are occasionally useful for alleviation of chest or abdominal wall pain, and bilateral sacrococcygeal rhizotomy may be effective for sacral or perineal pain.[49] Thoracic dorsal rhizotomies for refractory chest wall pain should be considered during a thoracotomy if one is performed for tumor resection, or, rarely, may be carried out as a separate procedure.[50]

Hypophysectomy may provide analgesia in patients with diffuse or multifocal pain (e.g. from bone metastases) through a mechanism that remains unknown. Hormonal ablation is not a prerequisite for analgesia, and pain relief can be achieved in patients with tumors that are not hormonally responsive.[51] Pain relief is attained in 73–93% of patients over a mean survival of 5 months.

Cingulotomy is most effective for treatment of musculoskeletal pain, often from widespread metastatic disease, but not for neuropathic pain. It has been suggested that the procedure is especially effective in patients in whom the component of anxiety, depression, and emotional suffering is significant and overwhelming. Cingulotomy is performed bilaterally, guided by MRI stereotaxis, and is associated with minimal risks of cognitive and behavioral dysfunction. The results of cingulotomy describe pain rating decreases of 46% and activity level increases of 55% in the initial postoperative period, and as many as half of patients report moderate to complete pain relief at 3 months.[52] Bilateral cingulotomy can be performed noninvasively by means of precision stereotactic radiosurgery, for example with a Gamma knife.

For patients unsuited for cordotomy with pain in the head and neck region, stereotactic medial thalamotomy is an alternative. The targets for lesioning are the center median, parafascicular, and intralaminar nuclei, representing the rostral extension and terminus of the spinothalamic tract. Medial thalamotomy can produce bilateral analgesia with unilateral lesions and does not result in an identifiable sensory loss. Medial thalamotomy has an advantage over midbrain tractotomy in that it avoids the risks of visual complications and is associated with lower overall morbidity.[53] Lesions of the pulvinar are an extension of medial thalamotomy. It has been suggested that extending the lesion of medial thalamotomy to the pulvinar improves the effectiveness of pain relief. Pain recurrence or loss of effectiveness over time are inherent drawbacks of the procedure. Discrete thalamic lesions for the relief of pain can be performed noninvasively by means of stereotactic Gamma knife irradiation.[54,55] The application of stereotactic radiosurgery for pain in general and pain of malignancy is limited and deserves further evaluation with systematic and prospective trials.

CONCLUSION

Optimal pain management is achieved with a multidisciplinary approach consisting in oncological strategies, pharmacotherapy, and anesthetic and neurosurgical modalities in concert with psychological and supportive care. From the neurosurgical perspective, intraspinal and cerebroventricular drug therapy is the simplest to implement, is reversible, and is associated with low morbidity. Ablative procedures, in contrast, require special expertise, carry higher risks, and produce irreversible changes in the CNS and are therefore the last resort. To perform optimal ablations, neurosurgeons must be proficient in stereotaxis and electrophysiological monitoring and should perform pain procedures on a regular basis to maintain experience. It is the authors' belief that patients are better served by neurosurgeons who master and gain experience in two or three neurosurgical ablative procedures that cover most cancer pain (e.g. anterolateral cordotomy, mesencephalic tractotomy) rather than by neurosurgeons sporadically resorting to a wide gamut of procedures. With the current knowledge and understanding of pain and available pharmacological and interventional modalities it is truly possible today to provide adequate relief of pain for nearly all cancer patients with pain.

REFERENCES

1. Foley KM. The treatment of cancer pain. *N Engl J Med* 1985; **311:** 84–95.
2. Twycross RG, Fairfield S. Pain in far advanced cancer. *Pain* 1982; **14:** 303–10.
3. Zhukovsky DS, Gorowski E, Hansdorff J, *et al.* Unmet analgesic needs in cancer patients. *J Pain Symptom Manage* 1995; **10:** 113–19.
4. Vantafridda V, Tamburini M, Caraceni A, *et al.* A validation study of the WHO method for cancer pain relief. *Cancer* 1987; **59:** 851–6.
5. Schug SA, Zech D, Diefenbach C, Bischoff A. Cancer pain management according to WHO analgesic guidelines. *J Pain Symptom Manage* 1990; **5:** 27–32.
6. Gonzales GR, Elliot K, Portenoy RK, Foley KM. The impact of comprehensive evaluation in the management of cancer pain. *Pain* 1992; **47:** 141–4,.
7. Arner S, Arner B. Differential effects of epidural morphine in the treatment of cancer-related pain. *Acta Anaesthesiol Scand* 1985; **29:** 32–6.
8. Tasker RR. Surgical approaches to chronic pain. In: Portenoy RK, Kanner RM eds. *Pain Management Theory and Practice*. Philadelphia, PA: FA Davis, 1996: 290–311.
9. Arbit E. The nature and management of cancer pain. In: Gildenberg PL, Tasker RR eds. *Textbook of Stereotactic and Functional Neurosurgery*. New York, NY: McGraw-Hill, 1998: 1345–52.
10. Dennis GC, DeWitty RL. Long-term intraventricular infusion of morphine for intractable pain in cancer of the head and neck. *Neurosurgery* 1990; **26:** 404–8.
11. Onofrio BM, Yaksh TL. Long-term pain relief produced by intrathecal morphine infusion in 53 patients. *J Neurosurg* 1990; **72:** 200–9.
12. Lazorthes YR, Sallerin BA, Verdie JP. Intracerebroventricular administration of morphine for control of irreducible cancer pain. *Neurosurgery* 1995; **37:** 422–9.
13. Cramond T, Stuart G. Intraventricular morphine for intractable pain of advanced cancer. *J Pain Symptom Manage* 1993; **8:** 465–73.
14. DuPen SL, Williams AR. The dilemma of conversion from systemic to epidural morphine: a proposed conversion tool for treatment of cancer pain. *Pain* 1994; **56:** 113–18.
15. Gildenberg PL. Administration of narcotics in cancer pain. *Stereotact Funct Neurosurg* 1992; **59:** 1–8.
16. DeConno F, Caraceni A, Martini C. Hyperalgesia and myoclonus with intrathecal infusion of high-dose morphine. *Pain* 1991; **47:** 337–9.
17. Rosomoff HL, Carol F, Brown J, Sheptak P. Percutaneous radiofrequency cervical cordotomy: technique. *J Neurosurg* 1965; **23:** 639–44.
18. Arbit E. Anterolateral cordotomy. In: Arbit E ed. *Management of Cancer-related Pain*. Mount Kisko, NY: Futura, 1993: 321–32.
19. Tasker RR. Percutaneous cordotomy for persistent pain. In: Gildenberg PL, Tasker RR eds. *Textbook of Stereotactic and Functional Neurosurgery*. New York, NY: McGraw-Hill, 1998: 1491–505.
20. Taren JA, Davis R Cosby EC. Target physiologic corroboration in stereotaxic cervical cordotomy. *J Neurosurg* 1969; **30:** 569–84.
21. Cowie RA, Hitchcock ER. The late results of antero-lateral cordotomy for pain relief. *Acta Neurochir* 1982; **64:** 39–50.

22. Kanpolat Y, Deda H, Akyar S, Caglar S. CT-guided pain procedures. *Neurochirurgie* 1990; **36:** 394–8.
23. Lin PM, Gildenberg PL Polakoff PP. An anterior approach to percutaneous lower cervical cordotomy. *J Neurosurg* 1966; **25:** 553–60.
24. Tasker RR. Surgical approaches to chronic pain. In: Portenoy RK, Kanner RM eds. *Pain Management Theory and Practice*. Philadelphia, PA: FA Davis, 1996: 290–311.
25. Rosomoff HL. Bilateral percutaneous cervical radiofrequency cordotomy. *J Neurosurg* 1969; **31:** 41–6.
26. Smith MV, Hodge CJ Jr. Somatosensory response properties of contralaterally projecting spinothalamic and non-spinothalamic neurons in the second cervical segment of the cat. *J Neurophysiol* 1991; **66:** 83–102.
27. Gildenberg PL, Hirshberg RM. Limited myelotomy for the treatment of intractable cancer pain. *J Neurol Neurosurg Psychiatry* 1984; **47:** 94–6.
28. Hitchcock ER. Stereotactic cervical myelotomy. *J Neurol Neurosurg Psychiatry* 1970; **33:** 224–30.
29. Hitchcock ER. Stereotactic myelotomy. *J Roy Soc Med* 1974; **67:** 771–4.
30. Schvarcz JR. Stereotactic high cervical extralemniscal myelotomy for pelvic cancer pain. *Acta Neurochir* 1984; **33** (Suppl. C) 431–5.
31. Haring JW, Hewitt E, Westlund KN, Willis WD Jr. Surgical interruption of a midline dorsal column visceral pain pathway. *J Neurosurg* 1997; **86:** 538–42.
32. Frank F, Fabrizi AP, Gaist G. Stereotactic mesencephalic tractotomy in the treatment of chronic cancer pain. *Acta Neurochir* 1989; **99:** 8–40.
33. Voris HC, Whisler WW. Results of stereotactic surgery for intractable pain. *Confin Neurol* 1975; **37:** 86–96.
34. Amano K, Kawamura H, Tanikawa T. Long term follow up study of rostral mesencephalic reticulotomy for pain relief-report of 34 cases. *Appl Neurophysiol* 1986; **49:** 105–11.
35. Crue BL, Carregal EJA, Felsoory A. Percutaneous stereotactic radiofrequency trigeminal tractotomy with neurophysiological recordings. *Clin Neurol* 1972; **34:** 389–97.
36. Hitchcock E. Stereotactic spinal surgery. *Neurol Surg* 1977; **433:** 271–9.
37. Schvarcz JR. Stereotactic trigeminal nucleotomy for dysesthetic facial pain. *Adv Pain Res Ther* 1979; **3:** 331–3.
38. Fox JL. Percutaneous trigeminal tractotomy for facial pain. *Acta Neurochir* 1973; **29:** 83–9.
39. Kanpolat Y, Cosman ER. Special radiofrequency electrode system for computed tomography-guided pain-relieving procedures. *Neurosurgery* 1996; **38:** 600–3.
40. Kanpolat Y, Akyar S, Caglar S, *et al.* CT-guided percutaneous selective cordotomy. *Acta Neurochir* 1993; **123:** 92–6.
41. Kanpolat Y, Deda H, Akyar S, *et al.* CT-guided trigeminal tractotomy. *Acta Neurochir* 1989; **100:** 112–14.
42. Kanpolat Y, Atalag M, Deda H, Siva A. CT-guided extralemniscal myelotomy. *Acta Neurochir* 1989; **91:** 151–2.
43. Krol G, Arbit E. Percutaneous electrocoagulation of trigeminal nerve using computed tomography guidance. *J Neurosurg* 1988; **68:** 972–3.
44. Arbit E, Krol G. Percutaneous radiofrequency neurolysis guided by computed tomography for treatment of glossopharyngeal neuralgia. *Neurosurgery* 1991; **29:** 580–2.
45. Caraceni A, Portenoy RK. Pain management in patients with pancreatic carcinoma. *Cancer* 1996; **78:** 639–53.
46. de Leon-Casasola OA, Kent E, Lema MJ. Neurolytic superior hypogastric plexus block for chronic pelvic pain associated with cancer. *Pain* 1993; **54:** 145–51.
47. Patt RB. Anaesthetic procedures for the control of caner pain. In: Arbit E ed. *Management of Cancer-related Pain*. Mount Kisko, NY: Futura, 1993: 381–407.
48. Patt RB, Reddy S. Spinal neurolysis for cancer pain: indications and recent results. *Ann Acad Med Singapore* 1994; **23:** 216–20.
49. Onofrio BM, Campa HK. Evaluation of rhizotomy. Review of 12 years' experience. *J Neurosurg* 1972; **36:** 751–5.
50. Arbit E, Galicich JH, Burt M, Mallya K. Modified open thoracic rhizotomy for treatment of intractable chest wall pain of malignant etiology. *Ann Thoracic Surg* 1989; **48:** 820–3.
51. Levin AB. Hypophysectomy in the treatment of cancer pain. In: Arbit E ed. *Management of Cancer-related Pain*. Mount Kisko, NY: Futura, 1993: 281–95.
52. Hassenbusch SJ, Pillay PK, Barnett GH. Radiofrequency cingulotomy for intractable cancer pain using stereotaxis guided by magnetic resonance imaging. *Neurosurgery* 1990; **27:** 220–3.
53. Frank F, Fabrizi AP, Gaist G. Stereotactic mesencephalotomy versus multiple thalamotomies in the treatment of chronic cancer pain syndromes. *Appl Neurophysiol* 1987; **50:** 314–18.
54. Lexell L: Cerebral radiosurgery. I. Gammathalamotomy in two cases of intractable pain. *Acta Chir Scand* 1968; **134:** 585–95.
55. Young RF, Jacques DB, Rand RW, Copcutt B. Medial thalamotomy with the Lexell Gamma Knife for treatment of chronic pain. *Acta Neurochir* 1994; **Suppl. 62:** 105–10.

20

Complementary therapies for cancer pain

JACQUELINE FILSHIE AND ADRIAN WHITE

Complementary therapies are methods of treatment that lie to varying degrees outside mainstream medicine. Some are not far removed from it in having something of a scientific basis: this includes therapies such as the antioxidant vitamins, herbal remedies, and relaxation. Other therapies, such as crystal healing and reflexology, use concepts that are very different from conventional treatment and are likely to be considered implausible. This is reflected in the labels that are commonly used, which range from "integrative" through "complementary" to "alternative" medicine. The word "holistic" is commonly used to describe complementary therapists but should not be applied exclusively: good physicians are also aware of the importance of the therapeutic relationship and attention to every aspect of a person's physical and emotional needs, particularly at critical times in life such as after a diagnosis of cancer has been made.

Complementary medicine (CM) is increasingly popular among the general public, and cancer patients are no exception. A review of 26 surveys of use of CM by cancer patients in 13 different countries found that the use varied from 7% to 64%, with an average of about 30%.[1] The frequency of use among children was up to 50%. Patients often used more than one therapy. Patients who use CM tended to be younger and were more likely to be female and to come from a higher socioeconomic group than those who made no use of CM.[2] The same survey found that the most common therapies used by mixed oncology patients in the UK were healing, relaxation, visualization, diet, homoeopathy, vitamins, and herbal therapy.

VandeCreek *et al.*[3] recently surveyed CM use among breast cancer patients in the USA, using a rather inclusive definition of CM. The most popular therapy was prayer (76%), followed by exercise (38%), spiritual healing (29%), and megavitamins (25%).

All 141 health care professionals who work in two cancer centers in Ontario were asked to identify which nonpharmacological strategies for cancer pain they would like to learn more about. They were offered a list of 19 therapies and asked to state which five were of greatest interest and then rank the remaining 14 in order of interest.[4] The five of greatest interest were:

- acupuncture or acupressure;
- massage therapy;
- hypnosis or self-hypnosis;
- therapeutic touch (healing in the UK);
- biofeedback.

The rest, in descending order of interest, were meditation; music or art therapy; progressive muscle relaxation; cognitive therapy; visualization or imagery; support groups; autogenic training; chiropractic; transcutaneous nerve stimulation or Codetron; individual psychotherapy; radiation; surgery; operant conditioning; and prayer.

The reasons why patients turn to CM have been explored (e.g. Cassileth and Brown[5] and Cassileth and Chapman[6]). Fundamental, unsurprisingly, is the fact that orthodox medicine has not delivered a cure. The fact that interest in CM is increasing can be seen as part of the rise in consumerism, particularly the wish for self-empowerment and the desire to cope both physically and psychologically. Patients are looking for therapies that are natural and gentle and which emphasize caring, partly as a reaction to the perceived deficiencies of conventional medicine, which has become increasingly objective and technical. Further, CM is more widely available and accessible, and increased exposure in the media has made the general public more aware of different therapies. Not least, patients may have an underlying but unstated wish for a magical cure, which may leave them open to exploitation.

The attitude of medical, nursing, and allied professions toward CM is changing from antagonism to productive coexistence.[7,8] Many people working in the caring professions feel more comfortable with the role of touch, time, support, and care, in a wider, "holistic" approach to medicine in palliation. Far from continuing to reject all unconventional approaches, medical staff are increasingly willing to integrate therapies that seem to have something valuable to offer.[9] These include:

- therapies directed at control of symptoms: mainly pain, but also anxiety, nausea, and vomiting;
- mind–body therapies that help patients come to terms with their disease and adopt a positive approach;
- sensible nutritional, exercise, or relaxation therapies that improve general health;
- psychosocial support.

On the other hand, medical staff continue to be suspicious of other aspects of complementary or alternative therapies which have no supporting evidence and may be potentially harmful, including:

- severe dietary regimens, which are particularly damaging to debilitated patients;
- herbs, megavitamins, and food supplements which are promoted as cures, a "scam" which has a long history[5] (such cures may even sometimes be promoted by state authorities on anecdotal evidence, as in the "di Bella" episode[10]);
- spiritual or psychological interventions that emphasize the individual's emotions or behavior as the cause of cancer, and therefore create guilt and misery in patients;
- therapists who have little experience of dealing with cancer and who raise false hopes, believing they can correct "fundamental imbalances" (this is particularly likely to be misleading when their treatment happens to coincide with a remission due to conventional therapy).

ACUPUNCTURE

History/introduction

Acupuncture is widely thought to have originated in China around 2,000 years ago. *The Yellow Emperor's Classic of Internal Medicine* (Huang Ti Nei Ching), the first known text on the subject, was written about 200 BC and translated into English by Veith in 1972.[11] The Yellow Emperor wanted to record current knowledge of acupuncture for posterity. However, it has recently been suggested that acupuncture may have originated in the Eurasian continent at least 2,000 years earlier. Tattoos found on Ötzi, the European ice man whose body was preserved in a glacier for 5,200 years, correspond to acupuncture points that would be used for the arthritis, which was revealed by radiography of the spine.[12]

The ancient Chinese described an elaborate system of diagnosis and therapy, based on painstaking observations, which involved piercing the skin with needles at precise locations in order to effect a cure or improvement in symptoms. They did not have the benefit of detailed knowledge of anatomy and physiology, as we do today. The Yellow Emperor's treatise describes the harmonizing of "Yin" and "Yang," forces of opposite polarity which may represent what is now described as homeostasis. Circulation of vital energy (Qi or Chi, the life force) was believed to occur in deep and superficial channels (meridians) on the body surface. To help in forming the diagnosis, 12 pulses at the radial arteries were palpated in a special way and the tongue was examined for color changes. Concepts of circulation of Qi predated the knowledge of the circulation of blood and lymph.

Over the last 30 years there has been increasing interest in acupuncture in the West, partly because of supportive neurophysiological and neuropharmacological evidence and partly because of disenchantment with the side-effects of drug therapy. Increasing numbers of practitioners take a pragmatic view of acupuncture and no longer adhere strictly to the traditional Chinese methods of diagnosis or treatment. They use a combination of segmental acupuncture points together with trigger points and some of the better known traditional points. In this way, acupuncture can be used in the context of a conventional medical history, clinical examination, investigation, and diagnosis. However, use of the traditional methods of diagnosis does still persist. Several texts are available which summarize traditional Chinese acupuncture,[13] whereas others offer a more evidence-based scientific approach.[14,15]

There are many methods of treatment with acupuncture, as outlined below.

- Traditional Chinese acupuncture involves manual stimulation of the needles to elicit "De Qi," a strange sensation of heaviness and numbness. Needles are usually retained for about 20 min. Moxibustion, a thermal stimulation from burning a special herb, may be used in addition.[16]
- Western medical acupuncture is given as part of conventional medical treatment. The strength and duration of needling are very variable.
- Electroacupuncture at low frequency (2–4 Hz) or high frequency (50–100 Hz) can be used for pain relief in selected cases, and for acupuncture analgesia.[17]

- Laser therapy (using a low-power, nonthermal laser) does not involve needling, but can be used at acupuncture points with the aim of reducing pain and enhancing tissue healing.[18***]
- Auriculoacupuncture, or ear acupuncture, involves needling the richly innervated pinna for a variety of painful and nonpainful conditions. There are claims that the body is represented as an inverted homunculus on the pinna,[19] but this has not been established rigorously. Other "microsystems" have been described, such as scalp acupuncture,[20] and any benefit from needling these areas may be linked to their rich innervation.
- Ryodoraku is a Japanese form of acupuncture in which skin impedance is measured. Disease states are believed to be associated with reduced impedance and to be improved by appropriate electrical stimulation.[21]
- Acupressure (shiatsu) involves pressure on traditional acupuncture points and is often regarded as a weaker form of stimulation than needle acupuncture.

Acupuncture is first-line treatment for many painful and nonpainful conditions in China and is increasingly available in both primary and secondary care in the West. In the UK, about 85% of chronic pain services offer acupuncture.[22,23]

A typical course of treatment for noncancer chronic pain would be once weekly for 6 weeks (or twice weekly for 3 weeks) with further "top-ups" as necessary. For treating cancer pain, a more gentle approach is necessary and the "dose" should be modified depending on the patient's response. If there is no pain relief whatsoever after three treatments it is probably better to stop, though this does not apply to the management of noncancer pain.

The balance of evidence supports the role of acupuncture in the treatment of some painful conditions, including dental pain,[24***] experimental pain,[25***] and headache.[26***] Systematic reviews of acupuncture for low back pain have produced conflicting results.[27***,28***] Although this second systematic review of acupuncture for back pain did not support the positive conclusion, Berman stated that studies in which six or more treatments were given were more likely to have a positive outcome (B Berman, personal communication, 1999).

Considering postoperative or "acute" pain in cancer patients, two studies by Poulain and colleagues on patients undergoing major abdominal surgery are relevant. In an open, randomized controlled trial, 250 patients who received electroacupuncture before and during surgery needed lower doses of conventional analgesic drugs.[29**] In another double-blinded study in 42 patients, electroacupuncture given peroperatively produced superior analgesia to sham acupuncture (P Poulain, personal communication, 1993). Both studies also suggested that acupuncture enhanced postoperative recovery.

There have been no randomized controlled trials of acupuncture for cancer pain, but there have been some observational studies. As early as 1973, Mann *et al.*[30*] described short-lived pain relief in eight patients with intractable cancer pain. In Hong Kong, Wen[31*] described using several electroacupuncture sessions daily in patients with terminal cancer, gradually reducing the number of sessions once pain control was established. This treatment was successful in treating pain in patients who were resistant to opioids or who had pain and opioid toxicity.

Filshie and colleagues conducted two audits of the use of acupuncture for pain control in a heterogeneous cancer population whose pain had not responded to conventional pharmacological approaches.[32*,33*] The results from both studies are presented here, representing 339 patients who were given a course of at least three weekly treatments of manual acupuncture. Between 52% and 56% of patients had worthwhile long-lasting relief after three weekly sessions, though subsequent top-ups were necessary. The interval between treatments could usually be increased progressively. Relief from pain related to conventional treatment (postsurgical and irradiation) was more prolonged than that relief of pain due to metastatic disease. A further 21–30% had short-lived analgesia of up to 2 days and may have benefited from more frequent treatments. Between 18% and 22% had no significant pain relief. It was noted that the greater the tumor load, the briefer the relief. Patients who developed new metastatic disease often suddenly experienced a shorter duration of pain relief than they had previously enjoyed with acupuncture; once the metastasis was treated, the patients often responded to acupuncture again. Muscle spasm was particularly helped by acupuncture treatment, and mobility often increased substantially.

In a further audit of treatment for pain, the psychological profiles of breast cancer patients with pain associated with surgery, radiotherapy, or tumor in the chest, axilla, and arm were studied. After 1 month of treatment, statistically significant reductions were seen in average pain, worst pain, interference with lifestyle, distress, pain behavior, and depression.[34*]

Aung[35*] used acupuncture in 344 patients with cancers at various stages of advancement, adopting a more traditional, energetic approach. His aim was to relieve "total pain" and included treatment of primary pain, related discomfort, anxiety and depression, and lack of energy. The results overall were similar to those of Filshie and co-workers.[32*,33*] However, it is not easy to draw firm conclusions as the acupuncture was used in combination with Qi Gong relaxation and meditation therapy.

An audit of a palliative care physician's first year of acupuncture practice found that 31 of 50 (62%) complaints of pain showed a "good" or "excellent" response, as measured by a verbal rating scale.[36*]

The problem of maintaining the pain-relieving effects

of acupuncture in late-stage disease has been overcome by the use of semipermanent indwelling acupuncture needles inserted into a tender area in the ear.[37*] In a sample of 28 patients in a hospice setting, massaging the studs at times of intense pain resulted in a statistically significant reduction in pain.

Mechanisms of action

The neurophysiology of acupuncture is summarized in numerous articles and reviews (e.g. White,[25] Stux and Hammerschlag,[38] Bowsher,[39] and Lundeberg[40]):

- Many acupuncture points are richly innervated.[41]
- The effects of acupuncture are prevented by prior local anesthetic injection.[42,43**]
- Acupuncture analgesia appears to depend on Aδ-nerve fiber stimulation.[44*]
- There is little evidence to support the meridian theories. However, these theories may be explained by the referral patterns from trigger points, which are often similar to traditional Chinese meridians, e.g. the gallbladder meridian.[45] Another hypothesis being explored is rapid conduction of electrical signals via liquid crystal formation of collagen fibers, bypassing the nervous system.[46]
- Acupuncture releases β-endorphins, enkephalins, and dynorphins, which act on mu, delta, and kappa receptors respectively, though not specifically. At least 17 lines of evidence have been advanced to support the opioidergic theory of acupuncture analgesia.[38]
- Cholecystokinin is also released by acupuncture, yet is antagonistic to endogenous opioids. This may in part explain the phenomenon of tolerance to acupuncture.[47]
- Acupuncture may also act by diffuse noxious inhibitory control.[48]
- Serotonin, a neurotransmitter involved in analgesia and mood elevation, is released by acupuncture.[49]
- Oxytocin, which has both analgesic and anxiolytic properties in addition to its other functions, is released by sensory stimulation such as acupuncture.[50]
- Myofascial trigger points often overlap with acupuncture points,[51*] and treatment by dry needling is used for many myofascial pain syndromes.[52–54]
- Acupuncture has been found to release adrenocorticotrophic hormone (ACTH)[55**] and therefore has the potential to reduce inflammation.
- Acupuncture has widespread autonomic effects on blood flow, blood pressure, and gastric motility.[56,57]
- There is increasing evidence that changes in expression of inhibitory transmitters may contribute to the sustained effects of acupuncture[58] (W Zieglgänsberger, personal communication, 1999).

Acupuncture for cancer symptoms other than pain

Acupuncture at the traditional point PC6, which is near the wrist, was found to reduce nausea more than various control interventions in 27 out of 33 random controlled trials.[59***] Some trials included patients with nausea induced by chemotherapy. Transcutaneous nerve stimulation (TENS) was found to prolong the effects.[60**]

In a pilot study, acupuncture was shown to be effective for treating dyspnea in 14 out of 20 patients with advanced, cancer-related breathlessness.[61*] There was statistically significant subjective benefit as well as reduction in the respiratory rate, measured objectively. A significant reduction in anxiety accompanied the relief of breathlessness. Semipermanent indwelling studs were inserted to prolong relief.

Several studies have shown that acupuncture increases salivary flow in patients with Sjögren's syndrome or radiation damage to the salivary glands.[40**] Acupuncture has helped to heal radionecrotic ulcers, which normally have an extremely poor prognosis.[62] Hot flushes induced by tamoxifen were reduced by manual acupuncture, with the addition of indwelling acupuncture studs in resistant cases.[63] Preliminary work has also shown the benefit of acupuncture treatment for vasomotor symptoms induced by therapy of prostate cancer.[64*] For further details of other nonpain symptoms that may respond to acupuncture, refer to Thompson and Filshie.[65]

Complications and contraindications

Side-effects of acupuncture have been classified as follows:

- infective (single-use disposable needles should always be used);
- traumatic, e.g. pneumothorax (good anatomical knowledge is essential and particular care is necessary in cachectic patients);
- needle fracture;
- miscellaneous including syncope, bruising, and sedation.

Severe adverse effects are rare. There are some 300 reports of serious adverse events in the literature over 30 years.[66] In cancer patients, acupuncture should be avoided in any area of spinal instability, as it may reduce protective muscle spasm and expose the patient to the risk of cord compression or transection. It should also be avoided in moderate or severely lymphedematous limbs. Severely disordered clotting function is a further contraindication. Electroacupuncture should not be used in patients with a demand pacemaker.

Beneficial side-effects, such as coincidental alleviation of other long-standing symptoms, can often be an unexpected bonus.

HERBAL MEDICINE (PHYTOTHERAPY), VITAMINS, AND FOOD SUPPLEMENTS

Herbs are part of traditional medicine in most cultures throughout the world, and a variety of herbal, mineral, and animal products and combinations are frequently promoted for use in cancer. Some have been shown *in vitro* to have antitumor effects such as cytotoxicity and immunostimulation, and have been reviewed.[67] The majority of anecdotal reports describe success.

One of the most widely promoted herbs for cancer is mistletoe (commonly given as the preparation Iscador®), which was proposed by Rudolph Steiner, the founder of anthroposophical medicine. It contains several active chemicals, some of which have immunostimulating properties.[68]** A systematic review of controlled trials of mistletoe found considerable methodological shortcomings in the 11 studies that were identified.[69]*** Blinding is difficult as mistletoe is given as a series of subcutaneous injections which produce strong local reactions. Overall, all but one study showed prolonged survival; the effect on pain was not considered in this review. The reviewers concluded that the evidence for an effect of mistletoe was still anecdotal.

Essaic, a combination of burdock root, Indian rhubarb, sheep sorrel, and the inner bark of slippery elm, is well known in North America and is claimed to be effective in strengthening the immune system, improving appetite, and relieving pain, as well as in reducing tumor size and prolonging life in many types of cancer.[70]*** A review of evidence by the Task Force of the Canadian Breast Cancer Research Initiative found no controlled trials and concluded that there was "some weak evidence of its effectiveness and [Essaic is] … unlikely to cause serious side-effects when used as directed."[70]***

Chinese herbs are usually prescribed according to a complex traditional diagnosis. Li *et al.*[71]** reported a controlled study in which a mixture of Chinese herbs appeared to give relief of acute pain following abdominal surgery for liver cancer. However, the numbers were small, and details of the methods are sparse, so no firm conclusions can be drawn.

Herbal medicines are part of traditional medicine in many countries, and there is evidence of a positive effect on pain due to rheumatological conditions,[72]*** though there are no controlled investigations in cancer pain.

In view of the number and potency of the chemicals in plants, including those from which many current drug preparations are derived, it is hardly surprising that the side-effects of herbs can be common.[67]* Herbs may also interact with orthodox medication.[73]* For example, patients may self-administer Chinese herbs in order to reduce the side-effects of conventional hormone therapy for cancer, but if the herbs block estrogen receptors then they are possibly likely also to reduce the effectiveness of the treatment. Medical staff are advised to be alert to the possibility that their patients are using herbs or supplements and to question them routinely.

HOMEOPATHY

The homeopathic method of treatment was first described in 1790 by the physician Samuel Hahnemann in Germany. The practice of homoeopathy (homeo = similar, pathos = illness) rests on two fundamental principles: the first is "similia similibus curentur" or "let like be cured with like:" the toxic symptoms of a substance are carefully recorded, and that substance is then used as a remedy for patients who present with those symptoms. The second principle stated by Hahnemann was that repeated dilution of the remedy, with vigorous shaking, increases its power of action, a process called "potentization." Extreme dilutions may be used in which no molecules remain. Claims that diluting the material increases its strength appear biologically implausible. Homoeopathic consultations are prolonged, and this may contribute to the beneficial effects on patients.

Despite the misgivings of scientists, a meta-analysis of all randomized controlled trials of homoeopathy found an overall positive result, over and above the placebo effect.[74]*** A pilot study was reported in which 50 consecutive patients from the Royal London Homeopathic Hospital Cancer Clinic were given a package of complementary care including homeopathy.[75]* The patients' quality of life improved as measured by the Rotterdam Symptom Checklist. The review of Linde *et al.*[74]*** found no randomized controlled trials of homoeopathy for cancer pain, but its analgesic effect may be worth exploring as homoeopathy was effective for the pain of rheumatic diseases in four out of the seven studies that were included. Rigorous randomized controlled trials comparing homoeopathy with placebo preparations are increasingly common and the results are awaited with interest.

HYPNOSIS

Trance experiences have been described as far back as the time of the ancient Greeks, but hypnosis was first identified as a formal psychotherapeutic interest in the eighteenth century by Anton Mesmer, who used "animal magnetism" for a range of psychosomatic conditions.

Hypnosis is an altered state of consciousness that provides access to unconscious processes and a change in memory or perception. Spiegel and Moore[76] define it as a "a natural state of aroused, attentive local concentration coupled with a relative suspension of peripheral awareness" with three main components: absorption, dissociation, and suggestibility. When subjects are hypnotized they become so absorbed in the experience that there is a distortion of time awareness, thoughts, memories, and perception of activities around them. They experience a curious degree of dissociation from the environment, emotions, and sensations. Some of their critical faculty is bypassed so that suggestions implanted in this state can continue to affect them after the therapy, a phenomenon known as "posthypnotic suggestion." Hypnotizability is a stable and measurable state.[77,78] Approximately two-thirds of the normal adult population are hypnotizable and up to 10% highly responsive. There are numerous methods of directly inducing the hypnotic state, which rely more on the individual subject than the skill of the hypnotist.[79] An indirect method of inducing hypnosis with a gentle, permissive, and less power-implicit technique can be successful even in cancer patients with low susceptibility,[80,81] although Reeves *et al.*[82*] found poor results in a controlled trial using the "indirect" method of hypnosis for acute pain of hyperthermia treatment in cancer patients.

Numerous techniques are used to diminish or even abolish pain in the hypnotized state:

- numbing of the painful site, as produced by local anesthetic or glove anesthesia;
- substitution of stabbing pain with sensation of tingling or vibration;
- reduction in the numerical value of pain in the mind's eye or on an imagined screen;
- displacement of pain to another site of the body or even outside the body;
- inducing a change in temperature by asking the subject to imagine a hot bath or a cool icy place, especially if the individual finds either heat or cold soothing;
- distraction from the pain through pleasant imagery;
- altering the meaning of pain so that it is less important and debilitating, e.g. "although the pain is there it ceases to bother or disturb you," or "filtering out the hurt of the pain," i.e. increasing patient's tolerance to the pain;
- regression to an earlier, pain-free time;
- amnesia for previous pain experience.

All these techniques can be supplemented by prolonged relaxation, a boosting of self-esteem (so-called "ego strengthening"), psychological support, and improvement in body image. Additionally, hypnosis can be used to access and purge unpleasant memories which are inaccessible to the conscious mind but profoundly affect behavior. This technique requires great skill. Self-hypnosis can be taught in the hypnotized state to enhance self-control and to give the patient a degree of mastery over pain.

Hilgard and Hilgard,[77] reviewing the literature on hypnosis for cancer pain, suggested that researchers should:

- measure hypnotic responsiveness prior to treatment;
- carefully delineate and define indications and therapeutics;
- use more objective outcomes.

A distinguished panel of experts who assessed the efficacy of behavioral and relaxation approaches for the treatment of chronic pain and insomnia concluded that there was strong evidence for the use of hypnosis in alleviating pain associated with cancer and for the use of relaxation techniques in reducing chronic pain.[83] However, one critical review of treatment highlighted confusion over nomenclature and re-emphasized the need for clarity in trial methodology.[84] The term "hypnosis" can have negative connotations, as shown when an identical treatment was viewed differently by patients, depending on whether it was labeled hypnosis, relaxation, or passive relaxation with guided imagery.[85]

Hypnotic interventions have been reviewed by Stam,[86] and further details of hypnotic techniques for cancer pain control are outlined by Spira and Spiegel,[87] Chaves,[88] and Levitan.[89] Trijsburg *et al.*[90] have critically reviewed trial methodology for cancer patients undergoing psychological treatment.

Probably the best evidence to date of long-term efficacy of hypnosis for cancer pain comes from Spiegel and Bloom.[91**] A group of 34 women with metastatic breast cancer achieved a significant reduction in pain and suffering with hypnosis compared with a control group. In addition, long-term follow-up showed that the treatment group lived on average 36 months, compared with 18 months for the control group.[92**] However, part of the success was undoubtedly the skillful psychotherapy involved in the "supportive expressive group therapy" given in addition to the hypnosis.[76]

Syrjala *et al.*[93**] found that superior pain control for mucositis of bone marrow transplantation was achieved in patients treated with individualized hypnosis with imagery compared with an untreated control group, a group whose only treatment was their usual therapist contact, and a fourth group who were taught cognitive behavioral coping skills.

Pediatric procedure-related pain

In the UK, general anesthesia is used almost routinely for children requiring painful procedures such as lumbar punctures and bone marrow aspiration. In many parts of the world sedation is employed, but as this can sometimes be inadequate hypnosis has been used in addition. Many studies have shown that hypnosis is helpful in reducing the pain of such procedures in children with cancer. Zeltzer and LeBaron[94] and Zeltser *et al.*[95**] have shown that hypnosis can reduce procedure-related pain and chemotherapy-related distress in children. The whole field of hypnosis for children and adolescents with cancer has been reviewed by Steggles *et al.*,[96,97] Sutters and Miaskowski,[98] Ellis and Spanos,[99] and Genuis.[100] They include papers by Olness,[101*] Hilgard and LeBaron,[102*] Zeltzer and LeBaron,[103**] Kellerman *et al.*,[104*] Katz *et al.*,[105*] and Wall and Womack.[106**]

Other symptoms

Hypnosis can be helpful in alleviating chemotherapy-related nausea and vomiting.[107**] Genuis[100] and Steggles *et al.*[97] included the treatment of anxiety, stress, and chemotherapy-related nausea and vomiting in their reviews. Rapkin *et al.*[108*] found that hospital stay after head and neck surgery was shorter in patients treated by hypnosis than in those who received standard care. Hypnosis is also useful in the treatment of dissociative disorders, post-traumatic stress disorders, anxiety, and smoking. However, the use of hypnosis for forensic purposes has aroused controversy.[109,110]

Side-effects

A skillful hypnotherapist should be able to manage a catharsis as this can be very distressing if it occurs during therapy. One retrospective survey of the use of hypnosis for relaxation and coping in 52 palliative care patients found that 61% were able to cope better with their illness, whereas 7% had negative effects.[111] One of the three patients reported that coping was "more difficult," one found the hypnotherapy an "emotionally and physically disturbing experience," and one found it an "adverse experience."

Mechanisms

It is still far from certain how hypnosis works for pain reduction although the findings may be relevant:

- Hypnosis is an altered state of consciousness with electroencephalographic (EEG) patterns of alert wakefulness.[112]
- According to Spira and Spiegel,[87] the hypnotic state is more akin to intense concentration than to sleep.
- There is some evidence that hypnosis is not reversible by naloxone,[113] but this does not entirely rule out an endogenous opioid mechanism.
- Pederson[114] reviewed early experimental work which provided supporting evidence that the hypnotic state is a largely a right hemisphere-oriented task.
- Gruzelier[115] has shown that hypnosis is much more complex than initially thought, with highly susceptible hypnotic subjects showing asymmetry in favor of the left hemisphere before hypnosis, which is reversed by hypnosis. The opposite effects were seen in subjects who had low susceptibility to hypnosis. The author describes frontal inhibition and accentuation of posterior right-sided hemisphere functions in the hypnotic state.
- When hypnosis alters perception, there is evidence that it alters the event-related potentials to somatosensory stimuli.[92] When highly hypnotized subjects imagine that a visual stimulus is blocked, their visual cortical response to those stimuli is reduced, particularly in the right hemisphere.[116]
- Dissociation of sensory and affective components of pain occurs under hypnosis.[117]
- The specific pain dimension on which hypnotic suggestions act depends on the content of the instructions and is not a characteristic of hypnosis itself.[118]
- Positron emission tomography (PET) has shown changes in the activity of the anterior cingulate cortex associated with hypnotic suggestions designed to alter the unpleasantness, or affective component, of pain.[119]

With the increasing availability of imaging techniques such as PET and functional magnetic resonance imaging (MRI) scans for research purposes, further scientific evidence for the mechanisms of hypnosis is accumulating.

Hypnotherapy appears to have a positive role in treatment of pain and treatment-related pain in cancer patients and merits further clinical trials. The success of hypnosis may depend on skill and interaction of patient and therapist more than in many other treatments. Any nonhypnotizable subjects should be offered another form of supportive therapy.[87]

RELAXATION, DISTRACTION, AND VISUALIZATION

Relaxation and visualization are other "mind–body" approaches used in cancer patients. They can be considered to be on a continuum with hypnosis, but seem to be viewed by patients with less suspicion.[85] Distraction is used by almost every patient in some form, whether it is work, relationships, television, etc. Music is selected more often than comedy by cancer patients.[120] Children who are encouraged by their families to use their imagination have a greater ability to obtain help by magic and fantasy than those brought up to use intellect and reason, although the latter may respond better to a combination of relaxation and instruction.[121] Kuttner *et al.*[122**] compared three forms of treatment in children undergoing bone marrow aspiration. The first group received standard medical management using reassurance and support, the second group were taught a distraction technique, and the third group were encouraged to involve their imagination, becoming totally absorbed as in hypnosis. Imaginative involvement was more helpful for the 3- to 6-year-olds, whereas both distraction and imaginative involvement were helpful in the 7- to 10-year-olds. In the distraction group, coping skills needed to be learned over one or more sessions.

Visualization with guided imagery, such as imagining white blood cells killing cancer cells, was popularized by Simonton *et al.*[123] Claims that this method is effective have not been backed up by any convincing evidence.

While seemingly benign, any failure to control the disease might add to a patient's burden of unwarranted guilt.[76**]

A plausible mechanism for these psychological techniques exists in psychoneuroimmunomodulation.[124] Further clinical studies on interactions between the immune system and psychology studies are eagerly awaited.

MASSAGE AND AROMATHERAPY

The touch that massage offers may convey psychological messages such as caring and comfort and support to patients who are stressed and vulnerable. It is widely available in hospices and palliative care units.[125*] There are two main types of massage therapy. Massage (also known as Swedish massage) includes techniques from slow, gentle stroking to more vigorous movements such as friction, kneading/rolling movements (petrissage), and flicking/clapping movements (tapotement). Shiatsu massage is a more forceful form of treatment that aims to "release blocked energy" by strong, sustained pressure at specific points. It is not commonly used for cancer patients.

In addition to any psychological effects, massage may have physical effects including:

- relaxation;
- relief of muscle spasm;
- nociceptive inhibition through gate control theory;
- improvement of circulation;
- reduction of swelling including lymphedema (this is not discussed here; for a review see Ko *et al.*[126*]).

Aromatherapy includes the use of essential oils as therapeutic agents, usually by mixing a selection of oils with the almond carrier oil for massage. The oils can also be given by inhalation either by vaporizer or when bathing. The oils will be chosen according to the individual patient's symptoms and personality.[127*]

Cawley[128***] reviewed 14 research studies evaluating massage and makes useful recommendations for future investigations of this therapy. Sims[129*] found a reduction in symptom distress (not directly measuring pain) in six breast cancer patients who were given a simple 10-min back massage. Ferrell-Torry and Glick[130*] demonstrated that massage, focused particularly on trigger points and given on two consecutive days, led to short-term reduction in pain and anxiety in nine patients, with an accompanying reduction in heart rate, blood pressure, and respiratory rate. The overall benefit of aromatherapy was shown by Kite *et al.*[127*] in an uncontrolled study in cancer patients. Eleven out of the 16 patients in whom pain was a presenting problem experienced significant improvement and there was a significant fall in anxiety and depression (measured with the Hospital Anxiety and Depression scale).

Corner *et al.*[131**] studied the effect of massage, with or without aromatherapy, compared with no massage in 52 patients who had a broad range of stages and types of cancer. The massage experience was described in general as "overwhelmingly positive." Compared with the untreated control subjects, patients who received massage scored significantly greater reductions in both anxiety and pain scores. Aromatherapy oils did not add significantly to the effect.

In another randomized controlled trial, Weinrich and Weinrich[132**] compared the effect on pain of a single 10-min Swedish massage of the back with a "visitation" control who had no massage, in a relatively small sample of 28 patients. Massage was associated with a significant fall in pain scores in men immediately after treatment but not after 1 or 2 h; there was no significant pain relief in women. The initial pain scores were higher in men than in women. The sample size was too small for these results to be definitive, and the effects of repeated treatment in patients with moderate or severe pain are worth exploring further. The treatment in this study was given by senior nurses who had received only 1 h training in massage therapy, which may be insufficient.

There is a theoretical risk that massage could mobilize dormant cancer cells, although there are no reports of this happening. However, this possibility should be borne in mind when assessing the benefit–risk ratio for an individual patient. Clearly, massage should not be performed close to tumors or venous thrombosis, or in patients with grossly abnormal clotting function. Possible adverse effects of the essential oils include skin reactions.

Mechanisms of action

Massage and other forms of sensory stimulation release oxytocin, which is both anxiolytic[50**] and analgesic.[133] Perhaps this goes some way to explaining the analgesic and sedative qualities of massage.

THERAPEUTIC TOUCH (US), EQUIVALENT TO HEALING (UK AND ELSEWHERE)

Healing usually involves the practitioner passing his or her hands over the patient's clothed body, usually without making physical contact (despite the term "therapeutic touch"). Patients are not required to hold any particular form of faith or belief. They are often aware of tingling or warmth during the session and relief of symptoms afterwards. There have been no trials of the benefits of healing for cancer patients, despite its popularity. A recent rigorous trial in chronic pain patients showed that healing produced the same benefit as sham healing,[134] and it appears that the outcome may be due to expectation, relaxation, and other nonspecific effects. No adverse effects have been recorded.

CONCLUSION

Complementary therapies are becoming increasingly popular with the general public, including cancer patients. Conventional medical personnel are now less inclined than previously to dismiss the use of such approaches, and should be aware when their patients are using them. Patients should be advised when they are at risk from practitioners who raise false hopes, from therapies that may harm them directly, and from therapies that may interfere with conventional treatments. For cancer pain, hypnosis offers a variety of approaches and is probably the therapy that is best supported by expert consensus opinion as well as the limited experimental evidence that exists. There is also reasonable trial evidence that both hypnosis and the related technique of imagery can be useful for procedure-related pain, particularly in children. Other therapies such as acupuncture, massage, and aromatherapy have shown promise as useful techniques for the palliation of symptoms; more and better quality studies are awaited before they can be considered an integral part of management. There is also some evidence supporting the use of herbal preparations of mistletoe, but it is not conclusive. The value of approaches using diet, healing, or homoeopathy in the management of cancer pain is still not known.

REFERENCES

1. Ernst E, Cassileth B. The prevalence of complementary/alternative medicine in cancer. *Cancer* 1998; **83:** 777–82.
2. Downer SM, Cody MM, McCluskey P, *et al.* Pursuit and practice of complementary therapies by cancer patients receiving conventional treatment. *Br Med J* 1994; **309:** 86–9.
3. VandeCreek L, Rogers E, Lester J. Use of alternative therapies among breast cancer outpatients compared with the general population. *Alt Ther* 1999; **5(1):** 71–6.
4. ● Sellick SM, Zara C. Critical review of 5 nonpharmacologic strategies for managing cancer pain. *Cancer Prevention Control* 1998; **21:** 7–14.
5. Cassileth BR, Brown H. Unorthodox cancer medicine. *Cancer J Clin* 1988; **38:** 176–86.
6. Cassileth BR, Chapman CC. Alternative cancer medicine: a ten-year update. *Cancer Invest* 1996; **14:** 396–404.
7. Baum M. Quack cancer cures or scientific remedies. *J R Soc Med* 1996; **89:** 543–7.
8. Cosh J, Sikora K. Conventional and complementary treatment for cancer [letter]. *Br Med J* 1989; **298:** 1200–1.
9. Burke C, Sikora K. Complementary and conventional cancer care: the integration of two cultures. *Clin Oncol* 1993; **5:** 220–7.
10. Remuzzi G, Schieppati A. Lessons from the Di Bella affair. *Lancet* 1999; **353:**1289–90.
11. Veith I. *The Yellow Emperor's Classic of Internal Medicine*, 3rd printing. Berkley, CA: University of California Press, 1972.
12. Dorfer L, Moser M, Bahr F, *et al.* A medical report from the stone age? *Lancet* 1999; **354:** 1023–5.
13. *Essentials of Chinese Acupuncture*. Beijing: Foreign Languages Press, 1980.
14. ● Filshie J, White A eds. *Medical Acupuncture: a Western Scientific Approach*. Edinburgh: Churchill Livingstone, 1998.
15. ● Ernst E, White A eds. *Acupuncture: a Scientific Appraisal*. Oxford: Butterworth-Heinemann, 1999.
16. Birch S, Kaptchuk T. History, nature and current practice of acupuncture: an East Asian perspective. In: Ernst E, White A eds. *Acupuncture: a Scientific Appraisal*. Oxford: Butterworth-Heinemann, 1999: 11–30.
17. ● White A. Electroacupuncture and acupuncture analgesia. In: Filshie J, White A eds. *Medical Acupuncture: a Western Scientific Approach*. Edinburgh: Churchill Livingstone, 1998: 153–75.
18. de Bie RA, Verhagen AP, Lenssen AF, *et al.* Efficacy of 904 nm laser therapy in the management of musculoskeletal disorders: a systematic review. *Phys Ther Rev* 1998; **3:** 59–72.
19. Nogier PFM. *Treatise of Auriculotherapy*. Moulins-lès-Mets, France: Maisonneuve, 1972.
20. Yamamoto T, Yamamoto H. *Yamamoto New Scalp Acupuncture (YNSA)*. Tokyo: Axel Springer Japan Publishing, 1998.
21. Yoshino N, Yamashita K. *Ryokaraku Acupuncture*. Ryokaraku Research Institute, 1977.
22. Woollam CH, Jackson AO. Acupuncture in the management of chronic pain. *Anaesthesia* 1998: **53:** 593–5.
23. Clinical Standards Advisory Group (CSAG). *Services for Patients with Pain*. Department of Health Publication, 2000.
24. ◆ Ernst E, Pittler MH. The effectiveness of acupuncture in treating acute dental pain: a systematic review. *Br Dent J* 1998; **184:** 443–7.
25. ● White A. Neurophysiology of acupuncture analgesia. In: Ernst E, White A eds. *Acupuncture: a Scientific Appraisal*. Oxford: Butterworth-Heinemann, 1999: 60–92.
26. ● Melchart D, Linde K, Fischer P, *et al.* Acupuncture for recurrent headaches: a systematic review of randomized controlled trials. *Cephalalgia* 1999; **19:** 779–86.
27. ◆ Ernst E, White A. Acupuncture for back pain: a meta-analysis of randomized controlled trials. *Arch Intern Med* 1998; **158:** 2235–41.
28. ◆ van-Tulder MW, Cherkin DC, Berman B, *et al.* The effectiveness of acupuncture in the management of acute and chronic low back pain. A systematic review within the framework of the Cochrane Collaboration Back Review Group. *Spine* 1999; **2411:** 1113–23.
29. Poulain P, Pichard Leandri E, Laplanche A, *et al.* Electroacupuncture analgesia in major abdominal and pelvic surgery: a randomised study. *Acupuncture Med* 1997; **XV(1):** 10–13.

30. Mann F, Bowsher D, Mumford J, *et al*. Treatment of intractable pain by acupuncture. *Lancet* 1973; **ii:** 57–60.
31. Wen HL. Cancer pain treated with acupuncture and electrical stimulation. *Mod Med Asia* 1977; **13(2):** 12–15.
32. Filshie J, Redman D. Acupuncture and malignant pain problems. *Eur J Surg Oncol* 1985; **11:** 389–94.
◆ 33. Filshie J. Acupuncture and malignant pain problems. *Acupuncture Med* 1990; **8(2):** 38–9.
34. Filshie J, Scase A, Ashley S, Hood J. A study of the acupuncture effects on pain, anxiety and depression in patients with breast cancer [Poster]. Pain Society Meeting, Newcastle, April 1997.
35. Aung S. The clinical use of acupuncture in oncology: symptom control. *Acupuncture Med* 1994; **XII(1):** 37–40.
36. Leng G. A year of acupuncture in palliative care. *Palliative Med* 1999; **13:** 163–4.
37. Dillon M, Lucas CF. Auricular stud acupuncture in palliative care patients: an initial report. *Palliative Med* 1999; **13(3):** 253–4.
◆ 38. Stux G, Hammerschlag R. *Scientific Basis of Acupuncture*. Berlin: Springer-Verlag, 2000.
◆ 39. Bowsher D. Mechanisms of acupuncture. In: Filshie J, White A eds. *Medical Acupuncture: A Western Scientific Approach*. Edinburgh: Churchill Livingstone, 1998: 69–82.
◆ 40. Lundeberg T. Effects of sensory stimulation (acupuncture) on circulatory and immune systems. In: Ernst E, White A eds. *Acupuncture: a Scientific Appraisal*. Oxford: Butterworth-Heinemann, 1999: 93–106.
41. Dung HC. Anatomical features contributing to the formation of acupuncture points. *Am J Acupuncture* 1984; **12:** 139–43.
42. Chiang C-Y, Chang C-T, Chu H-L, Yang L-F. Peripheral afferent pathway for acupuncture analgesia. *Sci Sin* 1973; **16:** 210–17.
43. Dundee JW, Ghaly G. Local anesthesia blocks the antiemetic action of P6 acupuncture. *Clin Pharmacol Ther* 1991; **50:** 78–80.
44. Chung JM, Fang ZR, Hori Y, *et al*. Prolonged inhibition of primate spinothalamic tract cells by peripheral nerve stimulation. *Pain* 1984; **19:** 259–75.
◆ 45. Filshie J, Cummings M. Western medical acupuncture. In: Ernst E, White A eds. *Acupuncture: a Scientific Appraisal*. Oxford: Butterworth-Heinemann, 1999.
46. Ho MW, Knight DP. The acupuncture system and the liquid crystalline collagen fibers of the connective tissues. *Am J Chin Med* 1998; **26:** 251–63.
47. Han JS, Ding XZ, Fang SG. Cholecystokinin octapeptide (CCK-8): antagonism to electroacupuncture analgesia and a possible role in electroacupuncture tolerance. *Pain* 1986; **27(1):** 101–15.
48. Le Bars D, Villanueva L, Willer JC, Bouhassira, D. Diffuse noxious inhibitory controls (DNIC) in animals and in man. *Acupuncture Med* 1991; **IX(2):** 47–56.
49. Han J, Terenius L. Neurochemical basis of acupuncture analgesia. *Annu Rev Pharmacol Toxicol* 1982; **22:** 192–220.
50. Uvnas-Moberg K. Physiological and endocrine effects of social contact. *Ann NY Acad Sci* 1997; **807:** 146–63.
51. Melzack R, Stillwell DM, Fox EJ. Trigger points and acupuncture points for pain, correlations and implications. *Pain* 1977; **3:** 3–23.
● 52. Travell JG, Simons DG. *Myofascial Pain and Dysfunction. The Trigger Point Manual*. Baltimore, MD: Williams & Wilkins, 1983.
● 53. Baldry PE. *Acupuncture, Trigger Points and Musculo-Skeletal Pain*, 2nd edn. Edinburgh: Churchill Livingstone, 1993.
◆ 54. Hong C-Z, Simons DG. Pathophysiologic and electrophysiologic mechanisms of myofascial trigger points. *Arch Phys Med Rehabil* 1998; **79:** 863–72.
55. Roth LU, Maret-Maric A, Adler RH, Neuenschwander BE. Acupuncture points have subjective (needling sensation) and objective (serum cortisol increase) specificity. *Acupuncture Med* 1997; **XV(1):** 2–5.
● 56. Han JS. *The Neurochemical Basis of Pain Relief by Acupuncture*. Bejing: Bejing Medical University Press, 1987.
◆ 57. Filshie J, White A. The clinical use of, and evidence for, acupuncture in the medical systems. In: Filshie J, White A eds. *Medical Acupuncture: a Western Scientific Approach*. Edinburgh: Churchill Livingstone, 1998: 225–94.
58. Lee JH, Beitz AJ. The distribution of brain-stem and spinal cord nuclei associated with different frequencies of electroacupuncture analgesia. *Pain* 1993; **52:** 11–28.
◆ 59. Vickers AJ. Can acupuncture have specific effects on health? A systematic review of acupuncture antiemesis trials. *J R Soc Med* 1996; **89:** 303–11.
60. McMillan CM, Dundee JW. The role of transcutaneous electrical stimulation of Neiguan antiemetic acupuncture point in controlling sickness after cancer chemotherapy. *Physiotherapy* 1991; **77:** 499–502.
61. Filshie J, Penn K, Ashley S, Davis CL. Acupuncture for the relief of cancer-related breathlessness. *Palliative Med* 1996; **10:** 145–50.
62. Filshie J. The non-drug treatment of neuralgic and neuropathic pain of malignancy. In: Hanks GW ed. *Pain and Cancer*. Oxford: Oxford University Press, 1988: 161–93.
63. Towlerton G, Filshie J, O'Brien M, Duncan A. Acupuncture in the control of vasomotor symptoms caused by tamoxifen. *Palliative Med* 1999; **13:** 445.
64. Hammar M, Frisk J, Grimas O, *et al*. Acupuncture treatment of vasomotor symptoms in men with prostatic carcinoma: a pilot study. *J Urol* 1999; **161:** 853–6.
● 65. Thompson JW, Filshie J. Transcutaneous electrical nerve stimulation (TENS) and acupuncture. In: Doyle D, Hanks G, Macdonald N eds. *Oxford Textbook of Pallia-*

tive Medicine, 2nd edn. Oxford: Oxford Medical Publications; 1997: 421–37.

● 66. Rampes H and Peuker E. Adverse effects of acupuncture. In: Ernst E, White A eds. *Acupuncture: a Scientific Appraisal*. Oxford: Butterworth-Heinemann, 1999: 128–52.

● 67. Spaulding-Albright N. A review of some herbal and related products commonly used in cancer patients. *J Am Diet Assoc* 1997 **10** (Suppl. 2): S208–15.

68. Hajto T, Hostanska K, Frei K, *et al*. Increased secretion of tumor necrosis factor alpha, interleukin 1, and interleukin 6 by human mononuclear cells exposed to β-galactoside-specific lectin from clinically applied mistletoe extract. *Cancer Res* 1990; **50:** 3322–6.

● 69. Kleijnen J, Knipschild P. Mistletoe treatment for cancer. Review of controlled trials in humans. *PhytoMed* 1994; **1:** 255–60.

● 70. Kaegi E. Unconventional therapies for cancer. 1. Essaic. *CMAJ* 1998; **158:** 897–902.

71. Li Q-S, Cao S-H, Xie G-M, *et al*. Relieving effects of Chinese herbs, ear-acupuncture and epidural morphine on postoperative pain in liver cancer. *Chin Med J* 1994; **107:** 289–94.

● 72. Ernst E, Chrubasik S. Phyto-antiinflammatories: a systematic review of randomized, placebo-controlled, double-blind trials. In: Panush RS ed. *Bailliere's Best Practice and Research in Clinical Rheumatology*. Philadelphia, PA: WB Saunders, 2000: 13–27.

73. Boyle FM. Adverse interaction of herbal medicine with breast cancer treatment. *Med J Aust* 1997; **167:** 286.

● 74. Linde K, Clausias N, Ramirez G, *et al*. Are the clinical effects of homoeopathy placebo effects? A meta-analysis of placebo-controlled trials. *Lancet* 1997; **350:** 834–43.

75. Clover A, Last P, Fisher P, *et al*. Complementary cancer therapy: a pilot study of patients, therapies and quality of life. *Complement Ther Med* 1995; **3:** 129–33.

◆ 76. Spiegel D, Moore R. Imagery and hypnosis in the treatment of cancer patients. *Oncology* 1997; **118:** 1179–95.

● 77. Hilgard ER, Hilgard JR. *Hypnosis in the Relief of Pain*. Los Altos, CA: William Kaufmann, 1975.

78. Spiegel H, Spiegel D. *Trance and Treatment: Clinical Uses of Hypnosis*. New York, NY: Basic Books, 1978.

79. Orne MT. Hypnotic control of pain. Towards a clarification of the different psychological processes involved. In: Bonica JJ ed. *Pain*, vol. 58. New York, NY: Raven Press, 1980: 155–72.

80. Barber J, Gitelson J. Cancer pain: psychological management using hypnosis. *Ca: Cancer J Clin* 1980; **303:** 130–6.

81. Barber J. Incorporating hypnosis in the management of chronic pain. In: Barber J, Adams C eds. *Psychological Approaches to the Management of Pain*. New York, NY: Brunner/Mazel, 1984: 40–59.

82. Reeves JL, Redd WH, Storm FK, Minagawa RY. Hypnosis in the control of pain during hyperthermia treatment of cancer. In: Bonica JJ, Ventafridda V eds. *Advances in Pain Research and Therapy*, vol. 5. New York, NY: Raven Press, 1983: 857–61.

● 83. NIH Technology Assessment Panel on Integration of Behavioral and Relaxation Approaches into the Treatment of Chronic Pain and Insomnia. Integration of behavioral and relaxation approaches into the treatment of chronic pain and insomnia. *JAMA* 1996; **2764:** 313–18.

● 84. Jay SM, Elliott C, Varni JW. Acute and chronic pain in adults and children with cancer. *J Consult Clin Psychol* 1986; **545:** 601–7.

85. Hendler CS, Redd WH. Fear of hypnosis: the role of labeling in patients' acceptance of behavioral intervention. *Behavior Ther* 1986; **17:** 2–13.

● 86. Stam HJ. From symptom relief to cure. In: Spanos NP, Chaves JF eds. *Hypnosis: The Cognitive-Behavioral Perspective*. Buffalo, NY: Prometheus Books, 1989: 313–39.

● 87. Spira JL, Spiegel D. Hypnosis and related techniques in pain management. *Hospital J* 1992; **8** (**1–2**): 89–119.

88. Chaves JF. Recent advances in the application of hypnosis to pain management. *Am J Clin Hyp* 1994; **372:** 117–29.

89. Levitan AA. The use of hypnosis with cancer patients. *Psychiatric Med* 1992; **101:** 119–31.

● 90. Trijsburg RW, van Knippenberg FCE, Rijpma SE. Effects of psychological treatment on cancer patients: a critical review. *Psychosomatic Med* 1992; **54:** 489–517.

◆ 91. Spiegel D, Bloom JR. Group therapy and hypnosis reduce metastatic breast carcinoma pain. *Psychosomatic Med* 1983; **454:** 333–9.

◆ 92. Spiegel D, Bloom J, Kraemer HC, Gottheil E. The beneficial effect of psychosocial treatment on survival of metastatic breast cancer patients: a randomized prospective outcome study. *Lancet* 1989; **ii:** 888–91.

93. Syrjala KL, Cummings C, Donaldson GW. Hypnosis or cognitive behavioral training for the reduction of pain and nausea during cancer treatment: a controlled clinical trial. *Pain* 1992; **48:** 137–46.

● 94. Zeltzer L, LeBaron S. The hypnotic treatment of children in pain. In: Wolraich ML, Routh DK eds. *Advances in Developmental and Behavioral Pediatrics*, vol. 7. Greenwich, CT: JAI Press, 1986: 197–234.

95. Zeltzer LK, Dolgin MJ, LeBaron S, LeBaron C. A randomized, controlled study of behavioral intervention for chemotherapy distress in children with cancer. *Pediatrics* 1991; **881:** 34–42.

● 96. Steggles S, Fehr, R, Aucoin P. Hypnosis for children and adolescents with cancer: an annotated bibliography 1960–1985. *J Assoc Pediatr Oncol Nurses* 1986; **31:** 23–5.

● 97. Steggles S, Damore-Petingola S, Maxwell J, Lightfoot N. Hypnosis for children and adolescents with cancer: an annotated bibliography, 1985–1995. *Am J Clin Hyp* 1997; **393:** 187–200.

● 98. Sutters KA, Miaskowski C. The problem of pain in

children with cancer: a research review. *Oncol Nursing Forum* 1992; **193:** 465–71.

● 99. Ellis JA, Spanos NP. Cognitive-behavioral interventions for children's distress during bone marrow aspirations and lumbar punctures: a critical review. *J Pain Symptom Manage* 1994; **92:** 96–108.

100. Genuis ML. The use of hypnosis in helping cancer patients control anxiety, pain, and emesis: a review of recent empirical studies. *Am J Clin Hyp* 1995; **374:** 316–25.

101. Olness K. Imagery (self-hypnosis) as adjunct therapy in childhood cancer: clinical experience with 25 patients. *Am J Pediatr Hematol Oncol* 1981; **33:** 313–21.

102. Hilgard JR, LeBaron S. Relief of anxiety and pain in children and adolescents with cancer: quantitative measures and clinical observations. *Int J Clin Exp Hyp* 1982; **XXX(4):** 417–42.

◆103. Zeltzer L, LeBaron S. Hypnosis and nonhypnotic techniques for reduction of pain and anxiety during painful procedures in children and adolescents with cancer. *J Pediatr* 1982; **1016:** 1032–5.

104. Kellerman J, Zeltzer L, Ellenberg L, Dash J. Adolescents with cancer. Hypnosis for the reduction of the acute pain and anxiety associated with medical procedures. *J Adolesc Hlth Care* 1983; **42:** 85–90.

105. Katz ER, Kellerman J, Ellenberg L. Hypnosis in the reduction of acute pain and distress in children with cancer. *J Paediatr Psychol* 1987; **123:** 379–94.

106. Wall VJ, Womack W. Hypnotic versus active cognitive strategies for alleviation of procedural distress in pediatric oncology patients. *Am J Clin Hyp* 1989; **313:** 181–91.

107. Jacknow DS, Tschann JM, Link MP, Boyce WT. Hypnosis in the prevention of chemotherapy-related nausea and vomiting in children: a prospective study. *Develop Behav Pediatr* 1994; **154:** 258–64.

108. Rapkin DA, Straubing M, Holroyd JC. Guided Imagery, hypnosis and recovery from head and neck cancer surgery: an exploratory study. *Int J Clin Exp Hyp* 1991; **XXXIX(4):** 215–26.

109. Spiegel D. Uses and abuses of hypnosis. *Integr Psychiatry* 1989; **6:** 211–18.

110. Spiegel D, Cardena E. new uses of hypnosis in the treatment of posttraumatic stress disorder. *J Clin Psychiatry* 1990; **51** (Suppl. 10): 4–8.

111. Finlay IG, Jones OL. Hypnotherapy in palliative care. *J R Soc Med* 1996; **89:** 493–96.

112. Alman M, Lambrou P. *Self-Hypnosis: The Complete Manual for Health and Self-Change*, 2nd edn. London: Souvenir Press, 1993.

113. Spiegel D, Albert LH. Naloxone fails to reverse hypnotic alleviation of chronic pain. *Psychopharmacol Berl* 1983; **812:** 140–3.

◆114. Pedersen DL. Hypnosis and the right hemisphere. *Proc Br Soc Med Dent Hyp* 1984; **54:** 2–13.

●115. Gruzelier J. The state of hypnosis: evidence and applications. *Q J Med* 1996; **89:** 313–17.

116. Spiegel D, Cutcomb S, Ren C, Pribram K. Hypnotic hallucination alters evoked potentials. *J Abnorm Psychol* 1985; **943:** 249–55.

117. Meier W, Klucken M, Soyka D, Bromm B. Hypnotic hypo- and hyperalgesia: divergent effects on pain ratings and pain-related cerebral potentials. *Pain* 1993; **53:** 175–81.

118. Rainville P, Carrier B, Hofbauer RK, *et al.* Dissociation of sensory and affective dimensions of pain using hypnotic modulation. *Pain* 1999; **82:** 159–71.

119. Rainville P, Duncan GH, Price DD, *et al.* Pain affect encoded in human anterior cingulate but not somatosensory cortex. *Science* 1997; **277 (5328):** 968–71.

120. Rhiner M, Dean GE, Ducharme S. Nonpharmacologic measures to reduce cancer pain in the home. *Home Hlth Care Manage Practice* 1996; **82:** 41–7.

121. LeBaron S, Zeltzer L. Imaginative involvement and hypnotizability in childhood. *Int J Clin Exp Hyp* 1988; **XXXVI(4):** 284–95.

122. Kuttner L, Bowman M, Teasdale M. Psychological treatment of distress, pain, and anxiety for young children with cancer. *Develop Behav Pediatr* 1988; **96:** 374–81.

123. Simonton OC, Simonton MS, Creighton S. *Getting Well Again*. Los Angeles, CA: JP Tarcher, 1978.

124. Ader R, Cohen N, Felten D. Psychoneuroimmunology: interactions between the nervous system and the immune system. *Lancet* 1995; **345:** 99–103.

125. Wilkes E. *Complementary Therapy in Hospice and Palliative care*. Report for Trent Palliative Care Centre, 1992.

126. Ko D, Lerner R, Klose G, Cosini AB. Effective treatment of lymphoedema of the extremities. *Arch Surg* 1998; **133:** 452–8.

127. Kite SM, Maher EJ, Anderson K, *et al.* Development of an aromatherapy service at a cancer centre. *Palliative Med* 1998; **12:** 171–80.

●128. Cawley N. A critique of the methodology of research studies evaluating massage. *Eur J Cancer Care* 1997; **6:** 23–31.

129. Sims S. Slow stroke back massage for cancer patients. *Nursing Times* 1986; **82:** 47–50.

130. Ferrell-Torry AT, Glick OJ. The use of therapeutic massage as a nursing intervention to modify anxiety and the perception of cancer pain. *Cancer Nursing* 1993; **16(2):** 93–101.

131. Corner J, Cawley N, Hildebrand S. An evaluation of the use of massage and essential oils on the wellbeing of cancer patients. *Int J Palliative Nursing* 1995; **1(2):** 67–73.

132. Weinrich SP, Weinrich MC. The effect of massage on pain in cancer patients. *Appl Nursing Res* 1990; **3(4):** 140–5.

133. McCarthy MM, Altemus M. Central nervous system actions of oxytocin and modulation of behavior in humans. *Mol Med Today* 1997; **36:** 269–75.

134. Abbot N, Harkness EF, Stevinson C, *et al.* Spiritual healing as a therapy for chronic pain: a randomized, clinical trial. *Pain* 2001; **91:** 79–89.

21

Management of bone pain

PETER J HOSKIN

Bone pain secondary to cancer is an extremely common symptom, reflecting its prevalence in the common cancers, in particular breast, lung, and prostate cancer. Although the vast majority of patients with malignant bone pain have bone metastases, it is, of course, also a feature of primary bone tumors, both benign and malignant. The prevalence of bone metastasis at postmortem in various primary sites is shown in Table 21.1.[1*]

It is always important to consider other causes of bone pain in the cancer patient who presents with this symptom, as outlined in Table 21.2, particularly as the population in whom this typically occurs is elderly, with coexistent degenerative and osteoporotic bone disease in many cases.

ETIOLOGY AND PATHOPHYSIOLOGY

Bone pain due to tumor infiltration is usually a result of blood-borne metastasis. Rarely there may be direct infiltration of a bone when a tumor arises adjacent to that site, for example bone pain in the paravertebral region arising from a retroperitoneal sarcoma or pain in the head and neck region as a result of direct infiltration of tumor into the skull base.

The pathophysiology of bone metastasis has been well described.[2*] The series of events from a tumor cell arriving at the bone surface is coordinated through the release of chemical agents that activate osteoclasts within the bone. These include prostaglandins, kinins, substance P, and parathyroid hormone-related peptides, collectively termed osteoclast-activating factors (OAFs). The osteoclast activity results in bone destruction, allowing entry of the malignant cells into the bone substance, where they establish a colony. In response to this, probably mediated by various chemical growth factors, there occurs an osteoblastic reaction whereby the bone attempts to repair the damaged areas by laying down osteoid. The balance between osteoclast and osteoblast activity defines the morphological features of the bone metastasis; when osteoclastic activity predominates, lytic bone disease is the result, and when osteoblastic activity predominates osteosclerotic metastasis occurs.

The actual mechanism of pain as a result of this process is not well understood. Suggestions have included the effects of direct damage to the bone and the surrounding periosteum, where the principal sensory nerve fibers exist, changes in the intraosseous pressure, and a neurochemical effect due to the release of the various OAFs, several of which, in particular the kinins, prostaglandins and substance P, are recognized pain mediators.

CLINICAL PRESENTATION

Malignant bone pain may present in the context of a patient with a known primary tumor or as the initial presentation of either metastatic bone disease or a primary bone tumor.

Malignant bone pain is typically dull and persistent, occurring through the night as well as in the daytime, and worse on weight-bearing. On clinical examination the affected area is usually locally tender; in addition, there may be local swelling and, in the case of a particularly vascular tumor, an audible bruit over the bone metastasis, which is said to be typical of renal cancer.

Table 21.1 *Incidence of bone metastases based on postmortem data*

Primary site	Percentage of patients with bone metastases	Total number of bone metastases yearly (based on UK incidence rates)
Breast	73	60/100,000
Prostate	68	34/100,000
Thyroid	42	0.8/100,000
Bronchus	36	29/100,000
Kidney	35	2.5/100,000
Rectum	11	3/100,000
Esophagus	6	0.6/100,000

Table 21.2 *Causes of bone pain in cancer patients*

Metastases
Fracture
Degenerative bone disease, e.g. osteoarthritis
Bone marrow pain
Nonmetastatic hypertrophic osteoarthropathy (HPOA)
Other bone disease, e.g. Paget's

DIAGNOSTIC CRITERIA

The presence of malignant tumor within a bone may be detected by plain radiography, isotope bone scan, computed tomography (CT), or magnetic resonance imaging (MRI). It is usual to work up this hierarchy. Isotope bone scan has the advantage of demonstrating the overall distribution of bone metastasis but can be relatively nonspecific, and distinction between spinal metastasis and degenerative disease can be difficult. It is, however, far more sensitive than plain radiographs, except in the case of predominantly lytic disease, such as that seen in multiple myeloma, when the bone scan may be entirely negative because of the minimal osteoblastic response. CT and MRI will give far better definition of the anatomical extent of the bone tumor. MRI is superior to CT for imaging the spine and long bones, whereas CT often gives better definition of flat bones such as the pelvis and scapula.[3*,4*]

Biochemical tests such as measurement of serum alkaline phosphatase and acid phosphatase may provide supportive evidence but are rarely diagnostic, although a very high serum alkaline phosphatase should raise the possibility of Paget's disease as an alternative or coexisting diagnosis. In patients with prostate cancer, a raised serum level of prostate-specific antigen (PSA) (above 20 ng/ml) is associated in over 90% of cases with bone metastasis,[5*] a proportion of which may be occult at the time of initial diagnosis.

In a patient presenting with no known underlying primary tumor, histological confirmation of metastatic disease in the bone is required if the primary cannot be identified by subsequent investigations. In the light of the known distribution and frequency of bone metastasis (Table 21.1), in all patients the neck should be examined and chest radiography performed to exclude bronchial and thyroid cancer, in male patients the prostate should be examined and serum PSA measured, and in women the breasts and axillae should be examined with bilateral mammograms. If lesions are predominantly lytic, then serum should be sent for protein electrophoresis and urine for measurement of Bence-Jones proteins to exclude multiple myeloma, the other cause of predominantly lytic bone metastasis being renal cancer, which may be diagnosed on abdominal ultrasound.

It is essential that management of bone metastasis is always undertaken in the light of histological confirmation of the tumor type, the one exception to this being the patient with widespread osteoblastic metastasis with a serum PSA of >50 ng/ml, in whom a diagnosis of carcinoma of the prostate can be considered proven.

EVIDENCE-BASED EVALUATION OF MANAGEMENT

Pharmacological management of malignant bone pain

The pharmacological management of malignant bone pain using basic pharmacological techniques does not differ from the management of other types of cancer pain, using the World Health Organization (WHO) analgesic ladder (see Chapter Ca10). Anecdotally it is said that bone pain does not respond as well as soft-tissue pain to opioid analgesia, although undoubtedly many patients do gain good relief.

Nonsteroidal anti-inflammatory drugs (NSAIDs) have a major role in the management of musculoskeletal pain, in keeping with the recognized role of prostaglandins in the etiology of metastatic bone pain. Although this is a well-established principle in reviews and textbooks on the subject,[6*] objective data on their efficacy for metastatic bone pain are not so readily available. When used alone as the primary means of pain control, pain relief is seen in only 20% of patients.[7*] This is in keeping with data on the use of the WHO analgesic ladder, in which NSAIDs together with simple analgesics are classified as level 1 analgesia, found to be effective alone in only 11% of one series of 1,229 patients.[8*] There are no data to recommend one NSAID over any other, and choice will in general be based upon individual preference and tolerance of side-effects, of which gastrointestinal symptoms, dizziness, and drowsiness predominate. One study[9**] has suggested a dose–response for naproxen in metastatic bone pain comparing 550 mg 8-hourly with 275 mg 8-hourly, but more side-effects are seen at the higher doses.

In most patients with metastatic bone pain, NSAIDs will be used as an adjuvant alongside opioid analgesics and the additional measures described below, but considerable variability in the relative use of these modalities is seen. Data from recent radiotherapy randomized bone pain trials show a wide variation in analgesic use at the time of radiation treatment for bone pain with radiotherapy. In a large UK trial,[10**] 30% of patients required no analgesia and 13% needed only mild analgesics. In a Danish trial[11**] 9% and in a Dutch[12**] trial 12% of patients required no analgesia, with the corresponding figures for the proportion of patients requiring mild analgesics or NSAIDs being 25% and 38% respectively.

Radiotherapy

Although the use of analgesics and NSAIDs will form the initial management of the patient presenting with malignant bone pain, definitive treatment will often be required to achieve optimal pain relief. Details of the management of primary bone tumors is outside the scope of this chapter, but in general a combination of chemotherapy and local treatment, either surgery or radiotherapy, will be indicated for chemosensitive tumors such as osteosarcoma and Ewing's tumor, whereas the mainstay of treatment for chondrosarcoma is surgery.

Radiotherapy has a major role in the treatment of metastatic bone pain. Treatment may be delivered either by external beam radiotherapy or by the use of radioactive isotopes that accumulate selectively in bone. Different techniques are chosen depending on the distribution and sites of pain.

Localized bone pain

For localized sites of bone pain, simple external beam radiotherapy is the most effective and appropriate treatment. This should not be undertaken without definitive evidence of metastasis at the site of pain and without having excluded other causes, such as degenerative disease, as the primary source of the pain. It is also important in weight-bearing areas to have excluded pathological fracture, for which internal fixation will be indicated. Having confirmed metastatic bone pain, the choice of radiotherapy technique will aim to give a homogeneous radiation dose across the involved bone while, as far as possible, avoiding sensitive normal structures. This is a particular concern when treating ribs, to avoid damage to the underlying lung, and when treating the lumbosacral spine and pelvis, to safeguard the abdominal contents. The radiotherapy procedure follows a series of defined steps as follows.

Immobilization

It is important that the treated area is stable within the treatment beam without significant movement while the treatment is delivered. In general, this will require cooperation from the patient and a comfortable position. With this in mind, it is important when patients attend for radiotherapy that adequate analgesia is provided and in particular that they do not miss doses of analgesia while attending the radiotherapy department.

Localization

Localization refers to the need to delineate the painful site accurately, based on both clinical evaluation and radiographic evidence.

- In the case of superficial bones, palpation may be sufficient, so that, for example, a painful rib may be identified and the treatment area defined on the patient's skin.
- In the case of deeper bones, a treatment simulator that produces diagnostic radiographs simulating the therapy X-ray beam may be used to identify the sites of metastasis accurately and define the beam size and shape required to cover the area. Once defined, skin marks will be used to enable relocation of the beam on the treatment machine.

Planning

Planning is rarely complex when treating bone metastasis. Occasionally, in the case of a spinal metastasis with a paraspinal mass, two or three beams may be focused on the treatment area to enable accurate coverage, but otherwise, for the majority of bone metastases, single or matched opposed beams will be used.

For superficial bones, a beam with limited penetration may be chosen. In modern departments this will be achieved using an electron beam whose depth of penetration is defined by its energy, for example a 10-MeV electron beam will deliver a high dose to a depth of between 3 and 3.5 cm, which is adequate for most chest wall treatments. An alternative is to use a low-energy X-ray beam of 250–300 kV. However, this does not have such a sharp cut-off in its dose distribution and delivers a higher dose to deeper tissues, a particular disadvantage when treating ribs but rarely of clinical significance in a patient with advanced disease. Low-energy X-rays are in fact preferentially absorbed in bone, interacting with the tissue through different processes to those of electrons, and may for the same exposure give around 10% higher absorbed dose. However, as will be discussed below, this may be of little consequence in achieving pain relief.

In the case of other bones, such as the spine, long bones, and pelvis, high-energy X-ray beams from a linear accelerator of 4–6 MV or, if not available, a cobalt-60 gamma-ray beam should be used. In the case of the spine, a single beam directed at the appropriate area should be chosen; for other sites two beams opposing each other may be used to give an even distribution of dose across the bone.

Treatment delivery

Treatment delivery is a simple matter of transferring the above processes to the actual treatment machine. Delivery of radiotherapy to the patient is little different from a diagnostic X-ray exposure lasting only a few minutes, with no associated immediate side-effects.

Radiation dose and bone pain

Although the techniques for treating malignant bone pain with external beam radiation are fairly uniform, there is controversy and considerable variation regarding the optimum dose and fractionation (fractionation refers to the way in which a total dose may be divided into smaller daily doses spread out over a longer period). A major question is whether small doses of radiation delivered as single treatments are as effective as more prolonged treatments given over a week or two or even longer but which ultimately deliver a higher total biological radiation dose. This has been addressed in a number of prospective randomized trials, and, with the exception of one trial carried out in the late 1970s,[13*,14**] all trials have demonstrated that low-dose radiation with single doses, or at most two doses of treatment, are as effective as more prolonged schedules. This applies to all parameters of pain, including rate of onset and overall incidence of pain relief. With the results of the latest bone pain trial from the UK Collaborative Group[10**] it is now also possible to confirm that duration of pain relief up to 1 year after treatment is equivalent comparing a single dose of 8 Gy with a five- or 10-fraction treatment. There is therefore little justification in routine practice for patients receiving more than a single dose of 8–10 Gy delivered to the painful site. This evidence is summarized in Table 21.3, and Fig. 21.1 shows the incidence of pain relief over 1 year of systematic pain chart measurements after radiotherapy in the latest UK trial.

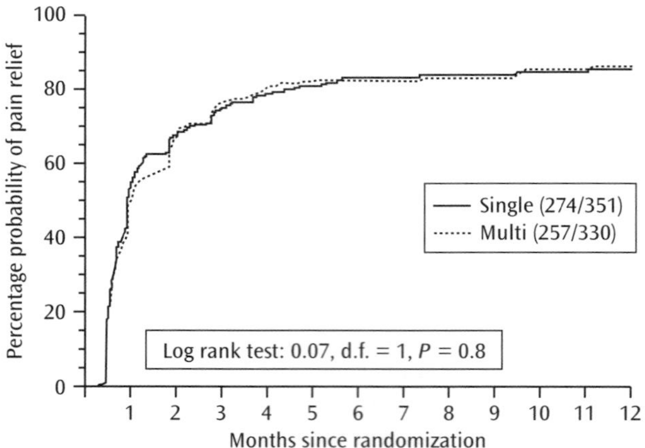

Figure 21.1 *Rate of onset of pain relief after localized radiotherapy for metastatic bone pain delivering either 8 Gy as a single dose or 30 Gy in 10 daily fractions (from Bone Pain Trial Working Party[10] with permission).*

Proponents of more lengthy treatment schedules have suggested that giving small doses daily is associated with less toxicity. In general, the toxicity from treating sites such as the cervical spine, ribs, and long bones is negligible, and the main issue focuses on whether treatments to the lumbosacral spine and pelvis are associated with more nausea, vomiting, and diarrhea when delivered as single doses than as multiple doses. The evidence base for treatment-related toxicity is less strong than for treatment effect in the randomized trials described in Table 21.3. However two of the trials[10**,15**] have now looked at this systematically, and in neither of these is there an obvious effect of treatment dose upon the incidence of toxicity. Again, therefore, the argument against single doses of radiation for malignant bone pain is no longer consistent with the current literature.

The one area where there does remain doubt which has not been addressed specifically by the above trials is that of neuropathic pain related to bone metastasis. This is currently the subject of a multicenter randomized trial in the UK and Australasia comparing single doses with multifraction doses. This may be the one area for which

Table 21.3 *Randomized controlled trials assessing the effect of single-fraction radiotherapy for metastatic bone pain*

			Pain response at 1 month[a] (%)	
Trial	**Single dose**	**Multidose**	**Single dose**	**Multidose**
Price *et al.*[15**]	8 Gy	30 Gy/10f	67	75
Cole[16**]	8 Gy	30 Gy/10f	85	82
Hoskin *et al.*[17**]	8 Gy vs. 4 Gy	None	44 (4 Gy) 69 (8 Gy)	
Gaze *et al.*[18**]	10 Gy	30 Gy/10f	84	89
Neilson *et al.*[11**]	8 Gy	30 Gy/10f	49	55
UK Collaborative Group[10**]	8 Gy	20 Gy/5f or 30 Gy/10f	55	54
Steenland *et al.*[12**]	8 Gy	24 Gy/6f	58	58[b]

a. None of the differences between single and multidose are statistically significant ($P > 0.05$).
b. Estimated from published actuarial graph.

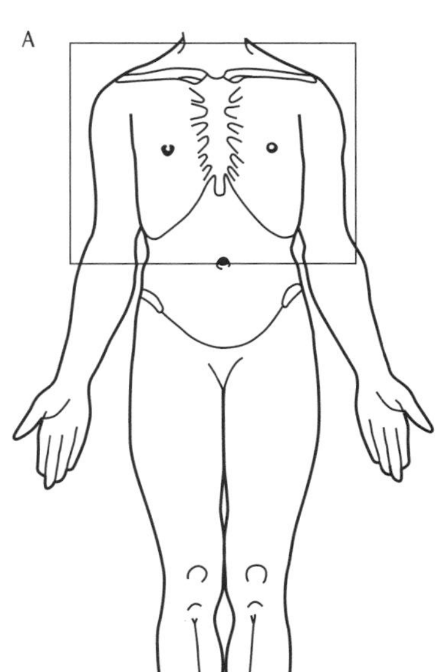

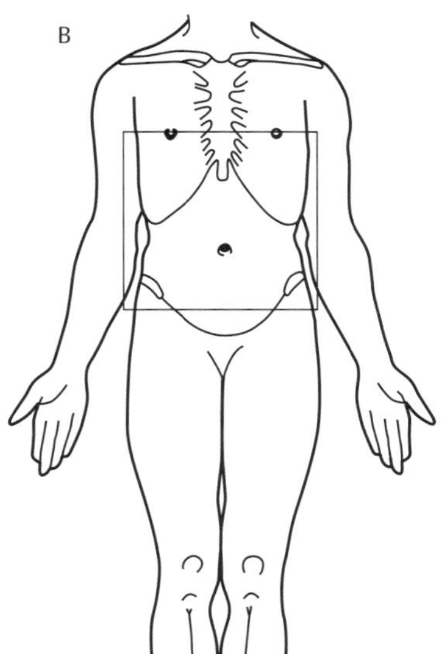

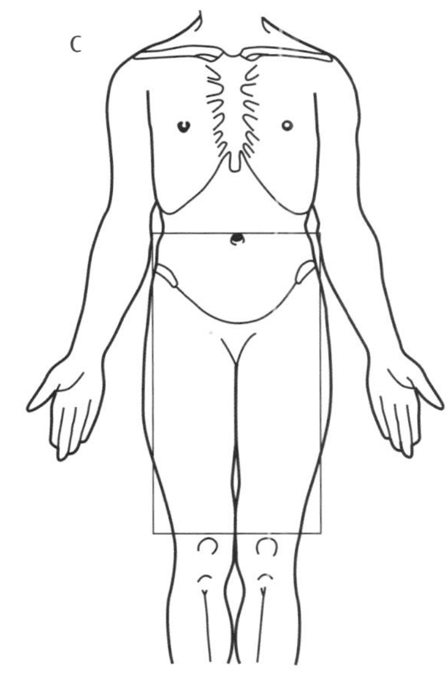

Figure 21.2 *Examples of hemibody radiation fields (A) to upper hemibody, (B) to mid-hemibody, and (C) to lower hemibody.*

prolonged radiation courses for cancer pain have some justification, in the absence of completed trial data evaluating single doses.

Bone pain in multiple sites

Because bone metastasis occurs by blood-borne spread, it usually affects multiple sites. Despite this, pain may occur in only one area, in which case local radiotherapy is appropriate. However, some patients will develop pain in multiple sites that cannot be treated with a single localized radiation beam covering one bone area. These patients can still be offered radiation therapy and, where possible, radiotherapy will remain the most effective treatment. In selected cases, which will be discussed below, chemotherapy or hormone therapy is also appropriate.

Wide-field irradiation

The technique of delivering wide-field irradiation is often described as hemibody radiotherapy, in recognition of the area that may be included in a radiation beam to deliver this type of therapy. The techniques are similar to those described above, but the radiation field is considerably larger and covers the region of the body where pain predominates. There are, however, limits to the extent that can be safely included because of the risks of bone marrow failure. Total body irradiation (TBI) is a valuable technique in association with bone marrow transplantation but is otherwise lethal because of the resultant bone marrow failure. It is, however, possible to target the upper, lower, or mid half-body, the choice of area depending on the predominant sites of pain, as illustrated in Fig. 21.2. One limitation may be the size of the X-ray beam that can be delivered from a linear accelerator, which is typically no bigger than 40 cm^2 on the patient's skin. This can be overcome by extending the treating distance so that the patient is further away from the beam, the size of the beam then increasing by simple geometry.

There is less controversy regarding dose fractionation with this technique and little argument against using single doses of radiation. The doses are limited to no more than 6 Gy to the upper half-body, more than this resulting in significant lung damage. Doses of up to 8 Gy to the lower half-body may be tolerated safely. These doses are targeted to the center of the body, i.e. midway between two beams, front and back, opposing each other to give equal dose distribution across the treated area. The dose must also be corrected for the increased transmission through lungs, ideally using a CT scan to determine the lung depth when the thorax is included.

There has been no randomized comparison of this technique against "best supportive care." Efficacy has been defined in single-arm studies,[19**–23*] and the results are very similar to those received with external beam radiotherapy. More rapid responses than with localized irradiation may be seen, often within 24 h, with up to 80% of patients reporting reduced pain at 1 month. However, there is undoubtedly an increased incidence of acute toxicity, as a result of which wide-field irradiation is perhaps underused. The principal toxicities are outlined in Table 21.4.

Radioisotope therapy

Radioisotope therapy is an alternative to wide-field irradiation. It involves the administration of a radioisotope, usually by intravenous injection. The isotope then circulates and is selectively taken up by bone, preferentially at sites of bone metastasis. The isotope delivers radiation by its natural decay. The ideal isotope will produce predominantly beta particle irradiation with a range of a few mil-

Table 21.4 *Toxicity of wide-field (hemibody) radiotherapy*

All sites
Bone marrow: transfusion requirements, measured falls in WBC and platelets
Upper body
Lungs: interstitial pneumonitis
Stomach: nausea
Liver: nausea, subclinical hepatitis
Lower body
Small and large bowel: diarrhea

limeters, depositing its energy within the bone metastasis in which it is localized. A small component of low-energy gamma irradiation is also of value as it can be detected by a gamma camera to give pictures analogous to a diagnostic bone scan showing the distribution of the isotope uptake.

Strontium

Strontium (^{89}Sr) is currently the most commonly used radioisotope for the treatment of metastatic bone pain. It decays entirely by beta emission and has a radioactive half-life of 50.5 days. Its beta-particles have an energy of 1.46 MeV, which means they will penetrate up to 8 mm in tissue. Chemically, strontium is similar to calcium and therefore taken up into bone in the same way and incorporated into hydroxyapatite. Areas of active mineralization will therefore concentrate strontium, and this will include all sites of osteoblastic response to bone metastasis.

One of the major advantages of strontium is its ease of administration, requiring a simple intravenous injection that can be given as an outpatient. Because it produces short-range beta irradiation, there are few if any major radiation hazards associated with its use and no acute toxicity. The only significant contraindication to strontium use is extensive bone marrow depression as its widespread uptake into bone results in a radiation dose being delivered to the bone marrow. Urinary incontinence is also a relative contraindication as strontium is excreted in the urine and, if there is spillage on to the patient's skin, clothing or bed, contamination can occur. However, provided incontinent patients are catheterized, this can be overcome. Advanced renal failure will prolong retention of strontium and may also be a relative contraindication.

The pattern of pain relief with radioactive strontium is different from that with external beam treatment and in general follows a longer time-course, with many patients taking up to 12 weeks to exhibit maximum response.[24*] For this reason, patients who have a life expectancy of less than this may benefit more from external beam treatment or appropriate pharmacological manipulations.

Strontium has been evaluated in both formal phase II dose escalation studies[25*] and a randomized, double-blind, placebo-controlled trial,[26**]in which it was found to be superior to placebo at its effective dose of 150 MBq. It has also been compared in a randomized trial with external beam radiotherapy,[27**] in which it was found to be equivalent. A case–control comparison with wide-field irradiation[28*] has shown equivalence for pain control but less associated toxicity and, in particular, fewer blood and platelet transfusion requirements after treatment.

Current licenced indications for strontium are restricted to prostate cancer, on which the initial evaluation was focused owing to the osteoblastic nature of its metastases. Activity in other primary tumor types has been demonstrated,[24*] and the indications will no doubt be broadened to include these as further evidence is accrued.

Although most patients will receive a single dose of strontium, there is limited experience of repeated doses,[25*] which appear to be as effective as the initial exposure and may be considered at 3- to 6-monthly intervals.

Samarium

Samarium (^{153}Sm) is available as an alternative to strontium. It is conjugated with a phosphonate compound (ethylenediaminetetramethylenephosphonate, EDMP) and thereby preferentially taken up after intravenous administration into sites of bone metastasis. Samarium is a beta-particle emitter with an average energy of 233 keV and a range of 3 mm in soft tissue. In addition, it produces low-energy gamma rays at 103 keV, which gives it the advantage that it can be imaged using a gamma-camera, as shown in Fig. 21.3. Administration is by single intravenous injection, and formal phase I and phase II dose escalation studies[29*] have shown optimal effect at a dose of 1 mCi/kg. It has been evaluated in randomized, placebo-controlled, double-blind trials[30**] and found to have demonstrable analgesic effect in hormone-resistant prostate cancer and also in breast cancer. As there is radiation dose to the bone marrow, some transient myelosuppression is seen, but this is rarely of clinical consequence, and multiple doses of samarium at 8-week intervals have been described.

Radioiodine

Radioactive iodine has a specific indication in bone metastasis from metastatic differentiated thyroid cancer. Up to 80% of such tumors retain the characteristics of thyroid tissue and avidly accumulate radioiodine. The ^{131}I isotope is used for therapeutic use.[31*] Again, this isotope produces both beta and gamma emissions and can therefore be imaged on gamma-camera scanning in addition to delivering a localized radiation dose through its beta emission. Although the use of radioiodine is well established in the management of thyroid cancer, it has in fact not been subjected to randomized controlled trial evaluation. Single-arm studies confirm lengthy survival in patients with metastatic thyroid cancer treated in this way and, indeed, radiographic remission of isotope concentrating metastases can be shown. Paradoxically, the

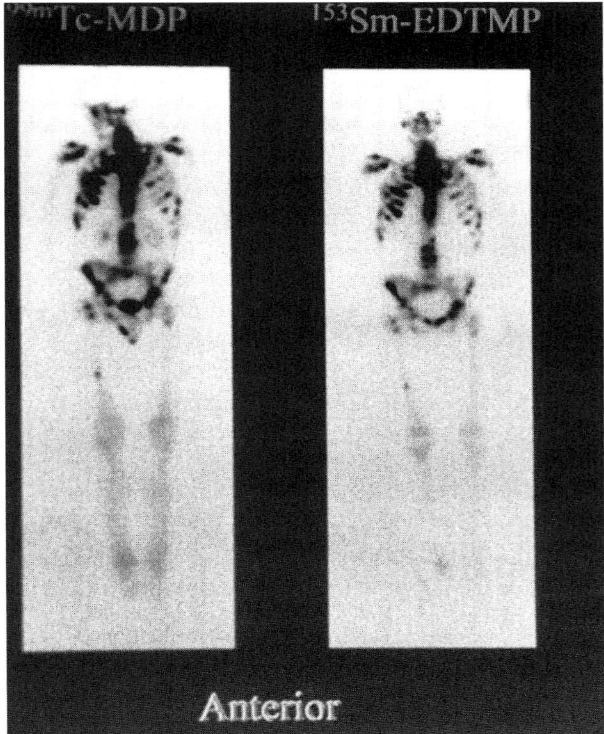

Figure 21.3 *Gamma camera pictures of (left) technetium uptake in diagnostic bone scan and (right) samarium uptake after therapeutic administration.*

effect on bone pain may be less striking, and one paper at least[32*] has suggested that external beam radiotherapy may be more effective than radioisotope therapy in this situation.

Phosphorus

The isotope ^{32}P has in the past been evaluated for the treatment of metastatic bone pain. Its primary use as a therapeutic agent is in the treatment of polycythemia as it is widely taken up in bone and suppresses bone marrow function. This is also its major disadvantage when used for the treatment metastatic bone pain, and with the development of more selective isotopes, including strontium and samarium, its use has largely fallen out of favor.

Rhenium

Rhenium (^{186}Re) has also been developed within a phosphonate compound analogous to the samarium compound. It has been less extensively evaluated and is not currently as widely available. Phase II studies[33*] suggest that it is similar to the other two major isotopes for relief of metastatic bone pain.

Chemotherapy

When metastatic bone pain is due to widespread disease, and particularly if, as may be the case, there is associated soft-tissue metastasis as well, systemic chemotherapy should be considered. The major limitations relate to the chemosensitivity of the primary sites commonly presenting with bone metastasis as shown in Table 21.5. From this it will be apparent that there are perhaps three major indications for chemotherapy in metastatic bone pain.

Table 21.5 *Chemosensitivity of primary tumors commonly metastasizing to bone*

Primary site	Sensitivity[a]
Myeloma	High
Breast	High
Prostate	Low
Thyroid	Low
Bronchus	High
Kidney	Low
Rectum	Mid
Esophagus	Mid/low

a. High = >50% response rate, mid = 25–50% response rate, low = <25% response rate.

Breast cancer has a greater than 50% response rate to most first-line chemotherapy.[34*] Many patients who present with bone metastasis will, however, have previously been exposed to adjuvant chemotherapy, and this will be an increasing problem as more adjuvant chemotherapy is used. In the majority of cases, however, the patient will be offered systemic chemotherapy, the drug combinations varying according to previous exposure. There are few published data on the efficacy of systemic chemotherapy in metastatic breast cancer specifically relating to bone pain relief. One review[35*] has suggested that response in bone metastasis lags some way behind that in soft tissue, with a median time to maximal response of 32 weeks, which is very different to the response to radiation therapy.

Small-cell lung cancer is a highly chemoresponsive disease. Patients presenting with metastatic disease will usually be offered some form of chemotherapy, specific drug combinations varying from time to time. A randomized trial reported by the Medical Research Council (MRC)[36*] has suggested that combination drug therapy may be better than single-drug therapy using etoposide, although the actual gains are relatively modest. The role of chemotherapy at relapse is a little more controversial, but one published randomized trial[37**] does support the use of second-line combination chemotherapy using drugs to which the patient has not previously been exposed, with better symptom control reported than in patients treated with "best supportive care."

Chemotherapy in *nonsmall-cell lung cancer* is less effective, but improvements in both quality of life and survival compared with best supportive care have been shown in phase III trials. Current best schedules use combinations of cisplatin or carboplatin with docetaxel, gemcitabine, or vinorelbine.[38*] Specific responses in bone pain are not reported, however, and there has been no randomized comparison with radiotherapy, but where multiple symptoms present this may be entirely appropriate.

Multiple myeloma is routinely treated with chemotherapy. First-line treatment involves the use of either oral melphalan or combination chemotherapy such as ABCM (adriamycin, BCNU, cyclophosphamide, melphalan).[39***] Response rates to this treatment are high in terms of both pain relief and suppression of the paraprotein, which is a useful marker of disease activity. However, few patients are cured, although some may be selected to proceed to even more intensive treatment with high-dose chemotherapy. At relapse the role of chemotherapy is less certain, but most patients are re-exposed to oral melphalan or cyclophosphamide or to high-dose dexamethasone-containing schedules,[40*] which can result in further remission in over 40% of patients. There is no randomized comparison of second-line chemotherapy against "best supportive care" in multiple myeloma.

Other primary sites may metastasize to bone, and in some of these also chemotherapy may be entirely appropriate. In general, hematological malignancies, including lymphomas, will be highly chemosensitive. Ovarian, bladder, and colorectal cancer are other less common sources of bone metastasis that may benefit.

Hormone treatment

Among the common cancers that metastasize to bone, breast and prostate are hormone sensitive, and this may result in dramatic improvements in pain control in responsive patients.

Prostate cancer

Prostate cancer in virtually all cases is androgen dependent at the time of presentation. Hormone therapy therefore aims to block androgen activity either pharmacologically, using oral antiandrogens such as cyproterone acetate or flutamide or gonadotrophin-releasing hormone analogs such as goserelin or leuprolide, or through surgical castration (orchidectomy). These individual methods of androgen ablation have been compared in multicenter randomized trials,[41**,42**] but no advantage for one over the other has emerged. Similarly, although some advocate "maximal androgen blockade," incorporating a central androgen blockade such as goserelin with peripheral androgen blockade using an oral antiandrogen drug, meta-analysis[43**] suggests there is no advantage for maximal androgen blockade in patients with metastatic disease. Single-agent therapy is therefore indicated, with response rates of 80–90% for pain relief, which may occur dramatically within 24 h of starting treatment. The duration of response to androgen therapy is limited, averaging 2–3 years, during which time clones of androgen-independent cells emerge and further exposure to second-line hormone therapy, although controversial, is in practice rarely of great value. It is in this group of "hormone-resistant" patients that wide-field irradiation and systemic isotope therapy have been widely evaluated.

Breast cancer

In many cases, breast cancer will also be hormone sensitive. This is particularly the case in post-menopausal women, of whom around 60% will have demonstrable estrogen receptors on the surface of their malignant cells; this proportion is approximately halved in premenopausal women.[34*] The standard treatment for hormone-responsive breast cancer has been tamoxifen. Increasingly, however, women are exposed to tamoxifen at the time of their primary presentation as adjuvant treatment. Women who have not been exposed to tamoxifen should have this at the time of relapse with bone metastasis; those who have had received previous adjuvant tamoxifen will be considered for second-line hormone therapy, which may be a progestogen such as medroxyprogesterone or megestrol or an aromatase inhibitor such as letrozole or anastrozole. There are no randomized data to suggest that any one of these approaches is superior to the other, and up to 50% of women may achieve a second response. Although this may be measured in terms of objective tumor shrinkage, the impact of such maneuvers upon pain control is less well documented and radiotherapy is often also required.

Endometrial cancer

Carcinoma of the endometrium is responsive to progestogens. Bone metastasis is in fact unusual in this tumor, but, when encountered, progestogens in the form of megestrol or medroxyprogesterone acetate may be of value for multiple sites of bone pain.

Renal cancer

Although, historically, renal cancer has been considered hormone sensitive, responding to progesterone exposure, more modern appraisal of the literature suggests that this is in fact a rare event, occurring in no more than 15% of patients,[44*] and possibly reflecting only those who would in any case experience spontaneous remission. Nonetheless, in the absence of any other effective systemic treatment, patients with renal cancer are often exposed to progesterone. The justification for this is the absence of significant side-effects for most patients and indeed often a positive benefit in terms of relief of nonspecific symptoms. In general, however, progesterone should not be relied upon for relief of metastatic bone pain, and alternative measures, in particular radiation therapy, should be considered.

Bisphosphonates

Bisphosphonates were originally developed for the treatment of metabolic bone disease such as osteoporosis and Paget's disease. The two agents most commonly used currently are clodronate and pamidronate, which have an increasing role in the management of metastatic bone disease. Their mode of action is through inhibiting the function of osteoclasts. As the initial response in the process of a bone metastasis is osteoclast activation, they have been proposed and investigated as a potential means of inhibiting the development of bone metastasis in patients who are at high risk. Data from phase III randomized, placebo-controlled trials support this effect in myeloma[45]** and breast cancer,[46]** although the magnitude of effect is relatively modest. One of the current limitations of the drugs available is that the oral formulation of clodronate is poorly and variably absorbed in many patients, while pamidronate needs to be administered by intravenous infusion on a 3-weekly basis. Newer, more potent drugs, such as ibandronate, are currently under evaluation with oral formulations. Undoubtedly, this class of drugs will have an increasing role in the early management of patients at high risk of bone metastasis and may influence the natural history of the disease and even survival.[47]**

A second role for bisphosphonates in the management of bone metastasis is in the treatment of established disease. Single-arm studies in patients with metastases predominantly from breast cancer and thyroid cancer have demonstrated radiological and biochemical responses with radiographic bone healing of lytic lesions and a reduction in markers of osteoclast activity[48]* such as urinary deoxypyridinoline, urinary calcium, and serum interleukin 6 (IL-6). It is also clear that a number of patients with metastatic bone pain have good pain relief with the use of bisphosphonate drugs. This has now been shown in both single-arm studies and double-blind, placebo-controlled trials[49]*** using clodronate or pamidronate. Although the greatest body of data comes from patients with breast cancer,[49a] several other sites have been included in these studies with no apparent difference in their response, albeit within small subgroups.

The relative role of bisphosphonates alongside the other measures for pain relief remains uncertain. There are obvious advantages over radiotherapy in their ease of administration without the need for a patient to be transferred to a center with radiotherapy facilities, and the development of more potent oral formulations will make this form of treatment increasingly attractive. It is unlikely that they will replace radiotherapy in the management of bone metastasis but they provide a further valuable treatment to complement definitive management of the underlying cancer.

Surgery

Surgery has an important role in the management of impending or actual pathological fracture associated with bone metastasis. Occasionally this may be the first presentation of the malignancy when diagnostic information from the bone biopsy at the time of fixation is also of vital importance.

Patients with advanced lytic disease are at high risk of fracture. Specific criteria for internal fixation to prevent fracture have been defined:[50]*

- lytic lesions > 2.5 cm in diameter;
- > 50% cortical destruction;
- diffuse lytic disease in a weight-bearing area.

In established pathological fracture of a long bone, internal fixation, where possible and appropriate, is undoubtedly the best management to produce early pain relief and mobility. The other indication for surgery in the management of bone metastasis is in vertebral collapse where there is associated compression of the spinal canal and spinal instability. In this setting radiotherapy alone is not adequate and anterior spinal stabilization and fusion are indicated.[51]*

Following surgery for pathological fracture, postoperative radiotherapy is generally recommended. Although

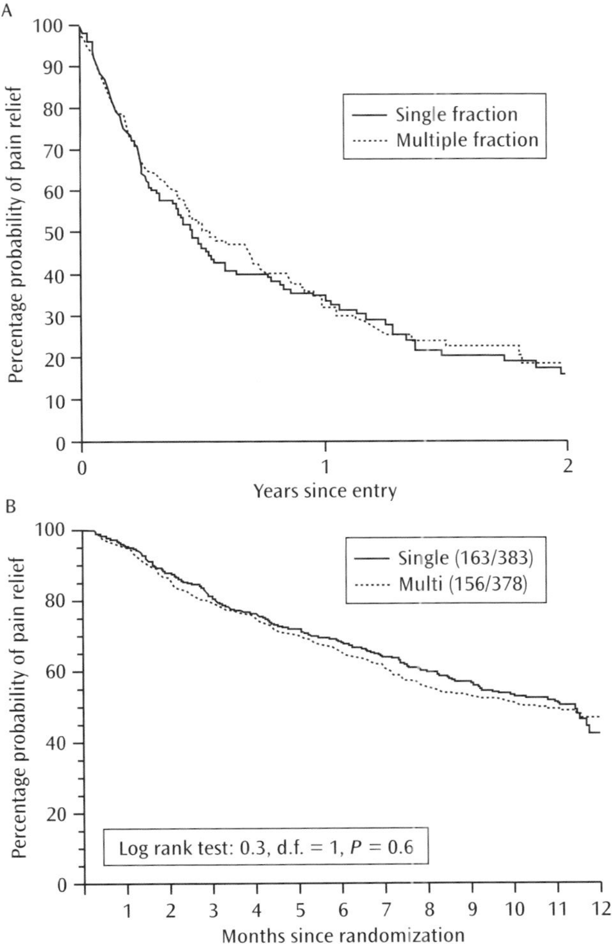

Figure 21.4 *(A) Survival curve for patients from time of localized radiotherapy for metastatic bone pain (from Price et al.[15] with permission). (B) Survival curve for patients from time of localized radiotherapy for metastatic bone pain in a population selected for a projected survival of at least 1 year from the time of treatment (from Bone Pain Trial Working Party[10] with permission).*

this is standard practice, there is limited evidence supporting its value.[52*] It is based on the hypothesis that surgery does not eradicate or even suppress residual tumor within the bone and anecdotal evidence that areas of internal fixation, left alone, are associated with subsequent complications and further bone destruction. In practice, postoperative radiotherapy is selected for patients with a life expectancy of more than 1 month following fixation.

PROGNOSIS

The prognosis for pain relief in patients with metastatic bone pain is relatively good, with over 80% experiencing pain relief and up to one-third achieving complete control of pain. The onset of pain relief with radiotherapy will be seen within 4–6 weeks, and in patients who survive prolonged relief for many weeks and months can be expected. There is also evidence that if pain returns retreatment with radiotherapy is of equal value to initial treatment.[53*]

The efficacy of radiotherapy in metastatic bone pain has been subject to a meta-analysis,[54**] which included all trials in which there was objective measurement of pain and recorded response rates. This has reported results in terms of the number of patients needed to treat for an effect (NNT) (http://www.jr2.ox.ac.uk/Bandolier/painpag/Chronrev/Cancer/CP073.html):

> Twenty-seven percent of patients had achieved complete pain relief one month after radiotherapy (NNT 3.9 (95% CI 3.5–4.4)), with half the patients taking 4 weeks to obtain relief. Additionally, 29% of patients had achieved at least 50% pain relief 1 month after radiotherapy (NNT 3.6 (95% CI 3.2–3.9)). Median duration of relief was 12 weeks.

In contrast, the prognosis for survival in patients with bone metastasis is poor, as shown by a representative survival curve of patients treated for bone metastasis in Fig. 21.4A. As these will also represent a selected sample of patients fit enough to attend for radiotherapy, it is likely that the actual survival of the entire population of patients with bone metastasis is even worse. This reflects the fact that symptomatic disease is a marker of widespread disseminated cancer often accompanied by soft-tissue disease and poor performance status, which in the absence of an effective systemic anticancer therapy results in death within a few months. The small number of patients surviving for a year or more are typically those with breast or prostate cancer who have not previously received hormone therapy. Even when patients are selected for longer survival, the actual survival is poor, as demonstrated in Fig. 21.4B from a trial in which the entry criterion was an expected survival of more than 1 year. It can be seen that even in this group the actual survival is poor.

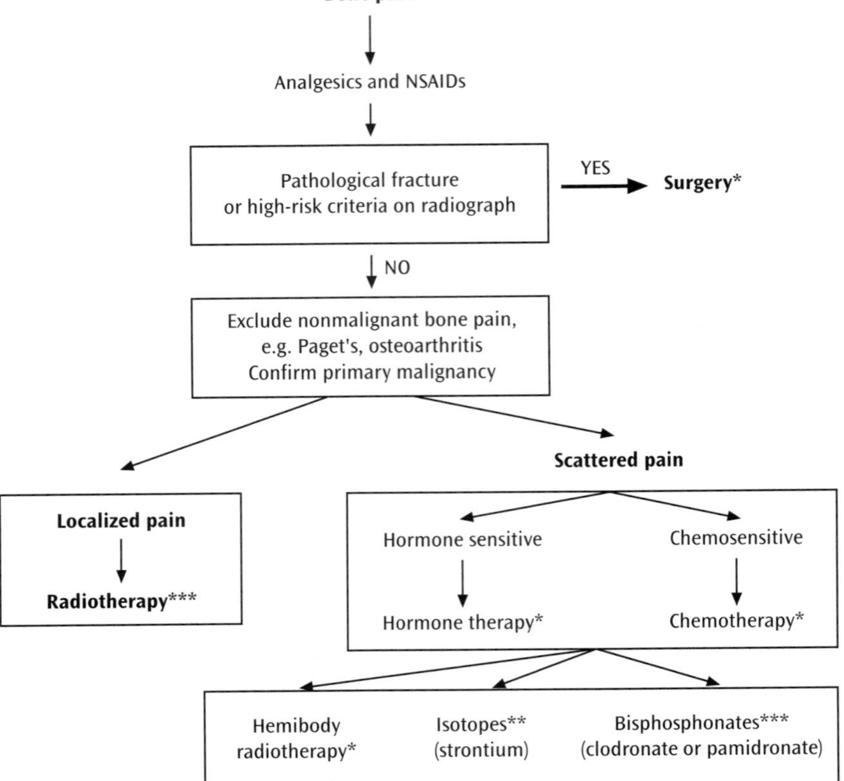

Figure 21.5 *Overview of the management of metastatic bone pain.*

SPECIAL COMMENTS

Bone metastases result in considerable morbidity. A range of treatments are available, which are largely complementary and should be considered as a comprehensive strategy to enable pain control and retain the performance status of the patient. This is illustrated in Fig. 21.5.

Finally, metastatic bone pain should not be considered in isolation. It is well established that few patients with advanced cancer have a single site or cause of pain, and this applies as much if not more so to bone metastasis as any other scenario. In particular, associated musculoskeletal pain, neuropathic pain, nerve compression with the associated problems of motor weakness, and degenerative bone disease must all be considered in the overall management of the patient.

REFERENCES

1. Abrams HL, Spiro R, Goldstein N. Metastases in carcinoma. Analysis of 1000 autopsied cases. *Cancer* 1950; **3:** 74–85.
2. Ross Garrett I. Bone destruction in cancer. *Semin Oncol* 1993; **20** (Suppl. 2): 4–9.
3. Cranston PE, Patel RB, Harrison RB. Computed tomography for metastatic lesions of the osseous pelvis. *J Comput Assist Tomogr* 1984; **8:** 582
4. Rimmer WD, Berquist TH, McLeod RA, *et al.* Bone tumours: magnetic resonance imaging versus computed tomography. *Radiology* 1985; **155:** 709–15.
5. Spencer JA, Chng WJ, Hudson E, *et al.* Prostate specific antigen level and Gleason score in predicting the stage of newly diagnosed prostate cancer. *Br J Radiol* 1998; **71:** 1130–5.
6. Rawlins MD. Non-opioid analgesics In: Doyle D, Hanks GW, MacDonald N eds. *Oxford Textbook of Palliative Medicine,* 2nd edn. Oxford: Oxford University Press, 1998: 355–60.
7. Coombes RC, Munro Neville A, Gazet J-C, *et al.* Agents affecting osteolysis in patients with breast cancer. *Cancer Chemother Pharmacol* 1979; **3:** 41–4.
8. McQuay H, Moore A. *An Evidence-based Resource for Pain Relief.* Oxford: Oxford University Press, 1998: 196.
9. Levick S, Jacobs C, Lonkas D, *et al.* Naproxen sodium in the treatment of bone pain due to metastatic cancer. *Pain* 1998; **35:** 253–80.
10. ◆ Bone Pain Trial Working Party. 8 Gy single fraction radiotherapy for the treatment of metastatic skeletal pain: randomised comparison with a multifraction schedule over 12 months of patient follow up. *Radiother Oncol* 1999; **52:** 111–21.
11. ◆ Nielsen OS, Bentzen SM, Sandberg E, *et al.* Randomized trial of single dose versus fractionated palliative radiotherapy of bone metastases. *Radiother Oncol* 1998; **47:** 233–40.
12. ◆ Steenland E, Leer J, von Houwelingen H, *et al.* The effect of a single dose versus fractionated palliative radiotherapy of bone metastases. *Radiother Oncol* 1999; **52:** 101–9.
13. Tong D, Gillick L, Hendrickson F. The palliation of symptomatic osseous metastases: final results of the study by the Radiation Therapy Oncology Group. *Cancer* 1982; **50:** 893–9.
14. ◆ Blitzer PH. Reanalysis of the RTOG study of the palliation of symptomatic osseous metastasis. *Cancer* 1985; **55:** 1468–72.
15. ◆ Price P, Hoskin PJ, Easton D, *et al.* Prospective randomised trial of single and multifraction radiotherapy schedules in the treatment of painful bony metastases. *Radiother Oncol* 1986; **6:** 247–55.
16. Cole DJ. A randomized trial of a single treatment versus conventional fractionation in the palliative radiotherapy of painful bone metastases. *Clin Oncol* 1989; **1:** 59–62.
17. ◆ Hoskin PJ, Price P, Easton D, *et al.* A prospective randomised trial of 4Gy or 8Gy single doses in the treatment of metastatic bone pain. *Radiother Oncol* 1992; **23:** 74–8.
18. Gaze MN, Kelly CG, Kerr GR, *et al.* Pain relief and quality of life following radiotherapy for bone metastases: a randomised trial of two fractionation schedules. *Radiother Oncol* 1997; **45:** 109–16.
19. ◆ Salazar OM, Rubin P, Hendricksen F, *et al.* Single-dose half body irradiation for palliation of multiple bone metastases from solid tumours. *Cancer* 1986; **58:** 29–36.
20. Hoskin PJ, Ford HT, Harmer CI. Hemibody irradiation (HBI) for metastatic bone pain in two histological distinct groups of patients. *Clin Radiol* 1989; **1:** 67–9.
21. Fitzpatrick PJ. Wide-Field irradiation of bone metastases. In: Weiss L, Gilbert HA eds. *Bone Metastasis.* Boston, MA: GK Hall, 1981: 83–113.
22. Qasim MM. Half body irradiation (HBI) in metastatic carcinomas. *Clin Radiol* 1981; **32:** 215–19.
23. Douglas P, Rossier Ph, Mirimanoff R-O, Coucke PA. Third-body irradiation as an effective palliative treatment for painful multiple bone metastases resistant to chemo- or hormonal treatment. *Radiother Oncol* 1993; **28:** 76–8.
24. Hoskin PJ. Strontium. In: Dollery C ed. *Drug Therapy Supplement 2.* Edinburgh: Churchill Livingstone, 1994.
25. ◆ Laing AH, Ackery DM, Bayly RJ, *et al.* Strontium-89 chloride for pain palliation in prostatic skeletal malignancy. *Br J Radiol* 1991; **64:** 816–22.
26. ◆ Lewington VJ, McEwan AJ, Ackery DM, *et al.* A prospective randomized double-blind crossover study to examine the efficacy of strontium-89 in pain palliation in patients with advanced prostate cancer metastatic to bone. *Eur J Cancer* 1991; **27:** 954–8.
27. ◆ Quilty PM, Kirk D, Bolger JJ, *et al.* A comparison of the

palliative effects of strontium-89 and external beam radiotherapy in metastatic prostate cancer. *Radiother Oncol* 1994; **31:** 33–40.

28. Dearnaley DP, Bayley RJ, A'Hern RP, *et al.* Palliation of bone metastases in prostate cancer: Hemibody irradiation or strontium-89. *Clin Oncol* 1992; **4:** 101–7.
◆ 29. Resche I, Chatal J-F, Pecking A, *et al.* A dose-controlled study of ^{153}Sm-ethylenediaminetetramethylenephosphonate (EDTMP) in the treatment of patients with painful bone metastases. *Eur J Cancer* 1997; **33:** 1583–91.
30. Serafini AN, Houston SJ, Resche I, *et al.* Palliation of pain associated with metastatic bone cancer using samarium-153 lexidronam: a double blind placebo-controlled clinical trial. *J Clin Oncol* 1998; **16:** 1574–81.
31. Tubiana M, Lacour J, Monnier MD, *et al.* External radiotherapy and radioiodine in the treatment of 359 thyroid cancers. *Br J Radiol* 1975; **48:** 894–907.
◆ 32. Brown AP, Greening WP, McCready VR, *et al.* Radioiodine treatment of metastatic thyroid carcinoma: the Royal Marsden Hospital experience. *Br J Radiol* 1984; **57:** 232–7.
33. Maxon III HR, Schroder LE, Hertzberg VS, *et al.* Rhenium-186(Sn)HEDP for treatment of painful osseous metastases: results of a double-blind crossover comparison with placebo. *J Nucl Med* 1991; **32:** 1877–81.
34. Honig SF. Hormonal therapy and chemotherapy In: Harris JR, Lippman M, Morrow M, Hellman S eds. *Diseases of the Breast*. Philadelphia, PA: Lippincott-Raven, 1996: 669–734.
35. Smith IE, Macaulay V. Comparison of different endocrine therapies in management of bone metastases from breast carcinoma. *J R Soc Med* 1985; **78** (Suppl. 9): 15–21.
◆ 36. Medical Research Council Lung Cancer Working Party. Comparison of oral etoposide and standard intravenous multidrug chemotherapy for small-cell lung cancer: a stopped multicentre randomised trial. *Lancet* 1996; **348:** 563–6.
◆ 37. Spiro SG, Souhami RL, Geddes DM, *et al.* Duration of chemotherapy in small cell lung cancer: a Cancer Research Campaign trial. *Br J Cancer* 1989; **59:** 578–83.
◆ 38. Schiller JH, Harrington D, Belani C, *et al.* Comparison of four chemotherapy regimens for advanced non small cell lung cancer. *N Engl J Med* 2002; **346:** 92–8.
● 39. Gregory WM, Richards MA, Malpas JS. Combination chemotherapy versus Melphalan and Prednisolone in the treatment of multiple myeloma: an overview of published trials. *J Clin Oncol* 1992; **10:** 334–42.
40. Alexanian R, Dimopoulos MA, Delasalle K, Barlogie B. Primary dexamethasone treatment of multiple myeloma. *Blood* 1992; **80:** 887–90.
41. Newling DWW. Anti-androgens in the treatment of prostate cancer. *Br J Urol* 1996; **77:** 776–84.
42. Galbraith SM, Duchesne GM. Androgens and prostate cancer: biology, pathology and hormonal therapy. *Eur J Cancer* 1997; **33:** 545–54.
43. Prostate Cancer Trialist's Collaborative Group. Maximum androgen blockade in advanced prostate cancer: an overview of 33 randomised trials with 3283 deaths in 5710 patients. *Lancet* 1995; **346:** 265–9..
44. Ramsay J. Immunotherapy and chemotherapy for carcinoma of the kidney. *Br J Urol* 1992; **70:** 465–8.
◆ 45. McCloskey EV, MacLennan ICM, Drayson MT, *et al.* for the MRC Working Party on Leukaemia in Adults. *Br J Haematol* 1998; **100:** 317–25.
◆ 46. Paterson AHG, Powles TJ, Kanis JA, *et al.* Double-blind controlled trial in patients with bone metastases from breast cancer. *J Clin Oncol* 1993; **11:** 59–65.
47. Diel IJ, Solomayer E-F, Costa SD, *et al.* Reduction in new metastases in breast cancer with adjuvant clodronate treatment. *N Engl J Med* 1998; **339:** 357–63.
48. Coleman RE, Houston S, Purohit OP, *et al.* A randomised phase II study of oral pamidronate for the treatment of bone metastases from breast cancer. *Eur J Cancer* 1998; **34:** 820–4.
● 49. Bloomfield DJ. Should bisphosphonates be part of the standard therapy of patients with multiple myeloma or bone metastases from other cancers? An evidence-based review. *J Clin Oncol* 1998; **16:** 1218–25.
49a. Pavlakis N, Stockler M. Bisphosphonates in breast cancer. *Cochrane Database Syst Rev* 2002; **1:** CD003474.
50. Harrington KD. Impending pathological fractures from metastatic malignancy: evolution and management. *Instr Course Lect* 1986; **35:** 357–81.
51. Siegal T, Siegal T. Surgical decompression of anterior and posterior malignant epidural tumours compressing the spinal cord: a prospective study. *Neurosurgery* 1989; **17:** 424–32.
52. Hardman PDJ, Robb JE, Kerr GR, *et al.* The value of internal fixation and radiotherapy in the management of upper and lower limb bone metastases. *Clin Oncol* 1992; **4:** 244–8.
53. Mithal NP, Needham PR, Hoskin PJ. Retreatment with radiotherapy for painful bone metastases. *Int J Radiat Oncol Biol Phys* 1994; **29:** 1011–14.
● 54. McQuay HJ, Carroll D, Moore RA. Radiotherapy for painful bone metastases: a systematic review. *Clin Oncol* 1997; **9:** 150–4.

22

Control of symptoms other than pain

NIGEL SYKES AND VICTOR PACE

This chapter reviews the management of some key symptoms other than pain that are encountered in cancer patients.

RESPIRATORY SYMPTOMS

Breathlessness

Breathlessness, defined as an uncomfortable awareness of the effort of breathing, is a complaint of nearly half of all cancer patients referred to a specialist palliative care service and almost 70% of those referrals with primary lung cancer.[1] The prevalence and severity rise as disease progresses and, although much can be done to ease the sensation of breathlessness, it remains a difficult symptom to control.[2]

Pathophysiology

It appears that a respiratory effort of more than a third of that of which the individual is capable produces breathlessness.[3] Hence, any impairment of respiratory capacity will tend to bring down the point at which breathlessness will be felt, until ultimately it may be experienced even at rest. Such impairment can arise from:

- reduced ventilation of gas exchange surfaces, e.g. asthmatic bronchoconstriction, bronchial obstruction by tumor;
- reduced area of gas exchange surfaces, e.g. compression or obliteration of alveoli by tumor, pleural effusion or ascites, occupation of alveoli by fluid, bronchiectasis;
- reduced perfusion of gas exchange surfaces, e.g. pulmonary embolism, anemia;
- increased lung stiffness, e.g. pulmonary fibrosis, emphysema, pulmonary edema;
- reduced respiratory muscle capacity, e.g. spinal cord compression, amyotrophic lateral sclerosis, pain.

In addition, there may be unusual respiratory demands, for instance in diabetic ketoacidosis or in thyrotoxicosis.

The symptom of breathlessness results from cortical perception of feedback from central and peripheral receptors and the emotional response that this generates. The receptors involved are:

- the juxta-alveolar J-receptors, which detect mechanical stimuli such as lung stiffness and also chemical stimuli;
- stretch receptors in the bronchial smooth muscle, which signal lung volume;
- irritant receptors in the bronchial epithelium, which in addition to being sensitive to chemical stimuli and being involved in the cough reflex also detect rate of change of lung volume;
- muscle receptors in the intercostal muscles and diaphragm, which detect the force and extent of respiratory muscular contraction;
- chemoreceptors in the carotid body, which detect arterial $P\text{O}_2$, and the aortic body, which are sensitive to $P\text{CO}_2$ via changes in $[\text{H}^+]$.

Clinical findings – history and examination

As with any cancer symptom, reversible causes must be discovered and dealt with. A past history of asthma, chronic obstructive pulmonary disease (COPD), or cardiac disease should prompt a check for signs of bronchoconstriction or pulmonary edema. COPD and lung cancer often coexist, and a trial of bronchodilator therapy should be considered. Anemia, especially a hemoglobin concentration below 8 g/dl, or a recent rapid fall in hemoglobin can be associated with breathlessness, which may then respond to transfusion. There may be a history and signs of a chest infection, and examination may reveal a pulmonary effusion or ascites.

The contribution of the cancer to the breathlessness needs to be assessed together with the possibilities of antineoplastic treatment. Further chemotherapy, say for small-cell lung cancer, may significantly improve breathlessness due to tumor obstruction. Conversely, specific treatments to alter the effects of the tumor, even if the cancer itself cannot be modified, may be valuable, e.g. bronchial stenting.

In making an assessment of breathlessness, the possible emotional component should not be overlooked. Breathing difficulty is frightening, and the fear that results worsens the perception of breathlessness further. Patients may worry that the dyspnea is further damaging their lungs and even that they might die in an episode of breathlessness. The symptom may be worsened by or be the result of hyperventilation; breathlessness that fluctuates rapidly, varies with social situations, is poorly linked with exertion, and is associated with marked fearfulness should suggest the possibility of hyperventilation. Getting the patient to overbreathe can then reproduce the symptoms and demonstrate their origin.

Investigations

A blood count is often useful as anemia is difficult to detect from the bedside, and blood glucose estimation and thyroid function tests may be indicated by history and examination. Chest radiography may be helpful in delineating effusions, confirming cardiac failure, or revealing lymphangitis carcinomatosa, which often presents few signs on auscultation. Often, however, cancer patients are breathless with no specific radiographic signs, and routine chest radiographs are not called for.

Management

The management options for breathlessness which will be described here cover the palliation of the symptom rather than the handling of reversible causes, which form part of general internal medicine.

Supportive care

Aside from medical interventions, there are certain supportive approaches to breathlessness which should underpin other types of management. These include:

- understanding and, if necessary, modifying the patient and his or her family's understanding of breathlessness and its causes and consequences;
- physiotherapy assessment of aids to mobilization, and breathing retraining, to demonstrate how most effective use can be made of remaining lung capacity and how the patient can exert some control over the rate and depth of respiration;
- use of a fan or open window;
- attention to social isolation;
- drawing up a simple, written plan of action in case of exacerbations of breathlessness.

This approach has informed nurse-led breathlessness clinics, which have proved beneficial to cancer patients in a controlled trial.[4**]

Specific management

Airway obstruction by tumor Chest radiography may suggest, and bronchoscopy confirm, that lung capacity is depleted by tumor obstructing a main bronchus. Radiotherapy can be given either by external beam or intraluminally. The external approach carries an increased risk of pulmonary fibrosis if the patient survives long enough. In a large series of breathless patients with bronchial obstruction treated with intraluminal radiotherapy, 60% of patients reported improvement and 46% of pulmonary collapses were alleviated. Retreatment for relapse provided similar rates of symptom relief, but only 7% of pulmonary collapses showed improvement.[5*] As a preliminary to radiotherapy, and for those are too ill to undergo it, a trial of steroids (dexamethasone 12–16 mg/24 h p.o. or s.c.) should be given, as reduction in peritumor edema can provide some symptomatic relief. In patients who are fit enough, an alternative to radiotherapy is the insertion of a metal wire stent, for which rapid symptomatic relief has been claimed.[6*]

Superior vena caval obstruction Superior vena caval obstruction (SVCO) from mediastinal malignancy, most often lung or lymphoma, includes breathlessness among its several distressing symptoms. The usual approach in patients with known advanced cancer is to give steroids (dexamethasone 16 mg *stat* p.o. or s.c.) and make urgent referral for radiotherapy. Good symptom relief was reported in 80% of a series of 125 patients with malignant SVCO.[7*] However, symptom relief is usually delayed 7–10 days, during which time symptoms may initially deteriorate despite steroids. In addition, some patients do not respond to radiotherapy because the superior vena cava is thrombosed. Expandable wire stents have been employed in SVCO; a retrospective comparison of stents and radiotherapy found advantage in the use of stents in the magnitude and speed of onset of symptom relief.[8*] Their use is often combined with that of thrombolytic therapy.[9*] However, breathlessness has been noted to be one of the more resistant symptoms, perhaps because of the effects of disease elsewhere in the lungs.[10]

Lymphangitis carcinomatosa This condition results from malignant infiltration of the lung lymphatic system, characteristically from a breast primary. The supposed etiology of the associated breathlessness is fluid retention in the lungs as a result of inadequate lymphatic drainage. With anecdotal but no research evidence, widespread practice in palliative medicine is to treat lymphangitis with dexamethasone 6–12 mg/24 h orally on the rationale that reduction in edema around the tumor deposits may assist lymphatic function.

Palliative therapies

The quantity of research evidence to support palliative therapies for breathlessness is limited.

Opioids

Despite the widespread caution exercised in the use of opioids in patients with respiratory impairment since it was established that they can cause respiratory depression,[11] these drugs are the cornerstone of palliation of breathlessness in patients with advanced cancer. The mechanism of their effectiveness in relief of breathlessness is not completely clear but involves a reduction in the sensitivity of the respiratory center and of the awareness of breathing, and on occasion an element of sedation and an easing of cardiac failure through a reduction in afterload.

Walsh[12] showed that morphine could safely be used for analgesia in patients with poor lung function without precipitating hypercapnia as long as the dose was proportionate to the level of pain. A small placebo-controlled single-dose trial of subcutaneous morphine in cancer patients already receiving opioids for pain and on continuous oxygen found a reduction in breathlessness and a marked patient preference for morphine over placebo (9 out of 10).[13**] An earlier uncontrolled trial had found a similar result, but noted that the duration of relief of breathlessness was less than that of pain, beginning to diminish after 75 min and back to baseline after 2.5 h.[14*] An uncontrolled trial of oral morphine for breathlessness differed in that most of the patients were opioid naive: 5 out of 18 patients withdrew because of drowsiness or dizziness, and only one reported definite improvement.[15*] The starting dose used was 20 mg morphine per day.

Thus, although morphine reduces breathlessness, it is less efficient in doing so than in relieving pain and with an increased likelihood of adverse effects. As with pain, the preference is to use morphine orally, and for the many patients who are already taking morphine for pain an increase of 25–50% in the analgesic dose is appropriate for persisting breathlessness. For those not currently taking morphine, the starting dose should be low and the titration gentle. Morphine solution 2.5 mg is suggested. Initially some will require this only on a p.r.n. basis, with a move to regular administration as the disease progresses. If breathlessness improves but morphine is poorly tolerated, an alternative opioid can be tried, as with pain. However, available preparations in some cases do not allow the low starting doses advisable, e.g. phenazocine, hydromorphone. Methadone solution offers flexibility of dosing, but the prolonged half-life of this drug means that it should be administered on an as required basis for at least a week after initiation.

Anxiolytics

Given the close association between breathlessness and anxiety, it is unsurprising that anxiolytics have found a role in its management. It is less clear whether they have any other mechanism of action, in particular through the muscle relaxant properties of the benzodiazepines. Diazepam has not been studied in cancer-associated breathlessness, but the results from patients with COPD are predominantly negative.[16**] However, clinical experience indicates that daily doses much lower than the 25 mg used in COPD can improve breathlessness in cancer patients. Often 2–5 mg t.i.d. have a worthwhile effect even in the context of considerable doses of morphine; because of the long half-life of diazepam this level of dose given only at night may eventually be sufficient. Furthermore, sublingual lorazepam (0.5–1.0 mg) has proved helpful for acute dyspneic episodes, and midazolam by subcutaneous infusion (initially 10–30 mg/24 h) is valuable in the control of breathlessness in the terminal phase.

There is limited evidence that phenothiazines can help breathlessness: promethazine was better than placebo in COPD[16] and the combination of chlorpromazine and morphine reduced breathlessness caused by extensive lung metastases.[17*] If a phenothiazine is required for subcutaneous infusion, levomepromazine is better tolerated than chlorpromazine.

Some dyspneic patients find either diazepam or chlorpromazine too sedating. An alternative that may be helpful is buspirone. This nonbenzodiazepine serotonin agonist has been found both to reduce breathlessness and to stimulate ventilation in subjects with nonmalignant lung disease.[18*] Its anxiolytic action may have a latency of onset of 7–10 days.

Oxygen

Oxygen is often the first recourse of medical staff for breathless patients. Once initiated, many patients are understandably reluctant to accept its withdrawal despite the unsightliness of the mask or nasal cannulae and the restrictions the equipment places on their freedom of movement. In a small series of severely hypoxic cancer patients, nearly all preferred oxygen to air,[19*] but in a somewhat larger series of cancer patients, of whom few were hypoxic, preferences were almost evenly divided, with those choosing oxygen not necessarily being the individuals who were hypoxic.[20**] Although oxygen should never be withheld from a patient who has previously found it useful or one who is acutely breathless and markedly hypoxic, it is reasonable to try alternative approaches to the palliation of breathlessness before commencing it. Even desaturation on pulse oximetry is a poor guide to which patients will benefit, and most palliative care physicians have seen patients who have ceased to depend on oxygen once given appropriate general support and the use of morphine and an anxiolytic.

Nebulized drugs

Other than bronchodilators in instances of reversible airways obstruction, there is little evidence that nebulized drugs are useful for breathlessness. In particular, nebulized lidocaine (lignocaine) is ineffective for breathlessness, although it may have a place in the control of severe cough.[21]* Although several case series claim benefit, the only controlled trial of nebulized morphine could not show a significant advantage over saline. Any improvement in breathlessness peaked after an hour, suggesting an effect from systemic absorption of morphine rather than locally.[22]** Nebulized morphine may be helpful to the individual patient, but there is no indication for its routine use.

Retention of secretions

Breathlessness at the end of life is often complicated by retained secretions, which produce a rattling sound that is distressing to relatives even if not to patients themselves. As a component of the retained fluid is often exudate from an infected chest, it is not always possible to eradicate the problem. However, addition of an anticholinergic drug to an opioid and an anxiolytic in a subcutaneous infusion can help. Hyoscine hydrobromide (0.8–2.4 mg/24 h) has been used most frequently and is usually somewhat sedative, although it can also produce paradoxical excitation. This is less likely with hyoscine butylbromide (60–200 mg/24 h) or glycopyrronium bromide (0.4–1.2 mg/24 h), as these drugs cross the blood–brain barrier less readily.

Key points

- Assess reversible causes of breathlessness and treat.
- Assess emotional contribution.
- Remember general principles of support, including good communication of information that is wanted, involvement of physiotherapy, and assistance in relaxation.
- If anxiety is prominent, commence palliation with diazepam.
- If anxiety is not prominent, commence palliation with oral morphine.
- Use morphine 2.5 mg either p.r.n. or 4-hourly initially, or an increase of 25–50% in the analgesic dose.
- Lorazepam 0.5–1.0 mg sublingually can be used for acute breathlessness.
- Breathlessness in the terminal stages can be managed by subcutaneous infusion of an opioid and midazolam, with the addition of hyoscine or glycopyrronium if there are retained secretions.
- Oxygen should be used as an adjunct to palliation, not its mainstay.

Cough

Cough may be voluntary or a reflex response to mechanical and chemical receptors in the airways, mediated via the cough center in the medulla and the phrenic, intercostal, and inferior laryngeal nerves.

Clinical findings – history and examination

In the context of a known diagnosis of cancer, the principal distinction to be made in the assessment of a complaint of cough is between a cough that is productive and one that is nonproductive. A cough that is of recent onset or exacerbation and is productive of yellow or green sputum accompanies lower respiratory tract infection. A dry, irritating cough suggests the stimulation of airways receptors by tumor. This may result not only from bronchial carcinomas but also from cancer affecting the larynx. Cough occurring principally at night may indicate asthma or cardiac failure, and in the latter case is usually associated with orthopnea.

Other than clarifying one of the general medical causes for cough, the value of investigations is limited unless the onset of cough suggests tumor recurrence. Sputum culture may guide antibiotic treatment of a chest infection, but can also reveal relapse of tuberculosis in a patient immunodeficient because of cancer.

Treatment

Palliative treatment of a dry cough is by suppression and for a productive cough aims to facilitate the expectoration of sputum and, if possible, reduce its production. The exception is at the very end of life, when it becomes appropriate to suppress even a productive cough.

Most cough suppressants are opioids, and there is evidence for a dose-related cough-inhibitory action of codeine, probably mediated via μ_2-receptors.[23] However, if morphine is already being taken for pain, it is more logical to titrate the dose further for troublesome cough rather than add a second opioid. Some patients find helpful the addition of a demulcent preparation such as simple linctus BP. If no opioid analgesia is in use, codeine, diamorphine, and methadone are all available as linctuses. The dose required to suppress cough may be less than that needed for analgesia, but nonetheless about 20% of cancer patients receiving dihydrocodeine for cough report drowsiness.[24] If sedation or constipation is a problem, it may be worthwhile using a drug such as pholcodine or dextromethorphan, which, although related to the opioids, act not via opioid receptors but on an alternative central mechanism.

Proprietary cough medicines often contain, as well as an opioid, other drugs such as antihistamines and low doses of emetic agents. Apart from sedation, any mode of antitussive action of antihistamines is unknown, and there is no evidence to support the claim that subemetic doses of drugs such as squill enhance expectoration.

Unless the patient has a favorite remedy, these combinations are best avoided.

There is some evidence that carbocisteine and methyl cisteine reduce the viscosity of saliva, but neither is available on National Health Service (NHS) prescription in the UK. Inhalation of steam, with or without addition of aromatic substances, or nebulized saline can be helpful in aiding expectoration of sputum. A trial of a bronchodilator may also be worthwhile in case reversible airways obstruction is exacerbating sputum retention.

Hemoptysis

The expectoration of blood is experienced as a particularly alarming symptom. Hemoptysis occurs in about 70% of lung cancers, usually through involvement of the bronchial arteries. Occasionally it is an overwhelming terminal event, particularly in association with cavitating squamous carcinomas of the bronchus.[25] Massive hemoptysis (over 500 ml/24 h) mostly causes death through asphyxia rather than blood loss. However, in the absence of lung cancer there are many nonmalignant reasons for coughing up blood and, indeed, up to 40% of cases remain undiagnosed. Upper or lower respiratory tract infections are by far the commonest causes, followed by bronchiectasis and tuberculosis.[26]

Clinical findings – history and examination

The principal fact to be established is that the blood actually originates in the lungs, rather than the stomach, mouth, or nose. Hemoptysis is generally bright red, frothy, or mixed with sputum. Blood from a gastric origin is dark and will be acidic on testing. The volume of blood is not necessarily helpful in diagnosis, but brief rather than prolonged episodes suggest a benign origin. A history of possible inhalation of a foreign body should be sought.

Acute onset of cough, pyrexia, and chest pain indicates lower respiratory tract infection or pulmonary embolism. Recurrent chest infections may originate from bronchiectasis, chronic bronchitis, or malignancy.

A key investigation is the chest radiograph with lateral view, for evidence of tumor, abscess, or tuberculosis. Radiological evidence of pneumonia may also indicate cancer, especially in an older person with hemoptysis extending longer than a week, and sputum should be sent for cytological and microbiological analysis. Bronchoscopy is advised in all those with recurrent hemoptysis and an abnormal chest radiograph, and in smokers even if they have a normal radiograph.

Treatment

Cancer-related hemoptysis responds well to radiotherapy, and this must be the treatment of choice. A review of 330 patients with lung cancer receiving radiotherapy found an 83% response rate for hemoptysis.[27*] Two fractions appear to be as effective as longer treatments.[28**] If radiotherapy is not available, there is clinical experience of improvement in hemoptysis following use of tranexamic acid (1 g t.i.d to 1.5 g q.i.d.), which is an antifibrinolytic, or the hemostatic agent ethamsylate (500 mg q.i.d.).[29*] A potential problem is that clots forming as a result of using these drugs may be unusually hard and, if they break loose, can in consequence be troublesome to expectorate.

GASTROINTESTINAL PROBLEMS

Oral problems

Up to 89% of hospice patients suffer from oral problems.[30] Often ignored, "minor" problems can hold the key to more major ones. Thus, a dry mouth easily becomes infected; it increases the likelihood of dental caries; the loss of taste can lead to anorexia; it makes tablets hard to swallow, leading to poor compliance; and it interferes with communication. Meticulous attention to detail makes all the difference.

Dry mouth

The salivary glands produce 1.0–1.5 l of saliva a day. Parotid and submandibular saliva is more serous, that from sublingual and minor salivary gland more mucous. Parasympathetic stimulation makes saliva more watery, while sympathetic stimulation slows down flow, reduces its amount, and increases the organic content. Vasoactive intestinal peptide (VIP) appears to play an important role in saliva regulation. Aldosterone has a similar effect on saliva to that on the kidneys.[31]

A dry mouth is a very common complaint in terminally ill patients (Table 22.1). Treatment is based on good oral hygiene, starting with meticulous mouthcare, up to 2-hourly in very weak patients. Fluid is encouraged, and medication reviewed. Having something in the mouth, for example fruit drops, stimulates salivary flow. Sucking pineapple chunks is said to increase moisture and clean up furring, because fresh pineapple contains the enzyme ananase.[34] Various artificial salivas are available, to be sprayed up to several times an hour underneath the tongue and swished in the mouth for a few seconds. Pilocarpine 5 mg t.i.d.,[35**] and possibly anethole-trithione, increase salivary flow, although this may take weeks.

Infections

Candidiasis is present in up to 89% of patients with terminal illness.[36] Risk factors for candidiasis include:

- elderly patient;
- dentures;
- dry mouth;

Table 22.1 *Common causes of dry mouth in palliative care*[32]

Reduced salivary secretion
Radiotherapy to head and neck
Drugs:[33] anticholinergics, tricyclic antidepressants, antihistamines, beta-blockers, diuretics, morphine
Tumor
Autoimmune disorders
Buccal mucosal damage
Cancer
Chemotherapy
Infection, e.g. herpes, *Candida*
Dehydration
Psychological
Depression
Anxiety

- malnutrition;
- diabetes;
- corticosteroids;
- antibiotics;
- head and neck radiotherapy;
- human immunodeficiency virus (HIV) infection.

Several species of *Candida* or other fungi may be involved; no antifungal is effective against all species.[37] *Candida* can present as pseudomembranous stomatitis (white plaques, easily scraped off, leaving an erythematous background) or as reddened smooth mucosa – chronic atrophic candidiasis; angular cheilitis may be present. Esophageal candidiasis produces pain on swallowing and is confirmed by gastroscopy or by barium swallow showing esophageal plaques. Nystatin often clears up oral infection, but its activity is impaired by chlorhexidine, which is present in many mouthwashes.[37] Its effectiveness in esophageal candidiasis or for prophylaxis in immunosuppressed patients has been questioned.[37] Fluconazole and itraconazole are easy to use, safe alternatives although drug interactions may be important, especially with itraconazole. Fluconazole has good oral bioavailability, so is very useful against esophageal or systemic *Candida*.[38] Ketoconazole can be hepatotoxic, is impaired by low gastric acid (e.g. H_2-blockers), and interacts with many medications. Amphotericin lozenges appear less effective. As Finlay[39] points out, candidal infection may be the result rather than the cause of mouth problems, and general oral hygiene in the terminally ill may be more important than antifungal medication.

Herpetic infections produce excruciatingly painful vesicles and often make the patient systemically unwell. Extension into the esophagus produces much more severe pain on swallowing than thrush does. Acyclovir, started early, aborts such infections.

Bacterial infections are frequently mixed, as xerostomia and immunosuppression cause an increase in Gram-negative flora. Treatment is with antibiotics and scrupulous oral hygiene. Severely dehydrated, ill patients can develop *infective parotitis* as a terminal event. Pus can be seen issuing from the parotid duct near the second upper molar tooth. Systemic antibiotics may be indicated, although death is usually very near and symptomatic measures are best.

Other oral problems

Mucositis may be due to chemotherapy (5-fluorouracil, methotrexate) or radiotherapy to the head and neck. It is time limited and is reduced by benzydamine oral rinse[40]** or sucralfate.[41]* Taste alterations are common and arise from a multitude of causes, dry mouth, chemotherapy, infection, and medication being some of the commoner ones. Treatment is directed at the underlying cause.

Dysphagia

Etiology

In one series of 800 palliative care patients dysphagia affected 12% of individuals.[42] Some causes of dysphagia in cancer patients include:

- mucositis
  - postradiotherapy/chemotherapy: mouth or esophagus
  - common oral problems: sepsis, dry mouth;
- masses in the lumen
  - head and neck tumors
  - carcinomas of esophagus or esophagogastric junction
  - food bolus blocking esophageal stent;
- masses in the wall
  - esophageal neoplasms
  - postradiotherapy or anastomotic strictures;
- extrinsic masses
  - mediastinal tumors
  - mediastinal lymphadenopathy;
- neurological problems
  - cranial nerve palsies (cerebral/head and neck tumors)
  - paraneoplastic syndromes: neuropathies, myopathies, e.g. Lambert–Eaton syndrome[43]
  - perineural tumor spread into the vagus nerve or sympathetic trunk.[44]

Clinical findings

Neurogenic dysphagia involves liquids initially and only later solids, whereas mechanical obstruction affects solids first. Mechanical obstruction often involves the esophageal phase; it may feel as if a lump of food refuses to go down on swallowing, or swallowing may be painful. Neurological problems are more likely to disturb the oropharyngeal phase of deglutition.[45] Patients can complain of difficulty or pain on chewing, aspiration, drooling, nasal regurgitation, and late regurgitation of undigested food.[45] Simple, easily remedied problems such as a dry mouth or insufficient mastication in edentulous patients can also cause dysphagia. Dentures may no longer fit as illness causes weight loss, but they can easily be relined by a dentist.

Investigation

Investigation by barium swallow, esophagogastroscopy for structural disorders and manometry, and video studies for neuromuscular disorders may be appropriate. An assessment by a skilled speech therapist can be invaluable both in elucidating pathology and in suggesting therapy.[46]

Management

Simple measures are important. Xerostomia must be relieved and teeth reviewed. Sauces and gravies help lubricate dry food. Food may need to be liquidized for patients with mechanical dysphagia. The underlying disease requires treatment. Benign strictures can be dilated, tumors intubated or lasered. Patients with esophageal tubes must masticate their food thoroughly and take fizzy drinks to wash away debris. Blocked tubes can indicate displacement, a food bolus wedged in the lumen that requires endoscopic removal, or tumor overgrowth, which is sometimes amenable to laser or reintubation.

In patients with neurogenic dysphagia, thickeners will help if thin liquids cause aspiration and drool from the mouth easily. Selected patients with head and neck problems do well with appropriate orthodontic prostheses and even resuspension surgery. Some patients after surgery or radiotherapy to the head and neck have a temporary loss of sensation in the mouth, which results in uncoordinated swallowing; very cold or warm food may help re-educate the swallowing mechanism.[47] In unilateral pharyngeal palsy, turning the head to the paralyzed side forces food to go through the sound side. The family needs to be re-educated with the patient.

Nausea and vomiting

In a series of 1,635 patients in a pain clinic, 40% suffered from nausea or vomiting.[48] Rational and effective therapy depends on a correct assessment of the gross anatomical and physiological disturbances and an appreciation of the neurotransmitters involved.

Clinical findings

Antiemetics are unhelpful in regurgitation (e.g. esophageal tumor), which is often mistaken for vomiting. A good history should differentiate easily between the two but also give vital clues to the etiology of vomiting.

- Gastric outlet obstruction tends, at least at first, to produce large-volume vomits, free of bile if the obstruction is complete, and episodes usually occur suddenly without preceding nausea (the only other common cause of this is vomiting from raised intracranial pressure). The patient may complain of hiccups and heartburn, and will often find undigested food in the vomit from meals taken more than 6 h previously.
- Squashed stomach syndrome, due to impaired gastric filling from extrinsic pressure, or from the rigid small stomach produced by linitis plastica, produces a similar picture; however, vomits are frequent and small volume as the stomach cannot fill to any appreciable extent.
- Intestinal obstruction is discussed in more detail below.
- Radiotherapy-induced nausea and vomiting can be intense and last for a number of days.
- Recent chemotherapy, especially with highly emetogenic agents (cisplatin, dacarbazine, high-dose cyclophosphamide), is a well-known cause.
- Learned responses play an important role in anticipatory nausea and vomiting in patients who are having cytotoxics, such that even meeting persons associated with administration of treatment can bring on an attack.
- A detailed drug and alcohol history is essential, both because drugs may cause nausea and vomiting (Table 22.2) and to avoid retrying treatment that has already failed.

Management

Precipitating causes such as strong smells, movement, and anxiety should be addressed. Concurrent medication needs reviewing. Most patients will require one or more antiemetics.

During vomiting, a complex coordinated series of events takes place, with autonomic changes, retching, and hypersalivation, followed by abdominal and diaphragmatic muscle contraction simultaneously with relaxation of sphincters and closure of the epiglottis and nasopharynx as the vomit is expelled. These actions are coordinated by the vomiting center (whose existence as a discrete structure is disputed) in the medulla. The main neurotransmitters at the vomiting center are shown in Fig. 22.1. Antiemetics that block these receptors tend to be generally good all-round agents and are often useful when the cause of vomiting is unclear. They include hyoscine, antihistamines such as cyclizine[49]* and levomepromazine[50]* (Table 22.3). Levomepromazine, a phenothiazine, is a powerful antiemetic at much lower doses than previously thought, and 6.25–25 mg orally (or

Table 22.2 *Common causes of nausea and vomiting in advanced cancer*

Gastrointestinal
Gastritis (alcohol, nonsteroidal anti-inflammatory drugs)
Gastric outlet obstruction (tumor, fibrosis, functional)
Slow gastric emptying (autonomic gastropathy, functional, drugs)
Squashed stomach syndrome (hepatomegaly, ascites, linitis plastica)
Intestinal obstruction
Constipation
Drugs
Opioids
Digoxin
Theophyllines
Cytotoxics
Erythromycin
Metabolic
Renal failure
Hypercalcemia
Hyponatremia
Neurological
Raised intracranial pressure
Posterior fossa tumors
Meningeal infiltration
Skull metastases
Emotional
Anxiety
Anticipatory vomiting with chemotherapy
Other
Severe uncontrolled pain
Colic of any origin
Radiotherapy: especially to L1 region, high-dose brain radiotherapy, upper hemibody radiation
Cough, thick sputum, postnasal drip

half the oral doses subcutaneously) usually provides very satisfactory control of nausea and vomiting without the limiting side-effects of sedation and hypotension associated with higher doses.[51]

Most emetogenic chemical changes are detected by chemoreceptor trigger zones (CTZ), the main one being in the area postrema in the floor of the fourth ventricle, outside the blood–brain barrier. Suitable antiemetics here are phenothiazines (D_2 antagonists),[52] ondansetron, and other 5-HT_3 antagonists,[52a]*** and to a lesser extent metoclopramide or domperidone (through their D_2 antagonist activity). These are also the most useful agents for radiotherapy-induced sickness. Cortical sickness, for example from anxiety, responds to benzodiazepines or cannabinoids but above all to explanation, calm, and fostering a feeling of safety.

The other main pathway feeding into the vomiting center is via the vagus from the gastrointestinal tract, relaying stretch impulses and also responses from 5-HT_3 receptors to local serotonin release. Ondansetron's principal action is its antagonism of these 5-HT_3 effects.

Metoclopramide is useful in gastric stasis, some cases of incomplete gastric outlet obstruction, or functional bowel obstructions. Domperidone is similarly effective rectally,[53] but its poor oral bioavailability (15%)[54] somewhat limits its usefulness by this route. In the denervated gut (surgical denervation,[55] diabetic gastroparesis,[56] intestinal pseudo-obstruction[57]) erythromycin can work where other prokinetics have failed; it exerts a widespread action as a motilin agonist, which appears to be independent of neural input, but side-effects mean that a significant proportion of patients cannot tolerate it.[58] Most prokinetics, however, work ultimately through cholinergic pathways.

With newer antiemetics under development, such as neurokinin-1 antagonists, the possibilities of control of nausea and vomiting may be significantly extended.

Hypercalcemia

Hypercalcemia is a common cause of nausea and vomiting in late-stage cancer. It occurs in 8.5% of hospice patients.[59] It is a marker of poor prognosis, with about 80% of affected patients dying within a year.[60] Hypercalcemia occurs most commonly in patients with squamous cell carcinomas, breast cancer, and myeloma (40–50% at some time during their illness[61]).

Hypercalcemia is usually due to production of parathyroid hormone-related peptide (PTHrP) by the tumor, which mobilizes calcium from bone, although other mechanisms occur.[62] High PTHrP levels imply a worse prognosis and poorer response to treatment.[63]

Symptoms include nausea and vomiting, constipation, polyuria, thirst, lethargy, and confusion. Later the patient becomes unconscious; seizures may occur and eventually death.

Who to treat[64] (but assess individual clinical state)

In patients in whom corrected calcium levels are below 3.0 mmol/l, oral rehydration, with or without oral phosphates (cause nausea and diarrhea), may be sufficient. In patients in whom corrected calcium levels are over 3.0 mmol/l, dehydration, marked nausea or vomiting, or pronounced neurological symptoms require inpatient intravenous treatment.

A calcium level above 3.5 mmol/l carries an appreciably increased risk of cardiac arrest and should be treated even if the patient is asymptomatic.

In patients on digoxin treatment should be initiated at lower calcium levels, as hypercalcemia predisposes to toxicity.

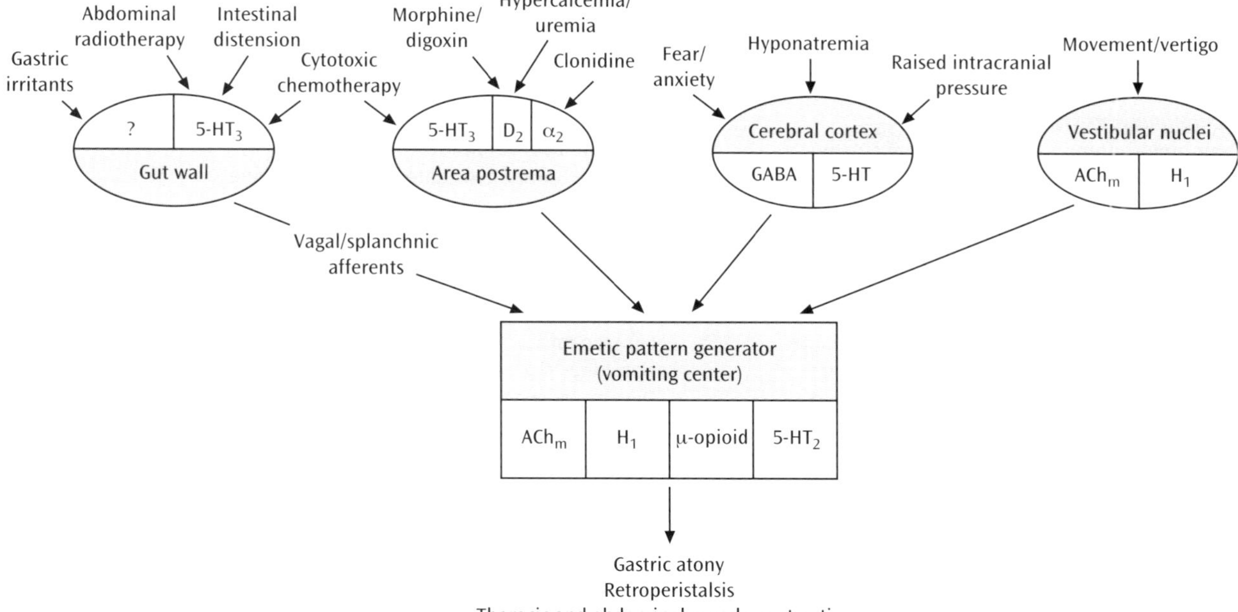

Figure 22.1 *Receptors involved in nausea and vomiting. (Reproduced with permission from Twycross R, Wilcock A, Thorp S.* Palliative Care Formulary. *Oxford: Radcliffe Medical Press.)*

Management

Diuretics and vitamin D and calcium supplements should be withdrawn if at all possible. Rehydrate the patient then give intravenous bisphosphonate (disodium pamidronate or clodronate). These measure should produce a clinical response in about 2 days, but it takes up to 2 weeks for calcium levels to return to normal.[65]**

The response rate to bisphosphonate can be up to 70–100%;[65,66] high levels of PTHrP predict resistance, but a test is rarely available. Gallium nitrate is associated with a response rate of 80% but requires infusion over 5 days and is nephrotoxic.

In resistant patients, try higher bisphosphonate doses or frequent infusion,[67] or plicamycin, a cytotoxic with a risk of marrow depression (no longer licensed in the UK).

In patients with dangerously high calcium levels, administration of calcitonin subcutaneously twice a day lowers the levels within hours, though not to normal; the effect is temporary unless treatment with longer acting drugs follows.[64]

Diuresis should *not* be used to treat hypercalcemia except under intensive care conditions. Diuresis worsens the dehydration caused by the vomiting and polyuria from high calcium levels and exacerbates nephrotoxicity due to hypercalcemia.

Intestinal obstruction in advanced cancer

Incidence

It is difficult to assess the incidence of bowel obstruction in patients with advanced cancer. Studies involve highly selected patients at selected times of their illness. Reported figures vary from 2.5% in home care patients[68] to 51% in an autopsy study of ovarian carcinoma.[69]

Pathophysiology

In advanced cancer the cause of bowel obstruction can be:[70]

- intraluminal, e.g. large bowel tumor;
- intramural, e.g. tumor spreading in the muscular layers can cause "intestinal linitis plastica," with a rigid, functionless bowel;
- extramural, e.g. mesenteric and omental masses and adhesions compress and kink the bowel;
- motility disorders – in addition to paralytic ileus (uncommon in this situation), patients can be affected by pseudo-obstruction due to infiltration of bowel muscle, mesentery, or nerve plexuses supplying the bowel, or as part of a paraneoplastic syndrome.

Other factors can also contribute, e.g. fecal impaction, change of bowel flora.

Clinical features

The classical features of bowel obstruction are colicky abdominal pain, vomiting becoming progressively feculent, abdominal distension depending on the level of obstruction, and absolute constipation. However, these may be altered in advanced cancer. Onset is often insidious, the course may be intermittent, bowel distension may be absent in extensive bowel infiltration, and diarrhea is not uncommon in incomplete obstruction. A con-

Table 22.3 *Classification of drugs used to control nausea and vomiting. (Reproduced with permission from Twycross R, Wilcock A, Thorp S.* Palliative Care Formulary. *Oxford: Radcliffe Medical Press.)*

Putative site of action	Class	Example
Central nervous system		
Vomiting center	Antimuscarinic	Hyoscine hydrobromide
	Antihistaminic, antimuscarinic[a]	Cyclizine, dimenhydrinate, prochlorperazine
	5-HT_2-receptor antagonist	Levomepromazine
Area postrema	D_2-receptor antagonist	Haloperidol, prochlorperazine, metoclopropamide, domperidone
	5-HT_3-receptor antagonist	Granisetron, ondansetron, tropisetron
Cerebral cortex	Benzodiazepine	Lorazepam
	Cannabinoid	Nabilone
	Corticosteroid	Dexamethasone
Gastrointestinal tract		
Prokinetic	5-HT_4-receptor agonist	Metoclopramide, cisapride
	D_2-receptor antagonist	Metoclopramide, domperidone
	Antimuscarinic	Hyoscine butylbromide, glycopyrrolate
	Somatostatin analog	Octreotide, vapreotide
Vagal 5-HT_3-receptor blockage	5-HT_3-receptor antagonist	Granisetron, ondansetron, tropisetron
Anti-inflammatory	Corticosteroid	Dexamethasone

a. The antihistamines and phenothiazines both have H_1-receptor antagonistic and antimuscarinic properties.

stant background abdominal pain is usually present in addition to the colic due to extensive tumor.

Management

Surgery needs to be considered in all cases. In about a third of patients, even those with advanced disease, obstruction has a benign cause.[71] In most cases, surgery is the only definitive treatment anyway. However, this has to be balanced against an overall mortality rate for operation for acute bowel obstruction of 20% in advanced cancer, rising to 69% in patients aged over 70 and 72% in the malnourished.[72] Thus, contraindications to surgical management include:

- obstruction at multiple sites (e.g. found at previous laparotomy);
- patient too ill for surgery;
- patient refusal.

"Drip and suck," indispensable in the short term as preparation for surgery, rarely leads to sustained symptom relief (Baines,[70] quoting figures of 0–14% from various authors). Symptoms are much better managed with a combination of drugs, usually given through a syringe driver:[73]

1 Diamorphine is given for the continuous element of the pain (prospective cohort and retrospective uncontrolled studies).
2 An antispasmodic, e.g. hyoscine butylbromide (Buscopan), is added for colic, starting at around 60 mg and titrating upwards (doses as high as 380 mg have been given).[74] Some preliminary data suggest that hyoscine butylbromide also lessens secretions in intestinal obstruction.[75]
3 Centrally acting antiemetics are used in most patients. Haloperidol 5–15 mg, cyclazine 100–150 mg, or methotrimeprazine, usually at 6.25–25 mg/24 h, are the usual doses, though one can go much higher. Metoclopramide was traditionally said to be contraindicated as it could worsen colic,[73] but it has been used at 60–240 mg/24 h and has a place in the treatment of incomplete proximal obstructions. Evidence for antiemetic effectiveness is based on some prospective cohort, but mostly retrospective, uncontrolled studies.
4 Octreotide, a long-acting analog of somatostatin, produces a marked reduction in the volume of nasogastric aspirate and in frequency of vomiting and nausea in patients with malignant bowel obstruction.[76*]
5 Steroids have been used to reduce obstruction through their anti-inflammatory effects. However, studies have been small, authors admitting to difficulty in extrapolating results,[77] and a meta-analysis, though suggesting improvement, showed no statistical significance at the 95% confidence level.[76***]
6 Stool softeners (e.g. magnesium hydroxide and liquid paraffin emulsion) are given for constipation, but bowel stimulants (e.g. senna, bisacodyl) are avoided as they can worsen colic. Occasionally antidiarrheal drugs are needed instead.
7 Patients are allowed to choose their own diet – most will opt for small, low-residue, often mainly fluid meals. Subcutaneous infusion of fluid, and less commonly the more problematic intravenous route, are

occasionally needed in patients who become dehydrated to the point they are symptomatic of it.

The symptoms of high obstructions (especially gastric outlet obstruction) are much more difficult to control than those of low obstructions. Venting percutaneous gastrostomies have been used in this context, though most trials are unsatisfactory.[76]

Results

Baines[70] quotes figures of 70–90% of patients becoming pain free with this regimen; nausea is often controlled but vomiting may be reduced to once or twice a day rather than totally abolished as this can at times only be done at the cost of severe drug adverse effects. Prognosis of up to 7 months has been reported with this regimen, though most patients die within a few weeks.

Constipation

Constipation is a complaint of about 10% of the general population and 50% of patients with cancer admitted to palliative care units. However, 63% of such patients require laxatives if they are not taking opioid analgesics and 87% if they are.[78] Constipation is thus a common symptom in cancer, especially if potent analgesia is required, and has been reported as causing more distress than pain in a population with advanced disease.

Pathophysiology

The normal gut transit time is 48–72 h in a Western population. Most of this time is spent in the colon. On a small number of occasions each day, peristaltic actions occur, which move colonic contents over considerable distances, and are associated with borborygmi and, sometimes, an urge to defecate. These mass movements are stimulated by gastric emptying and by physical activity, and in consequence the reduced food and fluid intake, and the physical debility, resulting from cancer are associated with constipation. In addition, drugs with anticholinergic effects, iron, cytotoxic chemotherapy agents such as vincristine, and opioid analgesics add to the problem.

Opioids have a range of effects which are likely to exacerbate constipation markedly, as follows:

- contraction of intestinal sphincters;
- reduction in frequency of peristaltic mass movements;
- reduction in net water secretion by gut mucosa;
- impairment of rectal sensation.

Clinical findings

The most important confusions to avoid in the assessment of constipation are malignant intestinal obstruction and spurious diarrhea secondary to impaction. As ever, the first step is a careful history, detailing the time of onset of the altered bowel habit, the stool frequency and extent of straining at defecation, and, if there is a complaint of loose motions or fecal leakage, whether this succeeded a period of constipation. Known abdominal malignancy increases the risk of obstruction.

Abdominal examination seeks to distinguish fecal masses in the line of the colon from tumor masses, which may be associated with obstruction. Rectal examination should reveal 90% of instances of fecal impaction.

Investigations

Investigations are rarely needed, but a plain abdominal radiograph may help distinguish obstruction from constipation. Constipation may precipitate vomiting, but both may be associated with hypercalcemia, which should not be overlooked.

Management

Good general symptom control, with encouragement of fluid intake and as high a dietary fiber content as is palatable, is likely to reduce the extent of constipation, although evidence is lacking. The constipating action of drugs should be anticipated and a laxative made available before the problem becomes established.

At least in advanced cancer, most patients will require a laxative. Most British patients prefer oral administration to enemas and suppositories. Clinically it is helpful to think of laxative agents as predominantly stool softening or predominantly gut peristalsis stimulating. Pharmacologically, the distinction is unsafe as any softening agent will increase the stool's bulk and so stretch the gut wall to cause reflex contraction, while a stimulant will reduce transit time and hence the time available for water absorption, so the stool will be softer.

However, there is evidence that in a model of constipation in human volunteers the combination of stimulant and softening drugs minimizes both medication burden and adverse effects compared with either class of agent used alone.[79**] This is one therapeutic area where the use of combination preparations can be valid. It is vital that the laxative dose is titrated adequately against the clinical response. All too often opioid-related constipation is treated ineffectively with a single agent in a dose that is too small.

The commonly used laxatives are tabulated below. Bulking agents, e.g. methyl cellulose, ispaghula, are inadvisable in cancer patients: they are relatively weak laxatives and also require to be taken with a significant volume of water, which can be intolerable to sicker patients. Reduction in the volume of water risks the formation of a viscous mass in the gut lumen, which can then precipitate or complete an obstruction.

Rectal laxatives may be needed for the clearance of fecal impaction, a sign that the oral laxative regimen requires review, or in the management of paraplegic patients who lack rectal sensation and anal sphincter tone. An alternative for the clearance of impaction is oral polyethylene glycol electrolyte solution, as long as the patient can cope with the volumes involved.[80*]

Commonly used laxatives and their method of action are listed in Table 22.4.

Key points

- Anticipate constipation, especially with opioids, and make a laxative available.
- Most patients receiving opioids will require a combination of stimulant and softening laxatives.
- Careful titration of laxative doses will minimize the need for rectal interventions.

Diarrhea

Diarrhea is much less common than constipation in cancer care, occurring in around 10% of admissions for palliative care.

Pathophysiology

The bowel receives about 9 l of fluid daily, 2 l from oral intake and the remainder from gastric, biliary, pancreatic, and intestinal secretions. All but some 150 ml of this total is reabsorbed. The difference between constipation and diarrhea amounts to 100 ml or so of water per day, indicating a remarkably fine control of fluid balance across the gut wall. This control is exercised via the myenteric neural plexus but is also subject to influence by luminal factors such as fatty acids and bile salts and also drugs such as opioids and some cytotoxic chemotherapy agents.[81]

Clinical findings

Although diarrhea is frequent evacuation of loose stool, patients may use the word to describe other situations such as an increase in frequency of any kind of stool, a single relatively loose bowel action per day, or fecal leakage or incontinence, any of which might represent constipation rather than true diarrhea. Therefore, a complaint of diarrhea must be elucidated by a careful history, including an account of drugs such as laxatives and elixir preparations, which might contain osmotically active sugars, and recent chemotherapy or radiotherapy. Abdominal and rectal examinations should also be performed, in order to exclude fecal impaction or loss of sphincter tone.

Investigations

In this patient group, investigations of diarrhea are not usually warranted because the cause emerges through history or examination, or because any infective cause is likely to be short-lived and self-limiting. However, if the patient is toxic or the diarrhea is continuing beyond about 3 days' duration, stool samples should be taken and cultured for pathogens such as *Clostridium difficile, Escherichia coli, Salmonella,* or *Shigella.* Prolonged diarrhea should also prompt monitoring and correction of fluid and electrolyte balance.

Management

The most common cause of diarrhea in palliative medicine is an excessive laxative dose.[82] However, an unduly long suspension of laxative therapy results in a pattern of alternating constipation and diarrhea; it is usually adequate to suspend the laxatives for 24 h and then resume a dose step down.

Specific therapies exist for certain causes of diarrhea (Table 22.5).

Most treatment for diarrhea is symptomatic. Available drugs are either absorbent or adsorbent, taking up water and toxins into or onto their structures, or are motility- and secretion-modifying agents (Table 22.6).

There is limited evidence for the efficacy of certain adsorbent and absorbent substances in acute diarrhea (e.g. pectin[83*] or attapulgite[84**]). The most effective general antidiarrheals are the opioids, of which loperamide is the most specific, as in adults it has an oral bioavailability close to 1% and hence its effects are limited almost exclusively to the gut.[85]

Octreotide is a somatostatin analog that has to be given by subcutaneous injection or infusion. There are clinical reports of its effectiveness in otherwise intractable diarrhea secondary to gut resection, chemotherapy, or HIV disease.[86**]

Key points

- Laxatives are the most common cause of diarrhea in cancer patients receiving symptom control.
- Remember specific therapies, but most treatment in this group is symptomatic using an opioid.
- Octreotide has shown value in resistant diarrhea.

OTHER SYMPTOMS

Cachexia and anorexia

Cachexia is a constellation of weight loss, weakness, anorexia, and inanition, often accompanied by chronic nausea.[87] It is very common in some cancers (esophagus, stomach, pancreas, small-cell carcinoma of the bronchus) but not in others (breast cancer, ovarian cancer, sarcomas, testicular tumors). The cachexia syndrome also occurs with a number of noncancer illnesses [e.g. acquired immunodeficiency syndrome (AIDS), heart failure]. Its presence in both malignant and nonmalignant conditions implies a poor prognosis.[88,89] Cachexia becomes commoner with disease progression.[90] However, marked cachexia can be present at diagnosis[91] or even before, and the relationship with tumor bulk is unclear.

Table 22.4 *Commonly used laxatives and their methods of action*

Mode of action	Examples	Usual dose range	Comments
Predominantly softening			
Osmotic agents (retain water in gut lumen)	Lactulose	15–40 ml b.i.d.–t.i.d.	Active principally in the small bowel Latency of action 1–2 days
	Magnesium hydroxide Magnesium sulfate	2–4 g daily	Act throughout the bowel and may have pronounced purgative effect, possibly partly as a result of direct peristaltic stimulation. Latency of action 1–6 h (dose dependent)
	Polyethylene glycol (PEG)	1–3 sachets per day (up to eight sachets for treatment of fecal impaction)	125 ml of water required with each sachet
Surfactant agents (increase water penetration of the stool)	Docusate sodium Poloxamer (available only in combination with danthron)	Docusate 60–300 mg b.i.d.	Probably not very effective when used alone Latency of action 1–3 days
Lubricant agents	Liquid paraffin Glycerine (as suppositories) Arachis oil Olive oil (as enemas)		Paraffin is best used only in a 25% emulsion with magnesium hydroxide (Mil-Par)
Predominantly stimulant			
Direct stimulation of myenteric nerves to induce peristalsis. Reduce absorption of water from gut	Senna Danthron	7.5–30 mg b.i.d. 50–450 mg b.i.d.	Anthraquinone family. Danthron available only in combination with docusate or poloxamer – stains urine red/brown Latency of action 6–12 h
	Bisacodyl Sodium picosulfate	10–20 mg b.i.d. 5–20 mg b.i.d.	Polyphenolic family Latency of action 6–12 h
Combination stimulant/ softener preparations			
Codanthramer standard	Danthron 25 mg with poloxamer 200 mg per 5 ml or capsule		Suspension or capsule
Codanthramer forte	Danthron 75 mg with poloxamer 1 g per 5 ml or two capsules		Suspension or capsule
Codanthrusate	Danthron 50 mg with cocusate 60 mg per 5 ml or capsule		Capsule or suspension
Emulsion magnesium hydroxide and liquid paraffin (3:1 ratio)			Liquid only

Clinical findings and investigations

Patients lose considerable weight, with both adipose tissue and muscle being affected.[88] They may show signs of specific nutritional deficiencies, although this should lead one to look for particular causes. Hepatic synthesis of acute-phase proteins [e.g. C-reactive protein (CRP)] is increased but that of functional proteins such as albumin and transferrin is reduced. Cachectic patients therefore often develop hypertriglyceridemia, hypoalbuminemia, hypoproteinemia, glucose intolerance, anemia, and lactic acidosis[87] (Box 22.1).

Management

Cachexia requires a broad approach. The relationship between anorexia and the genesis of cachexia, if any, is unclear. Managing cachexia involves:

Table 22.5 *Specific antidiarrheal therapies*

Fat malabsorption – pancreatic enzyme replacement
Chologenic diarrhea – cholestyramine 4–12 g t.i.d.; calcium carbonate
Radiation-induced diarrhea – cholestyramine 4–12 g t.i.d.; aspirin
Carcinoid syndrome – cyproheptadine: initially 12 mg once daily (also consider octreotide; see Table 22.6)
Ulcerative colitis – mesalazine 1.2–2.4 g/day; steroids
Pseudomembranous colitis – vancomycin 125 mg q.i.d.; metronidazole 400 mg t.i.d.

- treating the underlying disease;
- controlling nausea;
- dealing with swallowing problems;
- adequate mouthcare;
- appropriate nutritional advice and support;
- adaptive changes in lifestyle;
- pharmacological treatment.

A number of drugs have been used.

Corticosteroids

Corticosteroids (e.g. dexamethasone 3–6 mg, methylprednisolone 30–125 mg daily) are effective in stimulating appetite and providing a sense of well-being.[93]** There is, however, no weight gain or increase in survival, and the effect disappears after a few weeks. This benefit has to be weighed against the often serious adverse effects of steroid use. Steroids should therefore be tried for a week, and if not clearly helping they should be stopped; stopping dexamethasone 6 mg abruptly after a week's treatment is safe, though this is the not the case for higher doses or longer courses. If there is benefit, the patient should be left on the lowest effective dose; once no longer effective, steroids should be stopped.[94]

Progestogens

Investigation of *megestrol acetate* in several randomized placebo-controlled trials[93] shows that:

- megestrol is significantly superior to placebo in increasing appetite, producing weight gain, and increasing patients' sense of well-being;
- weight gain is dose related (160–1,600 mg in various trials);
- weight gain is not due simply to fluid retention but mostly to an increase in adipose tissue;
- there is no increase in muscle mass (lean body mass);
- megestrol has an antinauseant effect.

In one trial of megestrol 160 mg t.i.d., an improvement was noted within 10 days. Responses were seen in 30–80% of patients; mean weight gain in one study on 480 mg daily was 5.4 kg at 12 weeks.[95] The authors of a dose-ranging study suggested that, although 800 mg/day was most effective, one should start on 160 mg/day and build up only if needed in view of the large number of tablets and high cost. *Medroxyprogesterone*, at doses of, say, 1 g/day, also increases food intake, resting energy expenditure, and adipose tissue mass but not fat-free mass.[96] Mechanisms of action are still being elucidated, but progestogens appear to inhibit the production of cachexia-producing cytokines.[97]

Table 22.6 *Symptomatic treatments for diarrhea*

Absorbent agents
Bulk-forming agents, e.g. methyl cellulose
Pectin
Adsorbent agents
Kaolin
Attapulgite
Motility- and secretion-modifying agents
Opioids
Codeine: 10–60 mg 4-hourly
(Morphine – usually if already in use for pain)
Diphenoxylate (combined with atropine): 10 mg *stat*, then 5 mg 6-hourly
Loperamide: 4 mg *stat*, then 2 mg after each loose stool up to 16 mg/24 h
Somatostatin analogs
Octreotide: 300 μg/24 h s.c. titrated up to 2,400 μg/24 h if necessary

Other drugs

Cyproheptadine, an antihistamine with antiserotonergic and anticholinergic properties, produces weight gain possibly through an effect on the regulation of growth hormone.[98] It has not been found to be significantly helpful in cachexia. *Hydrazine sulfate* interferes with gluconeogenesis by inhibiting phosphoenolpyruvate carboxykinase. It therefore affects the abnormal glucose and protein metabolism in cachexia. Three large recent randomized placebo-controlled trials concluded that it was ineffective: patients on hydrazine actually had shorter survivals and a poorer quality of life than those on placebo. The cannabinoid *Δ9-tetrahydrocannabinol* (THC) has been shown in open and retrospective studies to produce weight gain and improved appetite varying from "slight" in one study of patients with advanced cancer to a weight gain of 0.6 kg/month in a small group of AIDS patients. In animal studies, cannabinoid antagonists have been found to suppress appetite and induce weight loss.[99] The evidence is consistent but not strong, and there is a need for proper randomized trials. A recent study showed THC to be less effective than megestrol in producing appetite improvement and weight gain, and the addition of THC to megestrol conferred no additional benefit.[99a] The methylxanthine *pentoxifylline* suppresses TNF activity, and has been tried on very small groups of patients with encouraging initial results. *Ibuprofen* reduces resting energy expenditure and serum CRP levels in pancreatic cancer patients,[88] and may provide interesting leads. Another promising drug is *eicosapentaenoic acid*, a polyunsaturated fatty acid and cyclooxygenase inhibi-

Box 22.1 *Pathophysiology of cachexia*

Cachexia is not starvation!

- In starvation there is lack of substrates for energy production, so starvation is a low-output state aimed at conserving energy.
- In cachexia there is frequently an overabundant supply of substrates through breakdown of muscle and adipose tissue but utilization is inefficient through:
  - increased anaerobic glycolysis: energy inefficient
  - recycling of resultant lactate to glucose through Cori cycle: energy inefficient
  - marked insulin resistance
  - downregulation of lipoprotein lipase (which hydrolyzes circulating chylomicrons and triglycerides to increase adipose tissue stores): lipogenesis is therefore reduced
  - lipolysis is, however, unaffected.[87]

These changes are mediated by:

- Tumor factors: lipid- and protein-mobilizing factors (LMFs, PMFs), leukemia-inhibitory factor D (LIF-D), interleukin 6 (IL-6).[87]
- Host factors: tumor necrosis factor (TNF), interleukin 1 (IL-1), IL-6, interferon-gamma (IFN-γ).

The generally held view is that cytokines are the key determinants of this cachexia, but this has recently been challenged, with the role of mobilizing factors being emphasized. Cachexia is therefore frequently a high-output state – akin to metabolic response to trauma or sepsis.

As the problem is one of utilization, not supply:

Feeding alone will not reverse cachexia

tor, which appears to interact with LMFs and PMFs to damp down catabolism in cachexia.[99b] In pancreatic cancer patients, eicosapentaenoic acid stabilized fat and protein reserves and weight loss. A number of experimental *anticytokine therapies* (including anti-TNF and anti-IL-6 antibodies and suramin, which acts as an IL-6 receptor antagonist) appear to inhibit the cachectic process in animal studies.[100]

Through all this it is essential to remember that cachexia is a human rather than purely a medical problem. Patients and their families need much help in adapting to the greatly increased disability and their progressive difficulty with the day-to-day tasks that make up the stuff of life and relationships. Help has to be both practical (physiotherapy, occupational therapy, aids and devices, adequate attention to social care needs) and psychological, as patients' way of defining themselves, body image, etc. changes as they deteriorate.

Pruritus

Pruritus, or itch, occurs in 5% of patients with advanced cancer. It has a particular association with lymphoma and is present in over 80% of cases of cholestasis, of malignant cause or otherwise.

Pathology

Pruritus is related to pain in that both are mediated by the same peripheral nerves. However, the two sensations are presumably subject to different information handling in the CNS. No specific itch receptors have yet been identified. Locally, itching can be induced by histamine at H_1 receptors, by substance P, and by interleukin 2, and appears to be modulated by serotonin (at 5-HT_3 receptors), prostaglandin E_2, opioids at μ-receptors, and, possibly, vasoactive intestinal peptide (VIP). Pruritus is suggestible, revealing a contribution of central neural processing.

Dry skin is a potent cause of pruritus in cancer patients. Morphine may cause pruritus when given spinally or epidurally but rarely does so when administered orally. Uremia and cholestatic jaundice are other common cancer-related causes of itch, and pruritus can be the presenting feature of lymphoma. Beyond this, the full range of general medical and dermatological causes of pruritus may be present in the cancer population.

Clinical findings

Generalized pruritus should be distinguished from local, and itching should be distinguished from related sensations that could represent neuropathic pain. A history should elicit details of associated conditions and potential allergens, as well as symptoms suggestive of anemia or renal failure, which are also associated with pruritus.

Examination will reveal the extent of skin excoriation caused by scratching, and areas of local itching should be checked for evidence of fungal or mite infestation. The presence, distribution, and form of any rash will help distinguish between general allergic reactions, eczema, and locally provoked dermatoses. Signs of anemia or jaundice should be noted.

Investigations

Pruritus related to allergy or local infection or infestation may require specialist investigation. Clinical suspicion of anemia, renal failure, or cholestasis will stimulate performance of the relevant blood tests.

Management

No drug is specific for the relief of pruritus, and if possible the underlying cause should be treated, e.g. bile duct stenting for malignant obstructive jaundice. Alongside any pharmacological treatment a number of general measures should be undertaken (Table 22.7).

Treatments may be topical or systemic. Topical applications are inconvenient except for localized itching but may still be justified if the symptom is very severe.

Topical treatments

Counterirritants and local anesthetics, e.g. phenol 0.5–2%, menthol 0.25–2%, camphor 1–3%, provide anesthesia of cutaneous nerve endings or a cooling sensation. However crotamiton, often used in this way, has been shown to be ineffective.[101**]

Capsaicin 0.025% causes depletion of substance P in peripheral nerves and blocks C-fiber conduction but also gives rise to local burning sensations, which may need local anesthetics for their relief. Capsaicin has been found to be effective in relieving renal failure-associated itch.[102**]

Transcutaneous electrical nerve stimulation (TENS) provides an electrical equivalent of counterirritation to produce surround inhibition of transmission of pruritic stimuli. There are case reports of its successful clinical use.[103*]

Topical 5% sodium cromoglycate has been reported to be effective in Hodgkin's lymphoma itching after the failure of other therapies.[104*]

Systemic treatments

Some systemic treatments for pruritus are general and others are associated with particular diseases.

General H_1 antihistamines are most effective when there is evidence of a local histamine involvement in itching but are also often used in other conditions. It appears that efficacy is related to the degree of sedation caused, e.g. chlorpheniramine 4 mg 4-hourly.

About 30% of those with generalized pruritus have evidence of depression, but the claimed effectiveness of doxepin[105*] and paroxetine[106*] in pruritus of a range of etiologies is attributed to their modulation of histamine and serotonin systems.

Specific In *cholestasis*, cholestyramine may be effective but is unpalatable. Rifampicin 150 mg can be successful.[107*] The anabolic steroid stanozolol has also been reported to be useful in jaundice-related itch even though it may make the jaundice worse.[108*] Other than effective dialysis, *uremic itch* has been reported to respond to ondansetron, a 5-HT_3 antagonist antiemetic,[109*] and to erythropoietin.[110*]

Ondansetron has been reported to be effective in a randomized controlled trial in *epidural morphine-induced pruritus.*[111**]

Pruritus associated with *lymphoma* may respond to cimetidine or plasma exchange.

Table 22.7 *General measures for pruritus*

Avoid friction from clothing, towels, and bed linen
Avoid excessive heat
Use emulsifying ointment rather than soap for washing
Avoid vasodilators (which for some will include coffee and alcohol)
Allow gentle rubbing but discourage scratching
Topical steroids to inflamed areas
Diversion
Control of other symptoms

Sweating

Excessive sweating occurs widely in cancer but is reported particularly by patients with lymphomas, leukemia, or liver metastases. It is not necessarily associated with fever or with infection and may be worse at night.

Pathology

Human body temperature control is accurate and complex. It appears that the anterior hypothalamus integrates information from temperature sensors in the skin, CNS, and viscera to stimulate autonomic and behavioral thermoregulatory mechanisms in order to maintain the body temperature at a set point. This set point can be altered in a number of circumstances, including malignancy, sepsis, and dehydration. Blood transfusion, cytotoxics (such as bleomycin), and changes in estrogen balance can also induce fever.

Clinical findings and investigations

The principal aim is to identify any infection, but hormone-related sweating ("hot flushes") will be suggested by a menopausal history or hormonal manipulation for breast or prostate cancers.

Management

General measures are important:

- use of cotton rather than artificial fibers;
- availability of regular changes of clothing;
- provision of a fan;

- regular tepid sponging;
- regular washing;
- encouragement of oral fluids.

Infections causing systemic toxicity should be treated. Megestrol acetate starting at 40 mg/24 h is effective for hot flushes in both breast and prostate cancer, and does not appear to impair tumor control.[112*]

Acetaminophen (paracetamol) is worth using initially, although its effectiveness is said to be reduced in neoplastic fevers. Nonsteroidal anti-inflammatory drugs (NSAIDs) can be effective in malignancy-related sweating, with particular value being claimed for naproxen.[113**] However, if loss of efficacy occurs, a change to another NSAID may recover it. In a randomized controlled trial, megestrol acetate was significantly better than placebo for hot flushes and the accompanying sweating in patients with breast or prostate cancer.[114] There is case history evidence for the use of thioridazine, the limiting factor being sedation. Steroids may be helpful in leukemia or lymphoma.[115*]

PSYCHOLOGICAL AND PSYCHIATRIC PROBLEMS

In terminal illness no area of life remains untouched. This calls for massive adaptation while physical resilience is greatly diminished. Some patients have pre-existing psychiatric disorders. Unsurprisingly, psychological problems are frequent in this situation.

Depression

Depression is commoner in cancer patients than in the general population though no more so than in patients with other physical illnesses.[116] It can precede diagnosis.[117] Both depression and suicide risk are increased in the early stages of cancer[118] and are higher in some cancers, e.g. head and neck tumors,[119] and if pain or severe symptoms are present.[120,121] Disease progression and recurrence are again associated with increased psychiatric morbidity.

Diagnosis and prevalence

The diagnosis of depression in terminally ill patients is fraught with problems. Adjustment reactions and appropriate sadness have to be distinguished from true depression. Somatic features of depression (e.g. loss of interest in normal activities, psychomotor retardation, anorexia, and weight loss) in advanced cancer can be due entirely to the physical deterioration. This has led to attempts to replace the somatic criteria in the DSM classification with nonsomatic ones with greater discriminative power for cancer patients.[122,123] Alternatively, Cohen-Cole *et al.*[123] proposed ignoring anorexia and fatigue in the DSM criteria and using only the remaining criteria. It has also been suggested that the simple question "Are you depressed ?" carries a higher sensitivity and specificity[123a] than formal questionnaires, and doubt has been cast on the applicability of the Hospital Anxiety and Depression Scale in hospice patients,[124,125] though others dispute this.[126] With all these provisos in mind, the prevalence of depression has been reported as varying between 1% for acute leukemia and 50% for pancreatic cancer.[127] Most experts agree an overall prevalence of 10–25% for patients with terminal illness.[128]

The psychological or cognitive symptoms are therefore the mainstay of diagnosis (Table 22.8). Ideas of worthlessness, hopelessness, guilt, and suicidal ideation need to be explored.

Management

Psychotherapy (individual or group) and cognitive behavior therapy have important roles to play in treating depression in cancer patients. Fawzy *et al.*[129***] and Sellick and Crooks[130***] produce evidence for the effectiveness of various forms of psychotherapy in cancer patients.

These approaches often need to be supplemented by the use of drugs. Tricyclic antidepressants are highly effective but cause troublesome adverse effects such as postural hypotension, cardiac arrhythmias, and anticholinergic effects. Such adverse effects are less common with selective serotonin reuptake inhibitors (SSRIs), but these often produce nausea, diarrhea, and insomnia. Different SSRIs also inhibit different hepatic enzymes, increasing the potential for drug interactions.[131] However, SSRIs can usually be started at a therapeutic dose, unlike the tricyclics, which have to be built up over time. The selection of nonsedating antidepressants for agitated forms of depression appears to be less important than previously thought. Any antidepressant, whether tricyclic or SSRI, needs 2–3 weeks or longer to work. Suggestions that adding pindolol might reduce the time for a response have not been borne out by a recent meta-analysis. A systematic review of antidepressant drug treatment showed that just over four patients with physical illness would have to be treated to produce one recovery that would not have occurred using placebo [number to treat (NNT) of 4.2] (95% confidence interval 3.2–6.4).[132***]

Table 22.8 *Endicott substitution criteria. (Reproduced with permission from Endicott.[122])*

Physical/ somatic symptom	Psychological symptom substitute
Change in appetite, weight	Tearfulness, depressed appearance
Sleep disturbance	Social withdrawal, decreased talkativeness
Fatigue, loss of energy	Brooding, self-pity, pessimism
Diminished ability to think or concentrate, indecisiveness	Lack of reactivity

Suicide risk

Roth and Breitbart[133] list the following risk factors for suicide in cancer patients:

- advanced illness;
- concurrent psychiatric morbidity (major depression, delirium, adjustment disorder);
- uncontrolled pain;
- sense of helplessness and loss of control;
- fatigue of resources, physical, psychosocial, and spiritual;
- lack of a good support system;
- suicidal ideation or prior attempts.

In dealing with a potential suicide, once an empathic rapport with the patient is established and risk factors evaluated, distressing symptoms need to be controlled, psychiatric disorders treated (with specialist help), and the support system shored up. The aim is to take away from the patient the feeling of helplessness and hopelessness and to put them back in the driving seat. A psychiatric opinion is needed to assess legal competence; some patients will need to be sectioned while underlying psychiatric problems are treated.

Anxiety

Anxiety severe enough to disrupt day-to-day activity can be a feature of adjustment disorder or a condition in its own right. Again, DSM-IV somatic diagnostic criteria (muscle tension, aches or soreness; easy fatigability; shortness of breath or smothering sensations; dry mouth, dizziness, or diarrhea; trouble falling or staying asleep and irritability) can equally well be due to the cancer itself. Psychological symptoms have to be relied on more heavily than the somatic in making decisions about such patients' anxiety levels.

Prevalence

This depends on the cut-off points one chooses to make the diagnosis. Anxiety is about twice as common in persons with chronic medical conditions as in those with no physical illness, though whether it is commoner in cancer than in other illnesses is unclear. Noyes *et al.*,[134] reviewing various studies, quote a prevalence of 9–19% for cancer patients. Mixed anxiety–depression is common. Once again, anxiety symptoms and panic attacks can be premonitors of cancer.[135]

Etiology

Factors increasing risk of severe anxiety include:

- premorbid personality;
- more advanced disease;
- active treatment with surgery, chemotherapy, or radiotherapy;
- poorly controlled pain;
- physical factors, e.g. sepsis, hypoxia;
- medication: corticosteroids, phenothiazines or derivatives, e.g. metoclopramide (e.g. akathisia), sudden alcohol or smoking cessation.

Sex, age, marital status, and other demographic variables are less useful predictors for anxiety than in the normal population.[134] In the last weeks of life, patients who wanted more information than they had been given scored significantly higher on anxiety scales than those whose information needs were satisfied.[136]

Management

There is evidence that concurrent psychotherapy and drug treatment is superior to either modality alone in treating anxiety or depression.[137] Exploration of a patient's fears in a psychotherapeutic environment can reduce psychological distress and improve coping.[129] Cognitive behavior therapy is effective in reducing anxiety, and the effect persists for 12 months.[138]** Moorey *et al.*[139]** found cognitive behavior therapy to be superior to supportive nondirective psychotherapy in relieving anxiety, improving adjustment to cancer, and improving coping strategies; this effect remained at 4 months' follow-up. Drugs need to be used selectively. However, at the very end of life there is often no alternative. Benzodiazepines reduce anxiety; in some situations (e.g. acute frightening exacerbations of breathlessness) the amnesic properties of these drugs also come in useful. Buspirone has a role in some patients, but the effect is slow to develop. Antidepressants are also used successfully to control anxiety.[140] For most patients, the potency of information and a safe environment (e.g. a constant human presence in moments of acute severe breathlessness) in reducing anxiety or panic cannot be overstated.

Delirium

Acute confusional states, sometimes superimposed on background dementia, occur in 15–20% of palliative care patients,[141] though figures of up to 85% have been reported.[142]

Clinical features

Delirium is often preceded by prodromal restlessness, anxiety, sleep disturbance, and irritability. It follows a highly fluctuant course, with disturbances of attention, perception, psychomotor activity, orientation, memory, and thinking.

Causes of confusion in terminally ill patients

Causes of confusion in terminally ill patients are numerous and include:

- drugs e.g. opioids, anticholinergics, steroids, cytotoxics;
- biochemical, e.g. hyponatremia, hypercalcemia, hypoglycemia;
- neoplastic, e.g. brain primary or secondary tumor;
- paraneoplastic, e.g. nonmetastatic cerebral syndromes in small-cell lung cancer;
- organ failure: hepatic, renal, respiratory, cardiac;
- infection, e.g. chest, urinary;
- pain;
- alcohol or nicotine withdrawal;
- fear and extreme anxiety.

Management

Environmental manipulation can reduce the prevalence of delirium.[143]** Medication is needed only if the patient is distressed or a danger to self or others. Happily confused patients should be treated if the underlying cause is reversible or they have a good prognosis.

- Reduce risk to the patient:
  - ensure a safe environment (e.g. patient not isolated, not easily able to inflict self-injury);
  - use medication if necessary (see below);
  - very occasionally use physical restraint.
- Defuse sense of threat experienced by the patient:
  - quiet, well-lit room;
  - familiar objects and persons, e.g. family;
  - reduce the number of persons the patient sees;
  - take an empathic approach (sit on same level as patient, touch, keep calm).
- Assess, and if possible treat, the underlying cause:
  - but this is often not amenable to treatment in this patient group.
- Try to ground the patient into reality:
  - gently point out misperceptions.
- Work out management plan for future events.

Medication

In general, drugs should be used sparingly, as they may worsen confusion, and adequate time should be given for them to work. Haloperidol is effective at controlling agitation and paranoia.[144]** Small doses (0.5–1 mg) used every 45–60 min are very effective; the dose can be increased if necessary. Other psychotropics may offer no particular advantage. Benzodiazepines should generally be avoided as they may cause disinhibition and worsen confusion or behavioral problems.[144] However, they are the drugs of choice in substance withdrawal or if the patient is prone to fit, when major tranquilizers may further lower seizure threshold. However, short-acting benzodiazepines, e.g. midazolam, have found a definite place in palliative care, for example in controlling terminal agitated delirium.[145] The new antipsychotic agents (e.g. risperidone, olanzapine) have been used at low doses with success to treat delirium, but evidence for their effectiveness is still being built up.[145a]

END OF LIFE CARE

Death is not necessarily seen as unwelcome by patients in the late stages of cancer. It can be a consolation to patients to be told that their condition will not go on for much longer.

Some professionals find it very difficult to be asked by patients for an estimate of prognosis not only because any attempt at accuracy is likely to be misplaced, but also because they fear that the answer will cause the person to give up. Relatives are even more likely to take this view. However, there is evidence that the grounds for hope change as illness progresses,[146] from the hope that cure may be achieved to one that the disease may be slowed in its progression, to the achievement of particular practical goals, and ultimately to hope for relief of discomfort and for a peaceful end to life.

Prior involvement of a multiprofessional palliative care team with 24-h availability can facilitate the continuing care of the patient at home, where most terminally ill people wish to be.[147] As life becomes more difficult the proportion wishing to stay at home diminishes but still remains about 50%.[148] For a significant number of families there comes a point when they feel they can no longer look after the patient at home, despite practical assistance. In this the patient may agree, or there may be divergence of opinion.

Even if all are in agreement that admission is needed, family members may still be left with a sense of failure and of guilt that they have let their relative down. It is important for their response in bereavement that families receive reassurance about the quality of their caring efforts prior to the admission, and the appropriateness of seeking inpatient care now. It is also important that there are the facilities and encouragement to enable relatives to remain with the patient as death approaches, if that would be helpful to them.

Most bereaved people do not need specific bereavement care. For a minority, perhaps up to 25%, adjustment can be facilitated by specialist bereavement support. This is increasingly widely available, and in Britain can be accessed through CRUSE, the local hospice, or the social service department.

Symptom control

Good symptom control at the end of life requires preparedness. It is a wholly inadequate response to the onset of a distressing symptom if control has to wait on a doctor's order or the pharmacist's acquisition of the medication required. The following categories of drug are most often required:

- opioids;
- sedatives;
- antiemetics;
- anticholinergic agents.

Opioids

Many patients will require a change of route from oral to parenteral, although often only in the last 48 h of life. This can be accomplished by subcutaneous injections (made less uncomfortable if a plastic cannula is left in place to avoid repeated needle sticks) or, more conveniently, if the length of the prognosis appears to justify it, by a subcutaneous infusion delivered by a portable syringe driver. Alternatively, morphine or oxycodone can be given rectally; morphine, phenazocine, or buprenorphine (a partial opioid agonist) can be administered sublingually; and fentanyl is available as a transdermal patch.

An important consideration if there is a change of route of an existing opioid is to make an appropriate calculation of the equivalent dose. All such ratios are subject to individual variation, and resulting doses may require upward or downward adjustment according to response. A change to the sublingual or rectal route of the same opioid does not require a change in dose except in the case of oxycodone, the dose of which should be doubled in transferring from the oral to rectal route. Unless the opioid requirement is stable, fentanyl, although convenient to give, is a less satisfactory choice of parenteral opioid as dose titration is relatively difficult owing to the wide steps between patch sizes and the long delay (up to 23 h[149]) in achieving and recovering from steady-state blood levels.

A patient who has gained particular analgesic benefit from an NSAID can have it continued by suppository (e.g. in the form of naproxen or ketoprofen) or syringe driver. Ketorolac will mix in a syringe with diamorphine but if, as is usually the case, other drugs are also required it is more reliable to give the NSAID rectally.

Pain is not generally a problem at the end of life if it has been adequately controlled previously. In patients who can no longer indicate their feelings, carers interpret nonverbal signs of distress – for instance groaning, grimacing, or restlessness. Before increasing medication, it should be checked whether there are remediable causes of discomfort, particularly a full bladder or rectum.

Sedatives

A generalized restlessness, which may be due to pain but also to anxiety, has to be distinguished from focal myoclonic jerks, as these may be worsened by opioids, especially in the presence of phenothiazines. Rather than persist with opioid medication for restlessness it is more appropriate to use a benzodiazepine, either instead or in addition, for its anxiolytic and muscle relaxant properties. This may take the form of diazepam suppositories rectally or liquid via a gastrostomy, given p.r.n. or b.i.d.–t.i.d., or midazolam subcutaneously. Midazolam combines satisfactorily with diamorphine or anticholinergic agents in a syringe driver. An initial midazolam dose is 2.5 mg *stat* or 10 mg/24 h.

A principal role of benzodiazepines is in the palliation of breathlessness, when their action is complementary to that of opioids. In an acute deterioration in breathing associated with failing respiratory function it is appropriate to give a combination of morphine/diamorphine and diazepam/midazolam initially and then to titrate the doses of each. A phenothiazine can be used instead of the benzodiazepine, e.g. chlorpromazine or the more sedating levomepromazine. Both have an antiemetic effect, if this is important, and there is limited evidence that chlorpromazine can palliate breathlessness. Watch should be kept for myoclonic jerking, and the lowering of the fit threshold that these drugs induce is a relative contraindication in cerebral tumor. Levomepromazine can be given by subcutaneous infusion, but chlorpromazine causes too many skin reactions to be given by this route.

Antisecretory drugs

Any severely ill patient with reduced ability to cough can accumulate secretions in the upper airways, resulting in noisy breathing, which even if not distressing to the patient may well upset attending relatives. At the end of life this problem is one that is best anticipated, as it is not easy to get rid of secretions which have already gathered. A chest infection is likely to be present, producing purulent exudates; this cannot be prevented by anticholinergics, so that it is not possible to stop rattly breathing altogether. Hence, the first step in management is to explain to the patient's family the mechanism of the noisy breathing, what is being done, and what its limitations are, and to reassure them that by this stage of their illness the dying person is unlikely to be nearly as aware of the sounds as they are themselves.

Hyoscine hydrobromide is normally sedating, whereas hyoscine butylbromide and glycopyrronium bromide are more neutral. Any of these can be given subcutaneously by syringe driver in combination with diamorphine and midazolam or levomepromazine. In Britain, the first two are significantly cheaper than the third.

Dose ranges are:

- hyoscine butylbromide: 20 mg *stat* s.c., 60–240 mg/24 h by s.c. infusion;
- glycopyrronium bromide: 0.2–0.4 mg *stat* s.c., 0.6–1.2 mg/24 h by s.c. infusion;
- hyoscine hydrobromide: 0.4–0.8 mg *stat* s.c., 1.2–2.4 mg/24 h by s.c. infusion.

CONCLUSION

Care at the end of life is crucial because it provides some of the most powerful memories for those who are left behind. The future attitudes of the patient's family and friends toward severe illness in themselves or others, and toward death itself, will be molded by it. Good symptom control and good communication with the patient as long as this is possible, and with the family, are crucial not only for their direct benefit to the dying patient but also as a public health measure for all those left behind who have been close to the patient.

Key points

- Continuation of good symptom control to the end of life is important not only for the patient but also for his or her family.
- Most patients will remain on oral medication until the last 48 h of life.
- The method of choice for nonoral administration of medication is subcutaneous infusion by syringe driver.
- There is no evidence for a crescendo of pain at the close of life, but medication doses may need readjustment because of changes in metabolism or in the pattern of symptoms.
- Analgesia, sedation, antiemesis, and drying of secretions may all be required.
- Midazolam or methotrimeprazine will combine with morphine or diamorphine in a syringe driver, and an anticholinergic such as glycopyrronium can also be added.

REFERENCES

● 1. Krech RL, Walsh D, Curtis EB. Symptoms of lung cancer. *Palliative Med* 1992; **6:** 309–15.

◆ 2. Higginson I, McCarthy M. Measuring symptoms in terminal cancer: are pain and dyspnoea controlled? *J Roy Soc Med* 1989; **82:** 264–7.

3. Ganong WF. *Review of Medical Physiology*, 6th edn. Los Altos, CA: Lange, 1973: 500.

4. Bredin M, Corner J, Krishnasamy M, *et al.* Multicentre randomized controlled trial of nursing intervention for breathlessness in patients with lung cancer. *Br Med J* 1999; **318:** 901–4.

5. Gollins SW, Burt PA, Barber PV, Stout R. High dose rate intraluminal radiotherapy for carcinoma of the bronchus: outcome of treatment of 406 patients. *Radiother Oncol* 1994; **33:** 31–40.

6. de Souza AC, Keal R, Hudson NM, *et al.* Use of expandable wire stents for malignant airway obstruction. *Ann Thorac Surg* 1994; **57:** 1573–7.

7. Armstrong BA, Perez CA, Simpson JR, Hederman MA. Role of irradiation in the management of superior vena cava syndrome. *Int J Radiat Oncol Biol Phys* 1987; **13:** 531–9.

8. Nicholson AA, Ettles DF, Arnold A, *et al.* Treatment of malignant superior vena cava obstruction: metal stents or radiation therapy. *J Vasc Intervent Radiol* 1997; **8:** 781–8.

9. Kee ST, Kinoshita L, Razavi MK, *et al.* Superior vena cava syndrome: treatment with catheter-directed thrombolysis and endovascular stent placement. *Radiology* 1998; **206:** 187–93.

10. Chacon Lopez-Muniz JI, Garcia Garcia L, Lanciego Perez C, *et al.* Treatment of superior and inferior vena cava syndromes of malignant cause with Wallstent catheter placed percutaneously. *Am J Clin Oncol* 1997; **20:** 293–7.

11. Wilson RH, Hoseth W, Dempsey ME. Respiratory acidosis. I. Effects of decreasing respiratory minute volume with specific reference to oxygen, morphine and barbiturates. *Am J Med* 1954; **17:** 464.

12. Walsh TD. Opiates and respiratory function in advanced cancer. *Recent Results Cancer Res* 1984; **89:** 115–17.

13. Bruera E, MacEachern T, Ripamonti C, Hanson J. Subcutaneous morphine for dyspnea in cancer patients. *Ann Intern Med* 1993; **119:** 906–7.

14. Bruera E, Macmillan K, Pither J, MacDonald RN. Effects of morphine on dyspnea of terminal cancer patients. *J Pain Symptom Manage* 1990; **5:** 83–93.

15. Boyd KJ. Oral morphine as symptomatic treatment of dyspnoea in patients with advanced cancer. *Palliative Med* 1997; **11:** 277–81.

16. Woodcock AA, Gross ER, Geddes DM. Drug treatment of breathlessness: contrasting effects of diazepam and promethazine in pink puffers. *Br Med J* 1981; **283:** 343–6.

17. Ventafridda V, Spoldi E, De Conno F. Control of dyspnoea in advanced cancer patients. *Chest* 1990; **6:** 1544–5.

18. Craven J, Sutherland A. Buspirone for anxiety disorders in patients with severe lung disease. *Lancet* 1991; **338:** 249.

19. Bruera E, de Stoutz N, Velasco-Leiva A, *et al.* Effects of oxygen on dyspnoea in hypoxaemic terminal cancer patients. *Lancet* 1993; **342:** 13–14.

20. Booth S, Kelly MJ, Cox NP, Adams L, Guz A. Does oxygen help dyspnea in patients with cancer. *Am J Respir Crit Care Med* 1996; **153:** 1515–18.

21. Wilcock A, Corcoran R, Tattersfield AE. Safety and efficacy of nebulized lignocaine in patients with cancer and breathlessness. *Palliative Med* 1994; **8:** 35–8.

● 22. Davis C. The role of nebulized drugs in palliating respiratory symptoms of malignant disease. *Eur J Palliative Care* 1995; **2:** 9–15.

23. Kamei J. Role of opioidergic and serotonergic mechanisms in cough and antitussives. *Pulm Pharmacol* 1996; **9:** 349–56.

24. Luporini G, Barni S, Marchi E, Daffonchio L. Efficacy and safety of levodropropizine and dihydrocodeine on nonproductive cough in primary and metastatic lung cancer. *Eur Respir J* 1998; **12:** 97–101.

25. Miller RR, McGregor DH. Hemorrhage from carcinoma of the lung. *Cancer* 1980; **46:** 200–5.

26. Cooke N. Hemoptysis. In: Walsh TD ed. *Symptom Control.* Oxford: Blackwell Scientific Publications, 1989: 235–9.

27. Slawson RG, Scott RM. Radiation therapy in bronchogenic carcinoma. *Radiology* 1979; **132:** 175–6.
28. Rees GJ, Devrell CE, Barley VL, Newman HF. Palliative radiotherapy for lung cancer: two versus five fractions. *Clin Oncol* 1997; **9:** 90–5.
29. Dean A, Tuffin P. Fibrinolytic inhibitors for cancer-associated bleeding problems. *J Pain Symptom Manage* 1997; **13:** 20–4.
30. Jobbins J, Bagg J, Finlay IG, *et al.* Oral and dental disease in terminally ill cancer patients. *Br Med J* 1992; **304:** 1612.
31. Ganong WM. *Review of Medical Physiology,* 19th edn. Stamford, CT: Appleton & Lange, 1999: 467–8.
32. Ventafridda V, Ripamonti C, Sbanotto A, De Conno F. Mouth care. In: Doyle D, Hanks GWC, MacDonald N eds. *Oxford Textbook of Palliative Medicine,* 2nd edn. Oxford: Oxford Medical Publications, 1998: 693.
33. Grad H, GrushkaM, Yanover L. Drug-induced xerostomia. *J Can Dent Association* 1985; **4:** 296–300.
34. Twycross RG. *Symptom Management in Advanced Cancer.* Oxford: Radcliffe Medical Press, 1997: 146.
35. Johnson JT, Ferretti GA, Nethery WJ, *et al.* Oral pilocarpine for post-irradiation xerostomia in patients with head and neck cancer. *N Engl J Med* 1993; **329:** 390–5.
36. Finlay I. Oral symptoms and candida in the terminally ill. *Br Med J* 1986; **292:** 592–3.
● 37. Finlay I. Oral fungal infections. *Eur J Palliative Care* 1995, **2** (2, Suppl.): 4.
38. Mangino JE, Moser SA, Waites KB. When to use fluconazole. *Lancet* 1995; **345:** 6–7
39. Finlay I. Oral symptoms and candida in the terminally ill. *Br Med J* 1986, **292:** 592–3.
40. Epstein EB, Stevenson-Moore P, Jackson S, *et al.* Prevention of oral mucositis in radiation therapy: a controlled study with benzydamine hydrochloride rinse. *Int J Radiat Oncol Biol Phys* 1989; **16:** 1571–5.
41. Solomon MA. Oral sucralfate suspension for mucositis. *N Engl J Med* 1986; **315:** 459–60.
42. Sykes NP, Baines M, Carter RL. Clinical and pathological study of dysphagia conservatively managed in patients with advanced malignant disease. *Lancet* 1988; **2:** 726–8.
43. Elrington G. The Lambert Eaton myasthenic syndrome. *Palliative Med* 1992; **6:** 9–17.
44. Carter RL, Pittam MR, Tanner NSB. Pain and dysphagia in patients with squamous carcinomas of the head and neck: the role of perineural spread. *J R Soc Med* 1982; **75:** 598–606.
45. Mattioli S. Dysphagia. In: Bianchi-Porro G, Cremer M, Kreis G, *et al.* eds. *Gastroenterology and Hepatology.* London: McGraw Hill, 1999: 20.
46. Leonard R, Kendall K. *Dysphagia Assessment and Planning: a Team Approach.* San Diego, CA: Singular Publishing Group, 1997.
47. Boyle JO, Kraus DH. Functional rehabilitation In: Close LG, Larson DL, Shah JP eds. *Essentials of Head and Neck Oncology.* New York, NY: Thieme, 1998: 369–78.
48. Grond S, Zech D, Diefenbach C, Bischoff A. Prevalence and pattern of symptoms in patients with cancer pain: a prospective evaluation of 1635 patients referred to a pain clinic. *J Pain Symptom Manage* 1994, **9:** 372–82.
49. Dundee JW, Jones PO. The prevention of analgesic-induced nausea and vomiting by cyclizine. *Br J Clin Practice* 1968; **22:** 379–82.
50. Higi M, Niederle N, Bierbaum W, *et al.* Pronounced aniemetic activity of the antipsychotic drug levomepromacine (L) in patients receiving cancer chemotherapy. *J Cancer Res Clin Oncol* 1980; **97:** 81–6.
● 51. Twycross RG, Barkby GD, Hallwood PM. The use of low dose levomepromazine (methotrimeprazine) in the management of nausea and vomiting. *Progr Palliative Care* 1997; **5(2):** 49–53.
52. Fortney JT, Gan TJ, Graczyk S, *et al.* A comparison of the efficacy, safety and patient satisfaction of ondansetron versus droperidol as antiemeics for elective outpatient surgical procedures. *Anaesth Analges* 1998; **86:** 731–8.
52a. Tramer MR, Reynolds DJM, Stoner NS, *et al.* Efficacy of 5-HT3 receptor antagonists in radiotherapy-induced nausea and vomiting: a quantitative systematic review. *Eur J Cancer* 1998; **34:** 1836–44.
● 53. Ramirez B, Richter JE. Promotility drugs in the treatment of gastro-oesophageal reflux disease. *Aliment Pharmacol Ther* 1993; **7:** 5–20.
54. Brunton LL. Agents affecting gastrointestinal water flux and motility; emesis and antiemetics; bile acids and pancreatic enzymes. In: Hardman JG, Limbird LE, Molinoff PB, Ruddon RW, Gilman AG eds. *Goodman & Gilman's The Pharmacological Basis of Therapeutics,* 9th edn. New York, NY: McGraw-Hill, 1996: 917–36.
55. Hill ADK, Walsh TN, Hamilton D, *et al.* Erythromycin improves emptying of the denervated stomach after oesophagectomy. *Br J Surg* 1993; **80:** 879–81.
56. Janssens J, Peeters TL, Vantrappen G, *et al.* Improvement of gastric emptying in diabetic gastroparesis by erythromycin. *N Engl J Med* 1990; **322:** 1028–31.
57. Armstrong DN, Ballantyne GH, Modlin IM. Erythromycin for reflex ileus in Ogilvie's syndrome. *Lancet* 1991; **337:** 378.
58. Cattnach SM, Fairclough PD. Erythromycin and the gut. *Gut* 1992; **33:** 397–401.
59. Kaye PM, Oliver DJ. Hypercalcaemia in advanced malignancy. *Lancet* 1985; **i:** 512.
60. Heath DA: Hypercalcaemia in malignancy: fluids and bisphosphonates are best when life is threatened. *Br Med J* 1989; **298:** 1468–9.
61. Warrell RP. Metabolic emergencies. In: De Vita *et al.* eds. *Cancer: Principles and Practice of Oncology,* 4th edn. Philadelphia, PA: Lipincott, 1993: 2128.
62. Ratcliffe WA, Hutchesson ACJ, Bundred NJ, Ratcliffe JG. Role of assays for parathyroid-hormone-related-protein in investigation of hypercalcaemia. *Lancet* 1992; **339:** 164–7.
63. Wimalawansa SJ. Significance of plasma PTH-rp in

patients with hypercalcaemia of malignancy treated with bisphosphonate. *Cancer* 1994; **73:** 2223–30.

64. Bilezikian JP. Management of acute hypercalcemia. *N Engl J Med* 1992; **326:** 1196–203.
65. Purohit OP, Radstone CR, Anthony C, *et al.* A randomized double-blind comparison of intravenous pamidronate and clodronate in the hypercalcaemia of malignancy. *Br J Cancer* 1995; **72:** 1289–93.
66. Plosker GL, Goa KL. Clodronate: a review of its pharmacological properties and therapeutic efficacy in resorptive bone disease. *Drugs* 1994; **47:** 945–82.
67. Judson I, Booth F, Gore M, McElwain T. Chronic high dose pamidronate in refractory malignant hypercalcaemia. *Lancet* 1990; **i:** 802.
68. Mercadante S. Bowel obstruction in home care patients: 4 years' experience. *Support Care Cancer* 1995; **3:** 190–3.
69. Dvoretsky PM. Richards KA. Angel C. *et al.* Survival time, causes of death, and tumor/treatment-related morbidity in 100 women with ovarian cancer. *Hum Pathol* 1988; **19:** 1273–9.
70. ● Baines MJ. The pathophysiology and management of malignant intestinal obstruction. In: Doyle D, Hanks GW, MacDonald N eds. *Oxford Textbook of Palliative Medicine*. Oxford: Oxford University Press, 1998: 526.
71. Walsh HPJ, Schofield PF. Is laparotomy for small bowel obstruction justified in patients with previously treated malignancy? *Br J Surg* 1984; **71:** 933–5.
72. ● Parker MC, Baines MJ. Intestinal obstruction in patients with advanced cancer. *Br J Surg* 1996; **83:** 1–2.
73. ◆ Baines MJ, Oliver DJ, Carter RL. Medical management of intestinal obstruction in patients with advanced malignant disease: a clinical and pathological study. *Lancet* 1985; **ii:** 990–3.
74. Ventafridda V, Ripamonti C, Caraceni A, *et al.* The management of inoperable obstruction in terminal cancer patients. *Tumori* 1990; **76:** 389–93.
75. De Conno F, *et al.* Continuous subcutaneous infusion of hyoscine butylbromide reduces secretions in patients with gastrointestinal obstruction. *J Pain Symptom Manage* 1991; **6:** 484–6.
76. ● Feuer DJ, Broadley KE, Tate AT. *Systematic Review of the Management of Intestinal Obstruction due to Advanced Gynaecological and Intestinal Cancer*. London: NHS Executive, 1998.
77. Hardy J, Ling J, Mansi J, *et al.* Pitfalls in placebo-controlled trials in palliative care: dexamethasone for the palliation of malignant bowel obstruction. *Palliative Med* 1998; **12:** 437–42.
78. Sykes NP. The relationship between opioid use and laxative use in terminally ill cancer patients. *Palliative Med* 1998; **12:** 375–82.
79. Sykes NP. A volunteer model for the comparison of laxatives in opioid-induced constipation. *J Pain Symptom Manage* 1997; **11:** 363–9.
80. Culbert P, Gillett H, Ferguson A. Highly effective oral therapy (polyethylene glycol/electrolyte solution) for faecal impaction and severe constipation. *Clin Drug Invest* 1998; **16:** 355–60.
81. ● Ippoliti C. Antidiarrheal agents for the management of treatment-related diarrhea in cancer patients. *Am J Health-System Pharmacy* 1998; **55:** 1573–80.
82. Twycross RG, Lack SA. Diarrhoea. In: *Control of Alimentary Symptoms in Far Advanced Cancer*. London: Churchill Livingstone, 1986: 208–9.
83. de la Motte S, Bose-O'Reilly S, Heinisch M, Harrison F. Double-blind comparison of an apple pectin–chamomile extract preparation [in German]. *Arzneimittel-Forschung* 1997; **47:** 1247–9.
84. DuPont HL, Ericsson CD, DuPont MW, *et al.* A randomized, open-label comparison of non-prescription loperamide and attapulgite in the symptomatic treatment of acute diarrhea. *Am J Med* 1990; **88** (Suppl. 6A): 205–35.
85. ● Ruppin H. Review: loperamide – a potent antidiarrhoeal drug with actions along the alimentary tract. *Aliment Pharmacol Ther* 1987; **1:** 179–90.
86. Harris AG, O'Dorisio TM, Woltering EA, *et al.* Consensus statement: octreotide dose titration in secretory diarrhea: Diarrhea Management Consensus Panel. *Dig Dis Sci* 1995; **40:** 1464–73.
87. ● Billingsely KG, Alexander HR. The pathophysiology of cachexia in advanced cancer and AIDS. In: Bruera E, Higginson I eds. *Cachexia–Anorexia in Cancer Patients*. Oxford: Oxford University Press, 1996: 1–22.
88. ● Tisdale MJ. Biology of cachexia. *J Natl Cancer Inst* 1997; **89:** 1763–73.
89. Anker SD, Panikowski P, Varney S, *et al.* Wasting as independent risk factor for mortality in chronic heart failure. *Lancet* 1997; **349:** 1050–3.
90. Bruera E, MacDonald N. Nutrition in cancer patients: an update and review of our experience. *J Pain Symptom Manage* 1988; **3:** 133–40.
91. Wigmore SJ, Plester CE, Richardson RA, Fearon KC. Changes in nutritional status associated with unresectable pancreatic cancer *Br J Cancer* 1997; **75:** 106–9.
92. ● Dunlop RJ, Campbell CW. Cytokines and advanced cancer. *J Pain Symptom Manage* 2000; **20:** 214–32.
93. ● Fainsinger R. Pharmacological approach to cancer anorexia and cachexia. In: Bruera E, Higginson I eds. *Cachexia–Anorexia in Cancer Patients*. Oxford: Oxford University Press, 1996: 128–40.
94. Twycross R. Corticosteroids in advanced cancer: if they are not working stop them. *Br Med J* 1992; **305:** 969–70.
95. Vadell C, Segui MA, Gimenez-Arnau JM, *et al.* Anticachectic efficacy of megestrol acetate at different doses and versus placebo in patients with neoplastic cachexia. *Am J Clin Oncol* 1998; **21:** 347–51.
96. Simons JP, Schols AM, Hoefnagels JM, *et al.* Effects of medroxyprogesterone acetate on food intake, body composition, and resting energy expenditure in patients with advanced, nonhormone-sensitive cancer:

a randomised, placebo-controlled trial. *Cancer* 1998; **82:** 553–60.

97. Mantovani G, Maccio A, Esu S, *et al.* Medroxyprogesterone acetate reduces the in vitro production of cytokines and serotonin involved in anorexia/cachexia and emesis by peripheral blood mononuclear cells of cancer patients. *Eur J Cancer* 1997; **33:** 602–7.
98. Sanders-Bush E, Mayer SE. 5-hydroxytryptamine (serotonin) receptor agonists and antagonists. In: Hardman JG, Limbird LE, Molinoff PB, *et al.* eds. *The Pharmacological Basis of Therapeutics.* New York, NY: McGraw Hill, 1996.
99. Colombo G, Agabio R, Diaz G, *et al.* Appetite suppression and weight loss after the cannabinoid antagonists SR 141716. *Life Sci* 1998; **63:** PL113–17.

99a. Jatoi A, Windschitl HE, Loprinzi, *et al.* Dronabinol versus megestrol acetate versus combination therapy for cancer-associated anorexia: a North Central Cancer Treatment Group study. *J Clin Oncol* 2002; **20:** 567–73.

99b. Islam-Ali B, Khan S, Price SA, Tisdale MJ. Modulation of adipocyte G-protein expression in cancer cachexia by a lipid-mobilizing factor (LMF). *Br J Cancer* 2001; **85:** 758–63.

100. Strassman G, Kambayashi T. Inhibition of experimental cancer cachexia by anti-cytokine and anti-cytokine receptor therapy. *Cytokines Mol Ther* 1995; **1(2):** 107–13.
101. Smith EB, King CA, Baker MD. Crotamiton and pruritus. *Int J Dermatol* 1984; **23:** 684–5.
102. Tarng DC, Cho YL, Liu HN, Huang TP. Hemodialysis-related pruritus: a double-blind, placebo-controlled, crossover study of capsaicin 0.025% cream. *Nephron* 1996; **72:** 617–22.
103. Monk BE. Transcutaneous electronic nerve stimulation in the treatment of generalised pruritus. *Clin Exp Dermatol* 1993; **18:** 67–8.
104. Leven A, Naysmith A, Pickens S, Pottage A. Sodium cromoglycate and Hodgkin's disease. *Br Med J* 1997; **2:** 896.
105. Smith PF, Corelli RL. Doxepin in the management of pruritus associated with allergic cutaneous reactions. *Ann Pharmacother* 1997; **31:** 633–5.
106. Zylicz Z, Smits C, Krajnik M. Paroxetine for pruritus in advanced cancer. *J Pain Symptom Manage* 1998; **16:** 121–4.
107. Price TJ, Patterson WK, Olver IN. Rifampicin as a treatment for pruritus in malignant cholestasis. *Support Care Cancer* 1998; **6:** 533–5.
108. Walt RP, Daneshmend TK, Fellows IW, Toghill PJ. Effect of stanozolol on itching in primary biliary cirrhosis. *Br Med J* 1988; **296:** 607.
109. Balaskas EV, Bamihas GI, Karamouzis G, Tourkantonis A. Histamine and serotonin in uremic pruritus: effect of ondansetron in CAPD-pruritic patients. *Nephron* 1998; **78:** 395–402.
110. Marchi S, Cechin E, Villalta D, *et al.* Relief of pruritus and decreases in plasma histamine concentrations during erythropoietin therapy in patients with uremia. *N Engl J Med* 1992; **326:** 969–74.
111. Borgeat A, Stirnemann HR. Ondansetron is effective to treat spinal or epidural morphine-induced pruritus. *Anesthesiology* 1999; **90:** 432–6.
112. Loprinzi CL, *et al.* Megestrol acetate for the prevention of hot flushes. *N Engl J Med* 1994; **331:** 347–52.
113. Tsavaris N, *et al.* A randomised trial of the effects of three non-steroidal anti-inflammatory agents in ameliorating cancer induced fever. *J Intern Med* 1990; **228:** 451–5.
114. Loprinzi CL, Michalak JC, Quella SK, *et al.* Megestrol acetate for the prevention of hot flashes. *N Engl J Med* 1994; **331:** 347–52.
115. Regnard C. Use of low dose thioridazine to control sweating in advanced cancer. *Palliative Med* 1996; **10:** 78–9.
116. Harrison J, Maguire P. Predictors of psychiatric morbidity in cancer patients. *Br J Psychiatry* 1994, **165:** 593–8.
117. Lishman WA. *Organic Psychiatry: The Psychological Consequences of Cerebral Disorder,* 3rd edn. Oxford: Blackwell Science, 1997: 744.
118. Harris EC, Barraclough BM. Suicide as an outcome for medical disorders. *Medicine* 1995; **73:** 281–96.
119. Moadel AB, Ostroff JS, Schanz SP. Head and neck cancer. In: Holland JC ed. *Psycho-oncology.* New York, NY: Oxford University Press, 1998: 314–23.
120. Spiegel D. Health caring: psychosocial support for patients with cancer. *Cancer* 1994; **74:** 1453–7.
121. McDaniel JS, Musselmann DL, Porter MR, *et al.* Depression in patients with cancer. *Archiv Gen Psychiatry* 1995, **52:** 89–99.

◆122. Endicott J. Measurement of depression in patients with cancer. *Cancer* 1983, **53:** 2243–8.

◆123. Cohen-Cole SA, Brown FW, McDaniel JS. Diagnostic assessment of depression in the medically ill. In: Stoudemire A, Fogel B eds. *Psychiatric Care of the Medical Patient.* New York, NY: Oxford University Press, 1993: 199–212.

123a. Chochinov HM, Wilson KG, Enns M, Lander S. "Are you depressed?" Screening for depression in the terminally ill. *Am J Psychiatry* 1997; **154:** 674–6.

124. Faull CM, Johnson IS, Butler TJ. The hospital anxiety and depression (HAD) scale: its validity in patients with terminal malignant disease. *Palliative Med* 1994; **8:** 69.
125. Urch CE, Chamberlain J, Field G. The drawback of the Hospital Anxiety and Depression Scale in the assessment of depression in hospice inpatients. *Palliative Med* 1998; **12:** 395–6.
126. Le Fevre P, Devereux J, Smith S, *et al.* Screening for psychiatric illness in the palliative care inpatient setting: a comparison between the Hospital Anxiety and Depression Scale and the General Health Questionnaire-12. *Palliative Med* 1999; **13:** 399–407.

127. Porter MR, Musselman DL, McDaniel JS, Nemeroff CB. From sadness to major depression: assessment and management in patients with cancer. In: Portenoy RK, Bruera E eds. *Topics in Palliative Care,* vol. 3. New York, NY: Oxford University Press, 1998: 193.

●128. Breitbart W, Chochinov HM, Passik S. Psychiatric aspects of palliative care In: Doyle D, Hanks GWC, MacDonald N eds. *Oxford Textbook of Palliative Medicine,* 2nd edn. Oxford: Oxford Medical Publications, 1998: 937.

●129. ◆ Fawzy IF, Fawzy NW, Arndt LA, Pasnau RO. Critical review of psychosocial intervention in cancer care. *Archiv Gen Psychiatry* 1995; **52:** 100–13.

●130. ◆ Sellick SM, Crooks DL. Depression and cancer: an appraisal of the literature for prevalence, detection, and practical guideline development for psychological interventions. *Psycho-oncology* 1999; **8:** 315–33.

●131. Kalash GR: Psychotropic drug metabolism in the cancer patient: clinical aspects of management of potential drug interactions. *Psycho-oncology* 1998; **7:** 307–20.

●132. Gill D, Hatcher S. Antidepressants for depression in medical illness. *Cochrane Database Syst Rev* 2000; **4:** CD001312.

133. Roth AJ, Breitbart W. Psychiatric emergencies in terminally ill cancer patients. *Haematology/Oncology Clin N Am* 1996, **10:** 235–59.

●134. Noyes R, Holt CS, Massie MJ. Anxiety disorders. In: Holland JC ed. *Psycho-oncology.* New York, NY: Oxford University Press, 1998: 551.

135. Passik SD, Roth AJ. Anxiety symptoms and panic attacks preceding pancreatic cancer diagnosis. *Psycho-oncology* 1999, **8:** 268–72.

136. Lloyd-Williams M, Friedman T, Rudd N. Information needs and levels of anxiety and depression in last weeks of life. *Psycho-Oncology* 1998; **7:** abstract no. 304.

●137. Twillman RK, Manetto C. Concurrent psychotherapy and pharmacotherapy in the treatment of depression and anxiety in cancer patients. *Psycho-oncology* 1998; **7:** 285–90.

◆138. Moorey S, Greer S, Watson M, *et al.* Adjuvant psychological therapy for patients with cancer: outcome at 1 year. *Psycho-oncology* 1994; **3:** 39–46.

139. Moorey S, Greer S, Bliss J, Law M. A comparison of adjuvant psychological therapy and supportive counselling in patients with cancer. *Psycho-oncology* 1998; **7:** 218–28.

140. Gelder M, Gath D, Mayou R, Cowen P. *Oxford Textbook of Psychiatry*, 3rd edn. Oxford: Oxford University Press, 1996: 169.

141. Santosh K, Chaturvedi MD, Prabha S, Chandra MD. Rationale of psychotropic medications in palliative care. *Progr Palliative Care* 1996; **4(3):** 80–4.

●142. Breitbart W, Cohen CR. Delirium. In: Holland JC ed. *Psycho-oncology.* New York, NY: Oxford University Press, 1998: 564.

◆143. Inouye SK, Bogardus ST, Charpentier PA, *et al.* A multicomponent intervention to prevent delirium in hospitalised *N Engl J Med* 1999; **340:** 669–76.

◆144. American Psychiatric Association Practice Guidelines: practice guideline for the treatment of patients with delirium. *Am J Psychiatry* 1999; **156** (5 Suppl.): 1–20.

145. McNamara P, Minton M, Twycross RG. Use of midazolam in palliative care. *Palliative Med* 1991; **5:** 244–9.

146. Herth K. Fostering hope in terminally ill people. *J Advanced Nursing* 1990; **15:** 1250–9.

147. Dunlop RJ, Hockley JM, Davies RJ. Preferred versus actual place of death – a Hospital Terminal Care Support Team experience. *Palliative Med* 1989; **3:** 197–201.

◆148. Hinton J. Which patients with terminal cancer are admitted from home care? *Palliative Med* 1994; **8:** 197–210.

●149. Portenoy RK, Southam MA, Gupta SK, *et al.* Transdermal fentanyl for cancer pain. *Anesthesiology* 1993; **78:** 36–43.

23

Painful procedures

COLIN CAMPBELL AND POLLY EDMONDS

Medical procedures are an increasing component in the investigation and treatment of malignant disease. This chapter will identify strategies for minimizing the distress caused by procedures such as intravenous cannulation, ascitic/pleural drainage, biopsies, bone marrow aspiration, and the dressing of malignant wounds.

BACKGROUND

Incidence of pain associated with procedures

There is evidence that procedure-associated pain is poorly managed and that this may contribute to the psychological distress associated with a diagnosis of cancer.[1–8] Between 30% and 80% of adults report that the level of analgesia provided for acute and postoperative pain is inadequate,[8–10] but the frequency of procedure-associated pain is less well documented. However, in a study of 190 patients undergoing lower gastrointestinal investigations, 85% reported moderate or severe pain during colonoscopy and 46% during double-contrast barium enema.[11]

In a pediatric oncology clinic, children also rated common procedures as moderately or severely painful: venipuncture (49%), lumbar puncture (62%), and bone marrow aspiration (73%) (Figs 23.1 and 23.2).[2] In the same study, only 25% of children reported that the disease itself was a source of severe pain.

Provision of analgesia

Procedure-associated pain may be compounded by a lack of provision of appropriate analgesia. In a national survey, 65% of 144 American practitioners in pediatric hematology/oncology reported they did not routinely use any premedication for bone marrow aspirations or biopsies.[5] In a further study of 29 Pediatric Oncology Group institutions, only 12% always used premedicating drugs before bone marrow aspirations, and only 7% for lumbar puncture.[12] In contrast, over 90% of all upper gastrointestinal endoscopies in the UK are conducted under intravenous sedation, usually with a benzodiazepine.[13] Sedation is also commonly used for radiological procedures such as nephrostomy insertion (76%) and biliary drainage (66%).[14]

DEVELOPING MANAGEMENT PLANS FOR PROCEDURE-RELATED PAIN

Table 23.1 outlines the common medical procedures that can cause pain and suggested interventions to manage that pain. A structured approach to managing procedural pain is outlined below and described in more detail in the text.

- *Assess* the potential for the procedure to cause pain and anxiety.
- *Assess* the needs of the individual patient.
- *Prepare* the patient (and parents, in the case of children).
- *Explain* what will happen in the procedure.

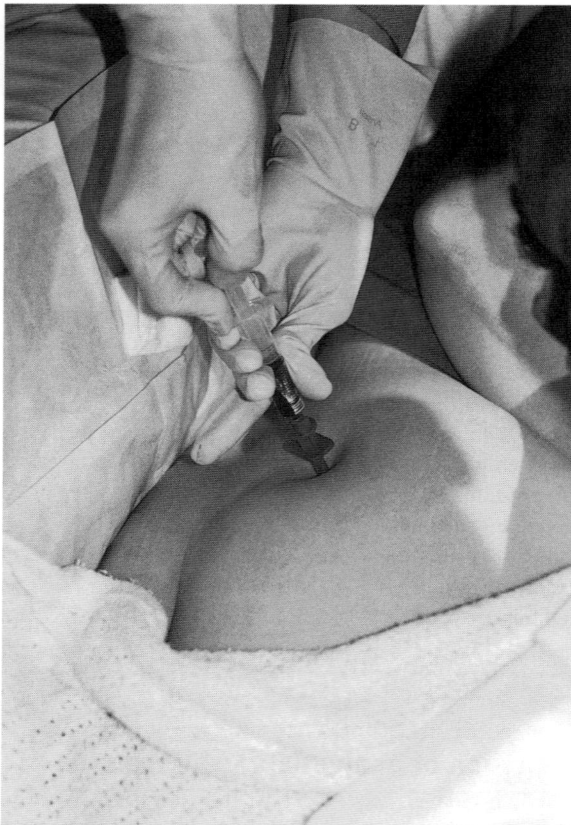

Figure 23.1 *Intrathecal administration of chemotherapy.*

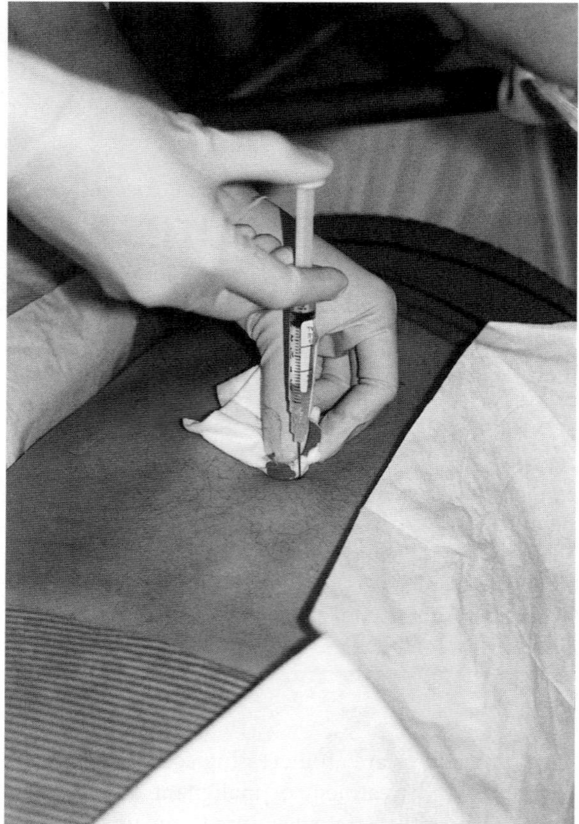

Figure 23.2 *Bone marrow aspiration.*

- *Consider nonpharmacological interventions.*
- *Consider pharmacological interventions.*

Assessing the needs of the individual patient

Although most procedures will cause a degree of pain, contributing factors to be considered include patient anxiety, relative anxiety, learned behavior from previous procedures, patient expectations, and staff experience. These are summarized in Table 23.2.

Preparing the patient and explaining the procedure

Explanation of a procedure has been shown to be beneficial in both adults and children.[15,16] Where procedures are likely to be repeated, appropriate management of pain and anxiety with the first procedure may reduce distress in subsequent procedures.[3,17] Other factors have been shown to be useful: preparing parents with a specific role is recommended for children,[15] and behavioral management techniques in adults have been shown to improve a number of postoperative variables, including pain, pain medication, negative affect, and overall patient satisfaction.[16] In many situations, a combination of pain management techniques will be required.[18] In particular, children should be matched to the most appropriate intervention for them, based on predictive factors such as age, coping style, or preference .[19]

Hierarchies of interventions that can be utilized to manage procedural pain are as follows:

- nonpharmacological interventions
  - relaxation
  - hypnosis
  - cognitive–behavioral therapy
  - distraction techniques
- local anesthetics
  - topical anesthesia
  - topical opioids
- nonsteroidal anti-inflammatory drugs
- conscious or deep sedation
  - sedative drugs
  - opioids.

NONPHARMACOLOGICAL INTERVENTIONS FOR PROCEDURE-ASSOCIATED PAIN

A number of nonpharmacological techniques have been used to reduce anxiety-related pain.[20,21] Broadly, these are

Table 23.1 *Common medical procedures causing pain in cancer patients*

Procedure	Suggested intervention
Mild to moderate pain	
Venipuncture	Topical anesthesia with EMLA or amethocaine
Intravenous cannula insertion	Topical anesthesia with EMLA or amethocaine
Arterial blood sampling	Intradermal infiltration with 1% lidocaine (lignocaine)
Fine-needle aspiration of breast lumps	Local anesthetic infiltration with 1% lidocaine
Abdominal paracentesis	Local anesthetic infiltration with 1% lidocaine
Pleural aspiration	Local anesthetic infiltration with 1% lidocaine
Urinary catheterization	Local anesthetic instillation with or without midazolam
Moderate to severe pain	
Lumbar puncture	Local anesthetic infiltration with or without nonpharmacological intervention; in children with or without conscious sedation with: midazolam + meperidine (pethidine) or OTFC or propofol + fentanyl
Bone marrow aspiration	Local anesthetic infiltration with or without nonpharmacological intervention; in children with or without conscious sedation with: midazolam + meperidine or OTFC or propofol + fentanyl
Gastrointestinal endoscopy (colonoscopy more painful than gastroscopy)	Conscious sedation with midazolam or propofol + meperidine, fentanyl or alfentanil. Titrate with additional boluses if required
Radiological interventions (urological/biliary)	Conscious sedation with midazolam or propofol + meperidine, fentanyl, or alfentanil. Titrate with additional boluses if required
Painful dressing (malignant wounds, pressure sores, debridement)	Conscious sedation with midazolam + meperidine with or without topical opioid or OTFC

As pain perception is influenced by many variables, it is unhelpful to give rigid guidelines. The suggested interventions reflect the authors' opinion of what constitutes practicable advice.
When using conscious sedation, there are recommended procedures regarding safety, including patient monitoring by a trained member of the team other than the person conducting the procedure. See text for details.
In children, anxious adults, and those in whom procedures will be repeated, aggressive analgesic interventions will be indicated earlier, including conscious sedation where appropriate.
OTFC, oral transmucosal fentanyl citrate.

Table 23.2 *Assessment of the individual patient*

Patient factors	Clinical relevance
Children	Ability to understand the procedure varies according to the child's developmental stage Dose and type of drug may vary according to age/weight[15] Parent/guardian's anxiety, and their role in supporting the child[17]
Elderly	Often coexisting medical conditions Multiple medications Declining renal function with potential for opioid accumulation
Repeated procedures	Tendency for increasing anxiety, especially if first procedure is distressing Potential for drug accumulation if short intervals between procedures Interference with feeding if fasting required before sedation
Psychological	Anticipation of pain heightens anxiety Fear associated with life-threatening illness Issues around sense of control

categorized as relaxation techniques, hypnosis, cognitive and behavioral therapy, and distraction.

Relaxation techniques

Successful relaxation is associated with decreased autonomic arousal and decreased skeletal muscle tension, which may reduce pain perception.[20] It is also a form of distraction. There is no universal method of inducing relaxation, or of defining what is a relaxation technique. In a meta-analysis of randomized controlled trials, relaxation had a beneficial effect on postoperative pain in three out of seven studies, but only 4 out of 12 studies showed an analgesic-sparing effect.[16***] A recent systematic review of randomized controlled trials involving 362 patients also suggested significant benefit in acute pain syndromes.[22***]

Hypnosis

Hypnosis is characterized by intense imaginative involvement (compared with relaxation alone). In children, it can reduce pain and anxiety associated with bone marrow aspiration and lumbar puncture.[23*] In adults, the evidence supporting efficacy is less clear: in a review of studies examining procedural pain, Spanos[24*] found that hypnotic interventions were more effective than no treatment for relieving pain. However, two studies comparing hypnotic with nonhypnotic suggestions failed to demonstrate that hypnosis was more effective.

Cognitive and behavioral therapy

Cognitive–behavioral therapy (CBT) treats internal thoughts as behavior that can be modified, which in turn may influence the perception of pain.[20] CBT may achieve an 18–50% reduction in procedure-related distress in children[25–27] but is of limited applicability to very young children (lower age limits 3–7) and in those with severe developmental delay.[28] A random-order crossover trial compared CBT with general anesthesia in 18 children with leukemia requiring repeated bone marrow aspirations. There were no significant differences between the treatments in self-reported fear or fearful anticipation of the next bone marrow aspiration.[19*]

Distraction techniques

Distraction focuses on stimuli other than pain, and may involve objects in the treatment area or bodily sensations.[12] Some form of distraction is an integral part of most procedures, but more innovative measures include the presence of a companion dog[29] and the playing of video films.[30] The efficacy of distraction remains unproven.

LOCAL ANESTHESIA AND TOPICAL ANALGESIA FOR PROCEDURAL PAIN

Local anesthetic infiltration

Local anesthetic infiltration will provide effective analgesia for many minor procedures. All local anesthetic agents exert their effect by causing a reversible block to conduction along nerve fibers.

Suitable preparations include lidocaine (lignocaine) 0.5%, 1%, and 2% and prilocaine 0.5%, 1%, 2%, and 4%.

Clinical tips

- Allow the liquid to reach room temperature, and allow 5–10 min after infiltration for optimum numbness.
- Toxicity initially results in light-headedness and sedation, but convulsions and cardiovascular collapse have been reported in cases of inadvertent intravenous injection. Severe toxic reactions are rare but constitute a theoretical risk following accumulation in procedures that require repeated local anesthetic.

Topical local anesthesia

These preparations can be useful for minimizing the pain of venipuncture and intravenous cannulation.

Preparations

EMLA® (Eutectic Mixture of Local Anesthetics) is an equal mix of the local anesthetics lidocaine and prilocaine, which form an oil at temperatures greater than 16°C (Fig. 23.3).[31] Table 23.3 summarizes the available evidence in support of its use.

- EMLA cream is effective in providing dermal anesthesia/analgesia.[32–35*,37–39]
- The cream is applied as a 2-mm-thick layer under an occlusive dressing
- EMLA requires at least 1 h of application to effect local anesthesia.
- In pretreatment topical analgesia, EMLA has a similar efficacy to ethyl chloride spray and lidocaine infiltration.[39]

EMLA should be avoided in infants because of the risk of methemoglobinemia.[37,40]

Amethocaine is available in the UK as a single-use 4% gel.[40] It has a faster onset and longer duration of action than EMLA.[41*,42*]

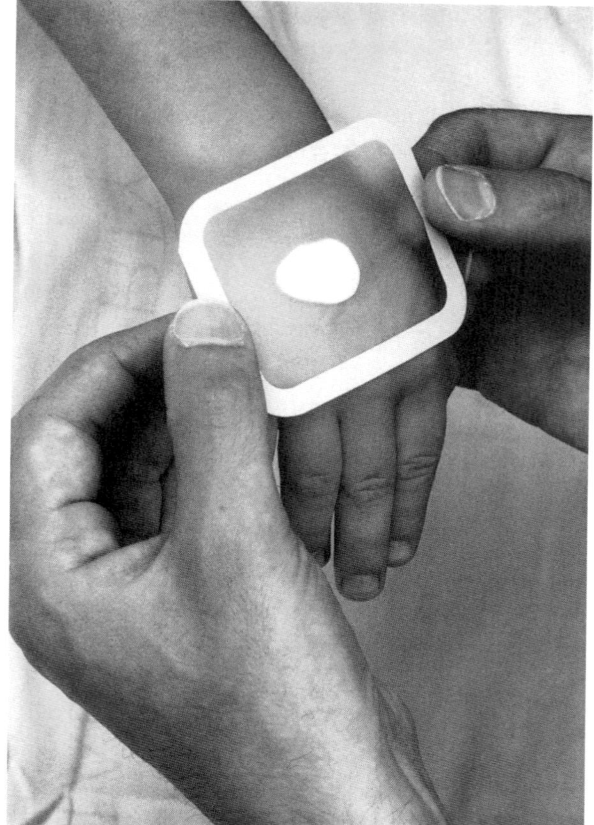

Figure 23.3 *EMLA patch.*

- Erythema, edema, and pruritus have been reported in association with its use.[41]
- Amethocaine requires 35–60 min for clinical effect.[41,42]

Clinical tips

Consider topical anesthesia:

- if the patient has a "needle phobia;"
- in children;
- if venous cannulation will have to be repeated regularly.

Points to consider

- Topical local anesthetics tend to cause vasodilation, facilitating systemic absorption, and therefore should be avoided in wounds and mucous membranes.

Topical opioids

There are case reports of the analgesic effects of topical opioids in the management of malignant wounds.[43,44] The opioid is added to a ready-mixed hydrogel wound dressing and applied daily. It is postulated that peripheral opioid receptors are activated by inflammatory changes in tissues.

NONSTEROIDAL ANTI-INFLAMMATORY DRUGS (NSAIDS) AND PROCEDURAL PAIN

Where procedural pain has an inflammatory component, NSAIDs may have a useful role. They may be considered before pleural aspirations and dressing malignant wounds, especially if sedation is not desired. In a systematic review of 35 trials of acute pain, ibuprofen showed a clear dose–reponse with a similar efficacy to diclofenac.[45]*** One out of every three patients treated with ibuprofen 400 mg will experience at least 50% pain relief compared with placebo, an analgesic effect that compares favorably with that of single-dose opioids.[46,47]***

CONSCIOUS SEDATION FOR PROCEDURAL PAIN

The principal aims of sedation are to relieve anxiety, to enable cooperation, and to produce some degree of amnesia.[48] Procedures that are likely to cause moderate to severe pain will require the concomitant use of analgesics. In conscious sedation, the patient maintains a response to physical stimuli and/or verbal command. The intended benefits are as follows:[15,17,49,50]

- Protective reflexes are maintained.
- The patient retains the ability to maintain a patent airway independently and continuously.
- Loss of consciousness should be unlikely with the drugs/techniques used.

The 1992 Joint Working Party of the Royal College of Anaesthetists and the Royal College of Radiologists of the UK recommend that, when any significant degree of sedation is likely, an appropriately trained assistant should monitor the patient and manage any complications of excessive sedation, including apneic episodes.[14]

Coexisting medical problems that may make conscious sedation hazardous include diabetes, morbid obesity, heart disease, old age, hepatic disease, renal disease, concurrent drug administration, and sedation within 2 h of eating.[18,49]

Serious complications of sedation are uncommon but there is no room for complacency. A survey by the American Society for Gastrointestinal Endoscopy found that, of 21,000 procedures, the incidence of serious cardiorespiratory complications and death with midazolam or diazepam was, respectively, 5.4 and 0.3 per thousand procedures.[51]

Route of drug administration for conscious sedation

The *intravenous* (i.v.) route has the following advantages:[17,18,53]

Table 23.3 *Clinical trials of EMLA for vinepuncture/cannulation*

Reference	No. of patients	Study design	Trial drug	Control drug	Pain assessment	Results
Maunuksela and Korpela[31]*	60 children	Double-blind	EMLA cream	Placebo	Child and anesthetist using verbal rating and two pictorial scales	Significantly better results with EMLA
Nilsson *et al.*[32]*	60 children	Open randomized	EMLA patch	EMLA cream	Patient (VAS), investigator (verbal rating scale)	No significant difference in pain between patch and cream
Hallen *et al.*[33]*	31 adults	Double-blind, randomized, crossover	EMLA cream	Placebo	10-cm VAS	28 out of 31 subjects had a reduction in VAS score with EMLA
Vaghadia et *al.*[34]*	51 adults	Randomized, double-blind	EMLA patch	Placebo patch	VAS	Significant analgesic benefit with EMLA
Molodeckas *et al.*[35]*	120 women	Double-blind	EMLA cream	Amethocaine cream	VAS	Good analgesic effect – no statistical difference between the two preparations
Lurngnateepate *et al.*[436]*	60 children	Randomized, double-blind	EMLA cream	Placebo cream	Investigator + two methods by children	No statistical difference in pain between EMLA and placebo (most children had mild or no pain with venipuncture)

- Onset of action is rapid.
- There is ease of access.
- In many hematological malignancies, thrombocytopenia prevents the use of other parenteral routes.
- An initial bolus can be followed by a top-up dose if required.
- Continuous background infusion can be given, titrated to patient response.

The main disadvantage is the narrow safety margin between adequate analgesia and toxic side-effects, necessitating close patient supervision.[18]

The *oral transmucosal* route has the advantage that it avoids a painful injection, and there is increasing interest in this route, particularly for children.

Precautions for monitoring conscious sedation are summarized in Table 23.4.

Sedative drugs for procedural pain

As yet, there is no consensus on which drugs to use in which procedure. A 1991 study of UK and Irish radiologists found that 71% used diazepam and 48% midazolam for procedure-related anxiety.[14] The use of diazepam was surprising as this drug's long half-life may delay emergence from procedural sedation.

The short-acting benzodiazepine drugs lorazepam and midazolam are useful for procedure-related anxiety, but they should not be seen as an alternative to analgesics.[52]

Midazolam reduces anxiety and, in therapeutic doses, provides amnesia. Coadministration with an opioid substantially increases the risk of producing respiratory depression compared with either drug alone.[17]

Lorazepam, 0.5–1 mg sublingually, is given 30 min to 1 h before a procedure, and usually does not impair cooperativeness.

Table 23.4 *Monitoring conscious sedation*

During the procedure[15,17,49,50]

All patient recordings and drugs administered should be documented

Continuous monitoring of oxygen saturation (e.g. pulse oximetry) and heart rate, and intermittent recording of respiratory rate and blood pressure are essential

After the procedure

The patient should be observed with the following equipment available:

- functioning suction apparatus
- a means of delivering >90% oxygen and positive-pressure ventilation, e.g. bag and mask
- laryngoscope for laryngeal intubation

Before being discharged, the patient should be easily rousable with protective reflexes intact

Propofol is a short-acting intravenous anesthetic agent and, after an initial bolus, the dose can be accurately titrated against response. It has been used to provide sedation along with fentanyl and midazolam in patients receiving extracorporeal lithotripsy for calculus therapy.[54]

In a prospective study of 274 patients undergoing gastrointestinal endoscopies, patients receiving propofol and fentanyl experienced better comfort and more sedation than those receiving midazolam and meperidine (pethidine).[55]

In a randomized trial of 66 patients, patients received either propofol and alfentanil in a patient-controlled pump or a single intravenous injection of diazepam and meperidine. Those using the patient-controlled sedation with propofol had lighter sedation and faster recovery times.[56]

Propofol has the advantage that induction is rapid and the patient emerges from sedation rapidly and with a clear head.[28] Its disadvantages are that published experience with the drug in this context still limited and it is associated with a higher incidence of transient apnea than ketamine.[57]

Strong opioids for procedural pain

Strong opioids are the drugs of choice for the more severe procedural pains and are probably underutilized. The ideal analgesic for procedural pain would have a rapid onset but short duration of action, consistent with many opioid analgesics. The main drawback to using opioids for procedural pain is the need to closely monitor and manage side-effects, especially respiratory depression.[15,18,49,50] This may be potentiated by the concurrent use of benzodiazepines.[49,50] Opioid-induced respiratory depression can potentially be reversed by administration of the opioid antagonist naloxone.

Meperidine (pethidine)

Meperidine is still used for many painful procedures, although there is a growing tendency to use the fentanyl group of opioids. Meperidine has a more rapid onset of action than morphine, and a short half-life of 2–3 h. It is less suitable for patients regularly taking high doses of strong opioids as the maximum recommended dose of meperidine will provide inadequate analgesia.

When using meperidine it is necessary to be aware of the following:

- Accumulation of the metabolite, normeperidine (norpethidine), can cause hyperexcitability, twitching, and convulsions. The risk is increased in patients with renal failure and with procedures that need to be repeated over a period of hours or days.
- Meperidine should be avoided in patients taking monoamine oxidase inhibitors because of the risk of precipitating a hypertensive crisis.

Fentanyl, sufentanil, and alfentanil

These synthetic opioids are more potent and selective for the μ-opioid receptor than meperidine.[58] Their lipophilic nature results in rapid uptake into the central nervous system (CNS). Whether given intravenously or by the oral transmucosal route, there is rapid onset of analgesia and sedation, with short duration of action. All the recommended precautions for conscious sedation are applicable.

A loading i.v. bolus dose of fentanyl or alfentanil is given pre-emptively, followed by either a continuous infusion (because of the short duration of action) or top-up doses, titrated to the patient response.

Oral transmucosal fentanyl citrate (OTFC) is produced in a sweetened matrix lozenge and sucked 30–60 min before the procedure. The lozenge comes in several strengths to accommodate different requirements. OTFC has been successfully used for many different painful procedures, including lumbar puncture, bone marrow aspiration,[59] and dermatological procedures.[60]

The advantages of OTFC are that injection is unnecessary, increasing patient tolerance, especially in children, and that it provides dose-related opioid analgesia and anxiolysis. It has the disadvantage[59–61] that vomiting is common (incidence 30–45%), although routine antiemetic medication may avoid this problem. In addition, pruritus during the induction period is common.

Dextromoramide (Palfium)

A potent agonist at the μ-opioid receptor and in clinical practice in cancer, dextromoramide has a more rapid onset of action and shorter duration of action than oral morphine.[62] Large interindividual variations in the absorption of the drug sublingually, with a half-life of up to 23 h, may limit its use.[63] Dextromoramide is available in 5- and 10-mg tablets, to be administered sublingually. It is useful for providing analgesia during painful wound dressings but tolerance to its analgesic effects may develop.

OTHER DRUGS USED FOR PROCEDURE-RELATED ANALGESIA

Nitrous oxide mixture (Entonox)

Entonox has been used during debridement of wounds and dressing changes,[64,65] during colonoscopy,[66] and during percutaneous liver biopsy.[67] Its advantages include:

- Onset and recovery are rapid.
- It produces analgesia approximately 20 s after the onset of inhalation, peaking at about 40 s to 2 min.[64]
- Cardiovascular effects are minimal.
- It is self-administered, so the mask will drop away if the patient becomes somnolent.[17]

The disadvantages of Entonox include:

- It causes excitability or drowsiness at higher concentrations.
- It is contraindicated in some pulmonary diseases. Because nitrous oxide diffuses into air-containing closed spaces, with a resulting increase in pressure, it should not be used in the presence of a pneumothorax, chronic pulmonary disease, or bullous lung disease.[17]
- It has the potential to induce bone marrow suppression, especially with chronic use.[64]

Ketamine

This is an anesthetic/analgesic agent that largely spares laryngeal reflexes.[68] It has been shown to have analgesic efficacy in subanesthetic doses for the management of painful burns dressings[64,69] and for painful procedures in pediatric cancer units,[68**,70*] and in accident and emergency units.[71*] Psychomimetic side-effects may be troublesome, especially in adults.[69] The advantages of ketamine include:

- It has a rapid onset of action and produces a state of conscious sedation in which patients respond to verbal commands and maintain airways reflexes but experience analgesia.[17]
- There is no need to avoid eating/drinking for long periods before or after the procedure.
- It does not cause respiratory depression in subanesthetic doses.[65]

Its disadvantages are:

- Tolerance to repeated doses develops rapidly.
- Potential psychomimetic emergence reactions on recovery from sedation occur in 0–30%.[68,69,71]

FUTURE DIRECTIONS

Within the last 10 years, there has been a heightened professional awareness of the need to provide effective analgesia for painful procedures. Yet practice still varies widely in different specialist centers, and even in units routinely offering pre-emptive analgesia/sedation there is no consistency in use of drugs or nonpharmacological interventions. There are still many unsatisfactory areas meriting research. In particular:

- What is the incidence and severity of pain experienced by adults undergoing different painful procedures?
- What are the factors hindering practitioners from ensuring good procedural analgesia?
- What are the optimum analgesic drug(s) for each of the common painful procedures?
- Is propofol going to supersede midazolam as the sedating drug of choice?

REFERENCES

1. Miser AW, Dothage JA, Wesley RA, Miser JS. The prevalence of pain in a paediatric and young adult cancer population. *Pain* 1987; **29:** 73–83.
2. McGrath PJ, Hsu E, Cappelli M, *et al.* Pain from pediatric cancer: a survey of an outpatient oncology clinic. *J Psychosoc Oncol* 1990; **8(2/3):** 109–24.
3. Weisman SJ, Bernstein B, Schechter NL. Consequences of inadequate analgesia during painful procedures in children. *Archiv Pediatr Adolescent Med* 1998; **152:** 147–9.
4. Klein ER. Premedicating children for painful invasive procedures. *J Pediatr Oncol Nursing* 1992; **9(4):** 170–9.
5. Bernstein B, Schechter NL, Hickman T, Beck A. Premedication for painful procedures in children: a national survey [Abstract]. *J Pain Symptom Manage* 1991; **6:** 190.
6. MacLellan K. A chart audit reviewing the prescription and administration trends of analgesia and the documentation of pain, after surgery. *J Advanced Nursing* 1997; **26:** 345–50.
7. Oates JDL, Snowdon SL, Jayson DWH. Failure of pain relief after surgery. Attitudes of ward staff and patients to postoperative analgesia. *Anaesthesia* 1994; **49:** 755–8.
8. Bostrom BM, Ramberg T, Davis BD, Fridlund B. Survey of post-operative patients' pain management. *J Nursing Manage* 1997; **5:** 341–9.
9. Kuhn S, Cooke K, Collins M, *et al.* Perceptions of pain relief after surgery. *Br Med J* 1990; **300:** 1687–90.
10. Owen H, McMillan V, Rogowski D. Postoperative pain therapy: a survey of patients' expectations and their experiences. *Pain* 1990; **41:** 303–7.
11. Steine S. Which hurts the most? A comparison of pain rating during double-contrast barium enema examination and colonoscopy. *Radiology* 1994; **191:** 99–101.
12. Hockenberry MJ, Bologna-Vaughan S. Preparation for intrusive procedures using noninvasive techniques in children with cancer: state of the art vs. new trends. *Cancer Nursing* 1985; **8(2):** 97–102.
13. Daneshmend TK, Bell GD, Logan RFA. Sedation for upper gastrointestinal endoscopy: results of a nationwide survey. *Gut* 1991; **32:** 12–15.
14. McDermott VGM, Chapman ME, Gillespie I. Sedation and patient monitoring in vascular and interventional radiology. *Br J Radiol* 1993; **66:** 667–71.
15. ● Zeltzer LK, Altman A, Cohen D, *et al.* Report of the subcommittee on the management of pain associated with procedures in children with cancer. *Pediatrics* 1990; **865:** 826–31.
16. ● Johnstone M, Vogele C. Benefits of psychological preparation for surgery: a meta-analysis. *Ann Behav Med* 1993; **15:** 245–56.
17. ● Agency for Health Care Policy and Research (AHCPR) 1992 Acute pain management: operative or medical procedures and trauma, part 2. *Clin Pharmacy* 1992; **11:** 391–413.
18. Justins DM, Richardson PH. Clinical management of acute pain. *Br Med Bull* 1991; **47:** 561–83.
19. Jay S, Elliott CH, Fitzgibbons, *et al.* A comparative study of cognitive behavior therapy versus general anesthesia for painful procedures in children. *Pain* 1995; **62:** 3–9.
20. ● Horn S, Munafo M. Interventions. In: Payne S, Horn S, series eds. *Pain: Theory, Research and Intervention.* Buckingham: Open University Press, 1997: 113–29.
21. DePalma MT, Weisse CS. Psychological influences on pain perception and non-pharmacologic approaches to the treatment of pain. *J Hand Ther* 1997; **10:** 183–91.
22. ● Seers K, Carroll D. Relaxation techniques for acute pain management: a systematic review. *J Advanced Nursing* 1998; **27:** 466–75.
23. Zeltzer L, LeBaron S. Hypnosis and nonhypnotic techniques for reduction of pain and anxiety during painful procedures in children and adolescents with cancer. *Behav Pediatr* 1982; **101:** 1032–5.
24. ● Spanos NP, Carmanico SJ, Ellis JA. Hypnotic analgesia. In: Wall PD, Melzack R eds. *Textbook of Pain,* 3rd edn. Edinburgh: Churchill Livingstone, 1994: 1349–66.
25. Jay SM, Elliott CH, Ozolins M, Pruitt C. Behavioral management of children's distress during painful medical procedures. *Behav Res Ther* 1985; **23:** 513–20.
26. Jay SM, Elliott CH, Katz ER, Siegel S. Cognitive-behavioral and pharmacologic interventions for children undergoing painful procedures. *J Clin Psychol* 1987; **55:** 860–5.
27. McCarthy AM, Cool VA, Hanrahan K. Cognitive behavioral interventions for children during painful procedures: research challenges and program development. *J Pediatr Nursing* 1998; **13:** 55–63.
28. Berde C. Pediatric oncology procedures: to sleep or perchance to dream? *Pain* 1995; **62:** 1–2.
29. Nagengast SL, Baun MM, Megel M, Leibowitz JM. The effects of the presence of a companion animal on physiological arousal and behavioral distress in children during a physical examination. *J Pediatr Nursing* 1997; **12:** 323–30.
30. Miller AC, Hickman LC, Lemasters GK. A distraction technique for control of burn pain. *J Burn Care Rehabil* 1992; **13:** 576–80.
31. Maunuksela E-L, Korpela R. Double-blind evaluation of a lignocaine–prilocaine cream (EMLA) in children. *Br J Anaesth* 1986; **58:** 1242–5.
32. Nilsson A, Boman I, Wallin B, Rotstein A. The EMLA patch – a new type of local anaesthetic application for dermal analgesia in children. *Anaesthesia* 1994; **49:** 70–2.
33. Hallen B, Carlsson P, Uppfeldt A. Clinical study of a lignocaine–prilocaine to relieve the pain of venepuncture. *Br J Anaesth* 1985; **57:** 326–8.
34. Vaghadia H, Al-Ahdal OA, Nevin K. EMLA (registered)

patch for intravenous cannulation in adult surgical outpatients. *Can J Anaesth* 1997; **44:** 798–802.

35. Molodecka J, Stenhouse C, Jones JM, Tomlinson A. Comparison of percutaneous anaesthesia for venous cannulation after topical application of either amethocaine or EMLA cream. *Br J Anaesth* 1994; **72:** 174–6.
36. Lurngnateetape A, Tritrakarn T. Placebo effect of lidocaine and prilocaine (EMLA) cream in reducing venepuncture pain in children. *Ann Acad Med Singapore* 1994; **23:** 465–9.
37. Russell SCS, Doyle E. A risk–benefit assessment of topical percutaneous local anaesthetics in children. *Drug Safety* 1997; **16:** 279–87.
38. Sims C. Thickly and thinly applied lignocaine–prilocaine cream prior to venepuncture in children. *Anaesth Intens Care* 1991; **19:** 343–5.
39. Buckley MM, Benfield P. Eutectic lidocaine/prilocaine cream. A review of the topical anaesthetic efficacy of a eutectic mixture of local anaesthetics (EMLA). *Drugs* 1993 July; **46(1):** 126–51.
40. Local anaesthesia. In: *British National Formulary*. London: BMA Books, 2002: 612–17.
41. Doyle E, Freeman J, Im NT, Morton NS. An evaluation of a new self-adhesive patch preparation of amethocaine for topical anaesthesia prior to venous cannulation in children. *Anaesthesia* 1993; **48:** 1050–2.
42. McCafferty DF, Woolfson AD. New patch delivery system for percutaneous local anaesthesia. *Br J Anaesth* 1993; **71:** 370–4.
43. Krajnik M, Zylicz Z. Topical morphine for cutaneous cancer pain. *Palliative Med* 1997; **11:** 325–6.
44. Krajnik M, Zylicz Z, Finlay I, *et al*. Potential uses of topical opioids in palliative care – report of 6 cases. *Pain* 1999; **80(1–2):** 121–5.
45. McQuay HJ, Moore RA. Oral ibuprofen and diclofenac in postoperative pain. In: *An Evidence-based Resource for Pain Relief*. Oxford: Oxford University Press, 1998: 78–93.
46. McQuay HJ, Moore RA. Dextropropoxyphene in postoperative pain. In: *An Evidence-based Resource for Pain Relief*. Oxford: Oxford University Press, 1998: 132–7.
47. McQuay H, Moore RA, Justins D. Treating acute pain in hospital. *Br Med J* 1997; **314:** 1531–5.
48. Reid E. Intravenous sedation for short procedures and investigations. *Nursing Standard* 1997; **12:** 35–8.
49. ● Bell GD, McCloy RF, Charlton JE, *et al*. Recommendations for standards of sedation and patient monitoring during gastrointestinal endoscopy. *Gut* 1991; **32:** 823–7.
50. ● Committee on Drugs. Guidelines for monitoring and management of pediatric patients during and after sedation for diagnostic and therapeutic procedures. *Pediatrics* 1992; **89:** 1110–15.
51. Arrowsmith JB, Gerstman BB, Fleischer DE, Benjamin SB. Results from the American Society for Gastrointestinal Endoscopy/U.S. Food and Drug Administration collaborative study on complication rates and drug use during gastrointestinal endoscopy. *Gastrointest Endosc* 1991; **37:** 421–7.
52. Ashburn MA. Burn pain: the management of procedure-related pain. *J Burn Care Rehabil* 1995; **16** (3 Pt 2): 365–71.
53. ● Maikler VE. Pharmacologic pain management in children: a review of intervention research. *J Pediatr Nursing* 1998; **13:** 3–14.
54. Hosking MP, Morris SA, Klein FA, Dobmeyer-Dittrich C. Anaesthetic management of patients receiving calculus therapy with a third generation extracorporeal lithotripsy machine. *J Endourol* 1997 SH; **11:** 309–11.
55. Koshy G, Nair S, Norkus EP, *et al*. Propofol versus midazolam and meperidine for conscious sedation in GI endoscopy. *Am J Gastroenterol* 2001; **95:** 1476–9.
56. Roseveare C, Seavell C, Patel P, *et al*. Patient-controlled sedation and analgesia, using propofol and alfentanil, during colonoscopy: a prospective randomised controlled trial. *Endoscopy* 1998; **30:** 768–73.
57. Galizia JP, Cantineau D, Selosse A, *et al*. Essai comparatif du propofol et de la ketamine au cours de l'anesthesie pour bain des grands brules. *Annales Francaises d'Anesthesie et de Reanimation* 1987; **6:** 320–3.
58. Chokhavatia S, Nguyen L, Williams R, *et al*. Sedation and analgesia for gastrointestinal endoscopy. *Am J Gastroenterol* 1993; **88:** 393–6.
59. Schechter NL, Weisman SJ, Rosenblum M, *et al*. The use of oral transmucosal fentanyl citrate for painful procedures in children. *Pediatrics* 1995; **95:** 335–9.
60. Gerwels JW, Bezzant JL, Le Maire L, *et al*. Oral transmucosal fentanyl citrate in patients undergoing outpatient dermatologic procedures. *J Dermatol Surg Oncol* 1994; **20:** 823–6.
61. Schutzman SA, Liebelt E, Wisk M, Burg J. Comparison of oral transmucosal fentanyl citrate and intramuscular meperidine, promethazine and chlorpromazine for conscious sedation of children undergoing laceration repair. *Ann Emerg Med* 1996; **28:** 385–90.
62. ● Hanks G, Cherry N. Opioid analgesic therapy. In: Doyle D, Hanks GWC MacDonald N eds. *Oxford Textbook of Palliative Medicine*. Oxford: Oxford University Press, 1993: 331–55.
63. Jones T, Morris RG, Saccoia NC, Thorne D. Dextromoramide pharmacokinetics following sublingual administration. *Palliative Med* 1996; **10:** 313–17.
64. Pal SK, Cortiella J, Herndon D. Adjunctive methods of pain control in burns. *Burns* 1997; **23:** 404–12.
65. Choiniere M. Pain of Burns. In: Wall PD, Melzack R eds. *Textbook of Pain,* 3rd edn. Edinburgh: Churchill Livingstone, 1994: 523–37.
66. Notini-Gudmarsson AK, Dolk A, Jakobsson J, Johansson C. Nitrous oxide: a valuable alternative for pain relief and sedation during routine colonoscopy. *Endoscopy* 1996; **28:** 283–7.
67. Castera L, Negre I, Samii K, Buffet C. Patient-administered nitrous oxide/oxygen inhalation provides safe and effective analgesia for percutaneous liver biopsy:

a randomized placebo-controlled trial. *Am J Gastroenterol* 2001; **96:** 1553–7.

68. Marx CM, Stein J, Tyler MK, *et al*. Ketamine–midazolam versus meperidine–midazolam for painful procedures in pediatric oncology patients. *J Clin Oncol* 1997; **15:** 94–102.
69. Kinsella J, Rae CP. Burn pain. *Bailliere's Clin Anaesthesiol* 1997; **11:** 459–71.
70. Parker RI, Mahan RA, Giugliano D, Parker MM. Efficacy and safety of intravenous midazolam and ketamine as sedation for therapeutic and diagnostic procedures in children. *Pediatrics* 1997; **99:** 427–31.
71. Dachs RJ, Innes GM. Intravenous ketamine sedation of pediatric patients in the emergency department. *Ann Emerg Med* 1997; **29:** 146–50.

PART III

Clinical management – special situations

24

Pediatric cancer pain

JOHN J COLLINS, MICHAEL M STEVENS, AND CHARLES B BERDE

The World Health Organization (WHO) has developed guidelines for the global application of the principles of pain management and palliative care for children with cancer.[1,2] The guidelines contain information on pain assessment, the administration of analgesics and adjuvant analgesics, and the application of nonpharmacologic pain interventions as applicable to children with cancer-related pain.[1,2] In effect, the WHO has established the principles of pain management and palliative care as a required standard of care for all children with cancer.

THE EPIDEMIOLOGY OF CANCER PAIN IN CHILDREN

Pain is a common symptom experienced by children with cancer. As part of the validation study of the Memorial Symptom Assessment Scale 10–18[3*] (MSAS 10–18), detailed information was acquired about symptom characteristics from a heterogeneous population of children with cancer aged 10–18 years at the Memorial Sloan Kettering Cancer Center, New York. The MSAS 10–18 is a 30-item multidimensional symptom assessment scale that records the prevalence and characteristics of a broad range of physical and psychological symptoms. Children were asked about their symptoms during the preceding week. Pain was the most prevalent symptom in the inpatient group (84.4%) and was rated as moderate to severe by 86.8% and highly distressing ("quite a bit to very much") by 52.8% of these children. Pain was experienced by 35.1% of the outpatient group, of whom 75% rated it as being moderate to severe and 26.3% rated distress as "quite a bit to very much."

A study of children with noncentral nervous system (CNS) malignancies at the National Cancer Institute[4] found that 62% presented to their practitioners with complaints of pain prior to the diagnosis of cancer. Pain had been present for a median of 74 days before definitive treatment was begun. The duration of pain experienced by patients with metastatic disease was not longer than that for patients without metastases. The majority of children had resolution of pain following the initiation of therapy directed at their cancer. Children with hematological malignancy had a shorter duration of pain following the institution of cancer treatment than those with solid tumors.[4]

Children with brain tumors often present to their practitioners with either symptoms consistent with raised intracranial pressure or abnormal neurological signs.[5] A retrospective review of children with spinal cord tumors showed that most children with spinal cord tumors present with a complaint of pain.[6] Back pain is more common than abnormal neurological signs as a sign of spinal cord compression in children,[7] and spinal cord compression due to metastatic disease is more likely to occur late in a child's illness.[7]

Tumor-related pain predominates at diagnosis and during the early treatment phase of treatment for childhood cancer and may recur at the time of relapse or when tumors become resistant to treatment. As multimodality cancer treatment protocols evolve for each patient, treatment-related, rather than tumor-related, causes of pain predominate.[8,9] Causes of treatment-related pain include mucositis, phantom limb pain, infection, antineoplastic therapy-related pain, postoperative pain, and procedure-related pain (e.g. needle puncture, bone marrow aspiration, lumbar puncture, removal of a central venous line).

Tumor-related pain frequently recurs in patients at the time of relapse and during the terminal phase of an illness. Palliative chemotherapy and radiation therapy, depending on tumor type and sensitivity, are sometimes instituted as modalities of pain control in terminal pediatric malignancy. Severe pain in terminal pediatric malignancy occurs more commonly in patients with solid tumors metastatic to spinal nerve roots, nerve plexus, large peripheral nerve, or spinal cord compression.[10*]

A variety of chronic pain conditions have been encountered in young adult survivors of childhood cancer as a consequence of cancer treatment.[11] These conditions include chronic regional pain syndrome of the lower extremity, phantom limb pain, avascular necrosis of multiple joints, neuralgia and mechanical pain due to failure of bony union after tumor resection, and postherpetic neuralgia. A proportion of these patients require opioids for the management of their nonmalignant pain.

NONPHARMACOLOGICAL METHODS OF PAIN CONTROL IN CHILDREN WITH CANCER

Nonpharmacological methods of pain control in children include a variety of techniques categorized as physical (e.g. massage, heat and cold stimulation, electrical nerve stimulation, acupuncture), behavioral (e.g. exercise, operant conditioning, relaxation, biofeedback, modeling, desensitization, art and play therapy), or cognitive (e.g. distraction, attention, imagery, thought stopping, hypnosis, music therapy, psychotherapy), according to whether the intervention is focused on modifying an individual's sensory perception, behaviors, or thoughts and coping abilities (see also Chapter P13).[12]

A quiet, calm environment conducive to reducing stress and anxiety, in a location separate from the child's room, is a nonpharmacological strategy arranged prior to performing a medical procedure in a child. Providing a combination of a description of the steps of a given procedure and of the sensations experienced is perhaps the most common intervention for the preparation of children about to undergo invasive medical procedures. Unexpected stress is more anxiety provoking than anticipated or predictable stress.[13,14]

The choice of which nonpharmacological method to use is based on factors such as the child's age, behavioral factors, coping ability, fear and anxiety, and the type of pain experienced.[12] Cognitive–behavioral techniques are most commonly used in the pediatric cancer patient to decrease distress and enhance a child's ability to cope with medical procedures. The decision to use a psychologic or pharmacologic approach or both depends on the knowledge of the procedure, the skill of the practitioner, the understanding of the child, and the expectations of pain and anxiety for that child undergoing that procedure.[13]

Similarly, the role of distraction techniques in reducing children's distress during procedures has been examined by several investigators and shown to be effective. Distraction was less effective for younger children in one study.[15] Another study enlisted the support of parents, and showed not only reduction in the children's behavioral distress but also lowering of the parent's anxiety.[16] Several investigators have examined and shown the effectiveness of cognitive–behavioral interventions comprising multiple components, which have included preparatory information, relaxation, imagery, positive coping statements, modeling, and/or behavioral rehearsal.[16–18] The effectiveness of hypnosis in the reduction of pain and anxiety during bone marrow aspiration and lumbar puncture in children has been confirmed by several reports.[19–21,22*]

PHARMACOLOGICAL MANAGEMENT OF CANCER PAIN IN CHILDREN

The need to improve pain management in children with cancer is demonstrated by recent data which indicate that pain is often not adequately assessed and treated effectively in this population.[23] Improvement in pain management will be dependent not only on advances in pediatric analgesic therapeutics but also on strategies to correct barriers to the adequate treatment of pain in these children. Few analgesic studies have been performed in children with cancer (Table 24.1).

The major difficulty in performing these studies in children with cancer relates to the heterogeneous nature of pain in this population. Solid tumors are less common in children than in the adult population, and it is less likely that children will have chronic cancer pain due to their tumor. Children often receive therapies directed at the control of their tumors until late in the course of their illnesses. These epidemiological and treatment variables make it less likely that a subpopulation of children with cancer exists that has a chronic stable pattern of pain amenable to evaluation in a trial.

In most analgesic studies performed in children with cancer, patient numbers have been low, and few have been controlled; in addition, only recently has self-report been used as an outcome measure for the effectiveness of analgesia. There have been no controlled clinical trials of adjuvant analgesic agents in children. Given the difficulties of performing analgesic studies in children with cancer, pediatric analgesic studies have usually been performed using a postoperative pain model. Although the pharmacokinetic and the major pharmacodynamic properties (analgesia and sedation) of most opioids have been studied in this manner in children, little information is available about oral bioavailability, potency ratios, and other pharmacodynamic properties.

Analgesics can be divided into three groups: (i) nonopioid analgesics, (ii) opioid analgesics, and (iii) adjuvant analgesics. The prescription of these drugs for children with cancer pain is based on the WHO analgesic ladder, which emphasizes pain intensity as the guide to choice of analgesic, rather than etiologic factors. In other words, the prescription of analgesics should be according to pain

Table 24.1 *Analgesic studies in children with cancer*

Reference	Indication for study	Sample size (*n*)	Age of subjects	Study duration	Analgesic study design	Analgesic outcome measures	Analgesic outcome results	Major findings
Miser *et al.*[24]	To test the safety and efficacy of continuous i.v .morphine infusions in a heterogeneous group of terminally ill patients	8	3–16 years	1–16 days	Survey	Composite impression from investigator, parents, and patients	Adequate to complete pain control	Intravenous morphine infusions were effective with minor side-effects recorded
Miser *et al.*[25]	To test the safety and efficacy of continuous s.c. morphine infusions in a heterogeneous group of terminally ill patients	17	2–22 years	0.25–30 days	Survey	Adequate analgesia defined as freedom from pain + absence of complaints of pain > 95% of the time	Satisfactory pain control	Subcutaneous morphine infusions were effective with mild side-effects recorded
Miser and Miser[26]	To test the safety and efficacy of p.o. methadone in a heterogeneous cancer population	19 (22 courses of methadone *in toto)*	4–23 years	2–267 days (median 24 days)	Open trial	Investigator's assessment using a visual analog scale	"Good" or "excellent" analgesia in 18 courses of methadone	"Adequate" pain control in 21 courses
Miser *et al.*[27]	To test the safety, efficacy, and tolerability of continuous i.v./s.c. morphine infusion in a heterogeneous cancer population	26 (30 infusions in toto)		0.75–154 days	Prospective survey	Investigator's assessment using a visual analog scale	"Good" or "excellent" analgesia in 20 courses of i.v./s.c. morphine	"Adequate" pain control in 29 courses
Miser *et al.*[28]	To test the safety, efficacy, and tolerability of i.v. fentanyl infusion in children and young adults with cancer	15 (20 fentanyl infusions)	Median age = 22 years (range 10–29)	0.5–33 days	Survey	Patient and investigator visual analog assessment of pain severity	Adequate analgesia in the majority of cases	Major toxicities included respiratory depression, acute aphonia, CNS toxicity

Table 24.1 *Continued*

Reference	Indication for study	Sample size (*n*)	Age of subjects	Study duration	Analgesic study design	Analgesic outcome measures	Analgesic outcome results	Major findings
Greene *et al.*[29]	To define the relationships between morphine pharmacokinetics in plasma and cerebrospinal fluid (CSF) in cancer patients receiving long-term i.v. infusions of morphine	Morphine infusions: $n = 17$ (21 infusions *in toto*) CSF specimens: $n = 5$			Pharmacokinetic study	Observer's assessment	Not recorded	Variable linear relationship between morphine infusion rate and plasma concentration
Kapelushnik *et al.*[30]**	To define the potential benefit of topical EMLA® prior to lumbar puncture in children with cancer	1 10 2 18	1 Mean age 9.2 + 3.9 years (range 5–15) 2 Mean age 6.1 + 2.1 years (range 4.5–11)		1 Double-blind placebo-controlled study 2 Open crossover study	1 Patient-rated visual analog scale 2 Patient-rated visual analog scale or faces scale	1 Favorable effect of EMLA® 2 Generally favorable effect of EMLA®. EMLA® inferior to placebo in two cases	Although the two studies suggested favorable effects of EMLA®, the need for placebo-controlled, randomized studies was emphasized
Mackie *et al.*[31]***	To compare patient-controlled analgesia (PCA) with continuous infusions for adolescents with prolonged oropharyngeal mucositis pain	20	12–18 years		Randomized controlled trial	Daily morphine intake; self-report pain intensity on visual analog scale	No difference in the pain intensity scores between the two groups	PCA group reported less sedation and less difficulty concentrating. Less morphine intake in the PCA group
Miser *et al.*[32]	To test the safety and efficacy of EMLA® for pain relief during central venous port access in children with cancer	47	3–21 years		Randomized, placebo-controlled double-blind crossover study	Self-report of pain intensity using a faces and visual analog scale	EMLA® superior to placebo	EMLA® provides effective superficial anesthesia

Collins *et al.*[33]**	To compare the efficacy, side-effect profile, and potency ratio of morphine to hydromorphone, and to obtain pharmacokinetic data on these drugs in children with cancer	10	8–19 years	10 days	Randomized, double-blind three-period crossover study	Self-report pain intensity on visual analog scale	No difference in analgesic and side-effect profile between the two drugs. A 6:1 hydromorphone–morphine ratio may be a more appropriate estimate	The clearance of hydromorphone and morphine was greater than in previous studies. Morphine pharmacokinetics were similar to previous studies
Collins *et al.*[34]*	Transdermal fentanyl in children with cancer pain: feasibility, tolerability, and pharmacokinetic correlates	12	7–18 years		Open-label study	Daily opioid "rescue" intake; self-report of pain intensity on visual analog scale	Excellent analgesia in the majority of patients	No major adverse event recorded. The clearance and volume of distribution were similar to that recorded in previous adult studies

severity, ranging from acetaminophen (paracetamol) and nonsteroidal anti-inflammatory drugs (NSAIDs) for mild pain to opioids for moderate to severe pain. The choice of analgesics is individualized to achieve an optimum balance between analgesia and side-effects.

Nonopioid analgesics

Acetaminophen

Acetaminophen (paracetamol) is one of the most commonly used nonopioid analgesics in children with cancer. It inhibits prostaglandin synthesis primarily in the central nervous system. Acetaminophen is not associated with the side-effects of gastritis and inhibition of platelet function found with aspirin and NSAIDs. It has a potential for hepatic and renal injury,[35] but this is uncommon in therapeutic doses. Unlike aspirin, acetaminophen does not have an association with Reye's syndrome. The antipyretic action of acetaminophen may be contraindicated in neutropenic patients, in whom it is important to monitor fever. Pediatric dosing of acetaminophen has been based on the dose–response for its antipyretic effect. Oral dosing of 15 mg/kg every 4 h is recommended, with a maximum daily dose of 90 mg/kg/day in children and 60 mg/kg/day in younger children. There are no data on the safety of chronic acetaminophen administration in children.

Aspirin and nonsteroidal anti-inflammatory drugs

Aspirin and NSAIDs are frequently contraindicated in pediatric oncology patients, who are often at risk of bleeding due to thrombocytopenia. In a comparative study of aspirin and ibuprofen in children with juvenile rheumatoid arthritis, the drugs were equally efficacious, but the drop-out rate caused by side-effects was significantly higher in the aspirin-treated group.[36*] In selected children with adequate platelet number and function, NSAIDs may be helpful analgesics, both alone and in combination with opioids.

Choline magnesium trisalicylate (Trilizate®) has been widely recommended because of reports in adults of minimal effects on platelet function *in vitro* and experimental studies showing minimal gastric irritation in rats, in contrast to aspirin.[37] Clinicians should view such data with caution because the studies do not include medically frail patients with thrombocytopenia or other morbidities.

Opioid analgesics

Pharmacokinetics and recommended starting doses of opioids commonly used in children with cancer are given in Tables 24.2 and 24.3 respectively.

Codeine

Codeine is a phenanthrene alkaloid derived from morphine. In children, codeine is commonly administered via the oral route, in combination with acetaminophen. It is prescribed for mild to moderate pain. In equipotent doses, codeine has a similar analgesic and side-effect profile to morphine. Codeine is typically administered in children over 6 months of age in oral doses of 0.5–1 mg/kg every 4 h.

Oxycodone

Oxycodone is a semisynthetic opioid. It is used for the treatment of moderate to severe pain in children with cancer. Oxycodone may be available only as an oral preparation in combination with acetaminophen in some countries. The total daily acetaminophen dose may be the limiting factor in dose escalation of these products. Oxycodone has a higher clearance value and a shorter elimination half-life ($t_{1/2}$) in children aged 2–20 years than in adults.[38,39] Oxycodone is available as a long-acting preparation in some countries.

Morphine

Morphine is one of the most widely used opioids for moderate to severe cancer pain in children. The binding of morphine to plasma protein is age dependent. In premature infants, less than 20% is bound to plasma proteins.[40,41] Within the neonatal period for term infants, the volume of distribution is linearly related to age and body surface area,[40–42] but after the neonatal period the values are approximately the same as in adults.[43,44]

Morphine is metabolized by the liver. The major metabolite of morphine, morphine 6-glucuronide, produces analgesia and side-effects similar to morphine with chronic dosing. Morphine 6-glucuronide may accumulate and exacerbate sedation in patients with renal insufficiency. Morphine clearance is delayed in the first 1–3 months of life. The half-life of morphine ($t_{1/2}$) falls from 10–20 h in preterm infants to 1–2 h in pre-school-children.[43,44] Thus, starting doses in very young infants should be reduced by approximately 25–30% on a per kilogram basis relative to dosing recommended for older children.

Following oral dosing, morphine undergoes significant first-pass metabolism in the liver. An oral to parenteral potency ratio of approximately 3:1 is commonly encountered during chronic administration.[45] A typical starting dose for immediate-release oral morphine in opioid-naive subjects is 0.3 mg/kg every 4 h. Typical starting intravenous infusion rates are 0.02–0.03 mg/kg/h beyond the first 3 months of life and 0.015 mg/kg/h in younger infants. Sustained-release preparations of morphine are available for children and permit oral dosing at intervals of either two or three times daily. Crushing sustained-released tablets produces immediate release

Table 24.2 *Opioid agonist drugs*

Drug	i.m.[a]	p.o.[a]	Half-life (h)	Duration of action (h)
Codeine	130	200	2–3	2–4
Dihydrocodeine		200	2–3	2–4
Oxycodone	15	30	2–3	2–4
Morphine	10	30 (repeated dose) 60 (single dose)	2–3	3–4
Hydromorphone	1.5	7.5	2–3	2–4
Methadone	10	20	15–190	4–8
Meperidine (pethidine)	75	300	2–3	2–4
Oxymorphone	1	10 (PR)	2–3	3–4
Levorphanol	2	4	12–15	4–8
Fentanyl (parenteral)	0.1	–	1–2	1–3
Fentanyl transdermal system[b]				48–72

a. Dose (mg) equianalgesic to 10 mg i.m. morphine.
b. Transdermal fentanyl 100 μg/h = ~ 4 mg/h.
Reprinted with permission from Cherney NI, Foley KM. Nonopioid and opioid analgesics pharmacotherapy. In: Cherney NI, Foley KM eds. *Hematol Clin N Am* 1996; **10:** 79–102.

Table 24.3 *Starting drug doses of commonly used opioids in pediatrics*

Drug	Usual i.v. starting dose (< 50 kg)	Usual i.v. starting dose (> 50 kg)	Usual p.o. starting dose (< 50 kg)	Usual p.o. starting dose (> 50 kg)
Morphine	0. 1 mg/kg q3–4 h	5–10 mg q3–4 h	0.3 mg/kg q3–4 h	30 mg q3–4h
Hydromorphone	0.015 mg/kg q3–4 h	1–1.5 mg q3–4 h	0.06 mg/kg q3–4 h	6 mg q3–4h
Oxycodone	NA	NA	0.3 mg/kg q3–4 h[b]	10 mg q3–4h
Meperidine[a]	0.75 mg/kg q2–3 h	75–100 mg q3 h	NR	NR
Fentanyl	0.5–1.5 mg/kg q1–2 h	25–75 mg/kg q1–2 h	NA	NA

a. Meperidine is not recommended for chronic use because of the accumulation of the toxic metabolite normeperidine.
b. Smallest tablet size is 5 mg.
NA, not available; NR, not recommended.
Reprinted with permission from Collins and Berde.[11]

of morphine. This limits their use in children who must chew tablets.

Hydromorphone

Hydromorphone is an alternative opioid when the dose escalation of morphine is limited by side-effects. Hydromorphone is available for oral, intravenous, subcutaneous, epidural, and intrathecal administration. Studies in adults suggest that intravenous hydromorphone is 5–8 times as potent as morphine. A double-blind, randomized, crossover comparison of morphine and hydromorphone using patient-controlled analgesia (PCA) in children and adolescents with mucositis following bone marrow transplantation showed that hydromorphone was well tolerated and had a potency ratio of approximately 6:1 relative to morphine in this setting.[33] Because of its high potency and aqueous solubility, hydromorphone is convenient for subcutaneous infusion. Little is known about the pharmacokinetics of hydromorphone in infants.

Fentanyl

Fentanyl is a synthetic opioid that is approximately 50–100 times more potent than morphine during acute intravenous administration. Fentanyl is eliminated almost entirely by hepatic metabolism. The half-life of this opioid is prolonged in preterm infants undergoing cardiac surgery,[46] but values similar to those observed in adults are reached within the first months of life.[47–50] The clearance of fentanyl appears to be higher in infants and young children than in adults.[49,50]

Fentanyl has a very rapid onset following intravenous administration because of its high lipid solubility and rapid entry into the brain. Its duration of action following intravenous bolus administration is much shorter than that for morphine. These features make fentanyl especially useful for procedures for which rapid onset and short duration are useful. Fentanyl may also be used for continuous infusion in selected patients who experience dose-limiting side-effects with morphine. Rapid administration of high doses of i.v. fentanyl may result in chest wall rigidity and severe ventilatory difficulty.

Oral transmucosal fentanyl produces a rapid onset of effect and escapes first-pass hepatic clearance. Schechter *et al.*[51]* described the use of oral transmucosal fentanyl for sedation/analgesia during bone marrow biopsy/aspiration and lumbar puncture. This formulation was found to be safe and effective, although the frequency of vomiting may be a limiting factor in its tolerability.

In a small study utilizing a clinical protocol, the utility, feasibility, and tolerability of transdermal fentanyl was demonstrated in children with cancer pain.[34] A larger study is required to confirm this finding. The mean clearance and volume of distribution of transdermal fentanyl are the same for both adults and children, but the variability is higher in adults.[34]

Meperidine

Meperidine (pethidine) has been used for the relief of procedural and postoperative pain in children. It is a synthetic opioid with a short half-life. It is eliminated more slowly in neonates than in children and young infants.[52–56] Normeperidine is the major metabolite of meperidine. This can cause CNS excitatory effects, including tremors and convulsions,[57] particularly in patients with impaired renal clearance. Meperidine is therefore not generally recommended for children with chronic pain but may be an acceptable alternative to fentanyl for short painful procedures. Meperidine in low doses (0.25–0.5 mg/kg i.v.) is effective for the prophylaxis and treatment of rigors following the infusion of amphotericin.

Methadone

Methadone is a synthetic opioid which has a long and variable half-life. Following single parenteral doses, its potency is similar to that of morphine. In children receiving postoperative analgesia, methadone produced more prolonged analgesia than morphine.[58,59] Because of its prolonged half-life, there is a risk of delayed sedation and overdosage occurring several days after initiating treatment with methadone.

The oral to parenteral potency ratio is approximately 2:1. Frequent patient assessment is the key to safe and effective use of methadone. If a patient becomes comfortable after initial doses, the dose should be reduced or the interval extended to reduce the likelihood of subsequent somnolence. If a patient becomes oversedated early in dose escalation, it is recommended to stop dosing, not just reduce the dose, and to observe the patient until there is increased alertness. Although "as needed" dosing is discouraged for most patients with cancer pain, some clinicians find this approach a useful way to establish a dosing schedule for methadone.[58,59] Methadone remains a long-acting agent when administered either as an elixir or as crushed tablets.

Routes and methods of analgesic administration in children with cancer

Oral

Oral administration of analgesics is the first choice for the majority of patients. Analgesics should generally be administered to children by the simplest, safest, most effective, and least painful route. Oral dosing is generally predictable and inexpensive, and does not require invasive procedures or technologies.

Topical

The eutectic mixture of local anesthetics (EMLA®) is a topical preparation that provides local anesthesia to the skin, dermis, and subcutaneous tissues if applied under an occlusive dressing for at least 1 h. It has been shown to be useful for procedural pain, including lumbar puncture[30] and central venous port access,[32] in children with cancer. Preliminary studies of topical amethocaine for percutaneous analgesia prior to venous cannulation in children have provided promising safety and efficacy data.[60,61]

Intravenous

Intravenous administration has the advantages of rapid onset of analgesia, easier opioid dose titration, improved bioavailability, and continuous effect when infusions are used. The intravenous route of administration is often an option in children with cancer as many have indwelling intravenous access. Typical starting i.v. morphine infusion rates are 0.02–0.03 mg/kg/h beyond the first 3 months of life and 0.015 mg/kg/h in younger infants.[24,62]

Subcutaneous

The subcutaneous route is an alternative route of administration for children with either no or poor intravenous access.[25] Solutions are generally concentrated so that infusion rates do not exceed 1–3 ml/h.[63] An application of a topical local anesthetic agent is recommended prior to the placement of a subcutaneous needle. A small catheter or butterfly needle (27 gauge) may be placed under the skin of the thorax, abdomen, or thigh and sites changed approximately every 3 days.

Intramuscular

Intramuscular administration is painful and may lead to the under-reporting of pain. This route of administration does not permit easy dose titration or infusion and should be avoided.

Rectal

Rectal administration is discouraged in the pediatric cancer population because of concern regarding infection and because of the great variability of rectal absorption of morphine.[64] Nevertheless, this route of administration may be useful in the home care of the dying child when there is no other route available. Slow-release morphine tablets can be administered via the rectum.

Patient-controlled analgesia

Patient-controlled analgesia (PCA) is a method of opioid administration that permits the patient to self-administer small bolus doses of opioid within set time limits. PCA caters for an individual's variation in pharmacokinetics, pharmacodynamics, and pain intensity. PCA allows appropriate children to have control over their analgesia and allows them to choose a balance between the benefits of analgesia versus the side-effects of opioids. In patients with severe mucositis, for example, opioid dosing can be timed with routine mouth care and other causes of incidental mouth pain. In postoperative use, PCA is widely used successfully by children aged 6–7 and above.

Patient-controlled analgesia has been used successfully for the management of prolonged oropharyngeal mucositis pain following bone marrow transplantation in children and adolescents.[31,33★★★,65] A controlled comparison of staff-controlled continuous infusion (CI) of morphine and PCA in adolescents with severe oropharyngeal mucositis found that the PCA group had equivalent analgesia but less sedation and less difficulty concentrating.[31]

Opioid dose schedules for children

Unless a child's episodes of pain are truly incidental and unpredictable, analgesics should be administered at regular times to prevent breakthrough pain. "Rescues" are supplemental "as needed" doses of opioid incorporated into the analgesic regimen to allow a patient to have additional analgesia should breakthrough pain occur. Rescue doses of opioid may be calculated as approximately 5–10% of the total daily opioid requirement and may be administered every hour.[45]

Opioid dose escalation (Box 24.1) may be required after opioid administration begins and periodically thereafter. The size of a dose increment may be calculated as follows:

- If more than approximately six "rescue" doses of opioid are given in a 24-h period, then the total daily opioid dose should be increased by the total of opioid given as "rescue" medication. For example, the hourly average of the total daily rescue opioid should be added to the baseline opioid infusion. An alternative to this method would be to increase the baseline infusion by 50%.[45]
- "Rescue" doses are kept as a proportion of the baseline opioid dose. This dose can be 5–10% of the total daily dose.[45] An alternative guideline for opioid infusions is between 50% and 200% of the hourly basal infusion rate.[45]

Box 24.1 *Case examples for opioid dose calculation and dose escalation*

A 4-year-old girl, weighing 20 kg, has severe continuous pain related to metastatic neuroblastoma. What is an appropriate opioid dose schedule?
Owing to the continuous nature of this patient's pain, an appropriate schedule would be to provide either regular dosing via the oral route or, alternatively, institute a continuous intravenous infusion. In addition, to provide relief from additional or "breakthrough" pain, the regimen should include supplementary opioid to be given when required.

Options
The recommended oral dose of morphine in a child is 0.3 mg/kg immediate-release morphine (IRM) every 4 h (i.e. 6 mg p.o. every 4 h). An appropriate "breakthrough" dose would be 3.5 mg IRM every hour (i.e. the total daily opioid dose is 36 mg and therefore 10% of this dose is approximately 3.5 mg morphine). If this regimen seems satisfactory with time, it may be reasonable to switch from IRM to slow-release morphine (SRM). An appropriate regimen would be 15 mg SRM twice a day. The "breakthrough" IRM dose remains the same. As an alternative, a loading dose of intravenous morphine (0.1 mg/kg) could be given, followed by a morphine infusion of 0.02 mg/kg/h (=0.4 mg/h morphine). An appropriate "breakthrough" dose could be 0.4 mg i.v. every hour.

During the next 24 h, six additional "breakthrough" doses of oral morphine were given. How should the opioid regimen be changed?
An additional 21 mg of oral morphine was given as "breakthrough" dosing (i.e. 6 × 3.5 mg = 21 mg). This dose could be divided and be given as additional SRM. An appropriate new regimen could be 25 mg SRM twice a day. The total daily dose of morphine is now 50 mg, and an appropriate "breakthrough" dose of IRM would now be 5 mg.

Opioid switching

The usual indication for switching to an alternative opioid is dose-limiting toxicity. This approach is recommended by the observation that a switch from one opioid to another is often accompanied by change in the balance between analgesia and side-effects.[66] A favorable change in opioid analgesia to side-effect profile will be experienced if there is less cross-tolerance at the opioid receptors mediating analgesia than at those mediating adverse effects.[67]

Following a prolonged period of regular dosing with one opioid, equivalent analgesia may be attained with a dose of a second opioid that is smaller than that calculated from an equianalgesic table, as shown in Table 24.3.[67] An opioid switch is usually accompanied by a reduction in the equianalgesic dose (approximately 50% for short half-life opioids). In contrast to short half-life opioids, the doses of methadone required for equivalent analgesia after switching may be of the order of 10–20% of the equianalgesic dose of the previously used short half-life opioid. A protocol for methadone dose conversion and titration has been documented for adults.[68]

Opioid side-effects

All opioids can potentially cause the same constellation of side-effects (Table 24.4). Children do not necessarily report side-effects voluntarily (e.g. constipation, pruritus, dreams) and should be asked specifically about these problems. An assessment of opioid side-effects is included in an assessment of analgesic effectiveness. If opioid side-effects limit opioid dose escalation, then consideration should be given to an opioid switch. Tolerance to some opioid side-effects (e.g. sedation, nausea and vomiting, pruritus) often develops within the first week of starting opioids. Children do not develop tolerance to constipation as an opioid side-effect, and concurrent treatment with laxatives should always be considered.

Adjuvant analgesics in children

Adjuvant analgesics are a heterogeneous group of drugs that have a primary indication other than pain but are analgesic in some painful conditions.[69] Adjuvant analgesics are commonly, but not always, prescribed with primary analgesic drugs. Common classes of these agents include antidepressants, anticonvulsants, neuroleptics, psychostimulants, antihistamines, corticosteroids, and centrally acting skeletal muscle relaxants.

Antidepressants

Data from adult studies have guided the use of antidepressants as adjuvant analgesics in children. Tricyclic antidepressants have been used for a variety of pain conditions in adults, including postherpetic neuralgia,[70***] diabetic neuropathy,[71***] tension headache,[72] migraine headache,[73] rheumatoid arthritis,[74] chronic low back pain,[75] and cancer pain.[76] Antidepressants are effective in relieving neuropathic pain. With very similar results for anticonvulsants, it is still unclear which drug class should be the first choice.[77***]

Baseline hematology and biochemistry tests (including liver function tests) and an electrocardiogram (EKG) to exclude Wolff–Parkinson–White syndrome or other cardiac conduction defects have been recommended prior to starting treatment with tricyclic antidepressants.[78] The measurement of antidepressant plasma concentration allows confirmation of compliance and ensures that optimization of dosage has occurred before discontinuing. An EKG is recommended periodically during long-term use, or if standard mg/kg dosages are exceeded.[79]

Psychostimulants

Dextroamphetamine potentiates opioid analgesia in postoperative adult patients,[80] and methylphenidate counteracts opioid-induced sedation[81] and cognitive dysfunction[82] in patients with advanced cancer. Psychostimulants may allow dose escalation of opioids in patients in whom somnolence is a dose-limiting side-effect.[69] The potential side-effects of methylphenidate include anorexia, insomnia, and dysphoria. The use of dextroamphetamine and methylphenidate was reported in a retrospective survey of 11 children receiving opioids for a variety of indications, including cancer pain.[83] Somnolence was reduced in these patients without significant adverse side-effects.

Corticosteroids

Corticosteroids may produce analgesia by a variety of mechanisms, including anti-inflammatory effects, reduction of tumor edema, and, potentially, by reducing spontaneous discharge in injured nerves.[84] Dexamethasone tends to be used most frequently because of its high potency, longer duration of action, and minimal mineralocorticoid effect. Corticosteroids may have a role in bone pain due to metastatic bone disease,[85] cerebral edema due to either primary or metastatic tumor,[86] and epidural spinal cord compression.[87]

Anticonvulsants

The mechanism of action of anticonvulsants in controlling lancinating pain is not known but is probably related to a reduction in paroxysmal discharges of central and peripheral neurons. Anticonvulsants are effective in relieving neuropathic pain. With very similar results for antidepressants it is still unclear which drug class should be the first choice.[77***] The use of phenytoin, carbamazepine, and valproate may be problematic in the pediatric cancer population because of the potential adverse effects of these drugs on the hematological profile. The novel anticonvulsant gabapentin is well tolerated and appears to have a benign efficacy to toxicity ratio in children[88] and may be useful for the treatment of neuropathic pain.[89]

Radionuclides

The use of other radionuclides for the treatment of pain-

Table 24.4 *Management of opioid side-effects*

Side-effect	Treatment
Constipation	1 Regular use of stimulant and stool softener laxatives (fiber, fruit juices are often insufficient) 2 Ensure adequate water intake
Sedation	1 If analgesia is adequate, try dose reduction 2 Unless contraindicated, add nonsedating analgesics, such as acetaminophen or NSAIDs, and reduce opioid dosing as tolerated 3 If sedation persists, try methylphenidate or dextroamphetamine 0.05–0.2 mg/kg p.o. b.i.d. in early morning and at midday 4 Consider an opioid switch
Nausea	1 Exclude disease processes (e.g. bowel obstruction, increased intracranial pressure) 2 Antiemetics (phenothiazines, ondansetron, hydroxyzine) 3 Consider an opioid switch
Urinary retention	1 Exclude disease processes (e.g. bladder neck obstruction by tumor, impending cord compression, hypovolemia, renal failure) 2 Avoid other drugs with anticholinergic effects (e.g. tricyclics, antihistamines) 3 Consider short-term use of bethanechol or Crede maneuver 4 Consider short-term catheterization 5 Consider opioid dose reduction if analgesia adequate or an opioid switch if analgesia inadequate
Pruritus	1 Exclude other causes (e.g. drug allergy, cholestasis) 2 Antihistamines (e.g. diphenhydramine hydroxyzine) 3 Consider an opioid dose reduction if analgesia adequate, or an opioid switch. Fentanyl causes less histamine release
Respiratory depression	
Mild–moderate	1 Awaken, encourage to breathe 2 Apply oxygen 3 Withhold opioid dosing until breathing improves, reduce subsequent dosing by at least 25%
Severe	1 Awaken if possible, apply oxygen, assist respiration by bag and mask as needed 2 Titrate small doses of naloxone (0.02 mg/kg increments as needed). Stop when respiratory rate increases to 8–10/min in older children or 12–16/min in infants. Do not try to awaken fully with naloxone **Do not give a bolus dose of naloxone as severe pain and symptoms of opioid withdrawal may ensue** 3 Consider a low-dose naloxone infusion or repeated incremental dosing 4 Consider short-term intubation in occasional patients in whom risk of aspiration is high
Dysphoria/confusion/ hallucinations	1 Exclude other pathology as a cause for these symptoms before attributing them to opioids 2 When other causes excluded, change to another opioid 3 Consider adding a neuroleptic such as haloperidol (0.01–0.1 mg/kg p.o./i.v. every 8 h to a maximum dose of 30 mg/day)
Myoclonus	1 Usually seen in the setting of high-dose opioids, or alternatively, rapid dose escalation 2 No treatment may be warranted, if this is infrequent and not distressing to the child 3 Consider an opioid switch or treat with clonazepam (0.01 mg/kg p.o. every 12 h to a maximum dose of 0.5 mg/dose) or a parenteral benzodiazepine (e.g. diazepam) if the oral route is not tolerated

Reprinted with permission from Collins and Berde.[11]

ful osseous metastases has been reported in adults.[90] One pediatric case report indicates the potential role of [^{131}I]meta-iodobenzylguanidine ([^{131}I]MIBG) for painful metastatic bone disease due to neuroblastoma.[91] The side-effects of [^{131}I]MIBG are thrombocytopenia and cystitis.

Neuroleptics

Methotrimeprazine, a phenothiazine, has been reported as being analgesic in the setting of adult cancer pain.[92] Methotrimeprazine is not considered to be a substitute for opioid analgesia. The mechanism by which methotrimeprazine produces analgesia and its role as an adjuvant agent in pediatric cancer pain is unclear. It may be useful as an adjuvant analgesic in a patient with disseminated cancer who experiences pain associated with anxiety, restlessness, or nausea.[69]

TOLERANCE, PHYSICAL DEPENDENCE, ADDICTION

Analgesic tolerance refers to the progressive decline in potency of an opioid with continued use, so that increasingly higher doses are required to achieve the same analgesic effect. Patients and parents are often reluctant to increase dosing because of a fear that tolerance will make opioids ineffective at a later date. Parents should be reassured that tolerance in the majority of cases can be managed by simple dose escalation, use of adjunctive medications, or perhaps by opioid switching in the setting of dose-limiting side-effects. Clinically relevant pharmacological tolerance is not usually an issue in cancer pain management.

Physical dependence is a physiologic state induced after dose reduction or discontinuation of an opioid, or administration of an opioid antagonist. Initial manifestations of withdrawal include yawning, diaphoresis, lacrimation, coryza, and tachycardia. Patients with cancer who have received opioids over a long period of time and in whom it is appropriate to either stop or reduce opioids should have the opioid dose reduced slowly.

Addiction is a psychological and behavioral syndrome characterized by drug craving and aberrant drug use. Some parents may fear that an exposure to opioids will result in their child subsequently becoming a drug addict. The incidence of opioid addiction was examined prospectively in 12,000 hospitalized adult patients who received at least one dose of a strong opioid.[93] There were only four documented cases of subsequent addiction in patients without a prior history of drug abuse. These data suggest that iatrogenic opioid addiction is an exceedingly uncommon problem,[93] an observation consistent with a large worldwide experience with opioid treatment of cancer pain.

SUMMARY

Pediatric cancer pain management should follow the logical, simple guidelines produced by the World Health Organization in combination with knowledge of the individual child and his or her family and an open mind about individual responses to analgesics.

REFERENCES

◆ 1. McGrath PA. Development of the World Health Organization Guidelines on Cancer Pain Relief and Palliative Care in Children. *J Pain Symptom Manage* 1996; **12(2):** 87–92.

● 2. World Health Organization. *Cancer Pain Relief and Palliative Care in Children*. Geneva: World Health Organization, 1998.

3. Collins JJ, Byrnes ME, Dunkel I, *et al.* The measurement of symptoms in children with cancer. *J Pain Symptom Manage* 2000; **19:** 363–77.

◆ 4. Miser AW, McCalla J, Dothage JA, *et al.* Pain as a presenting symptom in children and young adults with newly diagnosed malignancy. *Pain* 1987; **29:** 85–90.

5. Heideman R, Packer RJ, Albright LA, *et al.* Tumors of the central nervous system. In: Pizzo PA, Poplack DG, eds. *Principles and Practice of Pediatric Oncology*, 3rd edn. Philadelphia, PA: Lippincott-Raven, 1997.

6. Hahn YS, McClone DG. Pain in children with spinal cord tumors. *Child Brain* 1984; **11:** 36–46.

7. Lewis DW, Packer RJ, Raney B, *et al.* Incidence, presentation, and outcome of spinal cord disease in children with systemic cancer. *Pediatrics* 1986; **78:** 438–43.

◆ 8. Miser AW, Dothage JA, Wesley M, Miser JS. The prevalence of pain in a pediatric and young adult cancer population. *Pain* 1987; **29:** 73–83.

9. Elliott SC, Miser AW, Dose AM, *et al.* Epidemiologic features of pain in pediatric cancer patients: a co-operative community-based study. *Clin J Pain* 1991; **7:** 263–8.

10. Collins JJ, Grier HE, Kinney HC, Berde CB. Control of severe pain in children with terminal malignancy. *J Pediatr* 1995; **126:** 653–7.

● 11. Collins JJ, Berde CB. Management of cancer pain in children. In: Pizzo PA, Poplack DG eds. *Principles and Practice of Pediatric Oncology*, 3rd edn. Philadelphia, PA: Lippincott-Raven, 1997: 1183–99.

12. McGrath PA. Intervention and management. In: Bush JP, Harkins SW eds. *Children in Pain.* New York, NY: Springer-Verlag, 1991: 83–115.

13. Zeltzer L, Jay S, Fisher D. The management of pain associated with pediatric procedures. *Pediatr Clin N Am* 1989; **36:** 914–64.

14. Siegal LJ. Preparation of children for hospitalization: a selected review of the research literature. *J Pediatr Psychol* 1976; **1:** 26–36.

15. Kuttner L, Bowman M, Teasdale M. Psychological treatment of distress, pain and anxiety for children with cancer. *Dev Behav Pediatr* 1988; **9:** 374–81.

16. Manne S, Redd WH, Jacobsen P, *et al.* Behavioral intervention to reduce child and parent distress during venipuncture. *J Consult Clin Psychol* 1990; **58:** 565–72.

17. McGrath PA, DeVeber LL. The management of acute pain evoked by medical procedures in children with cancer. *J Pain Symptom Manage* 1986; **1:** 145–50.

18. Jay S, Elliott C, Ozolins M, *et al*. Behavioral management of children's distress during painful medical procedures. *Behav Res Ther* 1985; **5:** 513–20.
19. Katz E, Kellerman J, Ellenberg L. Hypnosis in the reduction of acute pain and distress in children with cancer. *J Pediatr Psychol* 1987; **12:** 379–94.
20. Hilgard J, LeBaron S. Relief of anxiety and pain in children and adolescents with cancer: quantitative measures and clinical observations. *Int J Clin Exp Hypn* 1982; **30:** 417–42.
21. Kellerman J, Zeltzer L, Ellenberg L, Dash J. Adolescents with cancer: hypnosis for the reduction of the acute pain and anxiety associated with medical procedures. *J Adolesc Hlth Care* 1983; **4:** 85–90.
22. Zeltzer L, LeBaron S. Hypnosis and nonhypnotic techniques for reduction of pain and anxiety during painful procedures in children and adolescents with cancer. *J Pediatr* 1982; **101:** 1032–5.
◆ 23. Ljungman G, Kreugar A, Gordh T, *et al*. Treatment of pain in pediatric oncology: a Swedish nationwide survey. *Pain* 1996; **68:** 385–94.
◆ 24. Miser AW, Miser JS, Clark BS. Continuous intravenous infusion of morphine sulfate for control of severe pain in children with terminal malignancy. *J Pediatr* 1980; **96:** 930–3.
25. Miser AW, Davis DM, Hughes CS, *et al*. Continuous subcutaneous infusion of morphine in children with cancer. *Am J Dis Child* 1983; **137:** 383–5.
26. Miser AW, Miser JS. The use of oral methadone to control moderate and severe pain in children and young adults with malignancy. *Clin J Pain* 1985; **1:** 243–8.
27. Miser AW, Moore L, Greene R, *et al*. Prospective study of continuous intravenous and subcutaneous morphine infusions for therapy-related or cancer-related pain in children and young adults with cancer. *Clin J Pain* 1986; **2:** 101–6.
28. Miser AW, Dothage JA, Miser JS. Continuous intravenous fentanyl for pain control in children and young adults with cancer. *Clin J Pain* 1987; **2:** 101–6.
29. Greene RF, Miser AW, Lester CM, *et al*. Cerebrospinal fluid and plasma pharmacokinetics of morphine infusions in pediatric cancer patients and rhesus monkeys. *Pain* 1987; **30:** 339–48.
30. Kapelushik J, Koren G, Solh H, *et al*. Evaluating the efficacy of EMLA in alleviating pain associated with lumbar puncture: comparison of open and double-blinded protocols in children. *Pain* 1990; **42:** 31–4.
◆ 31. Mackie AM, Coda BC, Hill HF. Adolescents use patient-controlled analgesia effectively for relief from prolonged oropharyngeal mucositis pain. *Pain* 1991; **46:** 265–9.
32. Miser AW, Goh TS, Dose AM, *et al*. Trial of a topically administered local anesthetic (EMLA cream) for pain relief during central venous port accesses in children with cancer. *J Pain Symptom Manage* 1994; **9:** 259–64.
33. Collins JJ, Geake J, Grier HE, *et al*. Patient-controlled analgesia for mucositis pain in children: a three-period crossover study comparing morphine and hydromorphone. *J Pediatr* 1996; **129:** 722–8.
34. Collins JJ, Dunkel IJ, Gupta SK, *et al*. Transdermal fentanyl in children with cancer: feasibility, tolerability, and pharmacokinetic correlates. *J Pediatr* 1999; **134:** 319–23.
35. Sandler DP, Smit JC, Weinberg CR, *et al*. Analgesic use and chronic renal disease. *N Engl J Med* 1989; **320:** 1238–43.
36. Giannini EH, Brewer EJ, Miller ML, *et al*. Ibuprofen suspension in the treatment of juvenile rheumatoid arthritis. *J Pediatr* 1990; **117:** 645–52.
37. Stuart JJ, Pisko EJ. Choline magnesium trisalicylate does not impair platelet aggregation. *Pharmatherapeutica* 1981; **2:** 547.
38. Poyhia R, Seppala T. Lipid solubility and protein binding of oxycodone in vitro. *Pharmacol Toxicol* 1994; **74:** 23–7.
39. Pelkonen O, Kaltiala EH, Larmi TKL, *et al*. Comparison of activities of drug metabolizing enzymes in human fetal and adult liver. *Clin Pharmacol Ther* 1973; **14:** 840–6.
40. McRorie TI, Lynn A, Nespeca MK. The maturation of morphine clearance and metabolism. *Am J Dis Child* 1992; **146:** 972–6.
41. Bhat R, Chari G, Gulati A, *et al*. Pharmacokinetics of a single dose of morphine in pre-term infants during the first week of life. *J Pediatr* 1990; **117:** 477–81.
42. Pokela ML, Olkkala KT, Seppala T. Age-related morphine kinetics in infants. *Dev Pharm Ther* 1993; **20:** 26–34.
43. Stanski DR, Greenblatt DJ, Lowenstein E. Kinetics of intravenous and intramuscular morphine. *Clin Pharmacol Ther* 1978; **24:** 52–9.
44. Olkkola KT, Maunuksela EL, Korpela R, Rosenberg PH. Kinetics and dynamics of postoperative intravenous morphine in children. *Clin Pharmacol Ther* 1988; **44:** 128–36.
● 45. Cherny NI, Foley KM. Nonopioid and opioid analgesic pharmacotherapy of cancer pain. In: Cherny NI, Foley KM eds. *Hematology/Oncology Clinics of North America*, vol. 10. Philadelphia, PA: Saunders, 1996: 79–102.
46. Collins C, Koren G, Crean P, *et al*. Fentanyl pharmacokinetics and hemodynamic effects in preterm infants during ligation of patent ductus arteriosus. *Anesth Analg* 1985; **64:** 1078–80.
47. Koren G, Goresky G, Crean P, *et al*. Unexpected alterations in fentanyl pharmacokinetics in children undergoing cardiac surgery: age related or disease related? *Dev Pharmacol Ther* 1986; **9:** 183–91.
48. Koren G, Goresky G, Crean P, *et al*. Pediatric fentanyl dosing based on pharmacokinetics during cardiac surgery. *Anesth Analg* 1984; **63:**577–582.
49. Johnson K, Erickson J, Holley F, Scott J. Fentanyl pharmacokinetics in the pediatric population. *Anesthesia* 1984; **61 (3A):** A441.
50. Gauntlett IS, Fisher DM, Hertzka RE, *et al*. Pharmaco-

kinetics of fentanyl in neonatal humans and lambs: effects of age. *Anesthesiology* 1988; **69:** 683–7.

◆ 51. Schechter NL, Weisman SJ, Rosenblum M, *et al.* The use of oral transmucosal fentanyl citrate for painful procedures in children. *Pediatrics* 1995; **95:** 335–9.

52. Tamsen A, Hartvig P, Fagerlund C, *et al.* Patient-controlled analgesic therapy. Part 1: pharmacokinetics of pethidine in the pre- and postoperative periods. *Clin Pharmacokinet* 1982; **7:** 149–63.

53. Hamunen K, Maunuksela EL, Seppala T, *et al.* Pharmacokinetics of iv and rectal pethidine in children undergoing ophthalmic surgery. *Br J Anaesth* 1993; **71:** 823–6.

54. Koska AJ, Kramer WG, Romagnoli A, *et al.* Pharmacokinetics of high dose meperidine in surgical patients. *Anesth Analg* 1981; **60:** 8–11.

55. Pokela ML, Olkkola KT, Kovisto M, *et al.* Pharmacokinetics and pharmacodynamics of intravenous meperidine in neonates and infants. *Clin Pharmacol Ther* 1992; **52:** 342–9.

56. Mather LE, Tucker GT, Pflug AE, *et al.* Meperidine kinetics in man: intravenous injection in surgical patients and volunteers. *Clin Pharmacol Ther* 1975; **17:** 21–30.

57. Kaiko RF, Foley KM, Grabinski PY, *et al.* Central nervous system excitatory effects of meperidine in cancer patients. *Ann Neurol* 1983; **13:** 180–5.

58. Berde CB, Sethna NF, Holzman RS, *et al.* Pharmacokinetics of methadone in children and adolescents in the perioperative period. *Anesthesiology* 1987; **67:** A519.

59. Berde CB, Beyer JE, Bournaki MC, *et al.* Comparison of morphine and methadone for prevention of postoperative pain in 3- to 7-year-old children. *J Pediatr* 1991; **119:** 136–41.

60. Van Kan HJM, Egberts ACG, Rijnvos WPM, *et al.* Tetracaine versus lidocaine–prilocaine for preventing venipuncture-induced pain in children. *Am J Health-Syst Pharm* 1997; **54:** 388–92.

61. Lawrie SC, Forbes DW, Akhtar TM, Morton NS. Comparison of lumbar plexus block versus conventional opioid analgesia after total knee replacement [see comments]. *Anaesthesia* 1991; **46:** 275–7.

62. Koren G, Butt W, Chinyanga H, *et al.* Postoperative morphine infusion in newborn infants: assessment of disposition characteristics and safety. *J Pediatr* 1985; **107:** 963–7.

63. Bruera E, Brenneis C, Michaud M, *et al.* Use of the subcutaneous route for the administration of narcotics in patients with cancer pain. *Cancer* 1988; **62:** 407–11.

64. Gourlay GK. Fatal outcome with use of rectal morphine for postoperative pain control in an infant. *Br Med J* 1992; **304:** 766–7.

65. Dunbar PJ, Buckley P, Gavrin JR, *et al.* Use of patient-controlled analgesia for pain control for children receiving bone marrow transplants. *J Pain Symptom Manage* 1995; **10:** 604–11.

66. Galer BS, Coyle NM, Pasternak G, Portenoy RK. Individual variability in response to different opioids. *Pain* 1992; **49:** 87–91.

● 67. Portenoy RK. Opioid tolerance and responsiveness: research findings and clinical observations. In: Gebhart GF, Hammond DI, Jensen TS eds. *Progress in Pain Research and Management.* Seattle. WA: IASP Press, 1994: 615–19.

68. Inturrisi CE, Portenoy RK, Max M, *et al.* Pharmacokinetic–pharmacodynamic relationships of methadone infusions in patients with cancer pain. *Clin Pharmacol Ther* 1990; **47:** 565–70.

● 69. Portenoy RK. Adjuvant analgesics in pain management. In: Doyle D, Hanks GWC, Macdonald N eds. *Oxford Textbook of Palliative Medicine.* Oxford: Oxford University Press, 1993: 187–203.

70. Watson CPN, Evans RJ, Reed K, *et al.* Amitriptyline versus placebo in postherpetic neuralgia. *Neurology* 1982; **32:** 671–3.

◆ 71. Max MB, Culnane M, Schafer SC, *et al.* Amitriptyline relieves diabetic neuropathy pain in patients with normal or depressed mood. *Neurology* 1987; **37:** 589–96.

72. Diamond S, Baltes BJ. Chronic tension headache treatment with amitriptyline – a double blind study. *Headache* 1971; **11:** 110–16.

73. Couch JR, Ziegler DK, Hassanein R. Amitriptyline in the prophylaxis of migraine: effectiveness and relationship of antimigraine and antidepressant effects. *Neurology* 1976; **26:** 121–7.

74. Frank RG, Kashani JH, Parker JC, *et al.* Antidepressant analgesia in rheumatoid arthritis. *J Rheumatol* 1988; **15:** 1632–8.

75. Ward NG. Tricyclic antidepressants for chronic low back pain: mechanisms of action and predictors of response. *Spine* 1986; **11:** 661–5.

● 76. Magni G. The use of antidepressants in the treatment of chronic pain. *Drugs* 1991; **42:** 730–48.

77. McQuay H, Moore A. Antidepressants in neuropathic pain. In: *An Evidence-based Resource for Pain Relief.* New York, NY: Oxford University Press, 1998.

● 78. Heiligenstein E, Gerrity S. Psychotropics as adjuvant analgesics. In: Schechter NL, Berde CB, Yaster M eds. *Pain in Infants, Children, and Adolescents.* Baltimore, MD: Williams & Wilkins, 1993: 173–7.

79. Biederman J, Baldessarini RJ, Wright V, *et al.* A double-blind placebo controlled study of desipramine in the treatment of ADD. II. Serum drug levels and cardiovascular findings. *J Am Acad Child Adolesc Psychiatry* 1989; **28:** 903–11.

80. Forrest WH, Brown BW, Brown CR, *et al.* Dextroamphetamine with morphine for the treatment of postoperative pain. *N Engl J Med* 1977; **296:** 712–15.

81. Bruera E, Miller MJ, Macmillan K, Kuehn N. Neuropsychological effects of methylphenidate in patients receiving a continuous infusion of narcotics for cancer pain. *Pain* 1992; **48:** 163–6.

82. Bruera E, Fainsinger R, MacEachern T, Hanson J. The

use of methylphenidate in patients with incident pain receiving regular opiates: a preliminary report. *Pain* 1992; **50:** 75–7.

83. Yee JD, Berde CB. Dextroamphetamine or methylphenidate as adjuvants to opioid analgesia for adolescents with cancer. *J Pain Symptom Manage* 1994; **9:** 122–5.
84. Watanabe S, Bruera E. Corticosteroids as adjuvant analgesics. *J Pain Symptom Manage* 1994; **9:** 442–5.
85. Tannock I, Gospodarowicz M, Meakin W, *et al.* Treatment of metastatic prostatic cancer with low-dose prednisone: evaluation of pain and quality of life as pragmatic indices of response. *J Clin Oncol* 1989; **7:** 590–7.
86. Weinstein JD, Toy FJ, Jaffe ME, Goldberg HI. The effect of dexamethasone on brain edema in patients with metastatic brain tumors. *Neurology* 1973; **23:** 121–9.
87. Greenberg HS, Kim J, Posner JB. Epidural spinal cord compression from metastatic tumor: results with a new treatment protocol. *Ann Neurol* 1980; **8:** 361–6.
88. Khurana DS, Riviello J, Helmers S, *et al.* Efficacy of gabapentin therapy in children with refractory partial seizures. *J Pediatr* 1996; **128:** 829–33.
89. Mellick GA, Mellick LB. [letter]. *J Pain Symptom Manage* 1995; **10:** 265–6.
90. Silberstein EB, Williams C. Strontium-89 therapy for painful osseous metastases. *J Nucl Med* 1985; **26:** 345–8.
91. Westlin JE, Letocha H, Jakobson S, *et al.* Rapid, reproducible pain relief with ^{131}iodine-meta-iodobenzylguanidine in a boy with disseminated neuroblastoma. *Pain* 1995; **60:** 111–14.
92. Beaver WT, Wallenstein S, Houde RW. A comparison of the analgesic effects of methotrimeprazine and morphine in patients with cancer. *Clin Pharmacol Ther* 1966; **7:** 436–46.
93. ◆ Porter J, Jick J. Addiction is rare in patients treated with narcotics [letter]. *N Engl J Med* 1980; **302:** 123.

25

Elderly cancer

MARGOT GOSNEY

There are many definitions of pain.[1,2] However, it must be remembered that pain is the most common symptom associated with cancer and often the most distressing one.[3] In addition, the meaning of pain is influenced by the individual's personal, social, and cultural experiences.[4]

Although most studies on the causes and management of pain are exclusively from the perspective of the patient, it is important, particularly in older patients, to consider the meaning of pain from the perspective of the patient, family, caregiver, and the health care professionals caring for the patient with cancer.[5*]

Although acute and chronic pain are defined by their duration, the traditional dichotomy between acute pain, with its recent onset and short duration, and chronic pain, which persists after an injury has healed, is increasingly untenable.[6] Acute pain associated with a new tissue injury might last for less than 1 month but, at times, for longer than 6 months.[7] Older people are more likely to suffer both acute and chronic pain[8*,9] and, although cancer pain in older sufferers may at times be considered to last for short periods because of limited survival, some authors never consider it to be chronic in nature,[10] although this is certainly not the finding when dealing with older patients with cancer pain.

> Pain, discomfort and suffering must not be equated with the process of normal ageing.[11]

However, in older people it may be difficult to distinguish between pain from unrelated pathology and pain due to malignant disease.

Pain is a frequent complaint of elderly people both in hospital and in the community,[12*] and researchers have developed conceptual models of the impact of pain on the dimensions of quality of life.[13*] This model depicts four domains of pain: physical well-being and symptoms, psychological well-being, social well-being, and spiritual well-being. The models do, however, fail to address many factors that are specific to older people, and this must be considered when analyzing response to therapy in this age group. Perhaps the most helpful definition of pain is that of McCaffery,[14] which, although not specific to pain in the elderly, states, "Pain is whatever the patient says it is and exists when he says it does." This concept needs to be borne in mind when dealing with older patients.

Worldwide, over three million people die each year with cancer, and seven million new cases of cancer are diagnosed, with over 50% of all cases occurring in patients aged 70 years or above. Between 50% and 80% of patients with cancer cite pain as a significant problem and feel that it disturbs overall quality of life,[15] with some studies suggesting that more than 50% of patients, many of whom are elderly, suffer unrelieved pain.[16–20,21**] A working party from the Royal College of Surgeons and College of Anaesthetists[22] reported that health care professionals working in acute pain management are ineffectual when attempting to establish suppression of this distressing symptom, with a 1997 study by Lynn *et al.*[23**] of 3,357 seriously ill and elderly patients reporting that 40% of the study subjects complained of being in severe pain in the last 3 days of life.

Ageist attitudes exist in most areas of clinical practice, and oncology and palliative care are no exception.

Patients and physicians alike often dismiss many symptoms attributable to cancer as being the normal consequence of aging. Bone pain is attributed to arthritis, abdominal pain to diverticulitis, and confusion is invariably considered to be the result of Alzheimer's disease.

Pain is related to the primary site of the tumor, to disease progression, and to the treatment that the patient receives. These facts are particularly pertinent in older patients, who in general have more advanced disease at presentation,[24] are less likely to receive active treatment,[25,26*,27*] and, in many cases, lack a definitive diagnosis, thus preventing definitive treatment.[28]

Breast and lung cancer are more likely to be associated with pain, and these are tumors that are predominantly found in older people. Although as many as 85% of patients with a primary bone tumor (common in young people) experience pain, there are few data on bony metastases, which are especially common in patients with primary breast, lung, or prostate cancers.

Uncontrollable pain is a reason for hospital admission and, when admitted, older patients do spend more time in hospital.[29] Unfortunately, despite the fact that over half of all terminally ill patients say they would prefer to die at home, 63% actually died in hospital.[30] Older patients with cancer are more likely to die in hospital, and this occurs for a variety of reasons. Firstly, the diagnosis of cancer is often made after an older patient presents in an atypical fashion. Thus, the older man who has "gone off his legs" actually has lung cancer with hypercalcemia, constipation, spurious diarrhea, and urinary retention. It may be during this admission that the patient dies from the new diagnosis of lung cancer. Secondly, it must be remembered that with medical advances older people not only have a prolonged active life expectancy, with the resultant terminal dependency being postponed, but also have a duration of terminal dependency that increases. Thus, it may be during this period of terminal dependency that the patient dies, with cancer being one of many diagnoses active at the time.[31]

Although it is easy to extrapolate that with increasing age, irrespective of diagnosis, older people are more likely to be admitted to hospital in the last year of their lives, it must be remembered that very elderly subjects, i.e. 85 years or older, are the least likely to be admitted to hospital in the last year of their lives, and generalizations must be avoided.[32]

IS PAIN DIFFERENT IN OLDER PEOPLE?

There is little doubt that older people complain less about pain than younger subjects do. This may be because they attribute pain to normal aging or are more stoical about pain, but there is also evidence that older people have altered tolerance to pain from various stimuli. Harkins[33] found that deep pain tends to become less frequent and less intense with age although superficial pain does not alter with increasing age. Evidence from studies of postoperative pain control shows that older patients achieve the same degree of pain control with less analgesic medication than younger patients,[34*] suggesting reduced pain experience in this group.

There may be difficulties in determining the etiology of pain in older people, as it is such a frequent finding. Brochet *et al.*[35*] found the prevalence of pain to be over 70% among community-living subjects over the age of 65 years. Although the etiology of the pain was unstated, the most commonly affected sites were limb joints and the back.

Of more concern is the finding by Vigano *et al.*[36*] that cancer patients aged 75 years or older, when compared with younger adults, received significantly lower amounts of opioid analgesia. They may or may not have had less pain, but they certainly received less analgesia.

In the case of renal dysfunction, due either to aging or to disease, there is evidence of increased potency of opioids.[37*,38**] As with the management of many diseases, older patients with pain are often not studied separately in a controlled and prospective fashion. This is particularly true for cardiovascular disease,[39**,40] although recently trials have been specifically designed to study older patients with cardiovascular disease.[41**,42,43**] Although some important information may be obtained from extrapolating existing knowledge, there are problems with this, and it may lead to suboptimal or dangerous therapy for older people.

In addition, it must be remembered that older patients may choose quantity over quality of life, and this may not be predictable from the person's clinical diagnosis. In a study by Tsevat *et al.*,[44*] 414 hospitalized patients aged 80–98 years were asked whether they would prefer to live for 1 year in their current state of health or less time in excellent health. They found that 69% of patients were unwilling to exchange 12 months of life in their present state of health for 1 month in excellent health. Thus, although we strive for quality of pain control, older people may have different goals to the physician or carer.

PAIN ASSESSMENT

It is vital to use instruments that are reliable and valid and are feasible in day-to-day clinical practice. There are three major areas for the assessment of pain. The first is a linear/visual analog scale (LAS or VAS),[45,46] the second a verbal-rated or categorical-rated scale (VRS or CRS),[47] and the third method, widely used for the assessment of quality of life in cancer clinical trials, is a patient daily diary card. It has been suggested that it is easier to explain to elderly patients verbal scales rather than the more abstract analog scales, but this remains to be formally tested[48*] and, although no study has prospectively followed older patients using daily diary cards, there is a suggestion that impaired vision and manual dexterity may make these more difficult to comply with over long periods of time.

Although it is clear that no one scale will be suitable for all patients, and particularly for older patients, it has been recommended that there is a universal adoption of a scale for clinical assessment of pain intensity in adults who are capable of responding to simple queries. This may be particularly valuable in the management of older patients with cancer pain.[49] It must, however, be remembered that all tools were designed for use with younger adults and therefore data regarding their appropriateness for older people remain preliminary.[50]

In pain assessment, as with assessment of other symptoms affecting quality of life, the use of a core questionnaire covering areas such as physical, psychological, and social well-being as well as a specific module relating to the primary tumor or topic under study, such as the approach of the European Organization for Research and Treatment of Cancer (EORTC), is required.[51]* This does little, however, to cover the spiritual aspect of palliative care and does not take account of other diseases that occur coincidentally with the primary cancer, as seen especially in older patients.

Pain affects social functioning, and in elderly patients this can be measured by the Katz Activities of Daily Living score, which is a standard instrument, validated for use in elderly patients with cancer.[52]

Although many of the effects of pain in elderly patients are also seen in younger patients, including depression, disrupted sleep, and impaired mobility, there are additional consequences that specifically affect activities of daily living (ADL) in older patients. For example, elderly patients experience an increased number of falls, one of the "giants of geriatric medicine," which may occur as a result of impaired mobility, cognitive dysfunction, or polypharmacy.[53,54]* In addition, the risk of malnutrition is increased when pain is poorly controlled, and poor nutrition in older patients is well described in both the cancer and noncancer literature.[55,56]* Delirium (acute confusion) may result from pain *per se* or occur as a result of drug therapy. In many older patients, polypharmacy is a problem prior to the introduction of analgesic drugs, with such drugs adding to an already complex list.

Measurement of pain relief is important in older patients, although the true benefit of the prescribed medication may not be fully apparent due to coexisting morbidity or even as a consequence of the newly prescribed drug. For example, the use of steroids may reduce pain but cause immobility due to muscle wasting, metabolic disturbances, or vertebral collapse as a result of osteoporosis. Thus, physical function or some global aspects of quality of life may not improve, or the added frustration of pain relief in the absence of improved mobility may worsen the patient's quality of life. Although pain assessment scales may be difficult to administer and interpret in older people, it is important not to abandon these in favor of easily recorded data such as analgesic consumption. This may be poorly recalled, but the poor compliance and undertreatment that occurs in older patients makes these data meaningless.

Although McGill Pain Questionnaires are well validated,[57] it is important that other self-reported measures of patients' ability to engage in functional activities are taken into account.[58] Although older patients can identify pain intensity on a visual analog scale (VAS) or a numerical rating scale (NRS), it has been found that nurses may be unable to identify patients in pain or choose an appropriate treatment.[59] Although increasing age has been associated with a higher frequency of incorrect responses to VAS,[60] this is not a consistent finding.[61] The use of body charts has been well validated in younger people; however, there are few data on their use in older patients with cancer.[62]

In summary, I would recommend the McGill Pain Questionnaire for those elderly patients with no cognitive impairment. However, for those with a mental test score of 7 or less, nurse observation of behavior in combination with the use of body charts provides a level of basic pain assessment.

PAIN CONTROL

Pain control is poorly achieved for a variety of reasons, which can be subdivided into patients and/or carer attitudes.[63,64]

Patients' attitudes

Patients of all ages with cancer have a reluctance to report pain.[65]* Yates *et al.*[66]* demonstrated that older people were more reluctant to express their pain and that the cause of such reluctance was multifactorial:[67,68]

- not wishing to be a nuisance;
- a belief that pain is a judgment and must be borne;
- a belief that pain is an inevitable part of cancer;
- not wishing to distract the doctor or nurse from treating the cancer;
- considering that nothing can be done to relieve pain.

Attitudes of health care professionals

Doctors

Studies of the management of cancer pain by doctors exist, but, although doctors from a wide variety of specialist areas are represented, most are hospital based.

Although these studies may help understand general principles, they fail to address the beliefs of doctors most likely to encounter patients with cancer, i.e. primary care physicians and medical oncologists.[69*,70*] Larue *et al.*[71*] studied 600 primary care physicians and 300 medical oncologists in France. A 12-min interview included both multiple choice and closed-ended questions on pain assessment as well as problems associated with morphine usage and included an assessment of the physicians' training in cancer pain management. Seventy-three percent of primary care physicians (PCPs) and 61% of medical oncologists (ONCs) reported never having received training in cancer pain management, and both PCPs (88%) and ONCs (90%) reported that they relied on their patients' claims to assess pain. Less than half of the 900 doctors studied prescribed morphine frequently or very frequently, and 30% of ONCs and 20% of PCPs reported problems with pharmacists when attempting to have morphine prescriptions filled. Only 27% of PCPs and 42% of ONCs knew that oral morphine could be prescribed daily to an adult without any upper limitation in dosage and 76% and 50.3%, respectively, expressed reluctance to prescribe morphine, with 40.2% of PCPs and 26.7% ONCs citing fear of side-effects as a reason. Almost one-fifth of doctors said that they would hesitate to prescribe morphine because there were other drugs as effective as morphine available. Although women doctors tended to prescribe morphine less frequently than male physicians, increasing age also resulted in less frequent prescription of morphine. The doctors who prescribed less frequently perceived the barriers to be risk of tolerance, availability of drugs as effective as morphine, constraints of the prescribing forms, and poor image of morphine in public opinion. The group of doctors who prescribed morphine more frequently reported a higher prevalence of pain among their patients, were more likely to rely on their patients to assess the pain, agreed that morphine could be prescribed at any stage of the disease, and perceived respiratory depression as a low concern.[71] Thus, education of doctors is essential to ensure that patients are not undertreated with opioids, particularly in the case of older patients, who complain less frequently.

Nurses

In 1983, McCaffery[72] reported that nurses seem to be responsible for controlling patients' expression of pain and that this may be accomplished by ignoring the patients' manifestations of pain. Indeed, Ferrell *et al.*[73] stated that nurses performed pain assessment rarely, poorly, or inconsistently. Despite this, there is little information available that identifies nurses' experiences and skills in managing pain specifically in older people with malignant disease, although Closs,[54] in her study of four clinical areas (cardiothoracic surgery, orthopedic surgery, general surgery, and care of the elderly wards), attempted to address this. Of the 55% of nurses who returned questionnaires, which were aimed at assessing knowledge, almost 84% reported that elderly people suffered more chronic pain than younger people. Although there is no evidence that pain and discomfort are unavoidable consequences of aging, more than half of the nurses in the sample felt this to be the case. Nurses from care of the elderly, in contrast to those from surgical units, correctly believed that there are differences in response to painful stimuli with age. In contrast, nurses from acute surgical areas were more likely to identify correctly that older patients were less likely to request pain relief. Some nurses were unaware that the duration of analgesic effect from a given medication differs between elderly and young patients, although higher grade nurses and those working on acute surgical wards more commonly answered this question correctly.

An important point raised by Closs[54] is that nurses should ask patients how the pain feels rather than whether they need anything for pain. The latter allows the patient to decline help regardless of how they actually feel whereas the former gives patients "permission" to ask for help to manage their pain.

MISCONCEPTIONS ABOUT ANALGESICS

Anxiety about the administration of opioids is exhibited by health care professionals, patients, and carers.[74] However, the proper use of opioids does not cause addiction,[75] and, although elderly people do experience higher peaks and a longer duration of action when given opioids, they do not experience the respiratory depression that many doctors and nurses predict.[76] Such inaccurate and widespread perceptions could undoubtedly lead to undermedication and ineffective pain control[54] when respiratory depression is in fact a rare occurrence and should present no problem when effective patient monitoring is in progress.[77,78*]

QUALITY OF LIFE ISSUES

The assessment of quality of life in older patients with cancer differs in many ways to the use of traditionally accepted quality of life scales in younger subjects. Clinicians must be aware that in the management of older patients with cancer there is often acceptance of potentially toxic treatment for a seemingly small survival benefit.[79*]

The older patient with cancer who is cared for at home may be at risk of suicide. Reasons for this include pain, helplessness, and exhaustion or poor contact with the health care system. In an Italian study of cancer patients cared for at home by palliative care teams, the five patients who committed suicide had a mean age of 55 years (range

50–76) and, despite their age and the apparent easy availability of drugs, only one took an overdose of morphine. Of the remaining four patients, two jumped from a window and two shot themselves.[80*]

CARER KNOWLEDGE AND EXPERIENCE

Many elderly patients with cancer are cared for not in hospitals, hospices, or nursing/residential homes but at home surrounded by family members. Although it is known that family members play an important role,[81,82,83*] it is fortunate that they can provide effective pain management despite not understanding the basic mechanisms of pain.[84*] If caregivers deny that the patient is in pain to avoid accepting that the disease process is progressing and the patient is close to death, this may result in the underadministration of analgesia. Many family members, in the absence of formal teaching of caregiving skills by health care providers, are left to administer pain relief by a process of trial and error.[85] Although previous studies have identified pain as a major source of concern, there has been very little focused research on caregivers and the management of pain. Ferrell *et al.*[74] identified the diversity of mean rating of patients' pain as assessed independently by caregivers and patients. Caregivers over-rated the pain; using a scale from 0 (no pain) to 100 (severe pain), the patients' mean rating of their pain was 45, whereas caregivers' mean rating of the patients' pain was 70.

Ferrell *et al.*[86*] developed and implemented a pain education program for patients and family caregivers. Information was delivered in a variety of formats. As the study was being undertaken in older patients, the booklet developed was reasonably short in length and printed in larger typeface and included illustrations. In addition, audiocassette tapes were produced and left with the patients at the conclusion of each of the first two education sessions. Older patients and their families endured pain from cancer for long durations. After education, the patients experienced a decrease in pain intensity and severity, a decrease in fear of addiction, and a subsequent increase in use of pain medication. The caregiver was also found to have an improved knowledge and a reduced fear of addiction or respiratory depression when using strong analgesia.

Ferrell *et al.*[13] assessed caregivers' knowledge in the care of 80 patients with cancer. Of a 14-item scale assessing carer knowledge and attitudes about pain, 10 items improved on retest as a result of educational intervention.

Ferrell *et al.*[87] suggested that caregivers' knowledge about pain management differed according to the settings where patients received care – an important consideration when elderly patients with cancer are likely to be treated in the hospital rather than the community.

If caregivers are to feel positive about their role it is important to consider which aspects of care are seen as positive experiences. When comparing mean scores obtained by caregivers and patients on selected aspects of quality of life and pain, family caregivers showed more positive scores in the domain of physical well-being. These included feelings of usefulness, strength, and appetite, and were in contrast to patients, who showed more positive results in the emotional aspects such as worry and sense of control.[13*] In five areas patients were more positive than their caregivers. These included patients being more likely to believe that pain could be relieved and that family members were useful helpers in pain management. The study also showed that family caregivers of elderly patients were less optimistic and more distressed by the pain experience than the patients' themselves.[13] Similarly, Yeager *et al.*[83] found that significantly higher levels of patient pain and significantly greater patient distress were reported by family caregivers than by patients themselves, and family caregivers experienced significantly more distress as a result of the patient's pain than the patient believed to be the case.

As well as the issue of education and caregiver burden, it is essential that we consider the demographics of such caregivers. In a study of caregivers by Ferrell *et al.*,[13] the median age of caregivers was 63.5 years; 76% were female and 66% were the spouse and 22% were the child of the index patient. Thus, older patients requiring informal care may be reliant on elderly spouses or daughters who are combining this caregiving with child care and paid employment. In the study, although the majority of caregivers lived with the patient (92%), over one-fifth (22%) were also employed outside the home and 10% were older than 74 years of age.

Clotfelter[88*] studied 36 subjects over 65 years of age with a diagnosis of cancer and randomized them to an experimental or a control group. The experimental group watched a 14-min video on managing cancer pain and also received written information. A follow-up assessment of their level of pain indicated that the study group had significantly less pain than the control group, and the author concluded that pain education is a central component in preventing and managing cancer pain in elderly people.

This highlights the need for close monitoring of both patient and caregiver, particularly with regard to education and false beliefs. If patients and caregivers interpret the pain experience differently, then management is based on inappropriate estimates of pain intensity.[89]

Nurses

Clinical research must be relevant to everyday clinical practice. This is particularly the case in nursing research, and different authors have suggested that problems such as lack of replication, lack of organization structure to support its integration, and lack of interest and understanding of research on the part of practicing nurses may be of paramount importance.[90] In order to avoid this problem it is important that practicing nurse clinicians identify a nursing practice problem, which is then further expanded and studied by researchers. Dufault *et al.*[91] found that nurses involved in the identification of key research-based areas who then participated in the development of the research improved not only their attitudes towards research but also their competency in research utilization. This results in better patient care in practice, developed from research knowledge.

Although most studies show that nurses generally underestimate patients' pain, Jandelli[92] found that the six nurses in her study overestimated the patient's pain in the majority of cases. In contrast to other studies, in which oncology patients' pain was found to be underestimated, studies by Marks and Sachar[93] of medical inpatients and by Cohen[94*] of surgical inpatients found pain to be overestimated. However, these patients were younger and had no communication problems. The nurses in Jadelli's study had all received Oncology or Care of the Dying Patient certificates, but this is not usually the case, which may at least partly explain the fact that pain is usually underestimated by nurses not experienced in or trained about pain management. Wakefield[95] found that nurses tend to categorize patients according to symptoms or overt pain behavior. She also found that nurses' knowledge regarding pain and pain management influenced the way in which they managed postoperative pain.

Nurses attribute significantly less pain to a patient with no physical pathology and more pain to a patient with symptoms of depression.[96] In addition, patient age influences management as nurses may be more willing to believe the reports of pain given by older patients than younger patients,[97] but less willing to administer opioid analgesia to such patients.[98]

Doctors

In a prospective study of patients with prostate cancer undergoing palliative therapy, symptoms were measured by means of patient- and physician-completed assessments. Although all patients were male and elderly, the data were not analyzed by age bands. Doctors tended to underestimate both nausea and pain and attributed a decreased performance status to the patient compared with the person's own self-assessments.[99**]

In a study in Italy of 148 physicians and 182 general practitioners, two-thirds of the sample agreed that, if more attention was paid to quality of life issues and pain control, euthanasia and physician-assisted suicide would be eliminated.[100*]

PATIENT KNOWLEDGE AND EXPERIENCE

In 1984, Jones *et al.*[101*] studied 82 patients with cancer to assess their knowledge about pain management. Although the compliance seen in these patients was high, patients were unaware of common side-effects of their drugs, and 11 of the 54 patients took medication as required even when it was prescribed on a regular basis. Patients' attitudes to cancer pain may also be affected by public attitudes: in a telephone survey of 496 adults, 57% felt that patients with cancer usually died a painful death and almost 50% viewed cancer pain to be severe.[102*]

To evaluate a pain education intervention, 80 patients with a median age of 67 years were recruited. Each patient received three education and two evaluation visits. Throughout the period of evaluation patients reported improvement in pain intensity and distress as well as an increase in pain relief. Both patients and health care providers found the pain education program to be beneficial and reported that it improved all aspects of quality of life.[103*]

PHARMACOKINETICS AND PHARMACODYNAMICS

Pharmacokinetics encompasses the movement of drugs through the body, including absorption, distribution, metabolism, and excretion. Thus, pharmacokinetics determines drug concentrations in plasma and tissues, in contrast to pharmacodynamics, which is the processes that determine the body's response to a given tissue or plasma concentration of a drug. Aging can affect either pharmacokinetics or pharmacodynamics, and on occasions will affect both.

Pharmacokinetics

Although there are now abundant data on the effect of age or aging on pharmacokinetics, most studies have been performed on healthy volunteers, with little reference to the frail elderly patient with multiple pathology. In older people, acid secretion is reduced and gastric emptying impaired, and the absorptive capacity of the small bowel and blood flow to the intestine are also reduced. The first-pass metabolism of some drugs declines significantly with age, and both the liver volume and hepatic blood flow are reduced with increasing age. Thus, the systemic concentration of drugs that undergo significant first-pass metabolism may be greatly increased in elderly subjects.

Distribution

In normal aging, both total body water and lean body mass decrease, resulting in a relative increase in body fat. The lipid solubility of a drug therefore determines the serum level with advancing age. Drugs that are water soluble, such as morphine, will tend to have a smaller volume of distribution, which results in a higher serum level. In older people, drugs such as benzodiazepines or barbiturates, which are lipid soluble, have a larger volume distribution and prolonged half-life.

Protein binding determines the levels of free drug available to cross plasma membranes. Acidic compounds bind principally to albumin. Thus, in older patients, who have a reduced level of serum albumin and hence reduced acid drug-binding capacity, the levels of free salicylic acid and benzodiazepines will be higher than in younger subjects for a given dose. In addition, α_1-acid glycoprotein, which binds to basic drugs, is increased by intercurrent illness, resulting in a higher level of plasma protein binding and reduced levels of free basic drugs.

Clearance of drugs from the body is primarily dependent on whether the compound is polar or nonpolar. Polar compounds are water soluble and thus are usually excreted unchanged through the kidneys. Normal aging is associated with a reduction in glomerular filtration rate, renal plasma flow, and tubular function, and thus renal excretion of drugs such as nonsteroidal anti-inflammatory agents is reduced in older patients. Drugs that are nonpolar are poorly soluble in water and must be metabolized before excretion. Hepatic clearance is reduced in the normal older person and this, together with alterations in conjugation, results in reduced clearance of acetaminophen and lorazepam.[104*,105*]

Although one may postulate that metastatic liver disease, particularly in older patients, would result in a reduction in liver metabolism, this has not been a consistent finding[106] perhaps because normal hepatic parenchyma is preserved as a result of hepatic enlargement.[107*]

Pharmacodynamics

The effect of drugs on the body is in essence pharmacodynamics. Although some clear-cut data regarding pharmacodynamics in older patients exist, there is a paucity of pharmacodynamic data in sick frail older people. Drugs of particular relevance in the management of pain in older patients include benzodiazepines, which may produce increased sedation and confusion and impaired postural righting reflexes,[108*,109*] and neuroleptics, which, used either for sedation or for their antiemetic effect, may result in tardive dyskinesia and Parkinsonism.[110,111*] In addition, drugs such as prochlorperazine are frequently prescribed to older people with dizziness and nausea although such agents have been documented to both increase postural sway and impair balance.

SIMPLE ANALGESICS

Nonopioid analgesics includes acetaminophen and nonsteroidal anti-inflammatory drugs (NSAIDs). Acetaminophen (paracetamol) does not cause gastric irritation and is more effective when used in combination with an NSAID than when given alone. It is the nonopioid analgesic of choice, particularly in the elderly[12] Acetaminophen may enhance the effect of warfarin in prolonged use, whereas the coadministration of metoclopramide increases the absorption and therefore the effectiveness of acetaminophen.[113]

Aspirin causes irreversible inactivation of both COX-1 and COX-2. It displaces a number of drugs from protein binding sites in the blood, and of particular relevance in older patients are drugs such as tolbutamide, chlorpropamide, and phenytoin. Coadministration of aspirin and warfarin results in an increased anticoagulant effect, partly by displacement of warfarin from protein binding sites and partly through a direct effect of aspirin on platelets. Recently, there has been an increase in the prescription of spironolactone for congestive cardiac failure among older patients, and this must be remembered when administering aspirin because aspirin reduces the pharmacological activity of spironolactone and may worsen cardiac failure in this group.[114]

Mild to moderate pain warrants the prescription of NSAIDs. Although NSAIDs are chemically unrelated to each other, they do share pharmacological properties and are used for their analgesic, anti-inflammatory, and antipyretic actions. The major advance in the use of NSAIDs in older people has been the differentiation between COX-1 and COX-2 inhibitors. Inhibition of COX-1 results in reduced renal function, gastric mucosal integrity, and platelet adhesiveness. However, COX-2 is expressed after tissue injury and augments inflammation and, thus, COX-2 inhibitors are not only efficacious but can be administered with a high level of safety to older people.[115**] NSAIDs are weak acids and are thus are well absorbed in the stomach. In the bloodstream, most NSAIDs are protein bound, and although a quarter of the drug is excreted in the urine unchanged, the remainder is oxidized or conjugated. Urinary excretion of NSAIDs is higher when the urine is acid and thus may be affected by the coadministration of other drugs. As renal function declines with age, the urinary excretion of NSAIDs must be carefully considered.

NSAIDs are responsible for almost one-quarter of all adverse drug reactions reported in the UK.[114] Upper gastrointestinal symptoms such as dyspepsia, nausea, and vomiting may occur in up to 20% of patients. Mucosal erosions, ulceration, or bleeding may be detected if the patient is symptomatic; however, slowly developing anemia may present atypically in the older patient. In a meta-analysis, ibuprofen was associated with the lowest incidence of gastrointestinal side-effects and piroxicam and ketoprofen with the highest incidence of gastric adverse effects.[116***]

NSAIDs cause both salt and water retention, resulting in hypertension and edema. This is particularly problematic in older patients, who may have some degree of cardiac failure or orthostatic leg edema. Thus, patients on diuretics or antihypertensive drugs should be carefully monitored if co-prescribed NSAIDs.

As all NSAIDs are highly protein bound, the free fraction of NSAIDs is increased in patients with hypoalbuminemia, and such subjects may also have a propensity to increasing peripheral edema. Poor mobility, pressure area instability, and falls may result from inability to wear footwear over edematous feet.

Although NSAIDs are well absorbed, an age-related decrease in gastric absorption may result in subtherapeutic levels. Alteration of hepatic enzymes with increasing age may also result in decreased levels of active agents such as fenbufen, a propionate that must be metabolized by the liver to yield active metabolites.

The half-life of aspirin and diclofenac is less than 6 h whereas naproxen and piroxicam have a longer half-life (10 h or greater). This should be considered particularly in older patients, in whom altered drug metabolism could further delay the establishment of a steady state. It may be more than a week after starting a drug with a long half-life before steady analgesic efficacy is noted, and clinicians must therefore be patient before dismissing NSAIDs as ineffective in older people.

NSAIDs may cause renal toxicity as a result of papillary necrosis or interstitial nephritis. Naproxen accumulates in patients with renal impairment, and its half-life is prolonged. Thus, older patients may need smaller doses and, as underpins all drug prescribing in older patients, drugs with a short half-life may be safer on the whole and prodrugs may be less nephrotoxic.[117] Careful monitoring of renal function is essential in all elderly patients receiving long-term treatment with NSAIDs because of the increased risk of interstitial nephritis, which in the early stages may be mistaken for physiological change.

Naproxen undergoes enterohepatic recycling, and any alterations in the gut flora may affect its excretion. The gut flora in older patients may be altered as a result of increased transit time or co-prescription of other drugs, including antibiotics.

Misoprostol is effective for the treatment of ulcers associated with the use of NSAIDs but is often poorly tolerated in the elderly because it causes diarrhea and abdominal pain. In a study of patients with ulcers or erosions in either the stomach or duodenum who required continuous NSAID therapy, omeprazole was compared with misoprostol. Eight weeks' treatment with 20 mg omeprazole or misoprostol resulted in successful treatment in 76% and 71% of patients respectively. Although the rate of gastric and duodenal ulcer healing was higher in the omeprazole-treated group than in those treated with misoprostol, misoprostol was more effective in healing erosions alone. After 6 months' maintenance treatment, 61% of patients in the ompeprazole group remained in remission compared with only 48% in the misoprostol-treated group ($P = 0.001$). In addition, there were more adverse events during the healing phase in the misoprostol group than in those treated with either 20 or 40 mg of omeprazole.[118]

The advent of proton pump inhibitors has been particularly useful for suppressing acid secretion in patients requiring regular NSAIDs. The ASTRONAUT study[119**] found omeprazole to be significantly more effective than ranitidine ($P < 0.001$) and, although many patients with cancer receive NSAIDs for only short periods of time, the finding of this study was that after 6 months' treatment omeprazole was also more effective than ranitidine in preventing ulcer formation.

In patients treated concomitantly with an NSAID and a corticosteroid, those receiving a total dose of steroid of over 140 mg of dexamethasone equivalent, or those with a previous history of peptic ulcer and advanced malignant disease, prophylaxis may be necessary to prevent ulcer formation. Research-based evidence suggests that misoprostol is the drug of choice for this indication.[120]

NSAIDs, especially aspirin, may precipitate bronchospasm and thus should be introduced cautiously in any older patient with a history of pulmonary disease.

OPIOIDS

Opioids are particularly useful in the management of moderate to severe pain.[112] Opioids act on injured tissue to reduce inflammation, in the dorsal horn to impede transmission of nociception, and supraspinally to activate inhibitory pathways that descend to the spinal segment. A further advantage of opioids in older patients is the variety of possible methods of delivery.

There are, however, problems associated with the introduction of opioids. Public awareness of the role of morphine in the treatment of cancer pain is well documented. A recent poll among members of the public found that 74% felt that morphine was dangerous and addictive, and a survey of general practitioners (GPs) found that patients were specifically concerned about addiction and dependency with morphine use, with 36% of GPs believing that the prescription of morphine signals that death is imminent. Although opioids are beneficial in the treatment of pain, a considerable amount of psychological support must be provided to patients when they are first administered.[121]

Weak opioids include codeine, dihydrocodeine, and dextropropoxyphene. However, cimetidine and fluoxetine, which may be co-prescribed in older patients, have both been reported to inhibit the enzyme that converts codeine into morphine, and thus their co-prescription may block the analgesic effect. Problems commonly seen with dextropropoxyphene are the enhancement of blood levels of carbamazepine resulting in drowsiness and increased anticoagulant effects of warfarin.

Drug combinations should, on the whole, be avoided in elderly patients. However, although codeine causes confusion and constipation, particularly in older subjects,[122***] Moore *et al.*[123***] found that the combination of codeine 60 mg and acetaminophen 600/650 mg is a more effective analgesic than acetaminophen 600/650 mg alone. The addition of codeine to acetaminophen increased the number of patients achieving at least 50% pain relief by 12%. This finding was confirmed by the Cochrane Systematic Review, which concluded that acetaminophen is an effective analgesic and is associated with a low incidence of side-effects. The addition of codeine 60 mg to acetaminophen produces additional pain relief even in single oral doses but may be accompanied by an increase in drowsiness and dizziness.[124***] Coproxamol, once the drug of choice combining acetaminophen and dextropropoxyphene, became unpopular after a large number of successful suicide attempts. In addition, it may cause confusion and drowsiness in older people because of its long elimination half-life.[125*] The Cochrane Systematic Review of dextropropoxyphene alone and in combination with acetaminophen focused on the effectiveness of the combination in relieving postoperative pain. It was found that single-dose dextropropoxyphene and acetaminophen were as effective as tramadol in the treatment of postoperative pain but were associated with a lower incidence of adverse effects. Although it was concluded that the same dose of acetaminophen combined with codeine appeared to be more effective than acetaminophen alone, there was an overlap in the 95% confidence intervals, allowing room for this conclusion to be challenged. It is, however, interesting that this review found that the number needed to treat was lower for ibuprofen than for either the combination of dextropropoxyphene plus acetaminophen or tramadol.[126***]

Strong opioids include morphine as well as some synthetic drugs, such as fentanyl. Tramadol and buprenorphine do not provide better analgesia than morphine but may cause fewer side-effects. Of particular note is fact that these drugs are associated with fewer gastrointestinal side-effects, respiratory problems, and urinary difficulties, all of which occur frequently in older people receiving opioids.[127]

In a randomized crossover study comparing transdermal fentanyl with sustained-release oral morphine, a significantly higher number of patients up to the age of 89 years preferred the fentanyl patches,[128] despite the fact that WHO performance status and EORTC Global Quality of Life scores indicated that there were significant difference in pain relief between groups.

It must be remembered that morphine, particularly if administered intrathecally, will inhibit detrusor contractions. This effect can be blocked by the administration of naloxone. Although published data are lacking, terminally ill elderly patients with an overactive bladder may respond well to the administration of morphine. This may in part explain the urinary retention frequently encountered in patients receiving morphine; although this effect traditionally is blamed on the coexistence of constipation, inhibition of detrusor contractions is a plausible alternative explanation.

The analgesic effect of opioids increases with increasing age. There is an inverse relationship between self-administered morphine consumption and age.[129*,130*] This is fortunate as older people are four times as sensitive to opioid analgesia as younger ones, a finding that has been attributed to slower metabolism and elimination of these drugs in elderly subjects.[131*]

Constipation is a major problem associated with opioid administration, and treatment with laxatives is mandatory as soon as opioids have been prescribed. In older people, opioid use results in a decrease in peristalsis and secretion, thus a combination of a softener and stimulant such as codanthrusate is the most appropriate approach. Gastric stasis is common and dose related and, together with nausea, is most frequently an initial side-effect of morphine. Campara *et al.*[132] reported an incidence of opioid-induced emesis of 28%.

Renal impairment may reduce the clearance of active metabolites of propoxyphene and morphine and, although morphine clearance is only minimally affected by mild or moderate hepatic impairment, it may be significantly reduced in patients with advanced disease.[133]

Although strong opioids are the top rung of the WHO analgesic ladder, many cancer patients continue to suffer pain and, even in cancer centers, documented evidence of morphine efficacy may be lacking.[134*]

Cherny *et al.*[135*] found that patients up to the age of 86 years referred to a pain service received a median of two different opioid drugs (range 1–8 different drugs), administered by a median of two different routes (range 1–4 routes), prior to their referral. Factors considered to be most important for selection of a specific opioid were that the drug had been used previously by the patient and was effective and well tolerated, or that the drug had been used without adverse effects or had not previously been tried. Thus, even patients with pain that is difficult to control often remain on oral opioid following referral to a specialist pain service.

Many older people wish to return to the community for their palliative care. The use of implantable ports and catheter systems permits ambulatory delivery of drugs when combined with electronic pumps. Although there is no evidence that these routes are more useful for elderly than other cancer patients, they may be particularly useful for older patients who wish to remain in either their own homes or in nursing homes, and intermittent attendance of a district nurse could enable adequate pain relief out of the hospital setting.[136]

Hydromorphone is a μ-selective full opioid agonist. It exerts similar pharmacological actions to morphine, and the oral analgesic potency ratio of hydromorphone to morphine is approximately 7.5:1. In a study that included patients up to the age of 81 years, sedation, constipation, and nausea were reduced with hydromorphone compared with morphine.[137] Those patients who were switched from morphine to hydromorphone because of uncontrollable side-effects experienced a 73% reduction in side-effects and an improvement in pain control as measured on the 10-cm visual analog scale.[138*] Therefore, patients with uncontrolled pain who develop side-effects with increasing doses of morphine may respond to conversion to hyromorphone.[139]

Oxycodone is a semisynthetic opioid derived from the naturally occurring opium alkaloid thebaine. The suggested oral potency ratio between oxycodone and morphine is between 2:3 and 3:4. However, because of the high oral bioavailability of oxycodone (up to 87%), a conservative approach to dose conversion is recommended, particularly in older people.[140] Another major advantage of oxycodone is its short half-life[141] and, in addition, there is some evidence that, compared with morphine sulfate tablets (MST), it causes less nausea, hallucinations, and disturbed sleep.[142**]

Fentanyl is a strong μ-agonist with potent analgesic action. Its delivery via a transdermal therapeutic system is particularly useful in older people. Although the usual dosing interval is 72 h, individual pharmacokinetic variability is large, and some patients may require dosing intervals to be as short as 48 h. Transdermal drug delivery is particularly beneficial in older patients who are unable to swallow because of impaired consciousness, severe mucositis, intractable nausea and vomiting, or dysphagia and in those who experience unacceptable side-effects with morphine preparations. In addition, the weight of evidence suggests that constipation is less common with fentanyl than with morphine. However, it must be remembered that older patients with chronic skin disorders and limited dexterity are not ideal candidates for the administration of fentanyl patches.[143]

Swallowing impairment may be due to a primary tumor or, in many elderly patients, a consequence of frailty or intercurrent disease such as stroke, motor neuron disease, or Parkinson's disease. Opioids suitable for continuous s.c. infusion must be soluble, well absorbed, and nonirritant. Continuous infusion has the advantage that it can be used to administer not only analgesics but also drugs to manage nausea. The addition of anxiolytic agents may be particularly helpful in older patients who are agitated as a consequence of an acute confusional state. Although neuroleptics may be administered in younger patients, their use in older people may precipitate Parkinsonian side-effects, which impair mobility, feeding, and other activities of daily living.

ADDITIONAL ANALGESIA

Antidepressants

Up to 12–15% of community-dwelling older people are diagnosed with depression.[144] Although the existence of a relationship between depression and pain in patients with cancer is well known, the influence of one upon the other is still poorly understood. In a study by Spiegel *et al.*[145*] that included older patients, the prevalence of depressive disorders was significantly higher among patients in the high-pain than among those in the low-pain group. The authors concluded that pain might play a causal role in producing depression, but their data could also have supported the opposite conclusion. Amitriptyline, a tricyclic antidepressant, is a commonly prescribed antidepressant but, although the main indication for tricyclic antidepressants among patients of all ages is neuropathic pain,[146***] many older patients with pain also have depression and difficulty sleeping. There is evidence of the analgesic efficacy of amitriptyline in older patients with trigeminal neuralgia and diabetic neuropathy,[147] although data in older patients with pain are lacking. The analgesic action of tricyclic antidepressants in neuropathic pain appears to be independent of their antidepressant effects as the speed of onset is faster and the effective dose is lower than for depression.[146] However, tricyclic antidepressants are difficult drugs to administer in older patients as they can result in postural hypotension, urinary hesitancy, and glaucoma, problems already common in the older population.

Anticonvulsant drugs

Like tricyclic antidepressants, anticonvulsants such carbamazepine and phenytoin are useful in the management of neuropathic pain. Unfortunately, phenytoin may result in sedation or confusion as well as dizziness and unsteadiness, particularly on standing. Similarly, carbamazepine may cause sedation and nausea, which results in a poor oral intake. Neutropenia and thrombocytopenia as well as aplastic anemia have been reported in patients receiving carbamazepine, and thus repeated full blood counts are necessary in older patients, especially those with bone marrow involvement or who have recently undergone chemotherapy or radiotherapy. Hepatotoxicity and congestive cardiac failure have also been reported, and older patients may be particularly at risk of hyponatremia due to inappropriate secretion of antidiuretic hormone (ADH). Clonazepam may cause ataxia, and for this reason must be cautiously used in an elderly person in whom mobility is already impaired and/or who is liable to falls. Extreme care must be exercised when withdrawing benzodiazepines because of the risk of seizures, which are troublesome in their own right but often lead to falls and bony injury in older people.[148]

Unfortunately, evidence for the efficacy of anticonvulsant drugs in relieving acute and chronic pain is somewhat lacking. Wiffen *et al.*[149***] investigate trials of anticonvulsant use in patients with acute and chronic pain but could find no trials comparing different anticonvulsants and only one study specifically of cancer pain. In addition, there is no evidence that anticonvulsants are effective in relieving acute pain, and in patients with chronic pain syndromes other than trigeminal neuralgia anticonvulsants should be withheld until other interventions have been tried.

Nonpharmacological

Nonpharmacological analgesia in the form of imagery, relaxation training, and hypnosis has been used successfully to treat procedure pain. In addition, many guidelines for the management of acute pain also mention relaxation and cognitive approaches. A study of 241 patients aged 18–92 years undergoing percutaneous vascular and renal procedures found that, although pain increased linearly with procedure time in the standard and the structured attention group, among the 82 patients in the hypnosis group (mean age 45, range 19–82, years) pain remained constant over time. Drug use in the standard treatment group was significantly higher than in either the structured attention or hypnosis group. With benefits for both economic considerations and patient comfort, the procedure times were significantly shorter in the hypnosis group than in the standard group.[150*]

Ferrell *et al.*[103] found that, before entering a pain management program, older patients rarely used nondrug interventions. However, on a scale of 0–4 (0 = not helpful, 4 = very helpful) heat was used by 68% of patients, with a mean effectiveness of 3.2, cold was used by 19% of patients, with a mean effectiveness of 2.9, massage was used by 64% of patients, with a mean effectiveness of 2.9, and distraction was used by 47% of patients, with a mean effectiveness of 3.3.

Massage

As for most complementary therapies there is a lack of sound research regarding the effectiveness of massage for pain relief, particularly among older people. Although Fraser and Kerr[151*] found that back massage reduced anxiety scores, the groups studied were small. A study by Ferrell-Torry and Glick[152*] of male patients up to the age of 77 found an average of 60% reduction in the level of pain perception and a 24% fall in anxiety after two consecutive evenings of 30 min therapeutic massage. Further research is needed to determine the benefit of massage as training is expensive and may at best provide no benefit and at worst have adverse effects if used inappropriately.[153]

Transcutaneous electrical nerve stimulation

In transcutaneous electrical nerve stimulation (TENS), surface electrodes connected to a small portable battery are used to stimulate large-diameter nerves in the skin and subcutaneous tissues. The advantages of the use of TENS in older patients are that the machine is compact, lightweight, easily portable and, if patients wish to purchase one, relatively inexpensive. For these reasons TENS can readily be used in the community and helps to maintain patients' mobility. It is difficult to predict which patients will respond to TENS, but it is effective in some patients. It must also be remembered that it is a technique with which many elderly patients may already be familiar for the treatment of noncancer pain.

Although skin irritation, burns, and allergy to the gel applied to the skin are rare, it is important that TENS should not be used in the area of the carotid sinus and the larynx as there is a risk of hypotension or laryngeal spasm. Of particular concern in older patients is that TENS is not appropriate in patients who have a cardiac pacemaker *in situ*.[154]

Radiotherapy

Radiotherapy for the palliation of painful bone metastases has been widely studied in a variety of age groups. On the whole, radiotherapy produces complete pain relief at 1 month in approximately 25% of patients and at least 50% relief in almost half of patients. Radioisotopes alone produce equivalent relief with a similar onset and duration to that provided by radiotherapy. However, following radioisotope treatment, patients report significantly fewer new sites of pain compared with control subjects who receive external irradiation alone.[155**] This may be particularly helpful in older patients and prevent frequent hospital attendances. A systematic review found little discernible difference in efficacy between fractionation schedules and between different doses of the same schedule, although the data were not subanalyzed by age.[156***] Cerebral metastases often cause intractable pain, and patients of all ages can be treated with radiotherapy.[157]

SPECIFIC PROBLEMS OF LATER LIFE

Dealing with patients who cannot respond verbally

Many elderly patients are unable to respond to questioning. These patients may have communication problems and be cognitively intact, or they may have cognitive impairment with no language barriers. Other communication difficulties may be exacerbated by distorted facial expression, such as occurs after a stroke, in patients with advanced Parkinson's disease, or as a result of facial dystonic movements. Communicating with such patients about food and drink or the need to be toileted is problematic, but determining patients' needs in these areas requires only crude levels of communication, whereas pain management is more complex and involves identification of pain and an assessment of response to treatment. Marzinsky[158] devised methods of assessing pain using nonverbal behavior but found none to be entirely suitable. Most documented pain behaviors have been described in patients with acute pain aged 65 or younger, and research on chronic pain is usually conducted in alert elderly people. The difficulty of developing such scales was highlighted by Hurley *et al.*,[159*] who, after devising a scale to measure discomfort based on nursing observation of patients with advanced Alzheimer's disease, found that only nine items from an original 26-item scale remained after reliability testing.

Simons and Malabar,[160*] in a study of three elderly care wards, used a combination of data sheet, pain assessment chart, and menu of observable pain behavior to identify those patients who were experiencing pain. They studied those patients who were able to communicate to validate nurses' observations. Although some nurses experienced difficulties using such a schema, it took about 8 min to carry out the initial assessment and 3 min for each reassessment. The authors concluded that pain management in the verbally unresponsive older patient was improved by the schema and that the combined documentation was both effective and easy to administer.

It must also be remembered that many ill or older people are silent when questioned about pain. This may not indicate the absence of pain but simply that the older person is trying to process the information that has been given.[161] There are guidelines *"Responding to patients who are silent"* which include elucidating the meanings of silence, its variability across cultures, and other factors that may be learned by patient observation.[162]

A recent study of patients with Down's syndrome indicated that this group are not insensitive to pain. However, they express pain or discomfort more slowly and in a less precise fashion than the general population. This study of 26 individuals lends further evidence that medical teams managing patients with communication problems should use pain control procedures even in the absence of obvious pain manifestations.[163*]

There is evidence that people who are profoundly cognitively impaired cannot express their pain verbally, and behavior and physiological indices may provide the only indications that they are in pain.[164]

Nursing or residential home patients

Many older people with cancer may be living in residential or nursing homes. These patients not only have cancer but are often frail and have multiple pathology, are being treated with numerous drugs, and, in many cases, have impaired cerebral function or communication problems, which compound the management of pain.

Although most authors do not study exclusively pain due to malignant disease, a high level of pain is seen in these patients. Over half of all nursing home residents report pain on a regular basis irrespective of cause, and a study of 49,971 nursing home residents found that 26% experienced pain daily.[165] In many residents, pain was associated with impairment in activities of daily living and mood. Even when pain was recognized, men, members of the racial minorities, and cognitively impaired patients had a higher risk of undertreatment. Indeed, only 25% of the residents experiencing daily pain were on appropriate medication.[166*] In a US study of 13,625 patients with cancer aged 65 or older, only 16% of those reporting pain received simple analgesia; 32% and 26% were given weak opioids and morphine respectively. Of particular concern is the fact that patients older than 85 who were in pain were about 50% less likely to receive analgesia than those aged 65–74, and this group are likely to be over-represented in a nursing home population. This study also confirmed that people from ethnic minority groups were less likely to receive analgesia, and for about 50% of the time there was a level of cognitive impairment in patients that made communication about pain difficult.[167**]

Yates *et al.*[60] conducted interviews in five large residential care settings in Brisbane, Australia, over a 3-month period. Although there has been little published on the use of focus groups in older patients, the 10 focus groups included people aged 65 or older. Three key areas emerged: first, a resignation to pain, i.e. pain is common in chronic and long-term elderly people; second, ambivalence about the benefit of action, i.e. that pain-relieving medication and other pain management strategies provide only limited pain relief; and, finally, a reluctance to express pain, with participants indicating that one should not bother others with one's pain, that staff are too busy to help, and that the willingness of staff to help varied.

Pain is a common and underdiagnosed feature in older patients with cancer. Its management is poorly studied and, where evidence exists, undertreatment is often exposed. Old patients pose particular problems, and until evidence exists best practice will be lacking.

REFERENCES

1. IASP Subcommittee on Taxonomy. Pain terms: a list with definitions and notes on usage. *Pain* 1980; **8:** 249–52.
2. Federation of State Medical Boards of the United States. *Model Guidelines for the Use of Controlled Substances for the Treatment of Pain*. Euless, TX: Federation of State Medical Boards of the United States, 1998.

● 3. Portenoy RK, Lesage P. Management of cancer pain. *Lancet* 1999; **353:** 1695–700.

4. Ferrell BR, Dean G. The meaning of cancer pain. *Semin Oncol Nursing* 1995; **11:** 17–22.

5. Ferrell BR, Taylor EJ, Sattler GR, *et al.* Searching for the meaning of pain: cancer patients', caregivers' and nurses' perspectives. *Cancer Pract* 1993; **1:** 185–94.

● 6. Carr DB, Goudas LC. Acute pain. *Lancet* 1999; **353:** 2051–8.

7. Katz B, Helme RD. Pain problems in old age. In: Tallis RC, Fillit HM, Brocklehurst JC eds. *Brocklehurst's Textbook of Geriatric Medicine and Gerontology*, 5th edn. London: Churchill Livingstone, 1998: 1423–30.

◆ 8. Ferrell BA, Ferrell BR, Osterweil D. Pain in the nursing home. *J Am Geriat Soc* 1990; **38:** 409–14.

9. Bowling A, Browne PD. Social networks, health, and emotional well-being among the oldest old in London. *J Gerontol* 1991; **46:** S20–32.

10. Merskey H, Bogduk N eds. *Classification of Chronic Pain: Descriptions of Chronic Pain Syndromes and Definition of Pain Terms.* Report by the International Association for the Study of Pain Task Force on Taxonomy, 2nd edn. Seattle, WA: IASP Press, 1994.

11. Harkins SW, Kwentus J, Price DD. Pain and suffering in the elderly. In: Bonica JJ ed. *The Management of Pain*, 2nd edn. Philadelphia, PA: Lea & Febiger, 1990: 552–9.

◆ 12. Brockopp D, Warden S, Colclough G, Brockopp G. Elderly people's knowledge of and attitudes to pain management. *Br J Nursing* 1996; **5:** 556–62.

◆ 13. Ferrell BR, Grant M, Chan J, *et al.* The impact of cancer pain education on family caregivers of elderly patients. *Oncology Nursing Forum* 1995; **22:** 1211–18.

14. McCaffery M. *Nursing the Patient in Pain*. Philadelphia, PA: JB Lippincott, 1972.

15. Anon. *Guideline No. 9*. Rockville, MD: Agency for Healthcare Policy and Research, 1994.

16. Bonica JJ. Treatment of cancer pain: current status and future needs. In: Fields JL, Dubner R, Cervero J eds. *Advances in Pain Research and Therapy*. New York, NY: Raven Press, 1985: 589–616.

17. World Health Organization. *Cancer Pain Relief.* Geneva: WHO, 1986.

● 18. Portenoy RK. Cancer pain, epidemiology and syndromes. *Cancer* 1989; **63:** 2298–307.

19. Bonica JJ, Loeser JD. Medical evaluation of the patient with pain. In: Bonica JJ, Loeser JD, Chapman CR, Fordyce WE eds. *The Management of Pain*, 2nd edn. Philadelphia, PA: Lea & Febiger, 1990: 563–80.

20. World Health Organization. *Cancer Pain Relief and Palliative Care*. Geneva: WHO, 1990.

◆ 21. Cleeland CS, Gonin R, Hatfield AK, *et al.* Pain and its treatment in outpatients with metastatic cancer. *N Engl J Med* 1994; **330:** 592–6.

22. Royal College of Surgeons and College of Anaesthetists Working Party (1990). *Commission on the Provision of Surgical Services*. Report of the Working Party on Pain after Surgery. London: Royal College of Surgeons and College of Anaesthetists, 1990.

23. Lynn J, Teno JM, Phillips RS, *et al.* Perceptions by family members of the dying experience of older and seriously ill patients. SUPPORT Investigators. Study to Understand Prognoses and Preferences for Outcomes and Risks of Treatments. *Ann Intern Med* 1997; **126:** 97–106.

24. Goodwin JS, Samet JM, Key CR, *et al.* Stage at diagnosis of cancer varies with age of the patient. *J Am Geriatr Soc* 1986; **34:** 20–6.

25. Samet JM, Hunt WC, Key CR, *et al.* Choice of cancer therapy varies with age of patient. *JAMA* 1986; **255:** 3385–90.

26. Greenfield S, Blanco DM, Elashoff RM, Ganz PA. Patterns of care related to age of breast cancer patients. *JAMA* 1987; **257:** 2766–70.

27. Markman M, Lewis JL, Saigo P, *et al.* Epithelial ovarian cancer in the elderly: the Memorial Sloan-Kettering Cancer Center experience. *Cancer* 1993; **71:** 634–7.

28. Watkin SW, Hayhurst GK, Green JA. Time trends in the outcome of lung cancer management: a study of 9,090 cases diagnosed in the Mersey Region, 1974–1986. *Br J Cancer* 1990; **61:** 590–6.

29. Henderson J, Goldacre MJ, Griffith M. Hospital care of the elderly in the final year of life: a population based study. *Br Med J* 1990; **301:** 17–19.

30. Dunlop RJ, Davies RJ, Hockley JM. Preferred *vs* actual place of death: a hospital palliative care support team experience. *Palliative Med* 1989; **3:** 197–201.

31. Stout RW, Crawford V. Active-life expectancy and terminal dependency: trends in long-term geriatric care over 33 years. *Lancet* 1998; **1:** 281–3.

32. Cartwright A. The role of hospitals in caring for people in the last year of their lives. *Age Ageing* 1991; **20:** 271–4.

33. Harkins SW. Geriatric pain. Pain perceptions in the old. *Clin Geriat Med* 1996; **12:** 435–59.

34. Bellville J, Forrest WH, Miller E, Brown BW. Influence of age on pain relief from analgesics: a study of post operative patients. *JAMA* 1971; **217:** 1835–41.

◆ 35. Brochet B, Michel P, Barberger-Gateau P, Dartigues JF. Population-based study of pain in elderly people: a descriptive survey. *Age Ageing* 1998; **27:** 279–84.

36. Vigano A, Bruera E, Suarez-Almazor ME. Age, pain intensity, and opioid dose in patients with advanced cancer. *Cancer* 1998; **83:** 1244–50.

37. Milne RW, McLean CF, Mather LE, *et al.* Influence of renal failure on disposition of morphine, morphine-3-glucuronide and morphine-6-glucurinide in sheep during intravenous infusion with morphine. *J Pharmacol Exp Ther* 1997; **282:** 779–86.

● 38. Davies G, Kingswood C, Street M. Pharmacokinetics of opioids in renal dysfunction. *Clin Pharmacokinet* 1996; **31:** 410–22.

39. Sacks FM, Pfeffer MA, Moye LA, *et al.* The effect of pravastatin on coronary events after myocardial infarc-

tion in patients with average cholesterol levels. Cholesterol and Recurrent Events Trial investigators. *N Engl J Med* 1996; **335:** 1001–9.

40. Rochon PA, Tu JV, Anderson GM, *et al.* Rate of heart failure and 1-year survival for older people receiving low-dose beta-blocker therapy after myocardial infarction. *Lancet* 2000; **356:** 639–44.
41. SHEP. Prevention of stroke by antihypertensive drug treatment in older persons with isolated systolic hypertension. Final results of the Systolic Hypertension in the Elderly Program. *JAMA* 1991; **265:** 3255–64.
42. Pitt B, Chang P, Timmermans PB. Angiotensin II receptor antagonists in heart failure: rationale and design of the evaluation of losartan in the elderly (ELITE) trial. *Cardiovasc Drugs Ther* 1995, **9:** 693–700.
43. Frost PH, Davis BR, Burlando AJ, *et al.* Serum lipids and incidence of coronary heart disease: findings from The Systolic Hypertension in the Elderly Program (SHEP). *Circulation* 1996; **94:** 2381–8.
44. Tsevat J. Dawson NV, Wu AW, *et al.* Health values of hospitalized patients 80 years or older. HELP Investigators. Hospitalized elderly longitudinal project. *JAMA* 1998; **279:** 371–5.
45. Scott J, Huskisson EC. Graphic representation of pain. *Pain* 1976; **2:** 175–84.
◆ 46. Carlsson AM. Assessment of chronic pain. Aspects of the reliability and validity of the Visual Analogue Scale. *Pain* 1983; **16:** 87–101.
47. Dalton J, Twomey T, Workman M. Pain relief for cancer patients. *Cancer Nursing* 1988; **11:** 322–8.
◆ 48. Ahmedzai S. palliative and terminal care. In: Fentiman IS, Monfardini S eds. *Cancer in the Elderly: Treatment and Research*. Oxford: Oxford Medical Publications, 1994: 152–68.
◆ 49. Dalton JA, McNaull F. A call for standardizing the clinical rating of pain intensity using a 0 to 10 rating scale. *Cancer Nursing* 1998; **21:** 46–9.
● 50. Gagliese L. Melzack R. Chronic pain in elderly people. *Pain* 1997; **70:** 3–14.
51. Aaronson NK, Bullinger M, Ahmedzai S. A modular approach to quality of life assessment in cancer clinical trials. *Recent Results Cancer Res* 1988; **111:** 231–49.
52. Beck-Friis B, Strang P, Eklund G. Physical dependence of cancer patients at home. *Palliative Med* 1989; **3:** 281–6.
53. Ferrell BA. Pain management in elderly people. *J Am Geriat Soc* 1991; **39:** 64–73.
54. Closs SJ. Pain and elderly patients: a survey of nurses' knowledge and experiences. *J Advanced Nursing* 1996; **23:** 237–42.
55. Hardy C, Wallace C, Khansur T, *et al.* Nutrition, cancer, and aging: an annotated review. II. Cancer cachexia and aging. *J Am Geriat Soc* 1986; **34:** 219–28.
56. McWhirter JP, Pennington CR. Incidence and recognition of malnutrition in hospital. *Br Med J* 1994; **308:** 945–8.
◆ 57. Melzack R. The McGill Pain Questionnaire: major properties and scoring methods. *Pain* 1975; **7:** 277–99.
58. Turk DC, Okifuji A. Assessment of patients' reporting of pain: an integrated perspective. *Lancet* 1999; **353:** 1784–8.
◆ 59. Carpenter JS, Brockopp D. Comparison of patients' ratings and examination of nurses' responses to pain intensity rating scales. *Cancer Nursing* 1995; **18:** 292–8.
◆ 60. Jensen MP, Karoly P, Braver S. The measurement of clinical pain intensity: a comparison of six methods. *Pain* 1986; **27:** 117–26.
61. Herr KA, Mobily PR. Comparison of selected pain assessment tools for use with the elderly. *Appl Nursing Res* 1993; **6:** 39–46.
◆ 62. Latham J. Assessment and measurement of pain. *Palliative Care* 1994; **3:** 75–8.
63. Cleary JF. Cancer pain in the elderly. In: Balducci L, Lyman GH, Ershler WB eds. *Comprehensive Geriatric Oncology*. Amsterdam: Harwood Academic Publishers, 1998: 753–64.
64. Forbes V. Management of cancer pain in elderly patients. *Prescribing* 1998; June: 21–8.
◆ 65. Ward SE, Goldberg N, Miller-McCauley V, *et al.* Patient-related barriers to management of cancer pain. *Pain* 1993; **52:** 319–24.
◆ 66. Yates P, Dewar A, Fentiman B. Pain: the views of elderly people living in long-term residential care settings. *J Advanced Nursing* 1995; **21:** 667–74.
◆ 67. Cherny NI, Catane R. Professional negligence in the management of cancer pain. *Cancer* 1995; **76:** 2181–5.
68. Redmond K, Aapro MS. The nursing care of the elderly with cancer. In: Redmond K, Aapro MS eds. *Cancer in the Elderly. A Nursing and Medical Perspective*. Scientific Updates, No. 2. Amsterdam: Elsevier, 1997: 63–78.
69. Cleeland CS, Cleeland LM, Dar R, Rinehardt LC. Factors influencing physician management of cancer pain. *Cancer* 1986; **58:** 796–800.
70. Von Roenn JH, Cleeland CS, Gonin R, *et al.* Physician attitudes and practice in cancer pain management: a survey from the Eastern Cooperative Oncology Group. *Ann Intern Med* 1993; **119:** 121–6.
◆ 71. Larue F, Colleau SM, Fontaine A, *et al.* Oncologists and primary care physicians' attitudes towards pain control and morphine prescribing in France. *Cancer* 1995; **76:** 2375–82.
72. McCaffery M. *Nursing the Patient in Pain*, 2nd edn. London: Harper and Row, 1983.
73. Ferrell BR, McGuire DV, Donovan MI. Knowledge and beliefs regarding pain in a sample of nursing faculty. *J Profess Nursing* 1993; **9:** 79–88.
74. Ferrell BR, Ferrell BA, Rhiner M, Grant M. Family factors influencing cancer pain management. *Postgrad Med J* 1991; **67** (Suppl. 2): S64–9.
75. Porter J, Jick H. Addiction is rare in patients treated with narcotics. *N Engl J Med* 1980; **302:** 123.

76. Kaiko RF. Age and morphine analgesia in cancer patients with postoperative pain. *Clin Pharmacol Ther* 1980; **28:** 823–6.
77. Watt-Watson JH. Nurses' knowledge of pain issues: a survey. *J Pain Symptom Manage* 1987; **2:** 207–11.
78. McCaffery M, Ferrell B, O'Neil-Page E, *et al*. Nurses' knowledge of opioid analgesic drugs and psychological dependence. *Cancer Nursing* 1990; **13(1):** 21–7.
79. Slevin ML, Stubbs L, Plant JH, *et al*. Attitudes to chemotherapy: comparing views of patients with cancer with those of doctors, nurses, and general public. *Br Med J* 1990; **300:** 1458–60.
80. Ripamonti C, Filiberti A, Totis A, *et al*. Suicide among patients with cancer cared for at home by palliative-care teams. *Lancet* 1999; **354:** 1877–8.
81. Given B, Given CW. Cancer nursing for the elderly. A target for research. *Cancer Nursing* 1989; **12:** 71–7.
82. Woods NF, Lewis FM, Ellison ES. Living with cancer. Family experiences. *Cancer Nursing* 1989, **12:** 28–33.
◆ 83. Yeager KA, Miaskowski C, Dibble SL, Wallhagen M. Differences in pain knowledge and perception of the pain experience between out-patients with cancer and their family caregivers. *Oncol Nursing Forum* 1995; 22: 1235–41.
84. Ferrell BR, Taylor EJ, Grant M, *et al*. Pain management at home: struggle, comfort, and mission. *Cancer Nursing* 1993; **16:** 169–78.
85. Grobe ME, Ilstrup DM, Ahmann DL. Skills needed by family members to maintain the care of an advanced cancer patient. *Cancer Nursing* 1981; **4:** 371–5.
86. Ferrell BR, Rhiner M, Ferrell BA. Development and implementation of a pain education program. *Cancer* 1993; **72:** 3426–32.
87. Ferrell BR, Rhiner M, Cohen MZ, Grant M. Pain as a metaphor for illness. Part 1: Impact of cancer pain on family caregivers. *Oncology Nursing Forum* 1991; **18:** 1303–9.
88. Clotfelter CE. The effect of an educational intervention on decreasing pain intensity in elderly people with cancer. *Oncology Nursing Forum* 1999; **26(1):** 27–33.
89. Rousseau P. Pain management in the terminally ill. *J Am Geriat Soc* 1994; **42:** 1217–21.
90. Stetler C. Research utilization: defining the concept. *Image: J Nursing Scholar* 1985; **17(2):** 40–4.
91. Dufault MA, Bielecki C, Collins E, Willey C. Changing nurses' pain assessment practice: a collaborative research utilization approach. *J Advanc Nursing* 1995; **21:** 634–45.
◆ 92. Jandelli K. A comparative study of patients' and nurses' perceptions of pain relief. *Int J Palliative Nursing* 1995; **1(2):** 74–80.
93. Marks RM, Sachar EJ. Under treatment of medical inpatients with narcotic analgesics. *Ann Intern Med* 1973; **78:** 173–81.
94. Cohen FL. Postsurgical pain relief: patients' status and nurses' medication choices. *Pain* 1980; **9:** 265–74.
95. Wakefield AB. Pain: an account of nurses' talk. *J Advanced Nursing* 1995; **21:** 905–10.
96. *Morrison* P. Psychology of pain. *Surg Nursing* 1991; **4(6):** 18–20.
97. Woodward S. Nurse and patient perceptions of pain. *Profess Nurse* 1995; **10:** 415–16.
98. Short LM, Burnett ML, Egbert AM, Parks LH. Medicating the postoperative elderly: how do nurses make their decisions? *J Gerontol Nursing* 1990; **16(7):** 12–17.
99. Fossa SD, Aaronson NK, Newling D, *et al*. Quality of life and treatment of hormone resistant metastatic prostatic cancer. *Eur J Cancer* 1990; **26:** 1133–6.
100. Grassi L, Agostini M, Magnani K. Attitudes of Italian doctors to euthanasia and assisted suicide for terminally ill patients. *Lancet* 1999; **354:** 1876–77.
◆101. Jones WL, Rimer BK, Levy MH, Kinman JL. Cancer patients' knowledge, beliefs, and behaviour regarding pain control regimens: implications for education programmes. *Patient Ed Counselling* 1984; **5(4):** 159–64.
102. Levin DN, Cleeland CS, Dar R. Public attitudes towards cancer pain. *Cancer* 1985; **56:** 2337–9.
◆103. Ferrell BR, Ferrell BA, Ahn C, Tran K. Pain management for elderly patients with cancer at home. *Cancer* 1994; **74:** 2139–46.
104. Greenblatt D, Allen MD, Locniskar A, *et al*. Lorazepam kinetics in the elderly. *Clin Pharmacol Ther* 1979; **26:** 103–13.
105. Wynne HA, Cope LH, Herd B, *et al*. The association of age and frailty with paracetamol conjugation in man. *Age Ageing* 1990; **19:** 419–24.
106. Preiss R, Matthias M, Sohr R, *et al*. Pharmacokinetics of adriamycin, adriamycinol and antipyrine in patients with moderate tumour involvement of the liver. *J Cancer Res Clin Oncol* 1987; **113:** 593–8.
107. Robertz-Vaupel GM, Lindecken KD, Edeki T, *et al*. Disposition of antipyrine in patients with extensive metastatic liver disease. *Eur J Clin Pharmacol* 1992; **42:** 465–9.
108. Castleden CM, George CF, Marcer D, Hallett C. Increased sensitivity to nitrazepam in old age. *Br Med J* 1977; **1:** 10–12.
109. Cook PJ, Flanagan R, James IM. Diazepam tolerance: effect of age, regular sedation, and alcohol. *Br Med J* 1984; **289:** 351–3.
110. Smith JM, Baldessarini RJ. Changes in prevalence, severity and recovery in tardive dyskinesia with age. *Archiv Gen Psychiatry* 1980; **37:** 1368–73.
111. Bateman DN, Darling DW, Boys R, Rawlins MD. Extrapyramidal reactions to metoclopramide and prochlorperazine. *Q J Med* 1989; **264:** 307–11.
◆112. Field GB, Parry J. Pain control: some aspects of day-today management. *Palliative Care* 1994; **3:** 79–86.
113. Cox S, Tookman A. Management of cancer and neuropathic pain. *Prescriber* 1998; March: 85–8.
114. Beaulieu J. Recommended analgesics in acute and chronic pain. *Prescriber* 2000; September: 63–74.

●115. Hawkey CJ. COX-2 inhibitors. *Lancet* 1999; **353:** 307–14.

116. Henry D, Lim LL, Garcia-Rodrigues LA, *et al.* Variability in risk of gastrointestinal complications with individual non-steroidal anti-inflammatory drugs: results of a collaborative meta-analysis. *Br Med J* 1996; **312:** 1563–6.

117. McCallion J, McLaren B, Blech JJF, Erwin L. Effects of fenbufen and indomethacin on renal function and prostaglandin synthesis in elderly patients. *J Clin Exp Gerontol* 1989; **11:** 97–105.

◆118. Hawkey CJ, Karrasch JA, Szczepanski L, *et al.* Omeprazole compared with mosoprostol for ulcers associated with nonsteroidal anti-inflammatory drugs. Omeprazole versus Mosprostol for NSAID-induced Ulcer Management (OMNIUM) Study Group. *N Engl J Med* 1998; **338:** 727–34.

◆119. Yeomans ND, Tulassay Z, Juhasz L, *et al.* A comparison of omeprazole with ranitidine for ulcers associated with nonsteroidal anti-inflammatory drugs. Acid Suppression Trial: Ranitidine versus Omeprazole for NSAID-associated Ulcer Treatment (ASTRONAUT) Study Group. *N Engl J Med* 1998; **338:** 719–26.

120. Ellershaw JE, Kelly MJ. Corticosteroids and peptic ulceration. *Palliative Med* 1994; **8:** 313–19.

121. Tookman A. Myths of morphine. *Palliative Care Today* 1996; 13.

●122. de Craen AJ, di Giulio G, Lampe-Schoenmaeckers JE, *et al.* Analgesic efficacy and safety of paracetamol/codeine combinations versus paracetamol alone: a systematic review. *Br Med J* 1996; **313:** 321–5.

●123. Moore A, Collins S, Carroll D, McQuay H. Paracetamol with and without codeine in acute pain: a quantitative systemic review. *Pain* 1997; **70:** 193–201.

●124. Moore A, Collins S, Carroll D, McQuay H. Single dose paracetamol (acetaminophen), with and without codeine, for postoperative pain. *Cochrane Database Syst Rev* 2000; **2:** CD001547.

125. Flanagan RJ, Johnston A, White AS, Crome P. Pharmacokinetics of dextropropoxyphene and nordextropropoxyphene in young and elderly volunteers after single and multiple dextropropoxyphene dosage. *Br J Clin Pharmacol 1989*; **28:** 463–9.

●126. Collins SL, Edwards JE, Moore RA, McQuay HJ. Single dose dextropropoxyphene, alone and with paracetamol (acetaminophen), for postoperative pain. *Cochrane Database Syst Rev* 2000; **2:** CD001440.

127. Livingstone H, Young J. Morphine. Appropriate use in older people. *Geriat Med* 2000; February: 33–6.

128. Ahmedzai S, Brooks D. Transdermal fentanyl versus sustained-release oral morphine in cancer pain: preference, efficacy, and quality of life. *J Pain Symptom Manage* 1997; **13:** 254–61.

129. Burns JW, Hodsman NB, McLintock TT, *et al.* The influence of patient characteristics on the requirements for post operative analgesia. *Anaesthesia* 1989; **44:** 2–6.

130. Zacharias M, Pfeifer MV, Herbison P. Comparison of two methods of intravenous administration of morphine for post-operative pain relief. *Anaesth Intens Care* 1990; **18:** 205–9.

131. Kaiko RF, Wallenstein SL, Rodgers AE, *et al.* Narcotics in the elderly. *Med Clin N Am* 1982; **66:** 1079–89.

132. Campara E, Merlin L, Pace M. The incidence of narcotic induced emesis. *J Pain Symptom Manage* 1991; **6:** 428–30.

●133. Cherny NI, Portenoy RK. Cancer pain management. Current strategy. *Cancer* 1993; **72:** 3393–415.

134. Zenz T. Palliative pain relief. *Lancet* 2000; **356:** 1273–4.

●135. Cherny NJ, Chang V, Frager G, *et al.* Opioid pharmacotherapy in the management of cancer pain. *Cancer* 1995; **76:** 1283–93.

◆136. Shaw HL. Treatment of intractable cancer pain by electronically controlled parenteral infusion of analgesic drugs. *Cancer* 1993 **72:** 3416–25.

137. MacDonald CJ, Smith AT, Smith KJ, *et al.* Opioid rotation: a place for hydromorphone. Poster Presentation, Pain Society of Great Britain and Ireland, 1997.

138. De Stoutz ND, Bruera E, Suarez-Almazor M. Opioid rotation for toxicity reduction in terminal cancer patients. *J Pain Symptom Manage* 1995; **10:** 378–84.

139. Ellershaw J. Hydromorphone: a new alternative to morphine. *Prescriber* 1998; February: 21–4.

140. Jones B, Finlay I. Oxycodone: alternative to morphine in cancer pain. *Prescriber* 2000; October: 43–50

141. Leng M. Oxycodone's place in pain in malignancy. *Prescriber* 2000; Suppl.: 9–12.

◆142. Kalso E, Vainio A. Morphine and oxycodone hydrochloride in the management of cancer pain. *Clin Pharmacol Ther* 1990; **37:** 639–46.

143. Edmonds P, Davies C. New approaches to the pharmacological management of pain. *Palliative Care Today* 1995; 32–4.

144. Beekman ATF, Copeland JRM, Prince MJ. Review of community prevalence of depression in late life. *Br J Psychiatry* 1999; **174:** 307–11.

◆145. Speigel D, Sands S, Koopman C. Pain and depression in patients with cancer. *Cancer* 1994; **74:** 2570–8.

146. McQuay HJ, Tramer M, Nye BA, *et al.* A systematic review of antidepressants in neuropathic pain. *Pain* 1996; **68:** 217–27.

147. Portenoy RK. Adjuvant analgesics in pain management. In: Doyle D, Hanks GWC MacDonald N eds. *Oxford Textbook of Palliative Medicine*. Oxford: Oxford University Press, 1993: 187–203.

148. Anon. Drug treatment of neuropathic pain. *Drugs and Therapeutics Bulletin* 2000; **38:** 89–93.

●149. Wiffen P, Collins S, McQuay H, *et al.* Anticonvulsant drugs for acute and chronic pain. *Cochrane Database Syst Rev* 2000; **3:** CD001133.

150. Lang EV, Benotsch EG, Fick LJ, *et al.* Adjunctive non-pharmacological analgesia for invasive medical procedures: a randomised trial. *Lancet* 2000; **355:** 1486–90.

151. Fraser J, Kerr JR. Psychophysiological effects of back

massage on elderly institutionalised patients. *J Advanced Nursing* 1993; **18:** 238–45.

152. Ferrell-Torry AT, Glick OJ. The use of therapeutic massage as a nursing intervention to modify anxiety and the perception of cancer pain. *Cancer Nursing* 1993; **16:** 93–101.

●153. Closs SJ. Pain in elderly patients: a neglected phenomenon? *J Advanced Nursing* 1994; **19:** 1072–81.

154. Sharma K. TENS and sensibility. *Hlth Ageing* 2001; April: 28–9.

155. Porter AT, McEwan AJ. Strontium-89 as an adjuvant to external beam radiation improves pain relief and delays the disease progression in advanced prostate cancer: results of a randomised controlled trial. *Semin Oncol* 1993; **20(3)** (Suppl 2): 38–43.

●156. McQuay HJ, Collins SL, Carroll D, Moore RA. Radiotherapy for the palliation of painful bone metastases. *Cochrane Database Syst Rev* 2000.

●157. Coia LR. The role of radiotherapy in the treatment of brain metastases. *Int J Rad Oncol Biol Phys* 1992; **23:** 229–38.

158. Marzinsky LR. The tragedy of dementia: assessing pain in the confused non-verbal elderly. *J Gerontol Nursing* 1991; **17(6):** 25–8.

159. Hurley AC, Volicer BJ, Hanrahan PA, *et al.* Assessment of discomfort in advanced Alzheimer patients. *Res Nursing Hlth* 1992; **15:** 369–77.

◆160. Simons W, Malabar R. Assessing pain in elderly patients who cannot respond verbally. *J Advanced Nursing* 1995; **22:** 663–9.

161. Murray R, Hueskoetter M. *Psychiatric/Mental Health Nursing*. Norwalk, CT: Appleton & Lange, 1987.

162. Davidhizar R, Giger-Newman J. When your patient is silent. *J Advanced Nursing* 1994; **20:** 703–6.

163. Hennequin M, Morin C, Feine JS. Pain expression and stimulus localization in individuals with Down's syndrome. *Lancet* 2000; **356:** 1882–7.

164. Abu-Saad HH. Challenge of pain in the cognitively impaired. *Lancet* 2000; **356:** 1867–8.

165. Ferrell BR, Ferrell BA. Easing the pain. *Geriatric Nursing* 1990; **11:** 175–8.

◆166. Won A, Lapane K, Gambassi G, *et al.* on behalf of the SAGE Study Group. Correlates and management of nonmalignant pain in the nursing home. *J Am Geriat Soc* 1999; **47:** 936–42.

◆167. Bernabei R, Gambassi G, Lapane K, *et al.* for the SAGE Study Group. Management of pain in elderly patients with cancer. *JAMA* 1998; **279:** 1877–82.

26

AIDS

MAEVE McKEOGH

Pain is a common and debilitating symptom in patients with human immunodeficiency virus (HIV) disease, occurring at all stages of infection from seroconversion to advanced disease. It is quite distinct from cancer pain and requires a different approach to its management. Most pain experienced by patients with acquired immunodeficiency syndrome (AIDS) is due to opportunistic infections rather than tumor, and these opportunistic infections can occur anywhere in the body, frequently on unusual sites such as the mucosal areas, the nerves, or the eye. It is not unusual for an AIDS patient to have a number of opportunistic infections and one or more tumors. A new pain may represent a new infection to be diagnosed and treated, and thus an etiological approach to pain is necessary. Pain in AIDS patients is inadequately treated, and opioid analgesics, in particular, are underutilized.

The natural history and clinical presentation of HIV disease varies between countries and between risk groups. AIDS is best regarded as a series of mini-epidemics in different risk groups, and the particular needs and priorities of each group must be addressed in management. The course of disease has altered substantially in developed countries in recent years as a result of the availability of HAART (highly active antiretroviral therapy). AIDS patients live longer and healthier lives as a result, but prescribing in AIDS has become more difficult because of the potential for significant drug interactions. An appreciation of the problems of particular risk groups, of the clinical presentation of AIDS in different settings, and of the likely underlying causes of pain, as well as some knowledge of the treatment regimens currently used, is essential to an integral approach to pain.

ANTIRETROVIRAL TREATMENTS

Palliative care physicians and pain specialists need to have an understanding of the mechanisms of action, side-effects, and potential for drug interactions of antiretroviral treatment[1] if they are to prescribe for symptom control in this group of patients. The potential for side-effects and unwanted drug interactions is high with the protease inhibitors and is a key issue for these patients.

The US Department of Health and Social Security guidelines summarize the problem as follows: "a major dilemma confronting patients and practitioners is that the antiretroviral regimens currently available that have the greatest potency in terms of viral suppression and CD4 T cell preservation are medically complex, are associated with a number of specific side-effects and drug interactions, and pose a substantial challenge for adherence."[2]

At the present time, four groups of drugs are licensed for use in the US and UK: nucleoside analogs, nucleotide analogs, non-nucleoside analog reverse transcriptase enzyme inhibitors, and protease inhibitors. These drugs are listed in Table 26.1.

The decision to stop antiretroviral treatment inevitably arises at some stage and should, if possible, involve the patient, the attending acute physician, and the palliative care physician. The management of pain in AIDS is considerably facilitated by terminating complex antiretroviral regimens when they are no longer helping both because these regimens can contribute to pain and because stopping them considerably widens the range of drugs available to use for symptom control.

Table 26.1 *Antiretroviral drugs licensed in the USA and UK at the end of June 2002*

Reverse transcriptase inhibitors			
Nucleoside analogs	**Nucleotide analogs**	**Non-nucleoside analogs**	**Protease inhibitors**
Zidovudine (AZT)	Tenovir	Nevirapine	Saquinavir
Didanosine (ddI)		Delaviridine	Hard gel
Zalcitabine (ddC)		Efaviranz	Soft gel
Lamivudine (3TC)			Indinavir
Stavudine (d4T)			Ritonavir
Abacavir			Nelfinavir
			Amprenavir
			Lopinavir

Nucleoside analogs

These drugs prevent viral replication by causing chain termination and/or blocking the reactive site of the enzyme reverse transcriptase, thus inhibiting retroviral cDNA synthesis. All are transformed in infected cells to the active triphosphate form. They are metabolized to differing extents by the liver, and both changed and unchanged drug is excreted in the urine.[3]

Zidovudine (AZT) has the greatest potential for interactions with drugs that influence liver metabolism. In an early study the concurrent use of acetaminophen (paracetamol) with zidovudine was associated with an increased incidence of myelotoxicity.[4] However, further research has not shown changes in the pharmacokinetic parameters of the two drugs.

Few drugs have been reported to alter the pharmacokinetics of didanosine (ddI), zalcitabine (ddC), and stavudine (d4T).

Didanosine is unstable at the pH found in the stomach. Therefore, it is supplied as a chewable/dispersible tablet with dihydroxyaluminum sodium carbonate, magnesium hydroxide, and sodium citrate as buffer to increase the pH of the stomach and thus its bioavailability. The presence of the buffer may interfere with the absorption of a number of drugs either by increasing the pH and reducing the solubility and absorption of acid-soluble drugs or by causing chelation of other drugs by the sodium and magnesium ions contained in the tablet formulation. To reduce the effect of didanosine on the absorption of other drugs they should be administered at least 2 h apart. Abacavir is a novel nucleoside reverse transcriptase inhibitor that is generally well tolerated with few significant adverse effects. The most important is a potentially fatal hypersensitivity in 3–5% of patients. Symptoms of this reaction may include skin rash, fever, nausea, abdominal pain, and severe tiredness.[4a]

The side-effects of nucleoside analogs are listed in Table 26.2 and significant potential drug interactions in Table 26.3.

Nucleotide analogs

Tenovir disoproxil fumarate is the first nucleotide analog approved for HIV-1 treatment. Nucleotide analogs are similar to nucleoside analogs: they are taken as masked prodrugs bearing labile lipophilic drug groups to facilitate penetration of target cell membranes. Subsequent unmasking by endogenous chemolytic enzymes releases a partially activated nucleoside analog metabolite. Tenovir has particular value because it has activity against many HIV viruses with mutations that render them insensitive to other nucleoside analogs.[4b,4c]

Non-nucleoside reverse transcriptase inhibitors

This group of drugs has been available for many years and its place in current treatment regimens is being redefined at the present time.[5] Drugs of this group are not as potent as drugs of the other two groups but are increasingly used in combination regimens as protease-sparing drugs, retaining the option of a protease inhibitor until later.

Currently, three non-nucleoside reverse transcriptase inhibitors – nevirapine, delaviridine, and efavirenz – are

Table 26.2 *Side-effects of nucleoside and nucleotide analogs[a]*

AZT	Bone marrow toxicity, anemia, neutropenia
ddI, ddC	Peripheral neuropathy, pancreatitis (ddC, thrombocytopenia 4%)
3TC	Peripheral neuropathy
d4T	Peripheral neuropathy, increases in hepatic transaminases
Abacavir	Severe hypersensitivity reaction in 3% of patients
Tenovir	Diarrhea, nausea, vomiting, flatulence

a. Lactic acidosis and hepatomegaly with steatosis (severe liver enlargement and excess fat in the liver) have occurred among patients treated with nucleoside and nucleotide analogs alone and in combination with antiretrovirals. These are severe and possibly fatal conditions.

Table 26.3 *Drug interactions of nucleoside analogs*

Drugs that can cause peripheral neuropathy should be used with caution in combination with ddI, ddC, and 3TC
Drugs that can cause pancreatitis should be used with caution in combination with ddI and ddC

Table 26.4 *Summary of pharmacokinetics of saquinavir*

Absorption	Low (*increased* by food)
Metabolism	Liver cytochrome P_{450}
Use is *contraindicated* with the following	Cisapride Terfenadine
Care should be taken with other drugs metabolized by CYP3A4	Nifedipine Midazolam
Subtherapeutic plasma concentrations of saquinivir may be caused by compounds that induce the enzyme. These agents should be *avoided* if possible	Carbamazepine Dexamethasone Phenobarbitone Phenytoin Rifabutin Rifampicin

available in clinical practice. Efavirenz may cause central nervous system symptoms (insomnia, somnolence, and disturbing dreams) that may overlap with those of analgesics but which usually disappear with time. Nevirapine induces the formation of the enzyme CYP3A4 and thus may affect the levels of drugs that are metabolized by this enzyme.

Protease inhibitors

Protease inhibitors are an extremely potent group of drugs with a complex range of significant interactions with other drugs and toxicities.[6,7] Hyperlipidemia, impaired glucose tolerance, and abnormal fat distribution (buffalo hump) may occur. In some patients, angina, myocardial infarction, and diabetes mellitus have been described.[8,9]

As the range of potential drug interactions of the protease inhibitors is enormous, only the interactions with drugs likely to be used by pain or palliative care physicians will be described. The interactions and toxicities described in the following tables are likely to be continually updated.

Saquinavir

Saquinavir is highly protein bound (approximately 98%), leading to negligible concentrations being found in the cerebrospinal fluid (CSF). Elimination is mostly nonrenal. Saquinavir is a weak inhibitor of the CYP3A4 isoenzyme and therefore has the potential to increase plasma concentrations of drugs that share this method of elimination. Its pharmacokinetics and drug interactions are summarized in Table 26.4, and its main toxicities, which are relatively few, in Table 26.5.

Indinavir

Indinavir has a similar drug interaction profile as saquinavir but is a more potent enzyme inhibitor. Not-

Table 26.5 *Toxicities of saquinivir*

Diarrhea 16%,
Abdominal discomfort 6%
Buccal mucosal ulceration 6%
Rash 4%
Headache 4%
Peripheral neuropathy 4%

Table 26.6 *Summary of pharmacokinetics of indinavir*

Absorption	Low (*reduced* by food)
Metabolism	Liver, isoenzyme CYP3A4, 20% renal excretion
Use is contraindicated with the following	Terfenadine Astemizole (cardiac) Cisapride (toxicity) Alprazolam Triazolam (sedation) Midazolam
Care should be taken with drugs with narrow therapeutic windows, e.g.	Carbamazepine Phenytoin Phenobarbital
Plasma concentrations of indinavir may be reduced with concomitant use of drugs that induce the CYP3A4 isoenzyme	Carbamazepine Dexamethasone Phenytoin Phenobarbital

Table 26.7 *Toxicities of indinavir*

Rash (19.1%)
Taste perversion (19.1%)
Dry skin (16.2%)
Nephrolithiasis (2–4%), (maintenance of adequate hydration essential)
Increases in mean cell volume, alanine aminotransferase, aspartate aminotransferase, indirect bilirubin, total serum bilirubin, decrease in neutrophils
Hematuria, proteinuria, and crystalluria

Table 26.8 *Toxicities of ritonavir*

At start of treatment	Nausea (47.5%) Diarrhea (44.9%) Circumoral (26.6%) and peripheral (15.4%) paresthesiae Vomiting (23.6%) Asthenia (22.3%) Headache (15.5%) Abdominal pain (11.6%) Taste perversion (11.4%)
Treatment is started at a low dose and increased	
Other side-effects	Hypertriglyceridemia Hypercholesterolemia Hyperuricemia Renal toxicity (monitor renal function)

Table 26.9 *Drugs* contraindicated *with ritonavir because large increases in their plasma concentration may lead to cardiac toxicity, profound sedation, seizures, or other serious adverse effects*

Isoenzyme inhibited	Drug affected
CYP3A4	Cisapride Terfenadine Midazolam Triazolam
CYP2D6	Meperidine (pethidine)
CYP2D4	Diazepam Flurazepam

Table 26.10 *Drugs known to undergo metabolism by the same cytochrome P_{450} isoenzyme and for which a* reduced starting dose *should be considered with ritonavir*

Azithromycin	Ketoconazole
Amitriptyline	Loratadine
Ca channel antagonists	Methadone
Carbamazepine	Metronidazole
Chloroquine	Nortriptyline
Clarithromycin	Paroxetine
Clindamycin	Prednisolone
Dexamethasone	Risperidone
Erythromycin	Sertraline
Fentanyl	Thioridazine
Fluoxetine	Tinidazole
Haloperidol	Tolbutamide
Imipramine	Trazadone
Itraconazole	Warfarin

Table 26.11 *Drugs whose plasma concentration have been found to be decreased when coadministered with ritonavir.* Increased *doses of these drugs may be needed*

Atovaquone
Ethinylestradiol
Morphine
Diamorphine
Codeine
Theophylline

Table 26.12 *Plasma concentrations of ritonavir may be decreased by enzyme inducers such as the following, which should be avoided if possible*

Carbamazepine
Dexamethasone
Phenytoin
Phenobarbital
Rifampicin

able side-effects are renal stones and hyperbilirubinemia. To reduce the incidence of renal stones it is recommended that patients should maintain adequate hydration of at least 1.5 l of fluid per 24 h. The pharmacokinetics and significant drug interactions of indinavir are summarized in Table 26.6 and its toxicities in Table 26.7.

Ritonavir

Ritonavir shares some of the pharmacokinetic properties of saquinavir, although it is a far more potent enzyme inhibitor than either saquinavir or indinavir. In addition to greater inhibition of the cytochrome P_{450} isoenzyme CYP3A4, it also inhibits isoenzymes CYP2D6 and CYP2C9, thus increasing the potential for drug interactions. It induces the enzyme glucuronyl transferase, resulting in increased metabolism of drugs such as morphine and diamorphine. Major toxicities of ritonavir are shown in Table 26.8.

The potential for significant drug interactions with ritonavir is vast, and only those drugs that are likely to be used in the pain setting have been included in Tables 26.9–26.12.

Nelfinavir

Nelfinavir is the fourth protease inhibitor to become commercially available and was the first to receive concomitant approval in the USA for both adults and children. Nelfinavir may be preferred over the other protease inhibitors because of its favorable toxicity profile. Its metabolism, drug interactions, and side-effect profile are similar to previous protease inhibitors. Diarrhea is the dose-limiting side-effect, occurring in 13–20% of patients. Elevated triglyceride and blood glucose levels have been observed.

Amprenavir

Amprenavir is a novel protease inhibitor. The major adverse effects observed in clinical usage have been gastrointestinal intolerance, skin rash, and perioral paresthesiae.[9a]

Lopinavir

Lopinavir is the sixth protease inhibitor licensed for use in adults and children more than 6 months of age with HIV. It is available as a coformulation of lopinavir and low-dose ritonavir. The subtherapeutic dose of ritonavir inhibits the metabolism of lopinavir, resulting in higher lopinavir concentrations than when the latter is administered alone. The side-effects associated with this combination are diarrhea, fatigue, headache, and nausea. As observed with other protease inhibitors, it may also be associated with serious adverse events, including increases in blood glucose, redistribution of body fat and potentially serious life-threatening drug interactions.[9b]

THE LITERATURE ON PAIN IN AIDS

HIV infection has a variable course, with a wide range of potential complications, rates of progression, and survival. Inevitably, this variability applies to pain in this patient group.

Most of the available data on pain in AIDS come from small studies on selected subpopulations of HIV-infected individuals, and the conclusions that can be drawn are limited. No large-scale epidemiological studies have been undertaken. Few studies consider the effects of stage of disease, transmission group, gender, or antiretroviral treatment on the incidence and presentation of pain. AIDS pain can only be understood in the context of the natural history of the disease and the evolution of its treatments. These factors, which are summarized in Table 26.13, must each be taken into account in any analysis of pain in AIDS.

Transmission group has an important effect on the natural history and presentation of disease, e.g. Kaposi's sarcoma and cytomegalovirus (CMV) retinitis are more common in homosexual men than in other risk groups. Pneumonia and pulmonary tuberculosis are more frequent in HIV-infected substance abusers than in other risk groups.[10,11] The syndrome of "crack lung" is associated with cocaine abuse and should be considered as a cause of chest pain in these patients.[12] In addition, fibromyalgia syndrome (FMS) is more prevalent in HIV-infected substance abusers than in other risk groups and is an important cause of rheumatic pain in these patients.[13]

Gender has an effect on the distribution of symptomatology, reflecting known gender differences in the prevalence of AIDS illnesses. Women experience a higher incidence of esophageal candidiasis and a lower incidence of Kaposi's sarcoma and CMV disease than men.[14]

Finally, the study period has an important bearing on the nature and prevalence of pain-related conditions. The introduction of *Pneumocystis* pneumonia (PCP) prophylaxis in 1989[15] and protease inhibitors[16] in 1996 are both significant landmark periods in the epidemic, changing the natural history of the disease and thus the nature and intensity of symptoms. The incidence of PCP, previously a significant cause of chest pain in some studies, has dropped dramatically since the introduction of prophylaxis and would now be an uncommon cause of chest pain where prophylaxis is available. The introduction of HAART in 1996 has transformed the natural history of the disease where these drugs are available, allowing AIDS patients to live longer and healthier lives.[16] Thus, all studies prior to 1996 need to be interpreted with caution as they do not reflect today's patient population. It is virtually certain that HAART has resulted in a dramatic change in both the nature and intensity of pain syndromes in AIDS, but as yet no work has been published on this key issue.

Table 26.13 *AIDS pain must be analyzed in context. Factors which influence the nature and presentation of pain in AIDS*

Transmission group
Setting – hospital, hospice, or outpatients
Stage of disease
Study period
1989 PCP prophylaxis
1996 protease inhibitors
Are participants on HAART?

The prevalence of pain in AIDS

Estimates of the prevalence of pain in hospitalized AIDS patients range from about 54% to 62%;[17,18] among outpatients, the reported prevalence in the USA,[19–21] France,[18] Denmark,[21a] and the UK[22] varies between 30% and 80%. One large prospective study in the USA reported a prevalence of 80% in outpatients with AIDS, but the methodology consisted in recording pain over the previous 6-month period.[23] Studies in hospice settings report higher prevalences of around 80%.[24,25] It seems clear that progression to AIDS is associated with a higher incidence of pain and that the prevalence of pain at the end of life can be high. In one retrospective study in a US hospice, 93% of patients experienced at least one 48-h period of pain and discomfort during the last 2 weeks of life.[26]

Studies from the USA have found similar prevalences of pain in intravenous drug users as in other transmission groups,[19,20] although intravenous drug users report more undertreatment of pain.[20] However, data from Europe conflict with this.[27] The prevalence of pain appears to be similar between genders,[19,21,25] although there is an association between female gender and specific pain syndromes.[25,28] Intensity of pain, however, has been associated with female gender and noncaucasian race as well as with more advanced disease.[19] The adverse impact of pain in AIDS on quality of life has been documented in a number of studies.[18,19,21,22,29]

There is limited research concerning pain in HIV-infected children and youths, but the studies available suggest that it is a frequently encountered symptom in this group also. One large observational US study over 4 years found the prevalence of pain to remain relatively constant, despite the introduction of HAART, during each year of observation, averaging 20%.[29a]

AIDS pain compared with cancer pain

The importance of classifying pains according to type, etiology, and syndrome has been well established in the treatment of cancer pain. The benefits include guidance for further diagnostic investigation, improved selection for therapeutic interventions, and more accurate prognostication. The seminal papers of Portenoy[30] and Elliott and Foley[31] have categorized cancer pain into somatic, visceral, and neuropathic, based on inferred pathophysiology, categorization that is clinically useful and widely accepted.

These definitions, however, are less useful in HIV disease. Firstly, AIDS is not a single process but a syndrome of profound immunosuppression resulting in a variety of opportunistic infections and, less commonly, tumors. Secondly, many of these infections occur in unusual sites such as the oral or genital mucosa. Treatment of the infection usually relieves any associated pain. Courses of analgesia may be appropriate pending diagnosis and treatment of the underlying problem.

Hence, the approach to AIDS pain must be etiological. All new pains should be investigated to establish their etiology, e.g. a new symptom of dysphagia could be due to *Candida*, CMV, or herpesvirus infection, Kaposi's sarcoma, or lymphoma. An endoscopy will, in most cases, provide the answer, and specific treatment of the cause will remove the pain. Thus, the management of patients with pain associated with HIV disease usually involves more liaison with referring hospitals than the management of patients with cancer pain. Pain, however, must be treated properly pending investigations and reassessed following treatment of the infection or tumor. The numbers of drugs for treatment and prophylaxis results in polypharmacy, with consequent potential for significant interactions, toxicity, and cost.

Some of the differences between AIDS patients and cancer patients relevant to the management of pain are summarized in Table 26.14.

Table 26.14 *AIDS patients compared with cancer patients*

AIDS patients are typically younger than cancer patients
AIDS is an infectious disease – whole families may be infected
AIDS has a predilection for particular risk groups, e.g. homosexual men, substance abusers
The underlying pathology in AIDS is immunosuppression with susceptibility to multiple infections and tumors
It is necessary to take an etiological approach to all new pains in AIDS patients – liaison with acute centers for investigation is essential
Polypharmacy with implications for interactions, toxicities, and cost
Susceptibility to adverse side-effects of drugs, e.g. dopamine antagonists
Caution with corticosteroids because of immunosuppression
Active management of some conditions up to death, e.g. CMV retinitis
Often keen to try alternative approaches, e.g. acupuncture
Infection control protocols are essential for transmissible infection, e.g. MDRTB, shingles, enteric diarrhea, e.g. *Salmonella*, *Shigella*, *Campylobacter*
AIDS patients more likely to have co-morbid psychiatric problems, especially substance abusers
The bereavement pattern in AIDS is unusual, e.g. multiple losses, loss of contact with family, hostility between family and partners
Stigma

AIDS services must be tailored to the particular needs and problems of the various risk groups. For example, substance abusers frequently have chaotic lifestyles and appropriate staff training is essential; the assessment of pain in substance abusers can be particularly difficult, and higher doses of pain relief, particularly opioids, may be required because of tolerance.

AIDS patients are more susceptible to extrapyramidal side-effects from antiemetic drugs such as prochlorperazine and metoclopramide, and all dopamine antagonists should be used with caution in these patients.[32,33] Patients with HIV dementia are particularly prone to side-effects of sedation and confusion on opioids,[34] and lower doses are often necessary.

Corticosteroids, although used as treatment in a variety of AIDS-related conditions, should be used with caution because of their immunosuppressive effects. They can cause worsening of candidiasis and herpes simplex and zoster infection, and one study has demonstrated an increased risk of CMV retinitis in patients with advanced disease treated with corticosteroids.[35] Protocols for the management of tumors in AIDS patients specify a reduced dose of corticosteroids.

Some conditions associated with AIDS may require active management until death. For example, it may be advisable to continue prophylaxis or treatment for severe recurrent candidiasis or herpes infections up to death to prevent recurrence of these painful and debilitating conditions. Similarly, active treatment for CMV retinitis may be continued in certain cases to prevent total blindness developing before death. Each case must be judged on its own merits. Prophylaxis for PCP is usually discontinued once the final stage approaches as infection has a slow and insidious onset and will not supervene suddenly.

AIDS patients often wish to be fully informed about their illness and treatments and frequently pursue alternative approaches. This is a reflection partly of their younger age but also of their level of education and affluence. Patient advocate groups have done much to change the doctor–patient relationship to a partnership of shared knowledge and decision-making. The pursuit of alternative approaches may also be a marker of anxiety, as has been demonstrated for a subgroup of cancer patients.[36]

Psychiatric disorders are common in patients with HIV infection, and high levels of both anxiety and depression have been found even within those HIV-infected populations that are physically asymptomatic.[37] Clearly, psychological disorders are likely to have a significant impact on the experience of pain. Equally, inadequately treated pain will contribute significantly to psychological morbidity. There is evidence that female gender[38] and ethnicity[39] are associated with a greater risk of psychological difficulties. Also, among risk groups, intravenous drug users have been found to have greater psychological morbidity than those in other transmission categories.[40,41]

The bereavement pattern in AIDS patients differs from cancer in that it frequently reflects multiple losses. Within families, individuals may have to deal with the death of more than one member or of deaths of different generations, including children. Guilt associated with transmission of the infection may be a contributory factor to a complex grief reaction.

Finally, the stigma associated with infection may result in denial, which has been a key factor in fueling the spread of the virus, especially in sub-Saharan Africa. Patients may not wish to share their diagnosis with family or partners and be reluctant to use interpreters because of concerns about confidentiality. This makes the provision of proper symptom control more difficult and may be a factor in the undertreatment of pain in AIDS.

The management of pain in AIDS

The evidence from both the USA and Europe is that pain in AIDS is both underdiagnosed and undertreated. In one large prospective study in the USA of ambulatory AIDS patients, nearly 85% were receiving inadequate analgesia therapy.[42] Less than 8% of the 110 who reported "severe" pain were prescribed a strong opioid. In a multicenter French study, doctors underestimated pain severity in 52% of patients reporting pain.[18] In that study, 57% of patients reporting moderate or severe pain did not receive any analgesic treatment. The US study found female gender, a lower level of education, and a transmission risk factor of intravenous drug use to be associated with inadequate analgesic therapy. In the French study, no association with transmission factor or gender was found, but identification of the source of pain by doctors was significantly associated with analgesic treatment.

Possible patient-related barriers were investigated subsequently by the US team, and those found to be connected to undertreatment of pain were the perceived addiction potential of pain medications and physical discomfort associated with opioid administration (e.g. injections) or their side-effects (nausea, constipation).[43] There was no association between undertreatment of pain and age, gender, or HIV transmission factor. However, noncaucasian patients and patients with lower levels of education endorsed more barriers to pain management than did caucasians. A study of physician-related barriers found that the most frequently endorsed barriers to pain management were lack of knowledge about pain management, lack of access to pain management experts, and concerns regarding potential substance abuse or addiction.[44] More experienced clinicians were less likely to cite these factors as barriers to pain management.

Thus, education of both physician and patient appears to be a key issue to improve the diagnosis and treatment of pain in AIDS. Part of the problem is a relative lack of integration of services for AIDS patients with palliative care services as the latter have traditionally developed to deal with cancer.[45] In the UK, specialist AIDS hospices offering palliative care to AIDS patients have been introduced as conventional cancer hospices have a variety of concerns about admitting AIDS patients, including infection control and fundraising. In the UK, hospices depend heavily on funding from local communities, and there are fears that this support could be eroded if their remit was widened to include patients with AIDS.[46] The principal reasons for the undertreatment of pain in AIDS are listed in Table 26.15.

All patients with AIDS should be routinely assessed for pain as an integral part of the examination. As in cancer, close collaboration of the health team is desirable in the investigation and management of pain. A careful history and physical examination may disclose an identifiable syndrome that can be treated appropriately. A standard

Table 26.15 *Some reasons for the undertreatment of pain in AIDS*

Patients often belong to marginalized risk groups who receive a lower standard of care
Stigma leads to denial and late accessing of services
Physician-related barriers, namely lack of education about pain problems in AIDS
Physicians reluctant to prescribe opioids, particularly to known substance users
Patient-related barriers, e.g. concerns about addiction potential of opioids, side-effects of medication, discomfort of injections, etc.
Lack of integration of AIDS care with palliative care services
Lack of development of palliative care services in countries most affected
Acute care prioritized over symptom control

pain history may provide clues to the underlying diagnosis and may disclose other treatable disorders.

Anecdotally, various physical and psychological therapies may prove useful in reducing the need for yet more drugs for the management of pain. Physiotherapy and occupational therapy can, by graded and regular exercises, alleviate musculoskeletal pain. A massage therapist is often of benefit in the relief of cramping muscular pains, particularly in the cachectic or bed-bound individual. Several psychological interventions are used to alleviate AIDS pain, including hypnosis,[46a] relaxation, and distraction techniques, such as biofeedback and imagery, and cognitive–behavioral techniques. Patient education is crucial, and partners and family may be taught techniques to implement at home.

The use of analgesics should follow the guidelines laid down for cancer. In the USA, the World Health Organization (WHO) approach to pain management, although not yet validated in AIDS, has been recommended by the Agency for Health Care Policy and Research (AHCPR) and clinical authorities in the field of pain management and AIDS.[47]

Thus, acetaminophen and nonsteroidal anti-inflammatory drugs (NSAIDs) are the drugs of choice for mild to moderate pain in AIDS. Some pains, for example headache due to intracerebral tumor, are frequently more responsive to acetaminophen than to strong opioids. Benefit is often obtained from continuing NSAIDs and acetaminophen alongside opioid drugs if they have proved useful for mild to moderate pain as their mechanism of action is quite different from that of the strong opioids. In addition, the use of these drugs reduces the total dose of strong opioid required.

In patients with AIDS who have marked loss of body fat, the starting dose of strong opioids may need to be smaller than used initially in cancer patients, for example morphine elixir 2.5 mg 4-hourly. This can then be titrated up as needed. No pain should be regarded as opioid insensitive until a trial of two strong opioids has been carried out. Methadone may be more effective than morphine or hydromorphone when a neuropathic component exists. Patients who complain of undue sedation and cognitive impairment on oral morphine may do better on oxycodone. In addition, opioid medication has useful effects on diarrhea in AIDS patients. In practice, lower doses of opioids are needed in the management of pain in AIDS compared with cancer patients, although there is no formal evidence to confirm this.

A small number of reports have described the use of opioids in the management of pain in AIDS patients.[48–50] The most important of these found that severe recalcitrant pain in 24 AIDS patients referred to a pain relief unit, some of whom had had uncontrolled pain for up to a year, proved to be completely controllable with regular round-the-clock opioid analgesia.[50] This suggests that the underutilization of opioids may be a key contributor to the undertreatment of pain in AIDS.

There are concerns regarding the prescription of opioids to current substance users,[51] but the evidence is that this group of patients suffer as much pain as other groups, and this should be treated properly. Higher opioid doses may be needed because of tolerance, and this must be allowed for without allowing users to escalate their intake far beyond reasonable estimates of what is likely to be necessary to relieve the pain. The multidisciplinary team should have knowledge of the approaches to substance abuse, a nonjudgmental attitude, and coordinated strategies in dealing with breaches of agreed rules of behavior.

Currently, there is very little research on the efficacy of analgesics other than opioids in pain syndromes in AIDS, e.g. adjuvant analgesics and neuropathic agents, or on the use of nerve blocks and epidural injections. Much more work needs to be done.

PAIN SYNDROMES IN AIDS

It is not possible to give an exhaustive account of all the possible causes of pain in AIDS given the wide diversity of possible problems, but a number of syndromes are consistently described. It is difficult to correlate the prevalence of these different syndromes from the few available studies as various classifications of pain are used in these studies, often together. Table 26.16 is an attempt to synthesize some of the data that are available. The tabulation is based on the most commonly used pain types in these studies and, as the methodology varies substantially between studies, it serves only to give a general overview of the relative frequencies of pain types in AIDS recorded in the literature.

NEUROLOGICAL PAIN SYNDROMES

HIV-1 is highly neurotrophic and is present in the central nervous system in the earliest stages of infection, well before significant immunosuppression.[53] Neurologic disease occurs both as a direct consequence of HIV-1 infection and as a result of the accompanying immunosuppression. The relationship of neurologic complications to CD4 count is illustrated in Fig. 26.1.

Neuropathic pain

Pain syndromes originating in the nervous system in patients with AIDS include painful peripheral neuropathies, radiculopathies, myelopathies, and headache.

Neuropathic pain syndromes occur in approximately 30% of AIDS patients with pain and constitute an important cause of pain in AIDS.[54] Several types of neuropathy have been described and are listed in Table 26.17. The commonest cause is the distal symmetrical axonal

Table 26.16 *Pain syndromes in AIDS. These studies were all conducted before the introduction of HAART*

Study	Setting and risk group	Neuro-pathic pain (%)	Rheumatic pain (%)	Visceral pain (chest, abdomen) (%)	Somatic pain (%)	Headache (%)
Leibovits *et al.*[17]	Single-hospital study (n = 134)	6	6	30	NG	13
Schofferman and Brody[52]	Single-hospice study (n = 100)	19	3	12	13	10
Moss[25]	Single-hospice study (n = 100)	22	Joint 7 Muscle 5	10	NG	8
Singer *et al.*[24]	Hospital outpatients (n = 191)[a]	18	NG	NG	NG	39
Hewitt *et al.*[28]	Hospital outpatients (n = 151) and ambulatory AIDS patients	28	Joint pain 31 Muscle pain 27	15	71	46
Larue *et al.*[19]	Multicenter hospital and outpatients study (n = 78)	13	Muscular pain 32 Joint or bone pain 20	15	NG	25
Kelleher *et al.*[26]	Single-hospice study (n = 118)[a]	19	11	25	12	11
Frich *et al.*[21a]	Hospital outpatient study (n = 95)	20	20	NG	NG	24

NG, data not given.
a. Fifty-nine male and 59 female patients; pain syndromes are combined in this table.

neuropathy, but most studies report a small percentage of patients with radiculopathies secondary to herpes zoster, lymphomatous nerve infiltration, autonomic dysfunction, and vasculitis.

Distal symmetrical axonal neuropathy

This predominantly sensory neuropathy is frequently painful and occurs in up to 30% of patients in the later stages of HIV infection. Pathological studies confirm that the main pathological feature is axonal damage with secondary demyelination. It is unclear whether it is a direct effect of HIV or mediated via cytokines or neurotoxins.

There is an association between plasma HIV-1 RNA levels and both the severity of pain and quantitative sensory test impairment in HIV-associated distal symmetrical axonal naeuropathy.[54a] There is, however, no formal evidence to demonstrate if aggressive use of antiretroviral drugs is of benefit to prevent or improve peripheral neuropathy.

Neuropathic pain is a challenge for clinicians because it is usually esistant to commonly prescribed analgesics such as acetaminophen, NSAIDs, and opioids. First-line therapy for neuropathic pain in conditions other than AIDS is either an older antidepressant such as amitriptyline or an anticonvulsant such as carbamezapine, sodium valproate, or gabapentin. In the author's experience, these drugs are all useful in sensory neuropathy in AIDS; however, there is no formal evidence supporting their use in AIDS. The evidence base for the management of neuropathic pain in AIDS is extremely limited. A randomized, double-blind trial of 145 patients assigned to receive either amitriptyline, mexiletine, or placebo showed no improvement in pain on either drug compared with placebo.[55] Similarly, a randomized, placebo-controlled, multicenter trial showed neither acupuncture nor amitriptyline to be more effective than placebo in relieving pain caused by HIV-related peripheral neuropathy.[56] A trial of peptide T for AIDS-related painful distal neu-

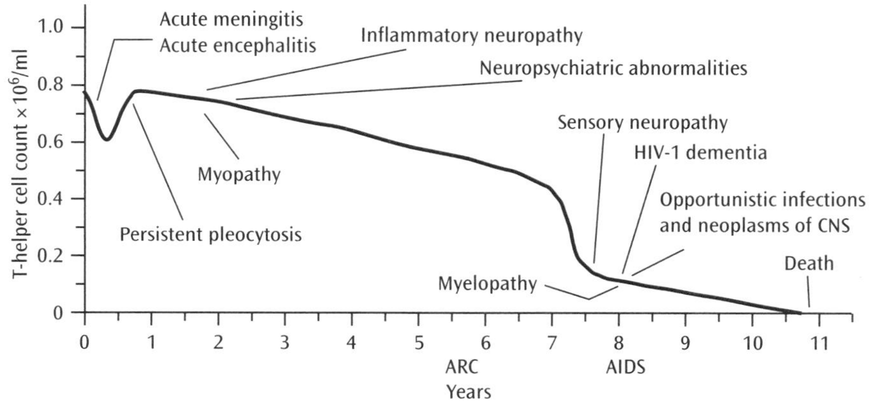

Figure 26.1 *Neurologic manifestations in AIDS and CD4 count.*

Table 26.17 *Neuropathies associated with HIV infection*

Cause	Clinical features	Diagnosis	Treatment
Distal symmetrical axonal polyneuropathy	Occurs in up to 30% of patients	EMG	Gabapentin Amitriptyline Sodium valproate
Inflammatory demyelinating neuropathies	Guillan–Barré or chronic demyelinating neuropathy	CSF analysis Electromyography	Steroids Plasma exchange
CMV radiculopathy	Progressive cauda equina syndrome	Lumbar puncture – CMV on microscopy	Ganclovir
		CMV on nerve biopsy	Foscarnet
Neuropathy secondary to drug treatment	Onset within weeks of starting drug treatment	Clinical history	Stop offending drug
Neuropathy not directly related to HIV infection, e.g. alcoholism, vitamin B_{12} deficiency	Relevant clinical history	Clinical history, low vitamin B_{12} levels, etc.	Appropriate medical management

ropathy found no benefit over placebo.[57] The successful use of ketamine has been described in one case report,[58*] and an uncontrolled trial showed improvement of pain in seven patients with HIV-related peripheral neuropathy with noninvasive electroacupuncture.[59] An open-label study found significantly improved pain symptoms in 200 patients with HIV-associated distal symmetrical polyneuropathy treated with recombinant nerve growth factor (NGF) over a period of 48 weeks.[59a]

Gabapentin is an important addition to the management of neuropathic pain syndromes in conditions other than AIDS, having been demonstrated to be effective for the treatment of neuropathic pain in diabetic neuropathy, postherpetic neuralgia,[59b] and neuropathic pain in cancer.[59c] Its lower rate of drug interactions and more favorable side-effect profile may make it drug of first choice in AIDS polyneuropathy. However, there is little reported evidence of its efficacy in AIDS-related neuropathic pain to date.[59d] If the use of the antidepressant and anticonvulsant drugs does not sufficiently relieve pain in this group of patients, a strong opioid should be tried in addition. Gabapentin has been shown to enhance the effect of morphine in healthy volunteers,[59e] although the clinical significance of this is not established.

Other causes of neuropathy in AIDS

The inflammatory demyelinating neuropathies Guillan–Barré syndrome (GBS) and chronic inflammatory demyelinating neuropathy (CIDP) have been described in association with HIV infection. The majority of cases are reported in asymptomatic patients with HIV rather than in patients with greater degrees of immunosuppression. The pathogenesis is unclear but is believed to be immune mediated. The natural history of the disease seems to be similar to that of idiopathic CIDP or GBS, and response to plasma exchange or steroids is recorded.

Cytomegalovirus infection is associated with a progressive cauda equina syndrome that frequently leads to death in a few months. Such patients often have CSF pleocytosis and may show some response to gancyclovir.

Isolated mononeuropathies are seen in a small percentage of HIV-positive individuals and are most frequent in the lateral cutaneous nerve of the thigh. This may progress to a more generalized neuropathy. There is one report of the successful treatment of a painful neuropathy of the lateral cutaneous nerve of the thigh with bupivacaine and triamcinolone in two patients.[60*]

Vasculitis is a rare cause of neuropathy in association with HIV. There is one report of the successful use of corticosteroids for this condition.[61*]

A number of antiretroviral drugs and other drugs used in the management of AIDS can cause peripheral neuropathy. These include ddI, ddC, dapsone, foscarnet, isoniazid, rifampicin, ethionamide, and metronidazole. Specifically, around 10% of patients receiving stavudine or zalcitabine and 1–2% of didanosine recipients may have to discontinue therapy with these agents because of neuropathy. Prompt withdrawal of these therapies enables gradual resolution of signs and symptoms in most patients, though a period of symptom intensification may occur shortly after withdrawal.[62]

Other etiologies that should be considered include vitamin B_{12} and other nutritional deficiency, toxins and alcohol-related nerve damage. Treatment for these is as for the general population.

Headache

Headaches are common in patients with HIV infection and increase in frequency with progression of disease. Several factors could lead to a higher prevalence of headache than in the general population:[63]

- HIV itself is a cause of headache though the mechanism for this is unknown.
- Many opportunistic infections and tumors of the central nervous system present with headache.
- The high prevalence of mood, anxiety, and adjustment disorders found in the HIV-infected population will contribute fo the occurrence of headache syndromes.
- Headaches can be caused by the use of, and withdrawal from, many recreational drugs. Several studies have found a relationship between the use of marijuana, opiates, and cocaine and headache.[64–66]
- The multiple medications, including analgesics, taken by most patients may contribute to headache.
- Any systemic infection causing high temperatures may be associated with headache.

The common causes of headache in HIV disease and their treatment are listed in Table 26.18.

Acute aseptic meningitis

Acute aseptic meningitis may appear during HIV seroconversion, presenting as fever, myalgias, headache, neck stiffness and, rarely, transient Bell's palsy. It has been estimated to occur in 1–2% of all primary HIV-1 infections. The headaches range from a febrile headache associated with the systemic viral infection to headaches associated with retro-orbital pain, photophobia, and meningeal signs reflecting an acute lymphocytic meningitis. CSF analysis shows lymphocytosis, moderately increased protein, normal glucose, and positive HIV culture. Clinical recovery generally occurs within 2 weeks, but the syndrome may recur periodically.

Late-stage headache

Up to 30% of HIV-1 carriers develop chronic tension-type headaches. These patients have a pleocytosis and may also have a CSF lymphocytosis that rarely exceeds 40 cells/mm^3.

Late-stage HIV headache without pleocytosis has been described in one series. All the patients had advanced disease, no mass lesions on computed tomography (CT), and sterile CSF. Complete resolution of headache occurred within 4 weeks in all but one patient,

Table 26.18 *Common causes of headache in AIDS*

Cause	Clinical features	Diagnosis	Treatments
Primary HIV-related headache			
Acute aseptic meningitis	Associated with seroconversion	Lumbar puncture – lymphocytosis and raised protein in CSF Positive HIV culture	Acetaminophen NSAIDs Amitriptyline
Chronic headache	No other features	Lumbar puncture and CT/MRI to exclude infection/tumor	As above
Secondary HIV-related headaches			
Toxoplasmosis	Headache, fever, seizures, focal signs	CT/MRI scan *Toxoplasma* IgG	Sulfadiazine Pyrimethamine Other anti-*Toxoplasma* treatment
Cryptococcal meningitis	Headache, fever Meningism not common Hydrocephalus may develop	CSF cryptococcal latex test	High-dose fluconazole Amphotericin B
Primary CNS lymphoma	Headache, confusion, focal signs	CT/MRI, brain biopsy	Whole-brain irradiation Steroids
Tuberculous meningitis	Headache, fever, cranial nerve signs	Presence of acid-fast bacilli in CSF	Quadruple therapy, adjuvant steroids
Progressive multifocal leukoencephalopathy	Hemiparesis, visual loss, dysphasia, ataxia	Hypodense lesions on CT CSF culture JC viral DNA	HAART[67]
Drug-induced headache, e.g. zidovudine		Clinical history	Stop offending drug

whose pain resolved after 6 weeks on 40 mg of amitriptyline.[68]* The cause of HIV-related headache is not known but may be related to viral load. If this is so, the introduction of HAART should result in a significant reduction in the prevalence of this symptom.

Opportunistic infections and tumors

The key issue for the clinician dealing with headache in an AIDS patient is whether it is a sign of an underlying infection or tumor. This is of crucial importance as some focal lesions, such as toxoplasmosis, can respond readily and completely to treatment if the diagnosis is made promptly.

In the vast majority of cases, opportunistic infections and tumors are associated with fever, meningeal signs, mental status changes, and focal deficits. If any of these features are present in a patient with headache he or she should be referred for CT or magnetic resonance imaging (MRI) scan and CSF examination for *Cryptococcus*, herpes zoster, *Mycobacterium tuberculosis*, and *Toxoplasma* serology and cytology. Two studies have analyzed the headache characteristics and associated symptomatology in HIV-infected patients presenting with an opportunistic infection or tumor. Headaches secondary to an opportunistic meningitis were constant, gradual in onset, and associated with fever, nausea, vomiting, and photophobia. Headaches secondary to mass lesions were variable in onset and quality, and associated with focal neurological deficits and confusion.[69,70] Occasionally, patients with severe cryptococcal meningitis can develop an obstructive hydrocephalus as a complication of the infection, the headache from which is relieved only by drainage of cerebrospinal fluid. This procedure may need to be repeated during convalescence when headache recurs.

The frequency of headache in different opportunistic infections, tumors, and neurological conditions of the brain is listed in Table 26.19.

HIV-infected patients are also susceptible to the same causes of headache as the general population and require the same treatments. However, sinusitis is commoner in AIDS and often more severe and should be treated with a full course of antibiotics. In advanced disease it can be difficult to clear and surgery may be necessary.

SOMATIC PAIN

Somatic nociceptive pain may arise from joints, muscle, skin, bone, and soft tissue. It is typically a well-localized "aching" or "gnawing" pain. In the context of AIDS this is a very broad category as it includes skin and mucosal areas, which are common sites for infection in this group of patients. Not all pathologies are directly related to HIV disease – gonorrhea, syphilis, and other sexually transmitted diseases may require attention.

Table 26.19 *Frequency of headache in opportunistic infections, tumors, and neurological HIV-related disease of the brain*

Diagnosis	Headache (%)
Cryptococcal meningitis	88[71]
Neurosyphilis	88[72]
Tuberculous meningitis	59[73]
Toxoplasmosis encephalitis	55[74]
Cytomegalovirus encephalitis	30[75]
Progressive multifocal leukoencephalopathy	23[76]
HIV-associated dementia	14[77]

Oral pain

Oral lesions can be identified in 40% of all HIV-infected patients and in over 90% of AIDS patients.[78,79] Not all of these lesions are necessarily painful. However, oral ulceration is usually extremely painful and occurs in an estimated 2–4% of patients with HIV infection.[80] Diagnosis of HIV-related oral pain is based primarily on clinical presentation in conjunction with routine smears and cultures. Biopsy is indicated for ulceration and masses. The common causes of oral pain in AIDS and their management are listed in Table 26.20.

Oral candidiasis

Over 90% of HIV patients experience oral candidiasis during the course of their disease, usually when the CD4 count falls below 400/mm^3. *Candida albicans*, part of the normal oral flora, is the most frequent pathogen, but other species have been identified.

The clinical variants of oral candidiasis include pseudomembranous (thrush), hyperplastic, and atrophic forms, and angular cheilitis.[81] Oral candidiasis may be asymptomatic or associated with pain, burning, or irritation of the mouth. Odynophagia or retrosternal pain with swallowing suggests esophageal involvement. Pseudomembranous candidiasis, the most common variant, is characterized by white or cream-colored plaques, which, when scraped by a tongue blade, reveal reddened or bleeding mucosa (Fig. 26.2). Multiple lesions may involve the buccal mucosa, dorsal tongue, gingiva, and hard and soft palates. It is distinguished from oral hairy leukoplakia in that the latter tends to occur on the posterior surface of the tongue and is not easily scraped off (Fig. 26.3). Oral hairy leukoplakia is usually painless.

Hyperplastic candidiasis, most often found on the buccal mucosa, manifests as white plaques (leukoplakia) that cannot be removed by scraping. Atrophic candidiasis is characterized by erythematous macular lesions of the buccal mucosa, hard palate, and dorsal surface of the tongue. Angular cheilitis presents as erythema, cracking, fissuring, and ulceration of the corners of the mouth.

The diagnosis is clinical but can be confirmed by

Table 26.20 *Common causes of oral pain in AIDS*

Cause	Clinical features	Diagnosis	Treatment
Atrophic candidiasis	Erythematous macular lesions	Clinical	Topical or systemic antifungals
Angular cheilitis	Fissuring and cracking of corners of mouth	Clinical	Topical or systemic antifungals
Herpes simplex infection	Small vesicles on erythematous base May ulcerate	Clinical	Acyclovir Famciclovir Valaciclovir
Herpes zoster infection	Painful vesicular eruption	Clinical	Antiviral drugs as above
CMV ulceration	Mucositis, large ulcers	Biopsy	Gancyclovir or foscarnet
Kaposi's sarcoma	Red or purplish macules or nodules	Biopsy	Excision, radiotherapy, or chemotherapy
Lymphoma	Firm, painless swelling anywhere in mouth	Biopsy	Excision, chemotherapy, or radiotherapy
Squamous cell carcinoma	Mass on lateral surface or undersurface of tongue		Local excision, radiation
Gingivitis and peridontitis	Erythema, ulceration of gingiva	Clinical, radiography	Scaling and root planing, antibiotic therapy
Warts	Sessile papular lesions	Clinical	Excision, cryosurgery, laser therapy
Aphthous ulceration	Painful shallow ulcers	Clinical, biopsy to confirm	Topical and oral steroids Topical GM-CSF Thalidomide
Idiopathic thrombocytopenic purpura	Bleeding, bullae	Platelet count	Steroids Splenectomy
Drug-related mouth ulceration	Clinical history	ddI or ddC	Stop offending drug

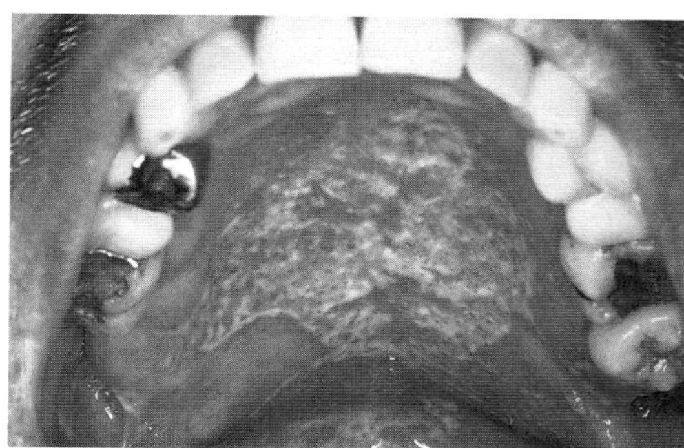

Figure 26.2 *Pseudomembranous candidiasis in an AIDS patient.*

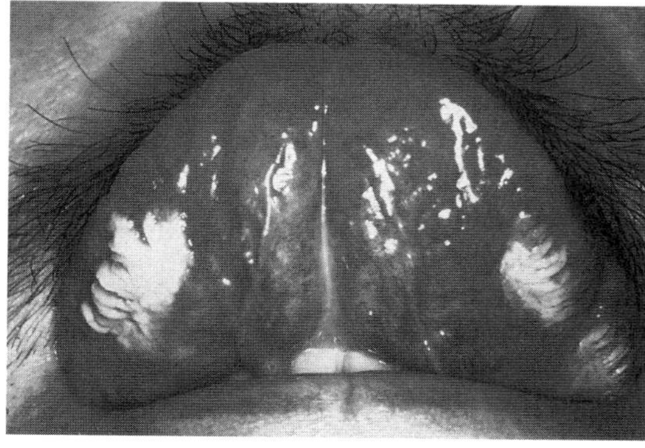

Figure 26.3 *Oral hairy leukoplakia in an AIDS patient.*

demonstration of budding yeast and pseudohyphae on smears examined with Gram's stain or potassium hydroxide. Treatment is with local and systemic antifungal agents. Mild thrush may respond to nystatin suspension and/or amphotericin lozenges. Systemic antifungals, their dosage, metabolism, side-effects, and potential drug interactions are summarized in Table 26.21.

A course of fluconazole, 50–100 mg/day for 5–7 days, is the commonest systemic treatment because of its efficacy, low risk of drug interactions, and lack of side-effects. In practice, higher doses of fluconazole up to 800 mg/day have been used without undue side-effects when necessary.

Oral candidiasis generally improves within a few days of initiation of treatment. In patients with frequent recurrences, prophylaxis should be considered. Azole resistance has become a problem, particularly in the late stages of disease,[83,84] but at the present time there is no consensus on whether continuous or intermittent antifungal therapy is to be preferred as both are associated with the development of resistance.[85]

Herpes simplex virus disease

Herpes simplex virus (HSV) (Fig. 26.4) produces painful ulcerations involving the oral mucosa (gingivostomatitis) or lips (herpes labialis) or both. Lesions appear

Table 26.21 *Systemic treatment for candidiasis*

Drug	Metabolism	Side-effects	Drug interactions
Fluconazole 50–100 mg/day for 5–7 days	Absorption unaffected by gastric pH Eighty percent excreted unchanged in urine	Nausea, diarrhea, abdominal discomfort, severe cutaneous reactions reported in AIDS patients	Dose reduction in renal impairment Care with nephrotoxic drugs
Ketoconazole 200–400 mg daily (cheaper than fluconazole)	Requires an acid environment for optimal absorption (take with acidic carbonated beverage, e.g. carbonated water or cola). Take with or after food Liver metabolism	Gastrointestinal disturbances as above Risk of hepatitis and fatal liver damage Monitor liver function clinically and biochemically	Note that all three azoles inhibit cytochrome P_{450} enzyme CYP3A4[a] – see below
Itraconazole capsules or suspension 200 mg daily for 15 days; maintenance 200–400 mg daily p.o.	Requires an acid environment for absorption (as above). Take with or after food[b] Liver metabolism	Gastrointestinal disturbances Raised liver enzymes and hepatitis, monitor liver function	As above
Amphotericin[c]	Monitor renal function closely, avoid rapid infusion (risk of arrhythmias)	Renal toxicity, cardiovascular toxicity, abnormal liver function, gastrointestinal disturbances, peripheral neuropathy	

a. All three azoles inhibit the cytochrome P_{450} liver metabolizing isoenzyme CYP3A4, leading to increased serum levels of many drugs (see Table 26.20). Concurrent administration of azoles with astemizole, terfenadine, and cisapride is contraindicated following reports of prolongation of the QT interval and fatalities. Phenytoin toxicity has been observed when fluconazole is added to the treatment regimen. The metabolism of ketoconazole, itraconazole, and fluconazole is accelerated by drugs that induce liver enzymes, such as rifampicin, rifabutin, and phenytoin. Poor treatment outcomes and clinical relapse have been reported in patients taking fluconazole and rifampicin. Carbamazepine and phenobarbital have also been shown to induce itraconazole metabolism. Isoniazid decreases plasma levels of ketoconazole and so may have the same effect on itraconazole levels.

b. Itraconazole elixir contains a buffer and is better absorbed in the fasted state. There is some evidence that the suspension is more effective than the capsules.[82]

c. A formulation of amphotericin encapsulated in liposomes is available and is apparently less toxic than the parent compound.

abruptly as solitary or multiple small vesicles on an erythematous base that rupture to form ulcerations. Herpes simplex virus infection frequently involves the hard and soft palate but may also involve the gingiva, floor of the mouth, and tongue. Labial lesions typically form large ulcerations that extend onto the facial skin. HIV-infected patients may have lesions that are atypical in appearance, aggressive, and persistent. Mucocutaneous HSV disease lasting longer than 4 weeks in this population meets the criteria for AIDS.

Diagnosis of HSV infection is made presumptively on clinical grounds and confirmed by culture or Tzanck smear, which shows multinucleated giant cells and viral inclusion bodies. Management consists of oral acyclovir, 200–800 mg five times a day; topical acyclovir is insufficient. Lesions generally clear within several days of initiation of therapy. If the response to oral therapy is inadequate, intravenous acylovir is indicated. Maintenance therapy at lower doses can be given in an effort to reduce the frequency of recurrent disease. Herpes simplex virus resistance to acyclovir has been described, and alternative agents such as famciclovir or valaciclovir and newer agents such as penciclovir cream, sorivudine,[86] and topical foscarnet cream[87] may be used instead.

Varicella-zoster virus

When varicella-zoster virus (VZV), the cause of shingles (Fig. 26.5), involves the second (maxillary) or third (mandibular) branches of the trigeminal nerve, the oral mucosa may be affected. VZV infection of the mouth produces unilateral pain and a vesicular eruption that leads to mucosal ulceration. Diagnosis of VZV infection is made clinically. Oral acyclovir, 800 mg daily, or, alternatively, famciclovir is used to expedite healing and to prevent dissemination. Famciclovir may reduce the incidence of postherpetic neuralgia, an important cause of morbidity, if instituted early.[88] Although recurrent VZV infection has been described in HIV-infected patients, maintenance therapy is generally not recommended.

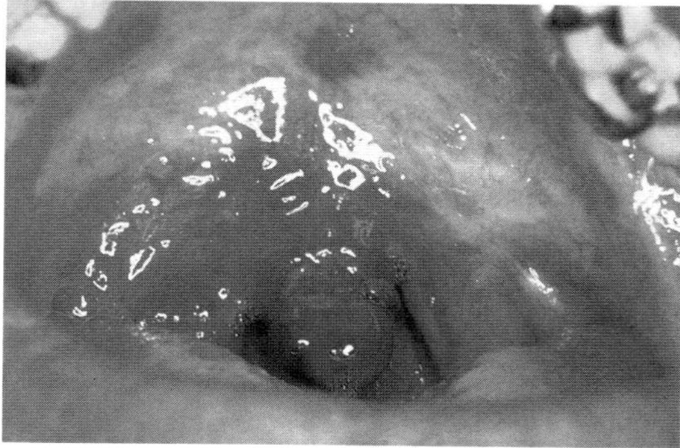

Figure 26.4 *Severe oral herpes simplex infection in an AIDS patient. The uvula has thrombosed. This painful complication has occurred because of inadequate initial treatment of the herpes simplex lesions.*

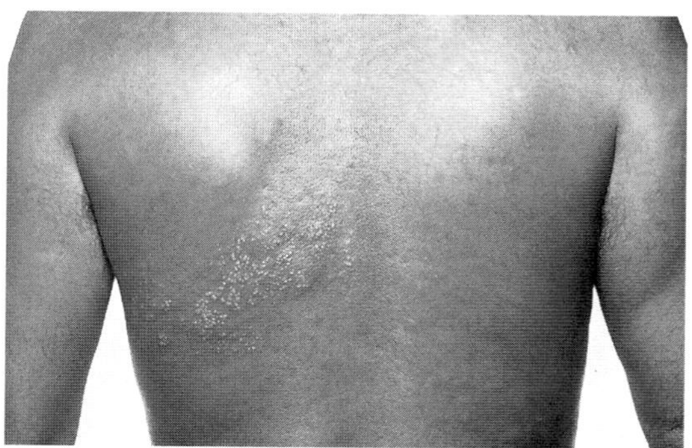

Figure 26.5 *Dermatomal shingles in an AIDS patient.*

Kaposi's sarcoma

More than 50% of AIDS patients have oral Kaposi's sarcoma (KS), which may occur with or without skin, visceral, and lymph node disease. In 10% of patients with KS, mouth lesions may be the only finding (Fig. 26.6). Lesions are especially common on the hard palate and gingival margins, and are occasionally painful. As lesions progress, they often ulcerate and bleed. Diagnosis of oral KS is by biopsy. Therapy is with surgical excision, laser or radiation therapy, or systemic chemotherapy, depending on the number and size of lesions and the presence of systemic disease. Lesions may recur following these treatments, but HAART (highly active antiretroviral treatment) often produces regression.[89]

Squamous cell carcinoma

Squamous cell carcinoma, usually on the lateral and undersurface of the tongue, has been described in HIV-infected patients. Treatment consists in local excision and radiation therapy.

Gingivitis and peridontal disease

HIV infection is associated with severe gingival and peridontal disease that differs from that seen in immunocompetent individuals in its atypical appearance and rapid progression. Although HIV-related gingivitis (HIV-G) and peridontitis (HIV-P) often involve the entire mouth, they can also present as discrete lesions adjacent to areas of healthy tissue.

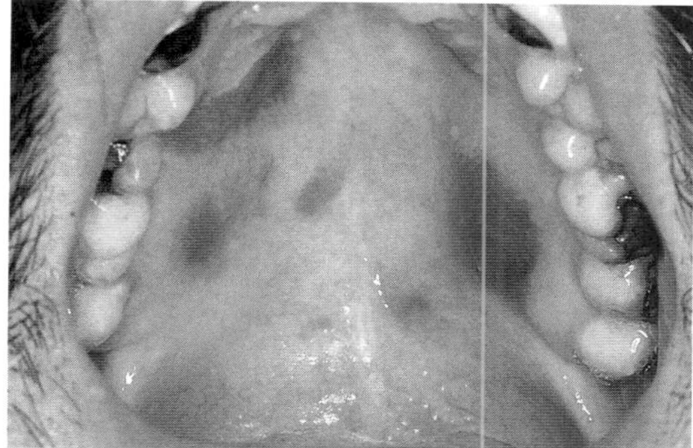

Figure 26.6 *Lesions of Kaposi sarcoma in the oral cavity in an AIDS patient. Patients may be unaware of their presence.*

HIV-G is a disease of the gingival margin, gingiva, and occasionally the alveolar mucosa that occurs in approximately 20% of HIV-infected patients. It is characterized by marked erythema of the gingiva, which may extend several millimeters away from the margin, and spontaneous or easy bleeding, ulceration, or necrosis of the interdental gingiva may be observed. HIV-G often responds poorly to conventional therapy and may progress to HIV-P.

HIV-related peridontitis presents with gingival erythema and ulceration, soft-tissue necrosis, and rapid destruction of the peridontal attachment. Deep pain, bleeding, and exposure of the underlying bone may be observed, with loss of more than 90% of the alveolar bone occurring within a few weeks. Significant tooth loosening is a common finding. Untreated HIV-P is rapidly progressive and results in tooth loss.

The management of HIV-G and HIV-P consists of removal of plaque and calculus by scaling and root planing, and debridement of necrotic tissue. Povidone-iodine solution and chlorhexidine may be useful adjunctively, as may antibiotic therapy with penicillin, metronidazole, or clindamycin. Extraction of involved teeth is often necessary.

Aphthous ulceration

Recurrent aphthous ulcerations are frequently associated with HIV infection and are usually extremely painful (Fig. 26.7). The diagnosis of aphthous ulceration is made when other causes such as CMV and Epstein–Barr virus infection have been ruled out. Although their etiology is unclear, trauma, systemic illness and viruses have been implicated as contributing factors. Small painful shallow ulcers on an erythematous base with a raised white

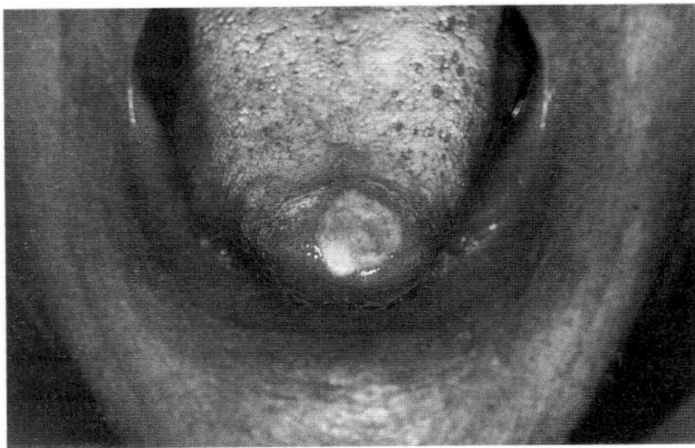

Figure 26.7 *A giant aphthous ulcer on the tongue in an AIDS patient.*

glistening margin are observed, and these may enlarge and become necrotic over time. Topical steroids or fluocinonide ointment 0.05% mixed with equal quantities of Orabase applied 3–6 times a day may be effective. Severe ulcers that do not respond to topical therapy may respond to a short course of oral corticosteroids.[90*] A double-blind, randomized, placebo-controlled clinical trial has confirmed the efficacy of thalidomide in the treatment of oral aphthous ulceration.[91**] However, the potential adverse effects of this drug, including somnolence, rash, and peripheral sensory neuropathy, can be serious, and patients must be monitored closely. The sensory neuropathy may prove irreversible despite stopping the thalidomide. A recent study has reported complete resolution of oral aphthous ulcerations in three patients treated with topical granulocyte–macrophage colony-stimulating factor (GM-CSF, 400 μg on 5% glucose 200 ml), a result that needs to be confirmed by controlled trials.[92*]

Cutaneous pain

The skin is affected in virtually all patients with HIV infection.[93] There is an association between cutaneous and oral diseases in HIV infection, and all the pathologies that commonly occur in the mouth may also involve the skin. In one cross-sectional study of HIV-positive outpatients, 93% had active oral conditions and 95% had active skin conditions including onychomycosis, dermatophytosis, seborrheic dermatitis, KS, folliculitis, xerosis, and molloscum contagiosum.[94]

However, cutaneous pain is not a common complaint, and only a proportion of cutaneous pathologies are painful, including both bacterial (e.g. *Staphylococcus*, *Histoplasma*), fungal (e.g. *Candida*), and viral (e.g. CMV, Epstein–Barr virus) infection. *Staphylococcus aureus* is a common cutaneous pathogen in HIV-infected patients. Cutaneous presentations of *Staphylococcus aureus* infection include folliculitis, impetigo, furuncles, carbuncles, cellulitis, pyomyositis, and toxic shock syndrome, all of which can be painful. *Staphylococcus aureus* may secondarily infect other skin lesions, such as those caused by herpesvirus infections and eczema. Treatment of folliculitis may prevent progression to furuncles, carbuncles, abscess, or cellulitis. Other causes of painful skin lesions include tumor, e.g. KS (Fig. 26.8) or squamous carcinoma, bed sores (Fig. 26.9), and, rarely, toxic epidermal necrolysis (Fig. 26.10). The additional causes of skin pain, not previously discussed, are listed in Table 26.22. As with other pain problems, the etiology should be sought, by biopsy if necessary, and appropriate treatment instituted. The WHO analgesic ladder should be followed in the management of pain.

Anal pain

All lesions that can cause oral pain also occur on the perianal area to cause pain in this region. In addition, squamous cell carcinoma of the anus and anorectal ulceration

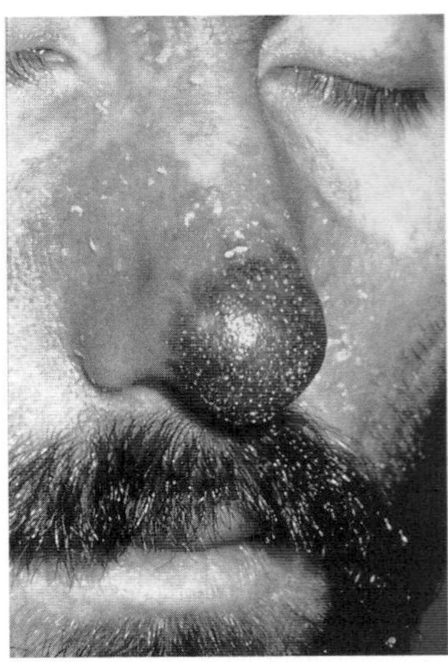

Figure 26.8 *Kaposi sarcoma on the tip of the nose. Lesions frequently occur in prominent positions such as this and should be referred early for treatment.*

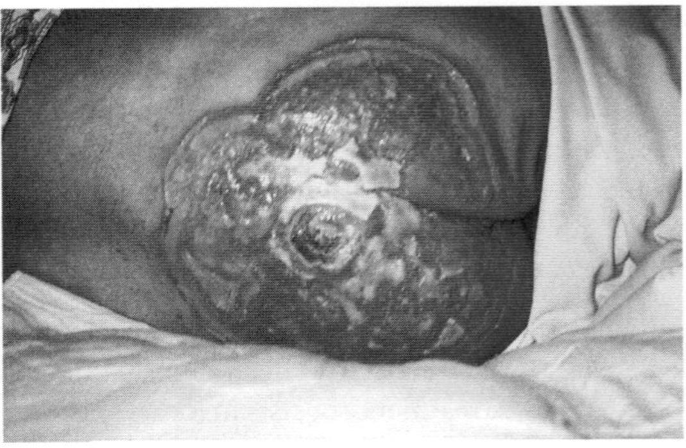

Figure 26.9 *Severe bed sore in an AIDS patient. This proved to be secondarily infected with herpes simplex and MAI. A search for infective etiologies should be made in all sores so that appropriate treatment can be given promptly.*

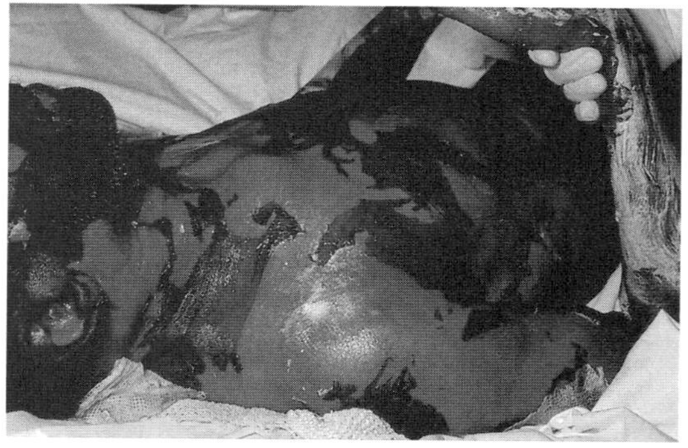

Figure 26.10 *Toxic epidermal necrolysis in an AIDS patient.*

are important causes of anal pain and will be considered here.

Squamous cell carcinoma of the anus

Squamous cell carcinoma of the anus accounts for 2–3% of all malignancies in the lower intestinal tract and there is a significantly increased incidence among homosexual men with AIDS.[95] The symptoms and signs of early-stage anal cancer in HIV-infected men often resemble those of other common anorectal diseases in homosexual men and there should be a high index of suspicion for possible malignancy and early biopsy.[96] Patients with early HIV disease respond well to conventional combined-modality treatment,[97,98] but AIDS patients suffer more adverse effects, including increased tissue damage with delayed healing.[99]

Anorectal ulceration

Causes of anorectal ulceration or anal fissure include viral infection, e.g. CMV, herpes simplex (Fig. 26.11), and herpes zoster infection, bacterial infection, e.g. histoplasmosis,[100] and tumors, e.g. squamous cell carcinoma, KS. All anal ulcers should be biopsied if their cause is not clear. Routine microscopic evaluation of anal ulcer tissue from AIDS patients is not the most accurate way to diagnose viral infection, and immunohistochemistry can improve the diagnostic accuracy and is a good confirmatory test for CMV inclusions.[101] A proportion of ulcers remain unexplained despite exhaustive investigation and are classified as idiopathic anal ulceration.[102]

Anal ulceration can cause severe and incapacitating pain. If medical treatment fails, persistent symptomatic ulcers should be treated operatively by excision with mucosal advancement.[103] One uncontrolled study reported good to excellent pain relief in 21 AIDS patients with anal ulcerations who underwent surgical debridement, biopsy, and intralesional steroids.[104*]

AIDS AND THE EYE

Ocular manifestations of HIV infection can be correlated with the CD4 cell count of the patient.[105] Allergic and immune-mediated conditions – sicca syndrome, allergic conjunctivitis, drug hypersensitivity reactions, and acute hypersensitivity reactions – tend to occur at CD4 counts of 200–500/μl. Opportunistic infections and neoplasms

Table 26.22 *Additional causes of skin pain in AIDS. See Table 26.20 for causes of oral pain, all of which may also affect the skin*

Cause	Clinical features	Diagnosis	Treatment
Warts (human papillomavirus)	Verrucous lesions	Clinical	Topical agents, blunt dissection cryosurgery
Molluscum contagiosum	Clusters of white umbilicated papules	Clinical, biopsy to confirm	Liquid nitrogen, curettage, topical tretinoin, electrodesiccation (painful procedure)
Folliculitis	Pustules affecting trunk, face or groin that heal without scarring	Gram's stain and culture of swab or biopsy lesions	Oral anti-staphylococcal penicillins and first-generation cephalosporins Consider rifampicin and topical mupirocin to clear nasal carriage
Eosinophilic pustular folliculitis	Acneiform, pruritic, papular or pustular eruption. Severe pruritus may be present	Culture negative Skin biopsy shows diagnostic follicular destruction with striking eosinophilic infiltration Etiology unknown	Ultraviolet B light treatments
Toxic epidermal necrolysis	Blistering skin rash, extensive mucosal ulceration, fever, pancytopenia	Clinical	Stop offending drug Consider i.v. immunoglobulin

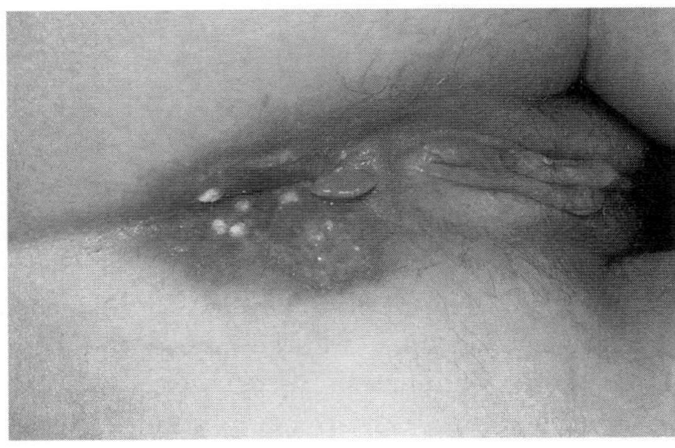

Figure 26.11 *Anal candidiasis and herpes simplex infection in an AIDS patient. Prompt treatment reduces the likelihood of ulceration.*

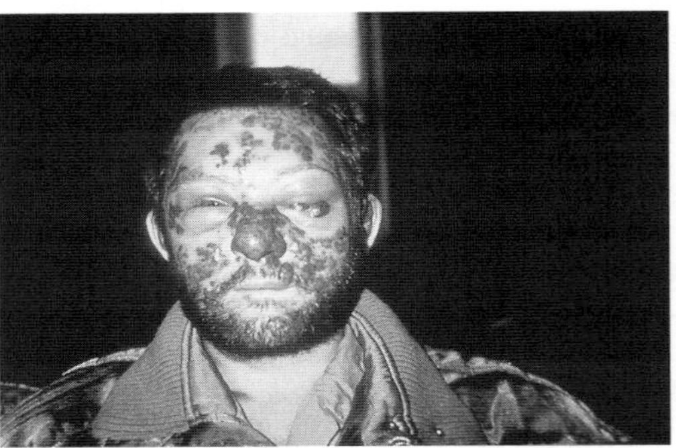

Figure 26.12 *Severe Kaposi sarcoma in an AIDS patient with pronounced periorbital swelling almost blocking vision. KS is frequently associated with considerable swelling of surrounding tissue.*

– CMV retinitis, herpetic retinitis, toxoplasmic retinochoroiditis, KS (Fig. 26.12), and intraocular lymphoma – become more common as the CD4 count falls below 100/μl. The causes of eye pain and their management are listed in Table 26.23. Liaison with an ophthalmologist is essential in the management of eye disease in AIDS.

RHEUMATIC PAIN IN AIDS

A number of rheumatologic disorders are associated with HIV disease, ranging from relatively benign arthralgia and fibromyalgia to potentially life-threatening conditions such as septic arthritis and systemic vasculitis. A variety of noninfectious articular syndromes, including Reiter's syndrome, psoriatic arthritis, and non-specific oligoarthritis, have also been associated with HIV infection, as has the development of autoantibodies.[106] Despite new treatments for HIV, reports of rheumatic diseases presenting in AIDS patients persist, especially HIV-associated arthritis, diffuse infiltrative lymphocytosis syndrome, HIV-associated vasculitis, and polymyositis.[106a] All are painful and can cause significant morbidity. There are no trials published on the use of analgesia for these conditions *in AIDS*, but the WHO analgesic ladder should be followed by using acetaminophen and a NSAID initially and adding a strong opioid if necessary. The commoner causes of joint pain in AIDS are listed in Table 26.24.

Table 26.23 *Eye pain in AIDS (reproduced with permission from McCluskey* et al.[105]*)*

Ocular site	Manifestation	Management
External eye	Kaposi's sarcoma	Radiotherapy, cryotherapy
	Molluscum contagiosum	Curettage, cryotherapy, excision
	Blepharitis	Lid scrubs, topical antibiotics, systemic vibramycin, lubricants
	Herpes zoster ophthalmicus	High-dose acyclovir
Anterior segment	Herpetic keratitis	Topical and systemic acyclovir
	Sicca syndrome	Ocular lubricants
	Microsporidial keratitis	Topical fumagillin
	Acute uveitis	Exclude posterior segment disease, HLA B27-related disease, rifabutin-induced uveitis, syphilis. Treat with topical corticosteroids and mydriatics
Posterior segment	Opportunistic infection	Appropriate antimicrobial therapy
	Intraocular lymphoma	Radiotherapy
	HIV microvasculopathy	No treatment necessary
Neuro-ophthalmic	Disk swelling	Neuroimaging to exclude space-occupying lesion. Consider optic nerve sheath fenestration or neurosurgical shunting
	Diplopia	Exclude cranial nerve palsy
	Field defect	Exclude intraocular cause
	Optic neuritis	Observe. Consider corticosteroids in selected patients

Table 26.24 *Common causes of joint pain in HIV disease*

Cause	Clinical features	Diagnosis	Treatments
Arthralgia	Joint pain without joint swelling	Clinical	Acetaminophen and NSAIDs
Fibromyalgia syndrome	Muscle pain with "trigger" points, sleep disturbance, depressive symptoms	Creatine phosphokinase normal	Low-dose tricyclic antidepressants and non-narcotic analgesics
Septic arthritis	Swollen hot joint Extremely painful	Synovial fluid white cell count and organisms	Systemic antibiotic therapy and adequate joint drainage
Reiter's syndrome	Arthritis, conjunctivitis, urethritis	Synovial fluid white cell count elevated. HLA B27 in 80%	NSAIDs, sulfasalazine, methotrexate rarely

Arthralgia

Arthralgia is the most common rheumatologic manifestation of HIV infection, with a prevalence ranging from 10% to 35% of unselected patients.[107] Transient arthralgias may occur at the time of HIV seroconversion or become part of a more chronic syndrome without the development of actual arthritis. Most often, arthralgia is intermittent and involves large joints such as the shoulders and knees. In practice, this pain responds well to nonsteroidal anti-inflammatory drugs (NSAIDs) although there are no formal trials to support this.

Fibromyalgia syndrome

Fibromyalgia syndrome (FMS) has been identified as a common cause of musculoskeletal symptoms, particularly in association with intravenous drug use.[13]

The reported prevalence of FMS in the setting of HIV infection ranges from 10% to 20%. The clinical presentation is of widespread pain and characteristic sites of muscle tenderness (trigger points). Its etiology is unknown but it has been linked to depression and chronic viral infection.

Septic arthritis

Joint infection due to a variety of pathogens, including *Staphylococcus aureus*, *Campylobacter* species, *Cryptococcus neoformans*, and *Sporothrix schenckii*, has been described in patients with HIV infection. The associated pain can be extremely severe.

Myositis

A variety of myopathies have been described in patients with HIV infection, including polymyositis, zidovudine-associated mitochondrial myopathy, and pyomyositis. Polymyositis in the setting of HIV infection presents with myalgias and proximal muscle weakness with elevated serum creatinine phosphokinase levels.

Osteonecrosis

Osteonecrosis (avascular necrosis) of the hip is an uncommon cause of hip pain in HIV-infected patients. The increased incidence of osteonecrosis in AIDS may be due to an increased frequency of risk factors previously associated with osteonecrosis such as hyperlipidemia, corticosteroid use, alcohol abuse, and hypercoaguability.[107a]

VISCERAL PAIN IN AIDS

Etiology and pathophysiology

Visceral pain results from infiltration, compression, distension, or stretching of thoracic or abdominal viscera and is typically poorly localized, a "deep," "squeezing," or "pressure" pain which may be associated with nausea, vomiting, or diaphoresis. It accounts for about 10–20% of pain in AIDS in most studies, a lower rate than that generally quoted for cancer. Most of this is due to infection, but tumors also contribute. In a few cases, pain may have a functional origin, and both the abdomen and chest are among the sites of complaints of psychogenic pain commonly associated with depressive symptoms in HIV disease.[108]

Chest pain in AIDS

The prevalence of chest pain in AIDS is not known. Pain may arise from the chest wall, lungs, heart, and gastrointestinal tract. Cardiac pain is uncommon in AIDS because of the young age of most of those infected, but coronary artery disease and thrombosis occur as a side-effect of the protease inhibitors.[7,9]

The lung is affected in more than 70% of AIDS patients at some time during the course of their illness.[109] A wide variety of infections account for the majority of lung pathology, but tumors such as KS and non-Hodgkin's lymphoma also contribute.

The likely cause of chest pain in AIDS is usually apparent from the clinical presentation and a chest radiograph. Chest pain is rarely the sole presenting feature. In most infections, the clinical picture is dominated by symptoms of pyrexia, cough, and breathlessness. The incidence of chest pain in different opportunistic infections and neoplasms of the chest is listed in Table 26.25.

The investigation of chest pain depends on the history and findings on clinical examination. Pulmonary symptoms will suggest the need for chest radiography and perhaps bronchoscopy, whereas a history of retrosternal pain suggesting an esophageal origin will necessitate upper gatrointestinal endoscopy.

There are no published data on pain relief for chest pain in AIDS. The WHO analgesic ladder should be followed, with acetaminophen and NSAIDs for mild to moderate pain and opioids for severe pain.

When the CD4 count falls below 200/μl the patient becomes at risk for opportunistic infections. *Pneumocystis carinii* is the most frequently recognized opportunistic pathogen (Fig. 26.13) and remains one of the two commonest AIDS index diagnoses in the USA despite the introduction of prophylaxis,[115] but a wide range of other protozoa, fungi, nontuberculous mycobacterial species, viruses, and unusual bacteria also cause illness in patients with advanced disease.

Bacterial pneumonia is commoner in AIDS than in the general population and is commoner in substance users than in other risk groups. Most patients have pleuritic chest pain at presentation. The commonest organisms responsible for community-acquired AIDS-related pneumonia are *Streptococcus pneumoniae*, *Hemophilus influenzae*, other *Streptococcus* species, and *Branhamella catarrhalis*.[116] Despite a rapid response to antimicrobial agents, many patients experience recurrences and bronchiectasis may develop.[117] Prophylactic antibiotics and immunizations should be considered for patients with recurrent infections.

Kaposi sarcoma

Postmortem studies have shown that most patients with KS have some pulmonary involvement, but relatively few are symptomatic.[118] Dyspnea, nonproductive cough, and fever are the most common symptoms on presentation. Hemoptysis and pain are reported less frequently (see Table 26.20). Physical examination is usually not revealing, although stridor suggests bulky lesions of the upper airways. Chest radiographic findings include bilateral interstitial or alveolar infiltrates, or both, often with poorly defined nodularity and accompanying pleural effusions. Definitive diagnosis of pulmonary KS usually requires open lung biopsy. Treatment is with cytotoxic chemotherapy though radiotherapy has also been used effectively for palliation of symptoms.[119] The pain of KS, both cutaneous and visceral, responds well to a strong opioid such as morphine elixir.

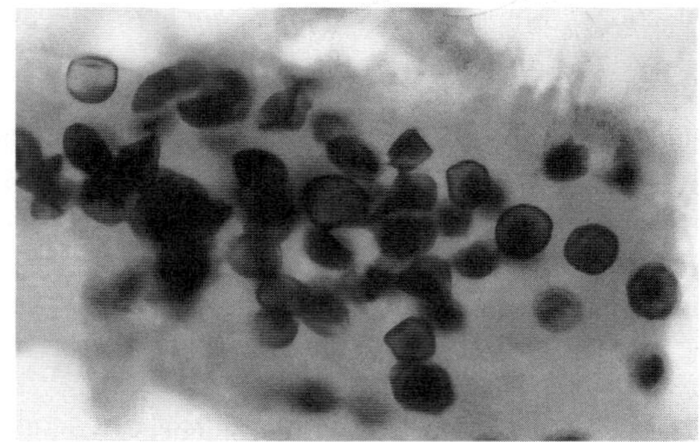

Figure 26.13 Pneumocystis *cysts in the sputum of an AIDS patient with* Pneumocystis carinii *pneumonia.* Pneumocystis *pneumonia can be complicated by pneumothorax, which should be considered if pleuritic chest pain develops.*

Painful swallowing

Odynophagia, or pain on swallowing, is an important cause of morbidity in AIDS and is associated with a poor prognosis. In one series 55% of patients died within 3.6 months of diagnosis.[120] This is because opportunistic infections causing odynophagia are associated with severe immunodeficiency and also because of the reduced nutritional intake associated with this symptom.

Esophageal candidiasis is the commonest cause of dysphagia and odynophagia in AIDS. It can occur in the absence of oral involvement and is characterized by white plaque-like lesions with associated erythema and ulceration. CMV infection of the esophagus is an important cause of esophageal ulceration in AIDS. Odynophagia is almost uniformly present and appearances are highly variable endoscopically.[121] Herpes simplex esophagitis is rare and appearances have not been well defined. Unusual causes of odynophagia include tumors, such as lymphoma or KS, and *Mycobacterium avium* complex infection. Epstein–Barr virus-associated esophageal ulcers in AIDS have also been described.[122]

Table 26.25 *The frequency of chest pain in association with pulmonary infections and tumors in AIDS*

Disease	Reference	Incidence of pain (%)
Pneumocystis pneumonia	Kovacs *et al.*[110]	23
Lung abscess	Furman *et al.*[111]	26
Pulmonary aspergillosis	Denning *et al.*[112]	24[a]
Pulmonary *Cryptococcus* infection	Meyohas *et al.*[113]	2
Pulmonary Kaposi's sarcoma	Gill *et al.*[114]	30

a. Chest pain associated with aspergillosis obstructing large airways.

A syndrome of large ulcerations of the esophagus has been described; esophageal perforation or severe gastrointestinal bleeding may ensue. These patients are markedly symptomatic with odynophagia and substernal chest pain. Despite biopsy evaluation, no identifiable cause is found. Patients with this disorder may respond to corticosteroids in the oral, intravenous, or intralesional form.[123*-125] Resolution of idiopathic esophageal ulceration in a series of seven patients was reported with misoprostol and viscous lidocaine.[126*] Thalidomide has been found to be effective in a large double-blind, randomized, placebo-controlled trial.[127**]

The causes of odynophagia in AIDS are listed in Table 26.26. The initial management is empiric fluconazole, but if improvement is not seen within 1 week upper gastrointestinal endoscopy should be performed.[128] The persistence of dysphagia or odynophagia despite appropriate therapy of esophageal opportunistic infections is recognized and may be secondary to a disorder of esophageal motility in these patients.[129]

ABDOMINAL PAIN IN AIDS

In the only large series available, severe abdominal pain occurred in 15% of 458 AIDS patients presenting to hospital over a 4-year period, and its presence was associated with a reduced survival.[130] The causes of abdominal pain in AIDS are different to those in the general population, with opportunistic infections predominating, although AIDS patients are also susceptible to the usual causes of abdominal pain seen in the immunocompetent host, such as appendicitis and cholecystitis.

The predominant site of pain has considerable predictive value in the diagnosis.[131] The causes of abdominal pain by site are illustrated in Fig. 26.14.

The investigation of abdominal pain depends on the clinical presentation. For upper abdominal pain, endoscopy and ultrasound are the most useful initial investigations, but endoscopic retrograde cholangiopancreatography (ERCP) has an important role in the diagnosis of AIDS-related sclerosing cholangitis. The patient with diffuse or lower abdominal pain is likely to have an infective cause for pain; proctoscopy and rectal biopsy and microbiological examination of the stools are essential. If microbiology and histology are negative and the patient satisfies the criteria for irritable bowel syndrome or constipation, then no further investigations are necessary. If the cause remains unclear, abdominal CT or MRI is appropriate.

The presentation of acute abdomen in AIDS presents particular problems. Severe abdominal pain may be seen in this population even in the absence of true surgical complications such as perforation, abscess formation, or obstruction. Localizing signs and symptoms are frequently misleading because of underlying immunosuppression, debilitation, and prior or current antibiotic use.[132] CT scanning can be useful in this setting for the characterization of disease and direction of therapy.[133] Emergency open laparotomy in AIDS patients is accompanied by a high mortality,[134] and a laparoscopic approach has been demonstrated to be safe and effective in the management of acute abdomen in AIDS patients.[135,136]

Treatment of abdominal pain is that of the underlying cause. Refractory abdominal pain may occur as a result of

Table 26.26 *Causes of odynophagia in AIDS*

Cause	Clinical features	Diagnosis	Treatment
Candidal esophagitis	Dysphagia, odynophagia in severe cases	May be oral candidiasis	Fluconazole, ketoconazole or itraconazole Amphotericin
Herpes simplex esophagitis	Severe odynophagia Extraesophageal herpes may be present	Endoscopy – superficial ulcerations, biopsy essential	Acyclovir Famciclovir Valaciclovir
CMV esophagitis	Severe odynophagia Severe immunosuppression – CD4 count $< 100/\mu l$	Endoscopy – appearances highly variable, multiple well-circumscribed ulcerations most common, biopsy essential	Ganciclovir or foscarnet
Aphthous ulceration	Severe odynophagia	Endoscopy – deep sharply demarcated ulcer craters with raised edges; may be single or multiple	Thalidomide Misoprostol and viscous lidocaine
Non-AIDS related, e.g. reflux esophagitis	No relationship to degree of immunosuppression. A previous history may be present	As in general population	Corticosteroids As in general population

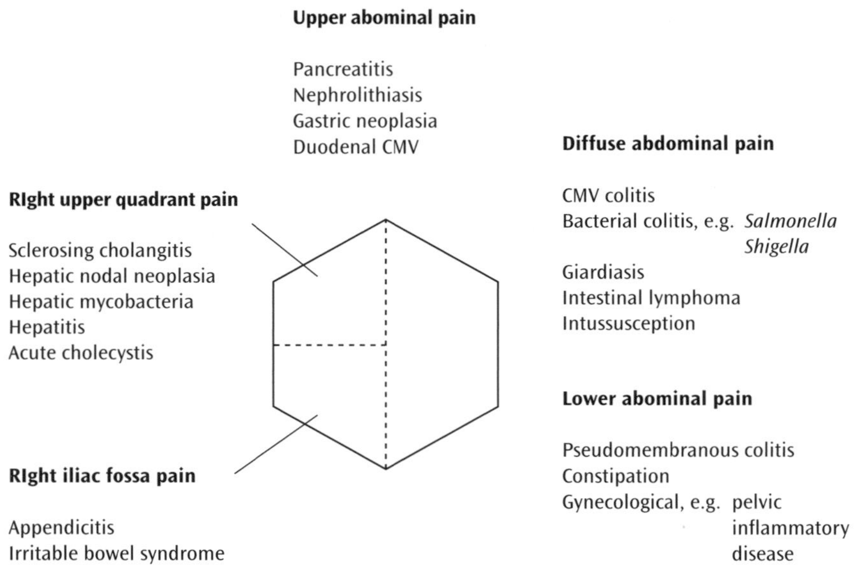

Upper abominal pain

Pancreatitis
Nephrolithiasis
Gastric neoplasia
Duodenal CMV

RIght upper quadrant pain

Sclerosing cholangitis
Hepatic nodal neoplasia
Hepatic mycobacteria
Hepatitis
Acute cholecystis

RIght iliac fossa pain

Appendicitis
Irritable bowel syndrome

Diffuse abdominal pain

CMV colitis
Bacterial colitis, e.g. *Salmonella* *Shigella*
Giardiasis
Intestinal lymphoma
Intussusception

Lower abominal pain

Pseudomembranous colitis
Constipation
Gynecological, e.g. pelvic inflammatory disease

Figure 26.14 *Abdominal pain in AIDS. Causes by location of pain.*

pancreatitis, sclerosing cholangitis, and tumor. One study reported complete relief of pain unresponsive to conventional analgesia in three patients with AIDS-related sclerosing cholangitis who underwent celiac plexus blocks.[137*]

Right upper quadrant pain

The commonest cause of right upper quadrant pain in AIDS is sclerosing cholangitis, which can involve either the common bile duct (CBD) alone, the CBD and ampulla, or the intrahepatic ducts alone. Patients generally present with right upper quadrant pain and an elevated alkaline phosphatase. The pain can be intractable and is poorly responsive to opiates.[138] Its exact cause is unknown. Endoscopic sphincterotomy can produce a dramatic improvement in the pain. In one large series a high incidence of associated pancreatic problems, notably chronic pancreatitis, was noted and may be responsible for some of the pain not relieved by biliary sphincterotomy.[139] Associated intrahepatic disease appears to progress rapidly and is relatively inaccessible to interventional therapy. Diagnosis is made by ERCP, and any significant strictures can be bypassed with an endoprosthesis at the time of the procedure. Cytomegalovirus and cryptosporidiosis may be detected on biopsy and should be treated. The synthetic bile salt urodeoxycholic acid has been reported to be useful in symptom relief.[140] Celiac plexus block should be considered for refractory pain.[137*]

Other causes of right upper quadrant pain include acute cholecystitis, hepatic disease, and biliary tract infections. Acute acalculus cholecystitis has been reported in AIDS patients, sometimes with systemic toxicity. Etiological agents include CMV, *Candida*, and *Cryptosporidium*. Diagnosis is by ultrasound scan. Urgent cholecystectomy may be necessary to prevent rupture of the gallbladder and peritonitis.

The spectrum of liver disease in AIDS is wide and includes infection with viral pathogens, e.g. viral hepatitis B, C, and D, cytomegalovirus, and herpes simplex, mycobacterial pathogens, e.g. *Mycobacterium avium* complex and *M. tuberculosis*, and fungal pathogens, e.g. *Cryptococcus*, *Candida*, and *Histoplasma*, as well as neoplasms, e.g. KS and lymphoma, and drug-related liver disease, for example secondary to sulfonamides, ketoconazole, isoniazid, etc. The history usually provides clues. If noninvasive diagnostic testing is unhelpful, liver biopsy for histology and culture may be necessary.

Right iliac fossa pain

Acute right iliac fossa pain in patients with AIDS patients is much less likely to be due to appendicitis than in patients without AIDS[141] and is frequently due to an opportunistic infection. In AIDS patients with signs of acute appendicitis, investigative strategies such as CT scan or laparoscopy should be performed before surgery is undertaken.

Irritable bowel syndrome does occur in AIDS patients but is proportionately less common and should not be diagnosed unless investigations have excluded infection as a cause of pain.

Constipation should not be forgotten as a possible cause of abdominal pain, particularly in substance users. In some series of AIDS patients it is commoner than diarrhea.

Upper abdominal pain

Causes of upper abdominal pain in AIDS include pancreatitis, renal stones, gastric neoplasia, and duodenal CMV infection. Chronic subacute abdominal pain with nausea, vomiting, early satiety, and weight loss is suggestive of an obstructive lesion caused by KS or lymphoma.

Acute pancreatitis is much more common in HIV-infected individuals than in the general population and has been reported as having an incidence in AIDS of 14%[142] to 22%.[143] Its presentation is similar to that in the general population, but there is a higher frequency of medication-associated pancreatitis, a low frequency of gallstones, and a high frequency of HIV-related causes.[144] Pancreatoxic medications used in AIDS patients include intravenous pentamidine, isoniazid, and the antiretroviral drugs ddI and ddC, and these drugs should be stopped immediately the condition supervenes. Opportunistic infections with *Cryptosporidium*, *Mycobacterium avium intracellulare* (MAI), and *Pneumocystis carinii* have been associated with pancreatitis in AIDS, as has intravenous drug use.[142,143] It has been reported that conventional predictors used to identify the severity of pancreatitis are not useful in this group of patients,[145] but other data conflict with this.[144,146] Management is as for the general population, including treatment of the underlying cause.

Urolithiasis occurs in 2–4% of patients on indinavir as a result of crystallization of the drug, which should be stopped when maintenance of an adequate fluid intake is not possible. Most patients present with flank pain and have microscopic hematuria. Pure indinavir cannot be seen on CT unless intravenous contrast is utilized. Mixed calcium and indinavir stones can occur and may be radio-opaque. Conservative treatment comprising intravenous hydration, narcotic analgesics, and temporary cessation of indinavir is successful in most cases.[147,148]

Lower or diffuse abdominal pain

Diffuse or lower abdominal pain suggests an infective cause. CMV colitis is a common cause of abdominal pain in most series and can be life-threatening. Treatment is with ganciclovir or foscarnet. Daily abdominal radiographs should be performed to allow early diagnosis of complications such as toxic megacolon or perforation and to enable early intervention (usually colectomy) when necessary. *Clostridium difficile* colitis is another important complication in AIDS because of the large numbers of antibiotics taken by these patients, and stools should be tested for the presence this organism in patients with unexplained abdominal pain with diarrhea. Other colonic manifestations of AIDS include infection with opportunistic pathogens, e.g. protozoa (*Giardia*, *Microsporidium*), mycobacteria (MAI, *M. tuberculosis),* or fungi (e.g. *Histoplasma*), typhlitis, idiopathic colonic ulcer, pneumatosis intestinalis, and neoplasms, e.g. KS and lymphoma.[149] Endoscopy plays an integral role in the management of many colonic disorders in AIDS patients.[150]

Intermittent cramping abdominal pain in an AIDS patient should raise suspicion of intussusception. Intussusception is commoner in this group than in the general population as AIDS-related gastrointestinal pathology (CMV, MAI, mesenteric lymphadenopathy, etc.) can provide lead points for its development.[151] It is diagnosed by CT scan.

Incapacitating pain due to bladder spasm and dysuria is uncommon in AIDS patients, but there is one report of the successful control of severe vesical pain by continuous infusion of intrathecal morphine and bupivacaine following the failure of both medical management and suprapubic urinary diversion to control the pain.[152]*

CONCLUSION

Pain in AIDS is inadequately treated, and opioid analgesics, in particular, are underutilized. Pain assessment and management needs to be more integrated into the total care of the AIDS patient. Its management presents at least as much a challenge as cancer pain and, in the light of its underlying heterogeneity, possibly more. It has its share of difficult pain problems, such as mucosal ulceration, sclerosing cholangitis, and neuropathic pain syndromes, but only when standard analgesic principles are implemented and monitored on a large scale will the true incidence of recalcitrant pain in AIDS be identified and the role of alternative strategies defined.

Currently, 40 million people are infected with HIV worldwide and, despite the advances in treatment, no cure is yet in sight. Over 70% of sufferers live in sub-Saharan Africa and do not have access to HAART. Thus, symptom control remains the mainstay of management for those infected. As HIV-infected men, women, and children become increasingly symptomatic, the challenge for palliative care teams worldwide is to implement strategies to minimize the potential for suffering on an enormous scale.

REFERENCES

1. Piscitelli SC, Flexner C, Minor JR, *et al.* Drug interactions in patients infected with human immunodeficiency virus. *Clin Infect Dis* 1996; **23:** 685–93.
2. Williams IG. HIV therapy guidelines (editorial). *Genitourin Med* 1997; **73:** 429–30.
3. ● Heylon R, Miller R. Adverse effects and drug interactions of medications commonly used in the treatment of adult HIV positive patients. *Genitourin Med* 1996; **72:** 237–46.
4. Richman DD, Fischl MA, Grieco MH, *et al.* The toxicity of azidothymidine (AZT) in the treatment of patients with AIDS and AIDS-related complex. A double-blind, placebo controlled trial. *N Engl J Med* 1987; **317:** 192–7.

4a. Saag MS, Sonnerborg A, Torres RA, *et al.* Antiretroviral effect and safety of abacavir alone and in combination with zidovudine in HIV-infected adults. Abacavir Phase 2 Clinical Team. *AIDS* 1998;**12(16):** F203–9.

4b. Squires KE. An introduction to nucleoside and nucleotide analogues. *Antivir Ther* 2001; **6** (Suppl. 3): 1–14.

4c. Gazzard BG. The potential place of tenovir in antiretroviral treatment regimens. *Int J Clin Pract* 2001; **55:** 704–9.

● 5. Havlir DV, Lange JM. New antiretrovirals and new combinations. *AIDS* 1998; **12** (Suppl.): S165–74.

● 6. Heylon R, Miller R. Adverse effects and drug interactions of medications commonly used in the treatment of adult HIV positive patients: part 2. *Genitourin Med* 1997; **73:** 5–11.

7. Flexner C. HIV-protease Inhibitors. *N Engl J Med* 1998; **338:**1281–92.

8. Carr A, Samaras K, Thorisdottir A, *et al.* Diagnosis, prediction and natural course of HIV-1 protease-inhibitor-associated lipodystrophy, hyperlipidaemia, and diabetes mellitus: a cohort study. *Lancet* 1999; **353:** 2093–9.

9. Henry K, Melroe H, Huebsch J, *et al.* Severe premature coronary artery disease with protease inhibitors. *Lancet* 1998; **351** (9112): 1328.

9a. Conway B, Shafran SD. Pharmacology and clinical experience with amprenavir. *Expert Opin Investig Drugs* 2000; **9:** 371–82.

9b. Hurst M, Faulds D. Lopinavir. *Drugs* 2000; **60:** 1371–9.

10. Selwyn PA, Feingold AR, Mantel D, *et al.* Increased risk of bacterial pneumonia in HIV infected intravenous drug users without AIDS. *AIDS* 1988; **2:** 267–72.

● 11. O'Connor PG, Selwyn PA, Schottenfeld RS. Medical care for injection drug users with human immunodeficiency virus infection. *N Engl J Med* 1994; **331:** 450–9.

12. Kissner DG, Lawrence WD, Selis JE, Flint A. Crack lung: pulmonary disease caused by cocaine abuse. *Am Rev Respir Dis* 1987; **136:** 1250–2.

13. Simes RW, Zerbini AF, Ferrante N, *et al.* Fibromyalgia syndrome in patients infected with human immunodeficiency virus. *Am J Med* 1992; **92:** 368–74.

14. Fleming PL, Ciesielski CA, Byers RH, *et al.* Gender differences in reported AIDS-indicative diagnoses. *J Infect Dis* 1993; **168:** 61–7.

◆ 15. Hoover DR, Saah AJ, Bacellar H, *et al.* Clinical manifestations of AIDS in the era of *Pneumocystis* prophylaxis. *N Eng J Med* 1993; **329:** 1922–6.

◆ 16. Jacobson MA, French M. Altered natural history of AIDS-related opportunistic infections in the era of potent combination antiretroviral therapy. *AIDS* 1998; **12** (Suppl. A): S157–63.

17. Lebovits AK, Lefkowitz M, McCarthy D, *et al.* The prevalence and management of pain in patients with AIDS. A review of 134 cases. *Clin J Pain* 1989; **5:** 245–8.

◆ 18. Larue F, Fontaine A, Colleau S. Underestimation and undertreatment of pain in HIV disease: a multicentre study. *Br Med J* 1997; **314:** 23–8.

19. Breitbart W, McDonald MV, Rosenfield B, *et al.* Pain in ambulatory AIDS patients. 1. Pain characteristics and medical correlates. *Pain* 1996; **68:** 315–21.

20. Breitbart W, Rosenfeld B, Passik S, *et al.* A comparison of pain report and adequacy of analgesic therapy in ambulatory AIDS patients with and without a history of substance abuse. *Pain* 1997; **72:** 235–43.

21. Vogl D, Rosenfeld B, Breitbart W, *et al.* Symptom prevalence, characteristics and distress in AIDS outpatients. *J Pain Symptom Manage* 1999; **18:** 253–62.

21a. Frich LM, Borgbjerg MD. Pain and pain treatment in AIDS patients: a longitudinal study. *J Pain Symptom Manage* 2000; **19:** 339–47.

22. Butters E, Higginson I, George R, *et al.* Assessing the symptoms, anxiety and practical needs of HIV/AIDS patients receiving palliative care. *Qual Life Res* 1992; **1:** 47–51.

23. Singer EJ, Zorilla C, Fahy-Chandon B, *et al.* Painful symptoms reported for ambulatory HIV-infected men in a longitudinal study. *Pain* 1993; **54:**15–19.

◆ 24. Moss V. Patient characteristics, presentation and problems encountered in advanced AIDS in a hospice setting. *Palliative Med* 1991; **5:** 112–16.

25. Kelleher P, Cox S, McKeogh M. HIV infection: the spectrum of symptoms and disease in male and female patients attending a London hospice. *Palliative Med* 1997; **11:** 152–8.

26. Kimball LR, McCormick WC. The pharmacologic management of pain and discomfort in persons with AIDS near the end of life: use of opioid analgesia in the hospice setting. *J Pain Symptom Manage* 1996; **11:** 88–94.

27. Martin C, Pehson P, Osterberg A, *et al.* Pain in ambulatory HIV-infected patients with and without intravenous drug use. *Eur J Pain* 1999; **3:** 157–64.

◆ 28. Hewitt D, McDonald M, Portenoy R, *et al.* Pain syndromes and aetiologies in ambulatory AIDS patients. *Pain* 1997; **70:** 117–23.

29. Rosenfeld B, Breitbart W, McDonald MV, *et al.* Pain in ambulatory AIDS patients. Impact of pain on psychological functioning and quality of life. *Pain* 1996; **68:** 323–8.

◆29a. Gaughan DM, Hughes MD, Seage GR, *et al.* The prevalence of pain in paediatric human immunodeficiency virus/acquired immunodeficiency syndrome as reported by participants in the Paediatric Late Outcomes Study (PPACTG 2). *Paediatrics* 2002; **109:** 1144–52.

● 30. Portenoy RK. Cancer pain: pathophysiology and syndromes. *Lancet* 1992; **339:** 1026–31.

31. Elliott KE, Foley KM. Pain syndromes in the cancer patient. *J Psychosoc Oncol* 1990; **8:** 11–44.

32. Edelstein H, Knight RT. Severe parkinsonism in two AIDS patients taking prochlorperazine. *Lancet* 1987; **2:** 341–2.

33. Rodgers C. Extrapyramidal side-effects of antiemetics presenting as psychiatric illness. *Gen Hosp Psychiatry* 1992; **14:** 192–5.

34. Factor SA, Podskalny GD, Barron KD. Persistent neuroleptic-induced rigidity and dystonia in AIDS dementia complex: a clinico-pathological case report. *J Neurol Sci* 1994; **127:** 114–20.

◆ 35. Nelson MR, Erskine D, Hawkins DA, Gazzard BG. Treatment with corticosteroids – a risk factor for the development of clinical cytomegalovirus disease in AIDS. *AIDS* 1993; **7:** 375–8.

36. Burstein HJ, Gelber S, Guadagnoli E, Weeks JC. Use of alternative medicine by women with early stage breast cancer. *N Engl J Med* 1999; **340:** 1733–9.

● 37. Jacobsberg L.B., Perry S. Psychiatric disturbances. Medical management of AIDS patients. *Med Clin N Am* 1992; **761:** 99–106.

◆ 38. Catalan J. The psychiatry of HIV infection. *Advanc Psychiatr Treat* 1997; **3:** 18–23.

39. Catalan J, Riccio M. Psychiatric disorders associated with HIV disease. *AIDS Care* 1990; **2:** 377–80.

40. Ceballos-Capitaine A, Szapoczemic J, Blakey N, *et al.* Ethnicity and emotional distress among HIV positive gay males. *Hispanic J Behav Sci* 1990; **12:** 135–52.

41. Gala C, Pergami A, Catalan J, *et al.* The psychosocial impact of HIV infection in gay men, drug users and heterosexuals: a controlled investigation. *Br J Psychiatry* 1993; **163:** 651–9.

42. Breitbart W, Rosenfield B, Passik S, *et al.* The undertreatment of pain in ambulatory AIDS patients. *Pain* 1996; **65:** 239–45.

43. Breitbart W, Passik S, McDonald MV, *et al.* Pain-related barriers to pain management in ambulatory AIDS patients. *Pain* 1998; **76:** 9–16.

44. Breitbart W, Kaim M, Rosenfeld B. Clinicians' perceptions of barriers to pain management in AIDS. *J Pain Symptom Manage* 1999; **18:** 203–12.

45. Masterson KJ. Suggestions for improving AIDS treatment in hospitals. *Leadersh Health Serv* 1996; **5(6):** 4–10.

◆ 46. Salt S, Wilson L, Edwards A. The use of specialist palliative care services by patients with human immunodeficiency virus-related illness in the Yorkshire Deanery of the Northern and Yorkshire region. *Palliative Med* 1998; **12:**152–160.

46a. Langenfeld MC, Cipanie, Borckardt JJ. Hypnosis for the control of HICV/AIDS related pain. *Int J Clin Exp Hypn* 2002; **50:** 170–88.

◆ 47. Jacox A, Carr D, Payne R, *et al. Clinical Practice Guideline Number 9: Management of Cancer Pain* (AHCPR publication no. 94-0592). Rockville MD: US Department of Health and Human Service, Agency for Health Care Policy and Research, 1994: 139–41.

48. Kaplan R, Conant M, Cundiff D, *et al.* Sustained-release morphine sulphate in the management of pain associated with acquired immune deficiency syndrome. *J Pain Symptom Manage* 1996; **12:** 150–9.

49. McCormack JP, Li R, Zarony D, Singer J. Inadequate treatment of pain in ambulatory HIV patients. *Clin J Pain* 1993; **9:** 247–83.

◆ 50. Anand A. Carmosino L, Glatt AE. Evaluation of recalcitrant pain in HIV-infected hospitalized patients. *J Acq Immune Def Syn* 1994; **7:** 52–6.

51. Morrison RE, Brint JM, Smith WR, *et al.* Appropriate and inappropriate prescribing of narcotics for ambulatory HIV-positive patients. *J Gen Intern Med* 1994; **9:** 301–5.

52. Schofferman J. Pain: diagnosis and management in the palliative care of AIDS. *J Palliative Care* 1988; **4(4):** 46–9.

● 53. Berger JR, Levy RM. The neurologic complications of human immunodeficiency virus infection. *Med Clin N Am* 1993; **77:** 1–23.

● 54. Winer JB. Neuropathies and HIV infection. *J Neurol Neurosurg Psychiatry* 1993; **56:** 739–41.

54a. Simpson DM, Haidich AB, Schifitto G, *et al.* Severity of HIV-associated neuropathy is associated with plasma HIV-1 RNA levsls. *AIDS* 2002; **16(3):** 407–12.

55. Kieburtz K, Simpson D, Yiannoustsos C, *et al.* A randomized trial of amitriptyline and mexiletine for painful neuropathy in HIV infection. AIDS Clinical Trial Group 242 Protocol Team. *Neurology* 1998; **51:** 1682–8.

◆ 56. Shlay JC, Chaloner K, Max MB, *et al.* Acupuncture and amitriptyline for pain due to HIV-related peripheral neuropathy: a randomized controlled trial. Terry Beirn Community Programs for Clinical Research on AIDS. *JAMA* 1998; **280:** 1590–5.

57. Simpson DM, Dorfman D, Olney RK, *et al.* Peptide T in the treatment of painful distal neuropathy associated with AIDS: results of a placebo controlled trial. The Peptide T Neuropathy Study Group. *Neurology* 1996; **47:** 1254–9.

58. Broadley KE, Kurowska A, Tookman A. Ketamine injection used orally. *Palliative Med* 1996; **10:** 247–50.

59. Galantino ML, Eke-Okoro ST, Findley TW, Condoluci D. Use of noninvasive electroacupuncture for the treatment of HIV-related peripheral neuropathy: a pilot study. *J Altern Complement Med* 1999; **5:** 135–42.

59a. Schifitto G, Yiannoutsos C, Simpson DM, *et al.* Long-term treatment with recombinant nerve growth factor for HIV-associated sensory neuropathy. *Neurology* 2001; **57:** 1313–16.

59b. Rose MA, Cam PC. Gabapentin: pharmacology and its use in pain management. *Anaesthesia* 2002; **57:** 451–62.

59c. Caraceni A, Zecca E, Martini C, De Conno F. Gabapentin as an adjuvnt to opioid analgesia for neuropathic cancer pain. *J Pain Symptom Manage* 1999; **17:** 441–5.

59d. Vadivelu N, Berger J. Neuropathic pain after anti-HIV gene therapy successfully treated with gabapentin. *J Pain Symptom Manage* 1999; **17:** 155–6.

59e. Eckhardt K, Ammon S, Hofmann U, *et al.* Gabapentin enhances the analgesic effect of morphine in healthy volunteers. *Anesth Analg* 200; **91:** 185–91.

60. Myers KG, George RG. Painful neuropathy of the lateral cutaneous nerve of the thigh in patients with AIDS: successful treatment by injection with bupivacine and triamcinolone. *AIDS* 1996; **10:** 1302–3.

61. Bradley WG, Verma A. Painful vasculitic neuropathy in HIV-1 infection: relief of pain with prednisone therapy. *Neurology* 1996; **47:** 1446–51.

● 62. Moyle GJ, Sadler M. Peripheral neuropathy with nucleoside antiretrovirals: risk factors, incidence and management. *Drug Safety* 1998; **19:** 481–94.

63. Holloway RG, Kieburtz MD. Headache and the human immunodeficiency virus type 1 Infection. *Headache* 1995; **35:**245–55.

64. Dhopesh V, Maany I, Herring C. The relationship of cocaine to headache in polysubstance abusers. *Headache* 1991; **31:** 17–19.

65. DeMarinis M, Janiri L, Agnoli A. Headache in the use and withdrawal of opiates and other associated substances of abuse. *Headache* 1991; **31:** 159–63.

66. El-Mallakh RS, Kranzler HR, Kamanitz JR. Headaches and psychoactive substance use. *Headache* 1991; **31:** 584–7.

◆ 67. Albrecht H, Hoffmann C, Degan O, *et al.* Highly active antiretroviral therapy significantly improves the prognosis of patients with HIV-associated progressive multifocal leucoencephalopathy. *AIDS* 1998; **12:** 1149–54.

● 68. Brew BJ, Miller J. Human immunodeficiency virus related headache. *Neurology* 1993; **43:** 1098–100.

69. Lipton RB, Feraru ER, Weiss G, *et al.* Headache in HIV-1 related disorders. *Headache* 1991; **31:** 518–22.

● 70. Goldstein J. Headache and acquired immunodeficiency syndrome. *Neurol Clin* 1990; **8:** 947–60.

71. Pons VG, Jacobs RA, Hollander H. Non-viral infections of the central nervous system in patients with acquired immunodeficiency syndrome. In: Rosenblum ML, Levy RM, Bredesen DE, eds. *AIDS and the Central Nervous System*. New York, NY: Raven Press, 1988: 263–83.

72. Katz DA, Berger JR, Duncan RC. Neurosyphilis. A comparative study of the effects of infection with human immunodeficiency virus. *Arch Neurol* 1993; **50:** 243–9.

73. Berenguer J, Moreno S, Laguna F, *et al.* Tuberculous meningitis in patients infected with the human immunodeficiency virus. *N Engl J Med* 1992; **326:** 668–72.

◆ 74. Porter SB, Sande MA. Toxoplasmosis of the central nervous system in the acquired immunodeficiency syndrome. *N Engl J Med* 1992; **327:** 1643–48.

75. Holland NR, Power C, Mathews VP, *et al.* Cytomegalovirus encephalitis in acquired immunodeficiency syndrome (AIDS). *Neurology* 1994; **44:** 507–14.

76. Karahalios D, Breit R, Dal Canto MC, Levy RM. Progressive multifocal leucoencephalopathy in patients with HIV infection: lack of impact of early diagnosis by stereotactic brain biopsy. *J Acquir Immune Defic Syndr* 1992; **5:** 1030–8.

77. Navia BA, Price RW. The acquired immunodeficiency syndrome dementia complex as the presenting or sole manifestation of human immunodeficiency virus infection. *Arch Neurol* 1987; **44:** 65–9.

78. Barr CE, Torosian JP. Oral manifestations in inpatients with AIDS or AIDS-related complex. *Lancet* 1986; **ii:** 288.

79. Engelbert AJ, Schulten JM, Reiner W, *et al.* Oral findings in HIV-infected patients attending a department of internal medicine: the contribution of intraoral examination towards the clinical management of HIV disease. *Q J Med* 1990; **76:** 741–5.

80. Zakrzewska JM, Robinson P, Williams IG. Severe oral ulceration in patients with HIV infection: a case series. *Oral Dis* 1997; **3** (Suppl. 1): S94–6.

81. Lewis MAO, Samaranyake LP, Lamey PJ. Diagnosis and treatment of oral candidosis. *J Oral Maxillofac Surg* 1991; **49:** 996–1002.

82. Cartledge JD, Midgely J, Gazzard BG. Itraconazole solution: higher serum drug concentrations and better clinical response rates than the capsule formation in acquired immunodeficiency syndrome patients with candidiasis. *J Clin Pathol* 1997; **50:** 477–80.

83. Tumbarello M, Caldarola G, Tacconelli E, *et al.* Analysis of the risk factors associated with the emergence of azole resistant oral candidiasis in the course of HIV infection. *J Antimicrob Chemother* 1996; **38:** 691–9.

◆ 84. Maenza JR, Keruly JC, Moore RD, *et al.* Risk factors for fluconazole-resistant candidiasis in human immunodeficiency virus-infected patients. *J Infect Dis* 1996; **173:** 219–25.

85. Revankar SG, Kirkpatrick WR, McAtee RK, *et al.* A randomized trial of continuous or intermittent therapy with fluconazole for oropharyngeal candidiasis in HIV-infected patients: clinical outcomes and development of fluconazole resistance. *Am J Med* 1998; **105:** 7–11.

86. Gnann JW, Crumpacker CS, Lalezari JP, *et al.* Sorivudine versus acyclovir for treatment of dermatomal herpes zoster in human immunodeficiency virus-infected patients: results from a randomized, controlled clinical trial. Collaborative Antiviral Study Group/AIDS clinical trials group, Herpes Zoster Study Group. *Antimicrob Agents Chemother* 1998; **42:** 1139–45.

87. Javaly K, Wohfeiler M, Kalayjian R, *et al.* Treatment of mucocutaneous herpes simplex virus infections unresponsive to acyclovir with topical foscarnet cream in AIDS patients: a phase I/II study. *J Acquir Immune Defic Syndr* 1999; **21:** 301–6.

88. Tyring SK. Efficacy of famciclovir in the treatment of herpes zoster. *Semin Dermatol* 1996; **15** (2 Suppl. 1): 27–31.

89. Lebbe C, Blum L, Pellet C, *et al.* Clinical and biological impact of antiretroviral therapy with protease inhibitors on HIV-related Kaposi's sarcoma. *AIDS* 1998; **12:** F45–9.

◆ 90. Chang Y. Cesarman E, Pessin MS, *et al.* Identification of Herpesvirus-like DNA sequences in AIDS-associated Kaposi's sarcoma. *Science* 1994; **265:** 1865–9.

◆ 91. Jacobson JM, Greenspan JS, Spritzler J, *et al.* Thalidomide for the treatment of oral aphthous ulcers in patients with human immunodeficiency virus infection. National Institute of Allergy and Infectious Diseases AIDS Clinical Trials Group. *N Engl J Med* 1997; **336:** 1487–93.

◆ 92. Herranz P, Arribas JR, Navarro A, *et al.* Successful treatment of aphthous ulcerations in AIDS patients with topical granulocyte–macrophage colony-stimulating factor. *Br J Dermatol* 2000; **142:** 171–6.

● 93. Porras B, Costner M, Friedman-Kien AE, Cockerell CJ. Update on cutaneous manifestations of HIV infection. *Med Clin N Am* 1998; **82:** 1033–80.

94. Mirowski GW, Hilton JF, Greenspan D, *et al.* Association of cutaneous and oral diseases in HIV-infected men. *Oral Dis* 1998; **4:** 16–21.

◆ 95. Melybe M, Cote TR, Kessler L, *et al.* High incidence of anal cancer among AIDS patients. The AIDS/Cancer working group. *Lancet* 1994; **343:** 636–9.

96. Forti RL, Medwell SJ, Aboulafia DM, *et al.* Clinical presentation of minimally invasive and in situ squamous cell carcinoma of the anus in homosexual men. *Clin Infect Dis* 1995; **21:** 603–7.

97. Chadha M, Rosenblatt EA, Malamud S, *et al.* Squamous cell carcinoma of the anus in HIV positive patients. *Dis Colon Rectum* 1994; **37:** 861–5.

98. Peddada AV, Smith DE, Rao AR, *et al.* Chemotherapy and low-dose radiotherapy in the treatment of HIV-infected patients with carcinoma of the anal canal. *Int J Radiat Oncol Biol Phys* 1997; **37:** 1101–5.

99. Harrison M, Tomlinson D, Stewart S. Squamous cell carcinoma of the anus in patients with AIDS. *Clin Oncol (R Coll Radiol)* 1995; **7:** 50–1.

100. Winburn GB, Yeh KA. Severe anal ulceration secondary to *Histoplasma capsulatum* in a patient with HIV disease. *Am Surg* 1999; **65:** 321–2.

101. Cohen SM, Schmitt SL, Lucas FV, Wexner SD. The diagnosis of anal ulcers in AIDS patients. *Int J Colorectal Dis* 1994; **9:** 169–73.

102. Wilcox CM, Schwartz DA. Idiopathic anorectal ulceration in patients with human immunodeficiency virus infection. *Am J Gastroenterol* 1994; **89:** 599–604.

103. Consten EC, Slors JF, Danner SA, *et al.* Local excision and mucosal advancement for anorectal ulceration in patients infected with human immunodeficiency virus. *Br J Surg* 1995; **82:** 891–4.

104. Modesto VL, Gottesman L. Surgical debridement and intralesional steroid injection in the treatment of idiopathic AIDS-related anal ulcerations. *Am J Surg* 1997; **174:** 439–41.

●105. McCluskey PJ, Hall AJ, Lightman S. HIV and eye disease. *Med J Austral* 1996; **164:** 484–6.

●106. Itescu S. Rheumatic aspects of acquired immunodeficiency syndrome. *Curr Opin Rheumatol* 1996; **8:** 346–53.

●106a. Reveille JD. The changing spectrum of rheumatic disease in human immundoeficiency virus infection. *Semin Arthritis Rheum* 2000; **30(3):** 147–66.

●107. Berman A, Espinoza LR, Diaz JD, *et al.* Rheumatic manifestations of human immunodeficiency virus infection. *Am J Med* 1988; **55:** 59–64.

107a. Scribner AN, Troia-Cancio PV, Cox BA, *et al.* Osteonecrosis in HIV: a case control study. *J Acquir Immune Defic Syndr* 2000; **25:** 19–25.

●108. Fukunishi I, Matsumoto T, Negishi M, *et al.* Somatic complaints associated with depressive symptoms in HIV-positive patients. *Psychother Psychosom* 1997; **66:** 248–51.

109. Miller AB, Hind CR. AIDS and the lung. *Hospital Update* 1991; March: 177–91.

◆110. Kovacs JA, Hiemenz JW, Macher AM, *et al.* *Pneumocystis carinii* pneumonia: a comparison between patients with the acquired immune deficiency syndrome and patients with other immunodeficiencies. *Ann Intern Med* 1984; **100:** 663–71.

111. Furman AC, Jacobs J, Sepkowitz KA. Lung abscess in patients with AIDS. *Clin Infect Dis* 1996; **22:** 81–5.

112. Denning DW, Follansbee SE, Scolaro M, *et al.* Pulmonary aspergillosis in the acquired immunodeficiency syndrome. *N Engl J Med* 1991; **324:** 654–62.

113. Meyohas MC, Roux P, Bollens D, *et al.* Pulmonary cryptococcosis: localized and disseminated infections in 27 patients with AIDS. *Clin Infect Dis* 1995; **21:** 628–33.

114. Gill PS, Akil B, Colleti P, *et al.* Pulmonary Kaposi sarcoma: clinical findings and results of therapy. *Am J Med* 1989; **87:** 57–61.

115. Forrest DM, Seminari E, Hogg RS, *et al.* The incidence and spectrum of AIDS defining illnesses in persons treated with antiviral drugs. *Clin Infect Dis* 1998; **27:** 1379–85.

116. Chaisson RE. Bacterial pneumonia in patients with human immunodeficiency virus infection. *Semin Respir infect* 1989; **4:** 133–8.

117. Verghese A, Al-Samman M, Nabhan D, *et al.* Bacterial bronchitis and bronchiectasis in human immunodeficiency virus infection. *Arch Intern Med* 1994; **154:** 2086–91.

●118. Millar AB. Respiratory manifestations of AIDS. *Br J Hosp Med* 1988; March: 204–12.

●119. White DA, Matthay RA. State of the art: Noninfectious pulmonary complications of infection with the human immunodeficiency virus. *Am Rev Respir Dis* 1989; **140:** 1763–87.

120. Martinez EJ, Nord HJ, Cooper BG. Significance of solitary and multiple esophageal ulcers in patients with AIDS. *South Med J* 1995; **88:** 626–9.

121. Wilcox CM, Straub RF, Schwartz DA. Prospective endoscopic characterization of cytomegalovirus esophagitis in AIDS. *Gastrointest Endosc* 1994; **40:** 481–4.

122. Kitchen VS, Helbert M, Francis ND, *et al.* Epstein–Barr virus associated oesphageal ulcers in AIDS. *Gut* 1990; **31:** 1223–5.

123. Sokol-Anderson ML, Prelutsky DJ, Westblom TU. Giant esophageal aphthous ulcers in AIDS patients: treatment with low-dose corticosteroids. *AIDS* 1991; **5:** 1537–8.

124. Kotler DP, Reka S, Orenstein JM, Fox CH. Chronic idiopathic esophageal ulceration in the acquired immune deficiency syndrome. Characterization and treatment with corticosteroids. *J Clin Gastroenterol* 1992; **15:** 284–90.

125. Slomianski A, Snyder M, Goldmeier P, *et al.* Concomi-

tant esophageal and penile ulcerations healed with steroid therapy in a patient with AIDS; case report. *Clin Infect Dis* 1992; **15:** 861–2.

126. Adeoti AG, Vega KJ, Dajani EZ, *et al.* Idiopathic esophageal ulceration in acquired immunodeficiency syndrome: successful treatment with misoprostol and viscous lidocaine. *Am J Gastroenterol* 1998; **93:** 2069–74.

◆127. Jacobson JM, Spritzler J, Fox L, *et al.* Thalidomide for the treatment of esophageal aphthous ulcers in patients with human immunodeficiency virus infection. National Institute of Allergy and Infectious Disease AIDS Clinical Trials Group. *J Infect Dis* 1999; **180:** 61–7.

128. Lai YP, Wu MS, Chen MY, *et al.* Timing and necessity of endoscopy in AIDS patients with dysphagia or odynophagia. *Hepatogastroenterology* 1998; **45:** 2186–9.

129. Fried RL, Brandt LJ, Kauvar D, Simon D. Esophageal motility in AIDS patients with symptomatic opportunistic infections of the esophagus. *Am J Gastroenterol* 1994; **89:** 2003–5.

◆130. Parente F, Cernuschi M, Antinori S, *et al.* Severe abdominal pain in patients with AIDS: frequency, clinical aspects, causes and outcome. *Scand J Gastroenterol* 1994; **29:** 511–15.

◆131. Thuluvath, Connolly GM, Forbes A, Gazzard BG. Abdominal pain in HIV infection. *Q J Med* 1991; **287:** 275–85.

132. Mueller GP, Williams RA. Surgical infections in AIDS patients. *Am J Surg* 1995; **169** (5A Suppl.): 34S–38S.

133. Wyatt SH, Fishman EK. The acute abdomen in individuals with AIDS. *Radiol Clin North Am* 1994; **32:** 1023–43.

134. Bizer LS, Pettorino R, Ashikari A. Emergency abdominal operations in the patient with acquired immunodeficiency syndrome. *J Am Coll Surg* 1995; **180:** 205–9.

◆135. Bouillot JL, Dehni N, Kazatchkine M, *et al.* Role of laparoscopic surgery in the management of acute abdomen in the HIV-positive patients. *J Laparoendosc Surg* 1995; **5:** 101–4.

●136. Endres JC, Salky BA. Laparoscopy in AIDS. *Gastrointest Endosc Clin N Am* 1998; **8:** 975–90.

◆137. Collazos J, Mayo J, Martinez E, *et al.* Celiac plexus block as treatment for refractory pain related to sclerosing cholangitis in AIDS patients. *J Clin Gastrol* 1996; **23:** 47–9.

138. Bird GL, Kennedy DH, Forrest JA. AIDS-related cholangitis: diagnostic features and course in four patients. *Scot Med J* 1995; **40:** 53–4.

◆139. Teare JP, Daly CA, Rodgers C, *et al.* Pancreatic abnormalities and AIDS-related sclerosing cholangitis. *Genitourin Med* 1997; **73:** 271–3.

●140. Libman H, Witzburg RA. *HIV Infection: a Clinical Manual*, 2nd edn. Boston, MA: Little, Brown, 1993: 157.

◆141. Savioz D, Lironi A, Zurbuchen P, *et al.* Acute right iliac fossa pain in acquired immunodeficiency: a comparison between patients with and without acquired immune deficiency syndrome. *Br J Surg* 1996; **83:** 644–6.

◆142. Dutta SK, Ting CD, Lai LL. Study of prevalence, severity and etiological factors associated with acute pancreatitis in patients infected with human immunodeficiency virus. *Am J Gastroenterol* 1997; **92:** 2044–8.

143. Dowell SF, Holt EA, Murphy FK. Pancreatits associated with human immunodeficiency virus infection: a matched case–control study. *Tex Med* 1996; **92(9):** 44–9.

144. Cappell MS, Marks M. Acute pancreatitis in HIV-seropositive patients: a case control of 44 patients. *Am J Med* 1995; **98:** 243–8.

145. Parithivel VS, Yousuf AM, Albu E, *et al.* Predictors of the severity of acute pancreatitis in patients with HIV infection or AIDS. *Pancreas* 1999; **19:** 133–6.

146. Manocha AP, Sossenheimer M, Martin SP, *et al.* Prevalence and predictors of severe acute pancreatitis in patients with acquired immune deficiency syndrome (AIDS). *Am J Gastroenterol* 1999; **94:** 784–9.

◆147. Sundaram CP, Saltzman B. Urolithiasis associated with protease inhibitors. *J Endourol* 1999; **13:** 309–12.

◆148. Kohon AD, Armenakas NA, Fracchia JA. Indinavir urolithiasis: an emerging cause of renal colic in patients with human immunodeficiency virus. *J Urol* 1999; **161:** 1765–8.

◆149. Chui DW, Owen RL. AIDS and the gut. *J Gastroenterol Hepatol* 1994; **9:** 291–303.

●150. Monkemuller KE, Wilcox CM. Diagnosis and treatment of colonic disease in AIDS. *Gastrointest Endosc Clin N Am* 1998; **8:** 889–911.

151. Wood BJ, Kumar PN, Cooper C, *et al.* AIDS-associated intussusception in young adults. *J Clin Gastroenterol* 1995; **21:** 158–162.

◆152. Jonson E, Coombs DW, Hunstad D, *et al.* Continuous infusion of intrathecal morphine to control acquired immunodeficiency syndrome-associated bladder pain. *J Urol* 1992; **147:** 687–9.

27

Pain management in the context of substance abuse

SHARON M WEINSTEIN

Among the most challenging problems in all of medicine is the management of cancer patients with pain who are also substance abusers (i.e. who suffer from psychological chemical dependence or addiction). A concurrent diagnosis of substance abuse (SA) complicates clinical pain management. Significant medicolegal and ethical considerations may arise.

The use of some substances (alcohol and nicotine) is known to increase the risk of cancer, and thus patients who are also substance abusers may be over-represented in the cancer population. Although a minority of all patients with cancer-related pain, this subpopulation requires careful management. Clinicians providing pain management and palliative care should be prepared for complex presentations. Substance abusers with cancer-related pain require closer supervision than patients without such dual diagnoses and utilize more health care resources. Unscheduled outpatient and emergency visits occur more often, and multidisciplinary staff meetings and family conferences may be required. When also socially disadvantaged, patients may require financial assistance, help with transport arrangements, housing, and legal aid. However, it is important to remember that SA is not restricted to patients in the lower socioeconomic stratum.

Although clinical reports and formal research in this area are limited, there is extensive literature on pertinent subjects, which include guidelines for therapeutic use of opioid analgesics; definitions and conceptualizations of addiction and related phenomena; treatment of chemical dependency; psycho-oncology; and quality of life.

Clinicians treating patients with cancer-related pain should be thoroughly familiar with the general principles of cancer pain management. The clinical use of opioid analgesics requires a thorough understanding of their physiological effects, including analgesia. The analgesic effect is due to the interaction of exogenously administered drug with complex neural networks that transmit and interpret nociceptive messages, through reversible binding to endogenous opioid receptors of several subtypes. Marked interindividual variability in opioid responsiveness is well recognized. The benefit-to-risk ratio of opioid therapy depends on various factors, foremost among which is the clinical condition with which pain is associated. Opioids are the mainstay of therapy for acute pain, cancer-related pain, and chronic pain associated with other life-limiting illnesses. Federal guidelines for the treatment of cancer-related pain were released in 1994.[1]*** The majority of cancer patients will achieve adequate pain control using oral opioids according to the World Health Organization three-step analgesic ladder.[2] In contrast to persons without pain seeking mood-altering effects of psychoactive substances, cancer patients with pain report dysphoria more commonly than euphoria as a side-effect of opioids. The risk of iatrogenic addiction in the setting of pain treatment is extremely low.

Over recent decades, understanding of addiction and SA has evolved considerably, although the interplay between heredity and environment is not fully understood. Neurotransmitter systems involved in reward circuits in the human brain are being discovered. It is noted that there may be overlap between the physiologic systems that mediate reward and analgesia although they are clearly distinct in many aspects. The two key components of the syndrome of substance abuse are: (1) use of a substance for its psychoactive effects despite the presence or potential for detrimental results ("use despite harm") and (2) inability to control substance use or behavior ("compulsive use"). The definition of substance dependence given in the *Diagnostic and Statistical Manual for Mental Disorders* vol. IV (DSM-IV) specifies physical dependence as a criterion. However, it is essential to recognize that the presence of physical dependence is not a useful criterion in the setting of pain treatment. Patients maintained on chronic opioid therapy will generally develop physical dependence, but that is rarely associated with psychological dependence and is not usually clinically problematic. The criteria for substance abuse emphasize the kinds of harm a patient may experience as a result of a maladaptive pattern of drug use.[3] Other authors have discussed a new nomenclature to be used in the settings of pain management and palliative care.[4]

It has been noted that health care professionals' knowledge deficits, fear of regulatory agencies, and exaggerated fear of patient addiction result in underprescribing of opioid analgesics.[5] Cancer pain patients who are also substance abusers are at even greater risk of undertreatment of their pain. There are limited data on which to base a nonabstinence model of treatment for cancer pain patients who are substance abusers. The treatment of SA in other settings usually includes psychological interventions and abstinence from the drug of abuse. It is difficult to find programs for patients needing both treatment for psychological dependence and ongoing medical therapy with psychoactive drugs.

Advances in the field of psycho-oncology have helped define the nature of psychological and psychiatric issues experienced by cancer patients. Contemporary psycho-oncology offers specific strategies for the provision of psychological support and psychiatric treatment of common diagnoses, such as depression, anxiety, and delirium. Quality of life research has emphasized the different components of distress or suffering in the cancer population, which include unrelieved physical symptoms and psychological concerns. Regardless of prognosis when managing pain with opioid analgesics, it is essential to distinguish worsening function from pain relief with improved function as outcomes of treatment. However, for patients with very advanced cancer, functional goals must be carefully established as physical capabilities decline as a result of disease progression. When patients are approaching death, there may not be sufficient time to offer in-depth psychotherapy for the treatment of SA, and psychological interventions may be mainly supportive to the patient and family.

The objectives of this chapter are to describe the impact of concurrent SA on cancer pain management; outline methods of patient assessment; describe a multidisciplinary approach to enhance compliance with pain treatment in cancer patients who are substance abusers; and outline issues for future investigation.

THE IMPACT OF SUBSTANCE ABUSE ON CANCER PAIN MANAGEMENT

The management of pain in the cancer patient is complicated by concurrent SA in several ways (Table 27.1). Firstly, trust is the basis of any therapeutic relationship. Trust is easily eroded when clinicians are expecting manipulative behavior from patients and patients have long-term experience with reluctant care providers. Pain assessment is difficult if it is assumed that patients cannot make distinctions between pain, anxiety, and other kinds of psychological distress. Patients who are substance abusers are more likely to have poor family and social support systems. They may be living with persons who are also substance abusers. The lack of control over use of a potentially addictive substance characterizes SA, and this can interfere directly with the implementation of effective pharmacologic therapy for pain. Overt illegal behaviors may further limit the prescription and use of controlled substances. Under these circumstances, pain may be left untreated, resulting in increased suffering and psychological distress and an ensuing vicious cycle. Care becomes chaotic and patients make erratic, ineffective use of health care resources.

PATIENT ASSESSMENT

Early identification of SA is important, as these patients are thought to be at increased risk for aberrant drug-taking during medical therapy with abusable drugs. Early identification also allows the coordinated engagement of clinical professionals who bring specific expertise (Table 27.2) to the management plan.

There are several ways in which SA may be recognized in the clinical practice setting (Table 27.3). Methods of prospective identification of patients with SA include routine medical history taking, physical examination, interviews of family members, and the use of self-administered questionnaires or more extensive structured interview tools. A simple yet specific method of screening for alcohol abuse may be easily incorporated in routine practice.[6] In the absence of a complete history, provider observations of patient behaviors may lead to the diagnosis. Body fluids screening is used more commonly after the clinical index of suspicion has been raised, or as part of the care plan after diagnosis (see below, Drug testing in pain management). Complete neuropsychological and

Table 27.1 *Substance abuse complicates pain management*

Assessment is based on trust, which may be eroded
Patients may not be able to distinguish analgesia from other psychoactive effects
Patients lack personal behavioral controls
Patients often live in "dysfunctional" settings
Legal and ethical issues arise

Table 27.2 *Suggested care team members*

Physician: pain specialist
Physician: addiction specialist
Physician: psychiatrist
Nurse: pain specialist
Nurse: psychiatric clinician
Nurse: addiction specialist
Social worker: mental health specialist
Social worker: addiction specialist
Psychologist: pain specialist
Psychologist: addiction specialist
Clinical pharmacist: pain specialist
Clinical pharmacist: addiction specialist

Table 27.3 *Patient assessment*

Medical history
Substance use history
Psychosocial history
Psychiatric history
Psychiatric examination
Physical examination
Family interview

psychiatric assessment are recommended when questions of psychiatric comorbidity are raised.

It is useful to consider types of aberrant drug-taking behavior.[7] Some medication requests ("drug-seeking" behavior) may reflect undertreatment of pain or "pseudoaddiction,"[8] whereas others may reflect true SA. Pseudoaddiction may be associated with increasing pain, inadequate management, or logistical problems such as lack of access to prescribed medications and nonpharmacologic therapies. Other more problematic behaviors demand immediate attention from the provider, such as confirmed criminal activity. A format for categorizing clinical problems is shown in Table 27.4.

The diagnosis of SA is made in the context of a thorough evaluation of the patient and their comorbidities, including full characterization of the underlying pathophysiology of the pain complaint(s). Clinicians should remember that many cancer patients experience neuropathic pain for which there may be no confirmatory diagnostic tests and which may require polypharmacy with several psychoactive medications (complex pharmacotherapy). Careful physical examination with detailed neurologic testing will often reveal neurologic dysfunction that is supportive of the clinical diagnosis of neuropathic pain.

MANAGEMENT GUIDELINES

At one busy tertiary cancer center, the University of Texas MD Anderson Cancer Center (MDACC), we developed a program to address the special needs of substance abusers with cancer pain while endeavoring to conserve our resources. This multidisciplinary program included institutional policy development, screening to identify patients at risk for aberrant drug-taking behavior, a multimodal approach to pain therapy, and incorporation of written agreements to facilitate outpatient treatment with opioids and other psychoactive drugs (Table 27.5). A broad institutional policy was first presented to and endorsed by the center's administration. A multidisciplinary management team and clinical resources in the community were identified. Rules for prescribing and documentation were established. Controlled prescribing was necessary at times and written agreements were utilized when routine written clinic guidelines were insufficient[9] (see below, Written care agreements).

We were interested in establishing screening procedures to identify patients at risk of aberrant drug use. When possible, cancer patients who were also substance abusers were identified on the first clinic evaluation by routine screening questions in the medical history, although at times diagnosis was delayed until a "crisis" situation arose. When the index of suspicion for concurrent SA was high, psychiatric and neuropsychological evaluations were instituted to enable comorbid conditions to be diagnosed more effectively.

Routine pain management practice utilizes an individual case-by-case determination of the need for and

Table 27.4 *Spectrum of active clinical problems*

Type of substance[a]	In recovery (Y/N)	Functional impairment[b] (Y/N)	Legal issue[c] (Y/N)
Alcohol			
Prescription drugs			
Illicit drugs			
Methadone maintenance			

a. Tobacco deliberately excluded.
b. Examples: no gainful employment, marital discord.
c. Examples: driving under the influence (DUI), drug trafficking, probation, incarceration.

Table 27.5 *Multidisciplinary program*

Institutional policy development
Hospital administration
Physician-in-chief
Pharmacy
Emergency department
Risk management
Ethics committee
Patient identification methods
Medical history
Self-report tool
Structured interview
Behaviors
Body fluids screening
Pain clinic program
Team structure
Community resources
Treatment program
Psychiatric/neuropsychological evaluation
Controlled prescribing
Monitoring of behaviors
Body fluids screening
Written care agreements

potential contraindications to opioid therapy. Initial comprehensive evaluation includes the use of standard pain assessment tools. World Health Organization and other guidelines for pharmacotherapy of cancer pain are followed. Patients with cancer pain who are also substance abusers are closely monitored for abuse behaviors, and prescribing schedules are modified accordingly. Nonpharmacologic approaches are utilized in conjunction with medications. Psychotherapy and cognitive/behavioral strategies are employed along with involvement of the patient's family and support systems. The use of social support services may at times be extensive.

A retrospective review of 2,100 MDACC Pain Clinic patient records revealed an incidence of SA of less than 5%, although it is clear that some substance abusers were not identified in the course of usual clinical practice. Of the 84 patients noted to be substance abusers, most were between the ages of 20 and 60, and the majority were male. Almost all patients had a diagnosis of cancer-related pain, and nearly all were prescribed opioids. Polysubstance abuse was noted in 33% and alcohol abuse alone in 14%; 9% had a positive family history of SA, and unsanctioned dose escalation occurred in 9%. There was a known criminal history in 5%, and a history of other prescription drug abuse in 2%. Two or more of these problems occurred in 28%. The majority had undergone a psychiatric evaluation, rendering an additional diagnosis of depression in 28%, anxiety in 11%, and personality disorder in 6%. Seventeen of these patients were managed with written care agreements. Overall, less than 5% of Pain Clinic patients were managed with written care agreements.[10] The results of our case series are described in Tables 27.6 and 27.7.

Unfortunately, the literature does not adequately address the impact of SA on the outcome of cancer treatment. In a retrospective review of a long-term cohort of 132 patients with genitourinary cancers and SA, survival was found to be unaffected compared with patients without SA (J Edwards, personal communication). At presentation, information regarding prior substance use was gathered via a structured interview tool as part of a comprehensive psychosocial assessment. Specific drugs used, amount and frequency of use, duration of use, and prior discontinuation or concurrent use at time of interview were recorded along with family history and the impact of substance use on personal relationships and job or school performance. This review revealed that, although SA may complicate pain assessment and treatment, it may not influence survival from cancer. Mortality, medical complications, time to disease recurrence, number of cancer relapses, and treatment courses to remission were similar in the sample identified with SA compared with the remainder of the study population.[10]

Table 27.6 *Case series* (n = *84)*

Age (years)	
0–20	1%
20–40	47%
40–60	47%
> 60	5%
Gender	
Female	42%
Male	58%
Pain diagnosis	
Cancer related	> 97%
Pain medications	
Opioids	> 98%
Characterization of problem	
Polysubstance use	33%
Alcohol abuse	14%
Family issues	9%
Dose escalation	9%
Criminal activity	5%
Prescription abuse	2%
Two or more of above	28%
Written contracts	17 (20%)
Psychiatric diagnosis	
Not evaluated/uncertain	44%
Depression	28%
Anxiety	11%
No diagnosis	11%
Personality disorder	6%

Table 27.7 *Outcomes of written care agreements (n = 17)*

Compliant, kept on contract	5
Compliant, went off contract	4
Dismissed	2/2 in process
Lost to follow-up	2
Referred for substance abuse treatment	1
Noncompliant/referred to hospice	1

PSYCHOSOCIAL SUPPORT GROUPS

Individual counseling and a pilot psychosocial support group were incorporated in a nonabstinence model program for SA patients at MDACC. Clinical impressions were that these interventions facilitated pain treatment and enhanced compliance in patients with psychosocial problems, psychiatric diagnoses, or illicit behaviors. It appeared that patients with SA can easily distinguish between analgesia and other psychoactive effects. Group therapy assisted them in coping with the many stresses of chronic pain, complex cancer treatment decisions, the threat of tumor progression or recurrence, and personal losses in many domains. Some patients responded positively to a more strictly structured approach to their pain management.[10] Based on this favorable experience, it is recommended that institutions consider establishing such groups and facilitating their functioning independently as peer support groups (see Table 27.8).

WRITTEN CARE AGREEMENTS

A written care agreement between patient and care provider may be indicated when SA complicates pain management. The written care agreement documents a detailed individualized agreement between patient and care provider, clearly setting out rules and expectations for both parties. Suggested criteria for initiating a written agreement are summarized in Table 27.9. At a minimum the agreement should include expectations for patient compliance with medication schedules and appointments for prescription refills, a medication replacement policy, and the patient's agreement to random screening of body fluids (Fig. 27.1). Such instructions are most useful when the consequences of noncompliance are outlined and may include a statement describing the likelihood of dismissal from treatment in the event of continued noncompliance. Written agreements serve as a communication tool for patient and provider, as well as a guide for different providers within the team and institution. This type of formally structured agreement also ideally addresses patients' problem behaviors, such as poor impulse control and "splitting" of staff, i.e. manipulative behaviors meant to cause conflict between staff members. Copies of the signed written agreement should be given to the patient and included in the record. Clear documentation is then assured in the event that it is necessary to dismiss a patient from care. It should be noted that the written care agreement is neither an informed consent document nor a legal contract.

Table 27.8 *Structure of pilot program*

Assessment
Group, individual, family therapy
Staff development
Multidisciplinary staff meetings for patient care
Documentation, including written patient care agreements
Prescription scheduling
Community interface
Monitoring of efficacy of program

Table 27.9 *Suggested criteria for initiating written care agreement*

Repeated acts of noncompliance with pain treatment
Evidence of ongoing illicit drug or excessive alcohol use
History of conviction or incarceration for a drug-related offense
Enrollment in a methadone maintenance program

Although most pain specialists practicing in the cancer setting will encounter patients with cancer-related pain and concurrent SA, dismissal from pain treatment is an infrequent outcome. In such cases, clinicians and their institutions must adequately document their decision that the benefit of continued pain treatment is outweighed by its risk. In most cases, consultation with clinical peers and institutional risk managers is highly recommended. For the most difficult circumstances, the practicing clinician may wish to consult with an institutional ethics committee.

ANALGESIC THERAPY

There is no consensus that any given opioid analgesic is less "addictive" than others in clinical use. Any drug preparation may be misused and/or diverted for illicit purposes. Controlled-release preparations of opioids may make it easier for patients to comply with medication schedules and may lessen the reinforcing aspects of pill-taking behavior. However, as pain intensity fluctuates, it is customary to prescribe immediate-release or short-acting medication for breakthrough pain when prescribing controlled-release preparations. Some substance abusers cannot adhere to complicated medication schedules and are less confused by immediate-release medication prescribed alone.

In the case of substance abusers receiving methadone maintenance therapy, Passik *et al.*[11] suggest that methadone being given for opioid dependency be titrated to

I understand that my pain treatment will consist of the following: _______ .

I agree to take medications at the dose and frequency prescribed. Any changes in the dose will be only at the direction of _______ or her/his designee _______ .

I will receive my prescriptions at the following interval: _______ .

I agree to come to all scheduled appointments. My next appointment is _______ .

I understand that prescriptions will only be supplied at my clinic visit. I will not request prescriptions by telephone.

I consent to random urine drug screening.

I will protect the safety of my medications. I will not give my medications to any other person.

I understand that lost or stolen medications will not be replaced. I agree to report stolen medications to the police.

I understand that if I have questions regarding pain or side-effects of medications, I am to call (telephone number) during regular business hours (specify).

I understand that a copy of this agreement is placed on my medical record.

I understand that a copy of this agreement is being sent to (primary physician).

I understand that failure to comply with this agreement may put at risk my continued pain treatment.

Patient (signature) Date _______

Physician (signature) Date _______

Other clinician (signature) Date _______

Renewal Date _______

Figure 27.1 *Sample content for written care agreement.*

analgesia. It is the author's preference to avoid disturbing the established use of methadone, instead regarding methadone as an endogenous opioid and administering a different opioid drug as the analgesic. Although this approach may be pharmacologically more complicated, it respects the legal restrictions on prescribing methadone for opioid maintenance, i.e. the requirement for special registration as a methadone clinic. It also allows for dosage titration of the analgesic without having to involve the methadone maintenance program in dosage changes. Periodic communication between the pain clinician and the methadone clinic staff is still strongly recommended to keep them informed of the specific agents prescribed and to discuss concerning behaviors. The need for repeated communication regarding analgesic titration is reduced when using an alternative to methadone for analgesia.

It is essential that psychiatric conditions such as depression and anxiety be treated as distinct clinical problems. Psychoactive medications prescribed for these indications may interact with analgesics. It is important that there is regular communication between prescribers, and periodic team conferences are recommended.

Comprehensive pain management includes nonpharmacologic as well as pharmacologic interventions. All nonpharmacologic means of controlling symptoms should be explored with cancer pain patients who are also substance abusers. Anesthetic or neurosurgical procedures to alleviate pain may reduce the need for analgesic medications, thus potentially simplifying therapy. Psychological and behavioral techniques should also be incorporated, although patients with high levels of distress and personality disorders may be less able to utilize these techniques successfully.

DRUG TESTING IN PAIN MANAGEMENT

Body fluid screening is useful to confirm the presence or absence of the prescribed controlled substances and nonprescribed drugs (licit or illicit). Patients must give consent for clinical tests, and it is unethical to perform such tests without the patient's knowledge. The limitations of most routine drug screening tests require that pain clinicians and laboratory staff collaborate to assure that the drugs of interest are screened. It is also important to know that detection thresholds for specific drugs are adequate in the tests performed. Generally, urine screening will be most readily available and is preferable for routine clinical purposes. Substance detection depends on many variables, such as the drug, dose, frequency of use, route of administration, individual metabolism, body weight, hydration status, and sensitivity of the detection method used. In addition, it should be recognized that there is poor correlation between analgesic dose and serum levels.[12] Given these variables and the possibility of laboratory error, it is advisable to obtain more than one test before results are incorporated in clinical decision making.

Test results should be discussed with the patient. The clinician's interpretation should be clearly communicated with specific reference to the pain management plan. If the screening tests result in significant changes in the management plan, these should be documented and an updated written agreement signed (see Table 27.10).

CASE EXAMPLE

A 54-year-old woman with malignant melanoma of the lower extremity was referred for pain and symptom management as a result of persistent thigh pain after groin tumor excision and femoral node dissection. Initial consultation revealed neuropathic pain with femoral deafferentation; chronic headaches; chronic pancreatitis; chronic obstructive pulmonary disease; anxiety disorder; history of tobacco, alcohol, and prescription drug abuse; a physically abusive alcoholic husband; chaotic family circumstances; and children with active illicit drug use. The patient was treated with antidepressant, benzodiazepine, and opioid analgesic medications. She was counseled by a psychiatric nurse clinician and social worker with credentials in the treatment of SA. She was referred to Alcoholics Anonymous. Repeated acts of noncompliance with general Pain Clinic rules led to strict prescribing and written care agreements. Nevertheless, at outpatient visits, the patient was unable to account for her medications and several urine screenings failed to detect her prescribed drugs. During a subsequent hospitalization, a strong suspicion arose that her opioid and benzodiazepine medications were being diverted. The patient's daughter had obtained the patient's outpatient prescriptions and was found unresponsive in the patient's hospital bathroom. On search of the hospital room, the patient's prescribed opioid was found in the daughter's purse with a syringe inserted. On the advice of institutional risk management staff, the police were informed. The patient was dismissed from the Pain Service with an explanation that we had determined that she was not taking her medications and we were concerned that her medications were being diverted to others. We remained available for inpatient consultation for the management of painful procedures or cancer treatment, and for outpatient reevaluation of changes in clinical condition.

Table 27.10 *Body fluids screening*

Patient communication
Specify test
Explain purpose of test and use of information to be obtained from test
Patient consent for testing
Repeat testing for confirmation
Written care agreements useful
Laboratory communication
Specify substances to be screened
Consider lowering thresholds for detection of substances of interest
Improve efficiency of testing and reporting

MEDICOLEGAL ISSUES

There are medicolegal considerations that arise in the management of patients with cancer pain who are also substance abusers that are largely beyond the scope of this chapter. Federal statutes, state laws, and state regulations recognize that the medical treatment of pain with opioid analgesics is essential, falling within the scope of good medicine. In practice, the documentation of diagnosis, treatment plan, and follow-up care should be every prescriber's routine.[13] Clinicians should consider obtaining legal counsel to address the use of information regarding a patient's illicit activities. When overt illicit behaviors are viewed as a contraindication to the prescribing of controlled substances, patient complaints of pain may be untreated. Prescribers' obligations and patients' rights may then come into conflict, resulting in ethical issues to be addressed.

RESEARCH

Many scientific and clinical questions remain. Can we differentiate distinct brain regions mediating analgesia versus reward using currently available functional brain imaging techniques? Do substance abusers with pain respond differently to opioid analgesics from pain patients who are not substance abusers? What is the relationship between the analgesic and mood effects of opioids in substance abusers compared with others? What is the role of psychological analgesic intervention for substance abusers with pain? How does SA impact on analgesic therapy and outcome from cancer treatment? Can we better define the clinical issues in treating pain in substance abusers? Do multidisciplinary programs for substance abusers with pain improve clinical outcomes and are they cost-effective? How can we balance individual rights and societal concerns in an ethical manner?

CONCLUSIONS

The majority of cancer patients will experience significant pain during their illness, and opioid analgesics are integral to cancer care. The prevalence of substance abuse in our society may be as high as 15%. The prevalence of SA in the cancer pain population may be even greater. Patients with a history of substance abuse and those with active abuse may engage in behaviors that complicate the assessment of pain as a subjective reported experience. The efficacy of therapeutic interventions may be difficult to measure in the patient using these agents for their psychoactive effects. In short, the therapeutic alliance is easily eroded, making pain treatment stressful for providers and patients alike. Legal problems may arise for the practitioner and institutions. Yet the standard approach to chemical dependency (detoxification and abstinence) may be inappropriate for those patients with severe persistent cancer-related pain.

Working with substance abusers with cancer-related pain provokes consideration of fundamental clinical and ethical questions. In the broad perspective, how the medical use of opioids relates to the problem of SA is still clouded in controversy, but meaningful dialog has begun to clarify these issues.[14,15] We must remain mindful of our assumptions and make efforts to structure clinical approaches for different practice settings.

It is important to recognize the exceptional care that substance abusers with cancer pain require.[16] Our aim should be to maintain the therapeutic alliance to the degree possible, by re-establishing trust and thus furthering the goals of pain relief and improved quality of life. Individuals without pain who require treatment solely for SA are best referred to dedicated SA treatment centers.

REFERENCES

◆ 1. Agency for Health Care Policy and Research, US Department of Health and Human Services. *Clinical Practice Guideline Number 9: Management of Cancer Pain.* Washington, DC: US Department of Health and Human Services, 1994.

◆ 2. World Health Organization. *Cancer Pain Relief and Palliative Care.* Geneva: World Health Organization, 1990.

3. American Psychiatric Association. *Diagnostic and Statistical Manual for Mental Disorders*, vol. IV. Washington, DC: American Psychiatric Association, 1994: 175–272.

● 4. Passik SD, Kirsh MS, Portenoy RK. Understanding aberrant drug-taking behavior: addiction redefined for palliative care and pain management settings. *Principles Pract Support Oncol* 1999; **2:** 1–12.

5. Weinstein SM, Laux LF, Thornby JI, *et al.* Physicians' attitudes toward pain and the use of opioid analgesics: results of a survey from the Texas Cancer Pain Initiative. *South Med J* 2000; **93:** 487.

6. Ewing JA. Detecting alcoholism: the CAGE questionnaire. *JAMA* 1984; **252:** 1905–7.

7. Passik SD, Kirsh KL, McDonald MV, *et al.* A survey of aberrant drug taking attitudes and behaviors in samples of cancer and AIDS patients. *J Pain Symptom Manage* 2000; **19:** 274–86.

8. Weissman DE, Haddox JD. Opioid psuedoaddiction – an iatrogenic syndrome. *Pain* 1989; **36:** 363.

9. Weinstein SM. Written contracts facilitate cancer pain treatment in the patient with substance use disorder. Thirteenth Annual Scientific Meeting of the American Pain Society, Miami Beach, FL, November, 1994.

10. Weinstein SM, Cunningham M, Edwards J. A Multidisciplinary program for cancer pain patients with substance use disorder. Twelfth Annual Scientific Meeting of the American Pain Society, Orlando, FL, November 1993.

11. Passik SD, Portenoy RK, Ricketts PL. Substance abuse issues cancer patients. Part 2: Evaluation and treatment. *Oncology* 1998; **12:** 729–34.

12. Cunningham M. Pain management in individuals with dual diagnosis: pain and substance use disorder. In: Kingdon RT, Stanley KJ, Kizior RJ eds. *Handbook for Pain Management.* St Louis, MO: Mosby, 249–93.

13. Weinstein SM, Thorpe DM, McCrory L. What the new board rules mean for your practice. *Texas Med* 1995; **91:** 36.

14. Savage SR. Pain medicine and addiction medicine: controversies and collaboration. *J Pain Symptom Manage* 1993; **8:** 265–78.

15. Portenoy RK, Payne R. Acute and chronic pain. In: Lowinson JH, Millman JG eds. *Substance Abuse: A Comprehensive Textbook.* Baltimore, MD: Williams & Wilkins, 1997: 691–721.

16. Hoffman M, Provatas A, Lyver A, Kanner R. Pain management in the opioid-addicted patient with cancer. *Cancer* 1991; **68:** 1121–2.

28

Pain in advanced nonmalignant disease[a]

JOHN J WELSH

Over the past 30 years there have been great strides forward in the clinical use of opioid analgesics to control pain in cancer patients. A large volume of research now justifies the guidelines which have been developed by many different sources.[1,2] In addition to advances in the clinical use of analgesics, there has been an explosion of pure scientific research into aspects of pain from both the physiological and pathophysiological point of view. There is an increasing tendency for clinicians and scientists to meet to compare observations and results obtained from studies in their own workplaces.

Much of this advance in the use of analgesia has been restricted to cancer patients, and even in that group of patients there are studies which suggest that control of pain is frequently suboptimal because of a lack of skill and lack of knowledge among prescribers and because of both health professionals' and patients' attitude toward the prescription of opioids.[3] However, it is now established that 70–80% of cancer patients' pain can be satisfactorily or well controlled by the application of simple analgesic prescribing guidelines.[4*]

PAINFUL NONMALIGNANT DISEASES

Pain is not the prerogative of those with cancer. There are a multitude of conditions that include pain as part of their symptomatology. Many of the conditions mentioned in this are discussed in specific chapters, to which the reader is referred for more detail. The incidence of stroke is 5% each year. Out of a population of 250,000, 12,500 people will present with new strokes each year, and 1,000 of those each year will have recurrent strokes.[5] Stroke patients may have co-morbid conditions that cause pain, or the stroke itself may produce pain. Stiffness and edema due to immobility of a joint or joints in the affected limb can result in pain. Seventy-two percent of stroke patients suffer from shoulder/hand syndrome.[6] Eight percent of stroke patients will suffer from central stroke pain.[7]

Ischemic heart disease causing intractable angina causes considerable pain, but there is controversy over the use of opioids in this situation.[8] It is argued that the use of strong analgesics in intractable angina may reduce the recognition of potentially fatal myocardial ischemia.

Fifty percent of multiple sclerosis patients have pain,[9] and up to 75% of those with motor neuron disease can be expected to experience pain. Multiple sclerosis pain syndromes may comprise musculoskeletal pain and spasticity, back pain, and paresthesia of the extremities or elsewhere. In motor neuron disease pains are described as paresthetic, lancinating, cramp-like, and aching.[10]

In children with neurological diseases, pain can be associated with contracture or muscle spasm or can be due to lack of movement of joints and general stiffness.[11] Pain secondary to sickle cell disease can be acute and exceedingly severe. In this case the pain is due to vaso-occlusion, leading to necrosis of bone marrow. More than 90% of hospital admissions among patients with sickle cell disease are the result of pain.[12] In such patients, more frequent pain episodes are associated with a poorer prognosis. In patients with acquired immunodeficiency syndrome (AIDS) the main symptom to be controlled is pain.[13,14] Approximately 50% of this pain is neuropathic in nature, with somatic pain occurring in 71% of patients.[15]

A survey of 26,000 patients in primary care across five

[a]Various aspects of long-term prescription of opioid analgesics for patients suffering from severely painful nonmalignant disease are discussed in this chapter. For a further in-depth discussion of this therapy the reader is referred to Chapter Ch15 and to the suggestion for practical guidelines for the management of such therapy, which are discussed in Chapter P7.

continents reported that 22% of patients had persistent pain which had been present over the previous year.[16]

Thus, there are many conditions, excluding cancer, which are associated with pain. And, as in the case of cancer, there is evidence that control of pain is suboptimal in patients with chronic nonmalignant pain.[17–20]

CONTROVERSY CONCERNING THE USE OF OPIOIDS

Although controversy over the use of opioids in chronic nonmalignant pain continues, over the last 10–15 years the use of these efficacious analgesics has increased. Opponents of the use of opioids put forward the following concerns:[21–24]

- Psychological dependence may occur with long-term use.
- Tolerance to the effects of opioids may develop.
- Patients treated with opioids exhibit reduced cognition.
- Opioid treatment is associated with a reduction in physical functioning.

In addition, much of the pain experienced by patients with chronic nonmalignant disease is neuropathic in nature, and there is a widespread belief that opioids are ineffective in alleviating this particular type of pain.[25,26]

Physical dependency on opioids is defined as the onset of usually adverse physical symptoms that occur when the drug is withdrawn. *Tolerance* occurs when increasing doses of a drug are required to achieve the same result. *Pseudoaddiction* is defined as a drug-seeking behavior driven by inadequate prescription of analgesics in the presence of pain and develops as a result of a physician's inability to treat the patient's pain state appropriately. With the increased use of opioids for chronic cancer pain, much research has been done in this area. In contrast, as a result of a reluctance by many to use opioids to treat noncancer pain, the amount of research involving the use of this class of drugs in chronic nonmalignant pain is small and generally not of high scientific quality.

An important question that must be answered is whether or not opioids are able to control the pain of chronic nonmalignant conditions and, if so, whether the use of these agents has long-term deleterious effects in terms of reduced functioning and lowered cognition. In addition, it is important to determine whether long-term use of opioids has effects on major organs within the body. The treatment goal of physicians is to reduce pain and, if possible, to achieve functional improvement. There is evidence that opioids are effective in alleviating neuropathic pain. This takes the form of anecdotes,[27] surveys,[28,29*] and uncontrolled studies;[30,31*] in addition, there have been two clinical controlled studies.[32**,33**]

Some studies have found evidence of a reduction in function among patients with noncancer pain who are treated with opioids.[34,35] However, other studies have reported an improvement in performance function and daily living activity.[35,36] A randomized controlled crossover trial of oral morphine found no evidence of a reduction in mood, functional status, perceived disability, cognition, or psychological status.[37] In addition, it was found that the incidence of depression was not correlated with long-term use of opioids. Concerns often raised about the use of opioids and evidence to allay such concerns are summarized in Table 28.1.

The greatest concern for physicians, patients, and families is the risk of psychological dependence. In one study, out of 11,882 hospitalized patients in whom opioids were instituted, only four subsequently became addicted.[38] Various studies have found that addiction is rare in patients with nonmalignant pain provided there is no previous history of addictive behavior.[31*,38,40]

The prevalence of psychological dependency is variously quoted as 0–2%.[31*,38] Other factors that predict a tendency toward addiction are psychosocial and genetic. In patients who have no history of chemical use or chemical dependency, the withdrawal of opioids used in the treatment of nonmalignant pain results in no long-term effects. This is also true for cancer patients.[22] However, in detoxified addicts there is a pattern of hypochondriasis, depression, and anxiety.

Nonmalignant pain patients do not show tolerance to analgesics.[31,32] There have been no reports of organ toxicity following the use of long-term opioids.[22]

Over the last 10 years in Denmark there has been a change in the indications for the prescription of opioids. Previously, most opioid prescriptions were for malignant pain. Now 90% of opioids are prescribed for nonmalignant pain.[41] Despite this change in prescribing practice there has been no increase in the addiction rate.

There have been a number of uncontrolled trials[42] and controlled trials[33] that support the use of a trial of opioids in carefully selected patients with nonmalignant chronic pain.

It seems therefore that the available evidence, although not extensive, points to the fact that opioids are efficacious for patients who have chronic nonmalignant pain and appear not to lead to psychological dependence. The exception is those patients who have a previous history of chemical abuse or dependency or come from families in which there is a history of chemical dependency or affective disorders. Severe major depression or alcoholism, antisocial behavior, and personality disorder should all alert the physician to a high propensity for the development of psychological dependency.[43]

Over the past 15 or so years there has been an increase in the use of opioids for chronic nonmalignant pain. In selected patients in whom prescribing principles derived from studies of cancer patients have been scrupulously applied, the use of opioids may be justified. There is no

Table 28.1 *Concerns about the use of opioids and evidence to counter such concerns*

Fears	Evidence
Fear of less efficacy against neuropathic pain	Shown to work in neuropathic pain in association with adjuvant treatments[30–32]
Reduced physical functioning	Better functioning demonstrated with good pain control[35,36]
Possible neurotoxicity long term	
Possible major organ toxicity	
Possible depression	No evidence of depression[37]
Reduced cognitive powers	No demonstrable reduction in cognition[37]
Psychological dependency	Minimal psychological dependency[38]
Tolerance will develop	Tolerance does not develop[31,45]

reliable test to determine whether chronic nonmalignant pain will respond to opioid treatment. Similarly, there are no clear-cut factors that predict whether a patient will become psychologically dependent upon the drug.

GUIDELINES

The increasing usefulness of opioids in the treatment of chronic nonmalignant pain is being more widely recognized, and guidelines to decrease the likelihood of drug abuse have been developed around the world.[47,48]

After careful assessment, which may involve psychological and cognitive screening and testing for contraindications in a patient's history (mentioned above), a selected patient with chronic nonmalignant pain may be given a trial of opioids providing certain conditions are met. Written protocols should be drawn up, and there should be written information material for patients to study. This information should include possible side-effects, toxicity, dangers of overdose, patient responsibilities, and potential withdrawal problems. In some protocols, there is a consent form to be signed.

Patients enter into a contract with their physician and should take the medication only as prescribed and contact their physician if any changes are to be made. They should obtain their prescriptions from one physician only, and that physician should be contacted if the patient at any time needs to consult another doctor. Patients must agree to inform the initial prescriber if they are given benzodiazepines or sedatives. Patients must agree to regular outpatient review and should always use the same pharmacy for obtaining prescriptions. A new prescription should not be given to a patient who runs out of medication early or claims to have lost pills. Patients must also agree to contact the police and physician if their medication is stolen. Some protocols require patients to agree to random checking of urine or blood for nonprescribed medication. It may be helpful to encourage patients to discuss problems arising with the physician before the situation becomes irredeemable. Patients should understand that if abuse of the above conditions occurs then the opioid may be withdrawn.[32] Very close supervision of these patients is required. In summary, guidelines for the use of opioids are as follows:

- The underlying cause of the pain should be carefully investigated.
- A history of substance abuse is a relatively strong contraindication to the use of opioids.
- A previous adequate but unsuccessful trial of non-opioid analgesics is mandatory.
- One physician only should provide opioids to any patient.
- Initially opioid treatment should be considered a trial. Effective therapy can be defined as meaningful partial analgesia with no adverse effects capable of compromising comfort or function.
- Frequent monitoring of analgesia, side-effects, and behavior consistent with substance abuse is required.[46]

CONCLUSION

In general, pain associated with chronic nonmalignant disorders is poorly assessed and poorly treated. In many cases, opioid prescription would be fully justified but is withheld because of politics, prejudice, or continuing ignorance.[47] This societal attitude prevents optimal opioid prescription in this patient group.

The limited findings of the studies that have been carried out on the use of opioids in patients with chronic nonmalignant pain suggest that these agents have a place in the treatment of noncancer pain. Ethical arguments support the nondiscriminatory use of analgesics known to ease suffering. It is vital that more research of a high methodological standard is carried out to provide incontrovertible evidence that will gradually sway both health professionals and the public of the benefits of the use of opioids in the treatment of nonmalignant pain. This societal shift will replicate the move over 30–40 years for the general public and increasingly health professionals to recognize the place of opioids in the treatment of cancer pain.

REFERENCES

1. WHO Guidelines. *Cancer Pain Relief*, 2nd edn. Geneva: World Health Organization, 1996.
2. SIGN. Publication No. 44: *Control of Pain in Patients with Cancer: A National Clinical Guideline*. Edinburgh: Scottish Intercollegiate Guidelines Network.
3. Von Roenn JH, Cleeland CS, Gonin R, Poandya KJ. *Results of Physicians' Attitude Toward Cancer Pain Management Survey by ECOG*. Philadelphia, PA: American Society of Clinical Oncology, 1991.
4. ◆ Zech DF, Grond S, Lynch J, *et al*. Validation of World Health Organization Guidelines for cancer pain relief – a 10 year prospective study. *Pain* 1995; **63:** 65–76.
5. Addington-Hall JM, Lay M, Altmann D, McCarthy M. Symptom control and communication with health professionals, and hospital care of stroke patients in the last year of life as reported by surviving family, friends and officials. *Stroke* 1995; **2612:** 2242–8.
6. Bohannon RW, Larkin PA, Smith MB. Shoulder pain in hemiplegia; statistical relationship to five variables. *Arch Phys Med Rehabil* 1986; **67:** 514–16.
7. Anderson G, Vestegaard K, Ingeman-Nielsen M, Jensen TS. Incidence of post-stroke pain. *Pain* 1995; **61:** 187–93.
8. Schoebel F C, Frazier OH, Jessurun GA, *et al*. Refractory angina pectoris in end-stage coronary artery disease: evolving therapeutic concepts. *Am Heart J* 1997; **143:** 587–602.
9. Moulin DE. Pain in multiple sclerosis. *Neurol Clin* 1989; **7:** 321–31.
10. O'Brien T, Kelly M, Saunders C. Motor neurone disease: a hospice perspective. *Br Med J* 1992; **304:** 471–3.
11. Hunt AM, Burne R. Medical and nursing problems of children with neurodegenerative disease. *Palliative Med* 1995; **9:** 19–26.
12. Fuggle P, Shand PA, Gill LJ, Davies SC. Pain, quality of life and coping in sickle cell disease. *Arch Dis Childh* 1996; **75:** 199–203.
13. Breitbart W. Pain management and psychosocial issues in HIV and AIDS. *Am J Hospice Palliative Care* 1996; **Jan/Feb:** 21–9.
14. Hewitt D, McDonald M, Portenoy R, *et al*. Pain syndromes and etiologies in ambulatory AIDS patients. *Pain* 1997; **70:** 117–23.
15. Bruera E, Neumann CM. In: Addington-Hall JM, Higginson IJ eds. *Palliative Care for Noncancer Patients*. Oxford: Oxford University Press, 2001: 73.
16. ◆ Gureje O, Von Korff M, Simon G, Gater R. Persistent pain and well-being: a World Health Organization study in primary care. *JAMA* 1998; **280:** 147–51.
17. Breitbart W, Rosenfeld BD, Passik SD, *et al*. The undertreatment of pain in ambulatory AIDS patients. *Pain* 1997; **72:** 235–43.
18. ● Elander J, Midence K. A review of evidence about factors affecting quality of pain management in sickle cell disease. *Clin J Pain* 1996; **12:** 180–93.
19. Farrell MJ, Katz B, Helme RD. The impact of dementia on the pain experience. *Pain* 1996; **67:** 7–15.
20. O'Brien T, Kelly M, Saunders C. Motor neurone disease: a hospice perspective. *Br Med J* 1992; **304:** 471–3.
21. McNairy SL, Maruta T, Ivink RJ, *et al*. Prescription medication dependence and neuropsychological function. *Pain* 1984; **18:** 169–77.
22. Turk DC, Brody MC, Okifuji EA. Physicians' attitudes and practices regarding the long-term prescribing of opioids for non cancer pain. *Pain* 1994; **59:** 201–8.
23. Martin WR, Jasinski DR, Haertzen CA, *et al*. Methadone: a re-evaluation. *Arch Gen Psychiatry* 1973; **28:** 286–95.
24. Bouckoms AJ, Masand P, Murray GB, *et al*. Chronic nonmalignant pain treated with long term analgesics. *Ann Clin Psychiatry* 1992; **4:** 185–92.
25. Portenoy RK. Chronic opioid therapy in non-malignant pain. *J Pain Symptom Manage* 1990; **5:** s46–s62.
26. ◆ Portenoy RK. Opioid therapy for chronic non-malignant pain: current status. In: Fields HL, Liebeskind JC eds. *Progress in Pain Research and Management*. Seattle, WA: IASP Press, 1994: 247–87.
27. McNairy SL, Maruta T, Ivnik RJ, *et al*. Prescription medication dependence and neuropsychological function. *Pain* 1984; **18:** 169–77.
28. Portenoy RK, Foley KM. Chronic use of opioid analgesics in non-malignant pain: report of 38 cases. *Pain* 1986; **25:** 171–86.
29. Pappagallo M, Raja SN, Haythornthwaite JA, *et al*. Oral opioids in the management of postherpetic neuralgia: a prospective survey. *Anaesth Analges* 1994; **1:** 51–5.
30. Taub A. Opioid analgesics in the treatment of chronic intractable pain of non-neoplastic origin. In: Kitahata LM, Collins D eds. *Narcotic Analgesics in Anaesthesiology*. Baltimore, MD: Williams & Wilkins, 1982: 199–208.
31. Zenz M, Strumpf M, Tryba M. Long-term oral opioid therapy in patients with chronic malignant pain. *J Pain Symptom Manage* 1992; **7:** 69–77.
32. Moulin DE, Lezzi A, Amireh R, *et al*. Randomised trial of oral morphine for chronic non-cancer pain. *Lancet* 1996; **347:** 143–7.
33. Arkinstall W, Sandler W, Goughnour B, *et al*. Efficacy of controlled-release codeine in chronic non-malignant pain: a randomised, placebo-controlled clinical trial. *Pain* 1995; **62:** 169–78.
34. Chabal C, Jacobson L, Chaney EF, Mariano AJ. Narcotics for chronic pain: yes or no? A useless dichotomy. *APS J* 1992; **1:** 289–91.
35. Schofferman J. Long-term use of opioid analgesics for the treatment of chronic pain of non-malignant origin. *J Pain Symptom Manage* 1993; **8:** 279–88.
36. Menefee LA, Pappagallo M, Quatrano-Piacentini AL, Haythornthwaite JA. Psychological effects of long-acting opioids in the treatment of failed back syndrome. Presented at the 14th Annual Meeting of the American Pain Society, 1995.
37. Pappagallo M, Campbell JN. The pharmacologic man-

agement of chronic back pain. In: Frymoyer JW, editor-in-chief. *The Adult Spine: Principles and Practice*, vol. 1, 2nd edn. Philadelphia, PA: Lippincott Raven, 1997: 275–86.

38. Porter J, Jick H. Addiction is rare in patients treated with narcotics. *N Engl J Med* 1980; **302:** 123.
39. Perry S, Heidrich G. Management of pain during debridement: a survey of U.S. burn units. *Pain* 1982; **13:** 267–80.
40. Chapman CR, Hill H. Prolonged morphine self-administration and addiction liability: evaluation of two theories in a bone marrow transplant unit. *Cancer* 1989; **63:** 1636–44.
41. Clausen TG. International opioid consumption. *Acta Anaesthesiol Scand* 1997; **41:** 162–5.
42. Portenoy R. Opioid therapy for chronic non-malignant pain. *Pain Res Manage* 1996; **1:** 17–28.
43. Pappagallo M, Heinberg LJ. Ethical issues in the management of chronic non-malignant pain. *Semin Neurol* 1997; **173:** 203–11.
44. Schug SA, Merry AF, Acland RH. Treatment principles for the use of opioids in pain of non-malignant origin. *Drugs* 1991; **42:** 228–39.
45. Anon. The use of opioids for the treatment of chronic pain: a consensus statement from the American Academy of Pain Medicine and the American Pain Society. *Pain Forum* 1997; **6:** 77–9.
46. Hagen N, Flynne P, Hays H, MacDonald N. Guidelines for managing chronic non-malignant pain. *Can Family Physician* 1995; **41:** 49–53.
47. McQuay H. Opioids in pain management. *Lancet* 1999; **353:** 2229–32.

Index

Page numbers in **bold** refer to tables or boxes; page numbers in *italic* refer to figures. Abbreviations: CNS, central nervous system; NSAIDs, nonsteroidal anti-inflammatory drugs; TENS, transcutaneous electrical nerve stimulation; WHO, World Health Organization.